Industrial
Microbiology

Industrial Microbiology

KL Benson

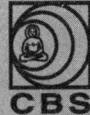

CBS Publishers & Distributors Pvt Ltd

New Delhi • Bengaluru • Chennai • Kochi • Kolkata • Mumbai • Pune
Hyderabad • Nagpur • Patna • Vijayawada

Industrial Microbiology

ISBN: 978-81-239-2914-9

Copyright © Publisher

First Edition: 2016

Published by Satish Kumar Jain and produced by Varun Jain for

CBS Publishers & Distributors Pvt Ltd

4819/XI Prahlad Street, 24 Ansari Road, Daryaganj, New Delhi 110 002, India.
Ph: 23289259, 23266861, 23266867   Website: www.cbspd.com
Fax: 011-23243014   e-mail: delhi@cbspd.com; cbspubs@airtelmail.in.
Corporate Office: 204 FIE, Industrial Area, Patparganj, Delhi 110 092
Ph: 4934 4934   Fax: 4934 4935   e-mail: publishing@cbspd.com; publicity@cbspd.com

Branches

- **Bengaluru:** Seema House 2975, 17th Cross, K.R. Road, Banasankari 2nd Stage, Bengaluru 560 070, Karnataka
  Ph: +91-80-26771678/79   Fax: +91-80-26771680   e-mail: bangalore@cbspd.com
- **Chennai:** 7, Subbaraya Street, Shenoy Nagar, Chennai 600 030, Tamil Nadu
  Ph: +91-44-26680620, 26681266   Fax: +91-44-42032115   e-mail: chennai@cbspd.com
- **Kochi:** Ashana House, No. 39/1904, AM Thomas Road, Valanjambalam, Eranakulam 682 018, Kochi Kerala
  Ph: +91-484-4059061-65   Fax: +91-484-4059065   e-mail: kochi@cbspd.com
- **Kolkata:** 6/B, Ground Floor, Rameswar Shaw Road, Kolkata-700 014, West Bengal
  Ph: +91-33-22891126, 22891127, 22891128   e-mail: kolkata@cbspd.com
- **Mumbai:** 83-C, Dr E Moses Road, Worli, Mumbai-400018, Maharashtra
  Ph: +91-22-24902340/41   Fax: +91-22-24902342   e-mail: mumbai@cbspd.com
- **Pune:** Bhuruk Prestige, Sr. No. 52/12/2+1+3/2 Narhe, Haveli (Near Katraj-Dehu Road Bypass), Pune 411 041, Maharashtra
  Ph: +91-20-64704058, 64704059, 32392277   Fax: +91-20-24300160 e-mail: pune@cbspd.com

Representatives

- **Hyderabad** 0-9885175004 • **Nagpur** 0-9021734563
- **Patna**   0-9334159340 • **Vijayawada** 0-9000660880

Printed at India Binding House, Noida, UP

Preface

Microbiology is the study of micro-organisms, which are unicellular or cell-cluster microscopic organisms. This includes eukaryotes such as fungi and protists and prokaryotes. Microbiology is a broad term which includes virology, mycology, parasitology, bacteriology and other branches.

Use of microbes to obtain a product or service of economic value constitutes industrial microbiology. Any process mediated by or involving micro-organisms in which a product of economic value is obtained is called fermentation. The terms industrial microbiology and fermentation are virtually synonymous in their scope, objectives and activities.

The microbial product may be microbial cells (living or dead), microbial biomass and components of microbial cells, intracellular or extracellular enzymes or chemicals produced by the microbes utilising the medium constituents or the provided substrate.

The services generated by micro-organisms range from the degradation of organic wastes, detoxification of industrial wastes and toxic compounds, to the degradation of petroleum to manage oil spills, etc. Industrial microbiology also encompasses activities like production of biocontrol agents, inoculants used as biofertilisers, etc.

Obviously, the scope and activities of industrial microbiology are too extensive as activities begin with the isolation of micro-organisms from nature, their screening for product formation, improvement of product yields, maintenance of cultures, mass culture using bioreactors, and usually end with the recovery of products and their purification. The subject matter of this reference textbook on Industrial Microbiology is accommodated in 27 chapters.

Chapter 1 open with a review of microbial taxonomy, metabolism and genetics. Chapter 2 focuses on yeasts which are eukaryotic micro-organisms classified in the kingdom fungi. Yeasts do not form a specific taxonomic or phylogenetic grouping, however, the term yeast is often taken as a synonym of *S. cerevisiae*. This chapter discusses in detail properties of yeasts, sexual reproduction and yeast cycles. Chapter 3 provides an in-depth knowledge of pure culture methods which includes general principles of culture maintenance and preparation, microbiological cultures, yeast cultures, pure culture, mould culture and pure culture techniques. Chapter 4 provides introduction to food microbiology. Micro-organisms have been used for centuries to modify food stuffs and fermented food and beverages, and thus constitute a major and extreme positive role in food industry. Micro-organisms can also effect desirable transformations in a way that is benefical. Because of the great variety of organic compounds in foods and the numerous kinds of micro-organisms that can decompose them, many different chemical changes are possible and many kinds of products can result. Considering this chapter 5 is devoted to chemical changes caused by micro-organisms. Chapter 6 covers milk and dairy products and discusses sources of milk, milk products and their processing operations. Chapter 7 explains bakery and cereal products along with their fermented aspects. Chapter 8 focuses on beer along with malting and brewery fermentations. The chapter also discusses role of enzymes in brewing. Chapter 9 deals with wine and cider. Chapter 10 explains distilled alcoholic beverages such as whisky, cognac, rum and allied products. Chapter 11 is devoted to flavoured spirits such as vodka, gin, liqueur and sake. Meat is animal flesh that is used as food. Most often, this means the skeletal muscle and associated fat, but it may also describe other edible tissues such as organs, livers, skin, brain, bone marrow, kidneys or lungs. Keeping this in mind chapter 12 focuses on meat and meat products and discusses spoilage of fresh meat, fermented meats, etc. Chapter 13 provides information about fish and seafood and explains microbiology of fish processing, spoilage of fresh fish, fermented fish, etc. Chapter 14 covers vegetables and fruit, their contamination, preservation and spoilage. Various methods of preservation of vegetables and fruits are discussed in detail. Chapter 15 deals with sugar and sugar products. Chapter 16 explores cocoa, tea, coffee, soya sauce and allied products. Chapter 17 focuses on miscellaneous foods such as fatty foods, salad dressing, essential oils, bottled soft drinks, spices, salt and nutmeats. Chapter 18 provides information about microbial biomass, single cell protein and other microbial products. Chapter 19 is devoted to production of baker's yeast. The baker's yeasts are strains of *S. cerevisine* and are propagated by pure culture methods in the laboratories of yeast producers. Chapter 20 focuses on enzymes in the food industry. Enzymes are added in food industries to bioconvert natural biochemicals in the foodstuffs into new food products with desirable colour, flavour, taste or texture. Chapter 21 provides information about citric acid which is a weak organic acid, and it is a natural preservative and is also used to add an acidic, or sour taste to foods and soft drinks. Various biochemical aspects of citric acid and their synthesis are discussed in detail. Amino acids are important substances which create life itself and are the oldest nutrients that have existed on earth. Amino acids are the principal building blocks of proteins and enzymes. Considering this chapter 22 is devoted to amino acids and discusses various types of amino acids and their manufacturing aspects. Chapter 23 provides basic information about vinegar and discusses types of vinegar and methods of manufacture along with its uses. Chapter 24 provides information about fermentation alcohol and algae for biofuels. Chapter 25 is devoted to food microbiology and public health. Food are complex mixtures of chemicals and often contain compounds that are potentially harmful as well as those that are beneficial. Various aspects related to significance of foodborne disease and risk factors associated with foodborne illness are discussed in detail. Chapter 26 concentrates on microbiology in food plant sanitation. The food industry sanitation is concerned with aseptic practices in preparation, processing and packaging of the food products of a plant, the general cleanliness and sanitation of plant and premises, and the health of employees. Finally chapter 27 deals with analytical techniques in food microbiology. The chapter discusses analysis of protein, lipid, carbohydrate, minerals and vitamins.

This reference textbook on *Industrial Microbiology* is designed to fulfil the requirements of undergraduates and postgraduates in the disciplines of industrial and environmental microbiology, industrial and environmental biotechnology, biotechnology and microbiology. The book will also useful for industrialists, scientists, researchers and professionals interested in exploring the role of micro-organisms in public health and allied fields.

The reference textbook is supported by a wealth of tables, figures, appendix and index which supplement the text. All the topics have been covered into a cogent and lucid style to help the reader grasp the information quickly and easily.

KL Benson

Contents at a Glance

Contents

Chapter 1

Microbial Taxonomy, Metabolism and Genetics: A Review

INTRODUCTION

Taxonomy is the science of classification, i.e. the assigning of objects to define categories. It has two functions: the first is to identify and describe as completely as possible the basic taxonomic units, or species; the second, to devise an appropriate way of arranging and cataloging these units.

All taxonomic concepts are manmade and, therefore, to certain extent arbitrary. This is especially true to classical approaches relying on macroscopic or microscopic observations because it is matter of opinion whether the difference in a particular character — say, a spore or the way in which it is formed.

SPECIES: THE UNITS OF CLASSIFICATION

The notion of a species is complex. Speaking broadly, a species consists of an assemblage of individuals (or, in micro-organisms, of clonal populations) that share a high degree of phenotypic similarity, coupled with an appreciable dissimilarity from other assemblages of the same general kind. The recognition of species would not be possible if natural variation were continuous, so that an intergrading series spanned the gap between two assemblages of markedly different phenotype. However, it became evident early in the development of biology that, among most groups of plants and animals, reasonably sharp discontinuities do separate the members of a group into distinguishable assemblages. Hence, the notion of the species as the base of taxonomic operation proved workable.

Every assemblage of individuals shows some degree of internal phenotypic diversity, because genetic variation is always at work. Hence, it becomes a matter of scientific tact to decide what degree of phenotypic dissimilarity justifies the breaking up of an assemblage into two or more species, or, to put the matter another way, how much internal diversity is permissible in a species. Opinions on this question vary. Taxonomists themselves can be broadly divided into two groups: 'lumpers', who set wide limits to a species, and 'splitters', who differentiate species on more slender grounds.

For plants and animals that reproduce sexually, a species can be defined in genetic and evolutionary terms. As long as a sexually reproducing population is free to interbreed at random, its total gene pool undergoes continuous redistribution, and new mutations, the source of phenotypic variation, are dispersed throughout the population. Such an interbreeding population may evolve in response to environmental changes, but it will evolve with reasonable uniformity. Divergent evolution, eventually leading to the emergence of new species, can occur only if a segment of the population becomes reproductively isolated in an environment that is different from that occupied by the rest of the population. Reproductive isolation is probably usually geographic in the first instance; a physical barrier of some sort (for example, a mountain range or a body of water) is interposed between two parts of the initially continuous population. Within each of these subpopulations, a common gene pool is maintained by interbreeding, but through chance mutation and selection, the two subpopulations are now free to evolve along different lines. They will continue to diverge, as long as the geographical barrier persists. Eventually, the cumulative differences become so great that physiological isolation is superimposed on geographic isolation; members of the two populations are no longer capable of interbreeding if they are brought together. Hence, even if the two populations subsequently commingle once more, their gene pools remain permanently separated; a point of no return has been reached. These evolutionary considerations lead to a dynamic definition of the species as a stage in evolution at which actually or potentially interbreeding arrays have become separated into two or more arrays physiologically incapable of interbreeding. This definition is, in fact, an explanation of the origin of specific discontinuities in nature. At the same time, it provides an experimental criterion for the recognition of species differences: inability to interbreed.

Because most micro-organisms are haploid, and reproduce predominantly by asexual means, the concept of the species that has emerged from work with plants and animals is evidently inapplicable to them. A microbial species cannot be considered an interbreeding population: the two offspring produced by the division of a bacterial cell are reproductively isolated from one another, and, in principle, they are free to evolve in a divergent manner. Genetic isolation is to some degree reduced by sexual or parasexual recombination in eucaryotic micro-organisms and by the special mechanisms of recombination distinctive of bacteria. However, it is very difficult to assess the evolutionary effect of these recombinational processes, because the frequencies with which they occur in nature are unknown. In bacteria the problem is further complicated by plasmid transfer which is relatively nonspecific, and permits exchanges of genetic material among bacteria of markedly different genetic constitution.

Since the dynamics of microbial evolution are so unlike the dynamics of evolution of plants and animals, there is no theoretical basis for the assumption that microbial evolution has led to phenotypic discontinuities that would justify the recognition of species. However, the experience of microbial taxonomists has shown that when many strains of a given microbial group are thoroughly analysed, they can usually be divided into a series of discontinuous clusters: it is such clusters of strains that the microbial taxonomist recognises empirically as species. Further insights into the dynamics of microbial evolution may eventually permit a formal definition of the microbial species; if so, this will most likely be different from the species definition applicable to plants and animals.

In bacterial populations, genetic change can occur so rapidly by mutation that it would be unwise to distinguish species on the basis of differences in a small number of characters, governed by single genes. Accordingly, the best working definition of a bacterial species is a group of strains that show a high degree of overall phenotypic similarity and that differ from related strain groups with respect to many independent characteristics.

Characterisation of Species

Ideally, species should be characterised by complete descriptions of their phenotypes or—even better of their genotypes. Taxonomic practice falls far short of these ideals; in most biological groups, even the phenotypes are only fragmentarily described, and genotypic characterisations are incomplete.

As a general rule, the phenotypic characters that can be most easily determined are structural or anatomical ones that can be directly observed. For this reason, biological classification is still based, at most levels, almost entirely on structural properties. Virtually the only exception is the classification of bacteria. The extreme structural simplicity of bacteria offers the taxonomist too small a range of characters upon which to base adequate characterisations. Hence, the bacterial taxonomist has always been forced to seek other kinds of characters—biochemical, physiological, ecological—with which to supplement structural data. The classification of bacteria is based, to a far greater extent than that of any other biological groups, on functional attributes. Most bacteria can be identified only by finding out what they can do, not simply how they look.

This confronts bacterial taxonomists with an additional problem. To find out what a bacterium can do, they have to perform experiments with it. The number of possible experiments that can be performed is extremely large, and although all will reveal facts, the facts so revealed will not necessarily be taxonomically significant ones, in the sense of contributing to a differentiation of the organism under study from related assemblages. Consequently, bacterial taxonomists can never be sure that they have performed the right experiments for taxonomic purposes; they may well have failed to perform certain experiments that would have shown them significant clustering in a collection of strains, and therefore erroneously conclude that they are dealing with a continuous series. There is no obvious way to get around this difficulty, except to make phenotypic characterisations as exhaustive as possible. However, an emerging alternative may soon resolve this dilemma; the molecular techniques for characterising bacterial genotypes provide a possible objective basis for defining a bacterial species. These techniques are discussed later in this chapter.

Naming of Species

According to a convention known as the binomial system of nomenclature, every biological species bears a latinised name that consists of two words. The first word indicates the taxonomic group of immediately higher order, or *genus* (plural, *genera*) to which the species belongs, and the second word identifies it as a particular species of that genus. The first letter of the genetic (but not of the specific) name is capitalised, and the whole phrase is italicised: *Escherichia* (generic name) *coli* (specific name). In contexts in which no confusion is possible, the generic name is often abbreviated to its initial letter: *E. coli*.

A rigid and complex set of rules governs biological nomenclature; the rules are designed to keep nomenclature as stable as possible. The specific name given to a newly recognised species cannot be changed unless it can be shown that the organism has previously been described under another specific name, in which case the older name is used because it has priority. Unfortunately, the same stability does not govern the generic half of the name, since the arrangement of related species into genera is an operation that can be carried out in different ways and that often changes in the course of time as new information becomes available. For example, *E. coli* has in the past been placed in the genus *Bacterium*, as *Bacterium coli* and in the genus *Bacillus*, as *Bacillus coli*. These three names are synonyms, since they all refer to one and the same species. This consequence of the binomial system can be very confusing, and taxonomic descriptions usually list all such synonyms in order to minimise the confusion. Binomial nomenclature is used for all biological groups except viruses. The virologists are currently divided over the best way to designate members of this group; some wish to extend the binomial system to the viruses, whereas others would prefer another system, which gives in coded form information about the properties of the organism.

In bacterial taxonomy, when a new species is named, a particular strain is designated as the type strain. Type strains are preserved in culture collections; if one is lost, a neotype strain, which resembles as closely as possible the description of the type strain, is chosen. The type strain is important for nomenclatural purposes, since the specific name is attached to it. If other strains, originally included in the same species, prove on subsequent study to deserve recognition as separate species, they must receive new names, the old specific name resting with the type strain and related strains.

In the taxonomic treatment of a biological group, the individual species are usually grouped in a series of categories of successively higher order: genus, family, order, class and division (or phylum). Such an arrangement is known as a hierarchical one, because each category in the ascending series unites a progressively larger number of taxonomic units in terms of a progressively smaller number of shared properties. It should be noted that the genus has a position of special importance, since according to the rules of nomenclature a species cannot be named unless it is assigned to a genus. The allocation of a species to a taxonomic category higher than the genus does not carry any essential nomenclatural information; it is merely indicative of the position of an organism, relative to other organisms, in the system of arrangement adopted.

PROBLEMS OF TAXONOMIC ARRANGEMENT

In dealing with a large number of different objects, some system of orderly arrangement is essential for purposes of data storage and retrieval. It does not matter what criteria for making the arrangement are adopted, provided that they are unambiguous and convenient. Books can be arranged in different ways: for example, by subject, by author, or by title. Different individuals tend to adopt different systems, depending on their particular needs and tastes. Such a system of classification, based on arbitrarily chosen criteria, is termed an artificial one. The earliest systems of biological classification were largely artificial in design. However, as knowledge about the anatomy of plants and animals increased, it became evident that these organisms conform to a number of major patterns or types, each of which shares many common properties, including ones that are not necessarily obvious upon superficial examination. Examples of such types are the mammalian, avian and reptilian types among vertebrate animals. The first system of biological classification that attempted to group organisms in terms of such typological resemblances and differences was developed in the middle of the eighteenth century by Linnaeus. The Linnaean arrangement was more useful than previous artificial arrangements, since the taxonomic position of an organism furnished a large body of information about its properties: to say that an animal belongs to the vertebrate class Mammalia immediately tells one that it possesses all those properties which distinguish mammals collectively from other vertebrates. Because Linnaean classification expressed the biological nature of the objects that it classified, it became known as a natural system of classification, in contrast to preceding artificial systems.

Phylogenetic Approach to Taxonomy

When the fact of biological evolution was recognised, another dimension was immediately added to the concept of a natural classification. For biologists of the eighteenth century, the typological groupings merely expressed resemblances; but for post-Darwinian biologists, they revealed relationships. In the nineteenth century the concept of a 'natural' system accordingly changed: it became one that grouped organisms in terms of their evolutionary affinities. The taxonomic hierarchy became in a certain sense the reflection of a family tree, and taxonomy suddenly acquired a new goal: the restructuring of hierarchies to mirror evolutionary relationships. Such a taxonomic system is known as a phylogenetic system.

Numerical Taxonomy

An alternative approach is an empirical one: the attempt to base taxonomic arrangement upon quantification of the similarities and differences among organisms. This was first suggested by Michel

Adanson, a contemporary of Linnaeus, and is known as Adansonian (or numerical) taxonomy. The underlying assumption is that, provided each phenotypic character is given explicit weighting, it should be possible to express numerically the taxonomic distances between organisms, in terms of the number of characters they share, relative to the total number of characters examined. The significance of the numerical relationships so determined is greatly influenced by the number of characters examined; these should be as numerous and as varied as possible, to obtain a representative sampling of phenotype.

Numerical taxonomy does not have the evolutionary connotations of phylogenetic taxonomy, but it provides an objective and stable basis for the construction of taxonomic groupings. Perhaps its greatest advantage is that it cannot be applied at all until a relatively large number of characters have been determined, so that its use encourages a thorough examination of phenotypes. The analyses are open to continuous revision and refinement as more characters in a given group are determined.

NEW APPROACHES TO BACTERIAL TAXONOMY

The growth of molecular biology has opened up a number of new approaches to the characterisation of organisms, which have had a profound impact on the taxonomy of bacteria. Of particular value are certain techniques that give insights into genotypic properties and thus complement the hitherto exclusively phenotypic characterisations of these organisms. Several kinds of analysis performed upon isolated nucleic acids furnish information about genotype: the analysis of the base composition of DNA, the study of chemical hybridisation between nucleic acids isolated from different organisms and the sequencing of nucleic acids.

Base Composition of DNA: Its Determination and Significance

DNA contains four bases: adenine (A), thymine (T), guanine (G) and cytosine (C). For double-stranded DNA, the base-pairing rules require that $A = T$ and $G = C$. However, there is no chemical restriction on the molar ratio $(G + C) : (A + T)$. Early in the chemical study of DNA, analyses showed that this ratio in fact varies over a rather wide range in DNA preparations from different organisms, and subsequent work has revealed that the base composition of DNA is a character of profound taxonomic importance, particularly among micro-organisms. Although DNA base composition may be determined chemically, after hydrolysis of a DNA sample and separation of the free bases, it can be determined more easily by physical methods, and these are now the ones principally used. The 'melting temperature' of DNA (i.e. the temperature at which it becomes denatured, by breakage of the hydrogen bonds that hold together the two strands) is directly related to $G + C$ content, because hydrogen bonding between GC pairs is stronger than that between AT pairs (a consequence of the fact that GC pairs form three hydrogen bonds, while AT pairs form only two). Strand separation is accompanied by a marked increase in absorbance at 260 nm, the absorption maximum of DNA, and this can be easily measured in a spectrophotometer. Physical methods of analysis also provide an indicating of the molecular heterogeneity of a DNA sample. If every molecule of DNA had the same $G + C$ content, both the thermal transition in a melting curve and the band position in a CsCl gradient would be extremely sharp.

Since no DNA preparation shows absolute molecular homogeneity, the $G + C$ content is always a mean value and represents the peak in a normal distribution curve.

Taxonomic Implications of DNA Base Composition

Two organisms with identical mean DNA base compositions may differ greatly in genetic constitution. This is evident from the very similar base ratio values for DNA from all plants and animals. Hence, major evolutionary divergence is not necessarily expressed by a divergence of mean base composition. When two organisms are closely similar in their DNA base composition, this fact can be construed as indicative of genetic and evolutionary relatedness only if the organisms also share a large number of phenotypic properties in common or are known to resemble one another in genetic constitution (e.g. different strains that belong to a single bacterial species). In such a case, near identity of DNA base composition provides supporting evidence for their genetic and evolutionary relatedness. Mean DNA base composition is a character of particular taxonomic value among bacteria, since the range for the group as a whole is so wide. Values have now been determined for large number of representative strains and species belonging to every major subgroup of procaryotes. Although the values for the constituents species in a genus differ somewhat, the total range within a bacterial genus is in general fairly narrow (rarely greater than 10 to 15 per cent), and can indeed be considered as an important character for the genus.

FUNGI

Like the protozoa, the fungi are nonphotosynthetic. Although some of the more primitive aquatic fungi show resemblances to flagellate protozoa, the fungi as a whole have developed a highly distinctive biological organisation that can be regarded as an adaptation to life in their most common habitat, the soil.

Most fungi are coenocytic organisms and have a vegetative structure known as a mycelium. The mycelium consists of a multinucleate mass of cytoplasm enclosed within a rigid, much-branched system of tubes, which are fairly uniform in diameter. Fungal growth is characteristically confined to the tips of the hyphae; as the mycelium extends, the cytoplasmic contents may disappear from the older, central regions. Usually, asexual reproduction occurs by the formation of uninucleate or multinucleate spores which are pinched off at the tips of the hyphae. Neither the spores nor the mycelium of higher fungi are capable of movement. However, the internal contents of a mycelium show streaming movements, which cannot be translated into progression over the substrate, because the cytoplasm is completely enclosed within its wall.

The fungi comprise three major groups: the Phycomycetes, the Ascomycetes and the Basidiomycetes. A fourth group, the Fungi Imperfecti, has been set aside to include those species for which the sexual stage, and hence the correct classification, is not yet known.

Phycomycetes

Although soil is by far the most common habitat of the fungi as a whole, many are aquatic. These fungi are known collectively as water moulds or aquatic phycomycetes. They occur on the surface of decaying plant or animal materials in ponds and streams; some are parasitic and attack algae or protozoa. It is these fungi which show the closest resemblances to protozoa; they produce motile spores or gametes, furnished with flagella, and in the simpler forms the vegetative structure is not mycelial. This description applies, for example, to many of the fungi known as *chytrids*.

The aquatic phycomycetes are a varied group with respect to their mechanisms of reproduction and life cycles. The range of this variation can be well illustrated by comparing a chytrid with another aquatic phycomycete, *Allomyces*. *Allomyces* shows a well-marked alternation of haploid and deploid generations.

Since the mycelium of phycomycetes is nonseptate, it is clear that these organisms are coenocytic. The regular occurrence of cross walls in the mycelium of other groups of fungi suggests, in contrast, that they are cellular organisms. This is not true, however. The cross walls do not divide the cytoplasm into a number of separate cells: each cross wall has a central pore, through which both cytoplasm and nuclei can move freely. There is thus just as much cytoplasmic continuity in the septate fungi as in the phycomycetes, and both groups are, in fact, coenocytic.

Ascomycota

The ascomycota are a division/phylum of the kingdom fungi, and subkingdom dikarya, whose members are commonly known as the sac fungi. They are the largest phylum of fungi, with over 30,000 species. Characteristically, when reproducing sexually, they produce nonmotile spores in a distinctive type of microscopic cell called an 'ascus' [from Greek: (*askos*), meaning 'sac' or 'wineskin']. These spores are called ascospores. However, some members of the ascomycota do not reproduce sexually and do not form asci or ascospores. These members are assigned to ascomycota based upon morphological and/or physiological similarities to ascus-bearing taxa, and in particular by phylogenetic comparisons of DNA sequences.

In ascomycetes, the diploid zygote develops into a saclike structure, the ascus, while the nucleus undergoes meiosis, often followed by one or more mitotic divisions. A wall is formed around each daughter nucleus and the neighbouring cytoplasm to produce four, eight, or more ascospores within the ascus (Fig. 1.1). Eventually the ascus ruptures and the enclosed spores are liberated.

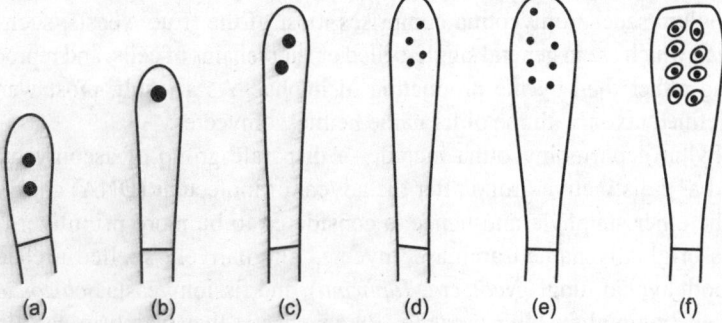

Fig. 1.1. Successive stages in the formation of an ascus: (a) binucleate fusion cell, (b) nuclear fusion, (c), (d), (e), nuclear divisions, and (f) ascospore formation.

This monophyletic grouping is an extremely significant and successful group of organisms. Familiar examples of sac fungi include morels, truffles, brewer's yeast and baker's yeast, dead man's fingers, cup fungi, and the majority of lichens (loosely termed 'ascolichens') such as Cladonia. Many plant-pathogenic fungi belong to the ascomycota. Commonly seen examples include apple scab, ergot, black knot and the powdery mildews. Species of ascomycetes are also popular in the laboratory. Sordaria fimicola, neurospora crassa and several species of yeasts are used in many genetics and cell biology experiments. Penicillium species on cheeses and in the antibiotic industry are examples of asexual taxa, otherwise known as anamorphs, that belong in the ascomycota. Prior to definitive phylogenetic research, moulds such as Penicillium were sometimes classified in an artificial phylum, called the deuteromycota.

Ascomycetes versus Ascomycota

In the past, before the recognition of the fungal kingdom, the sac fungi were considered to be a class, not a phylum. The original collective term for them was 'ascomycetes', a label first coined in the 1800s for a rankless nonlichenised taxon based upon the presence of asci. Ascomycetes was soon used to include lichenised taxa, and became the standard term, at the class level, for all ascus-bearing species, just as the term 'basidiomycetes' became used for their basidium-bearing counterparts. Elevation of the taxonomic rank of the ascomycetes resulted in the names ascomycetae, ascomycotina and finally ascomycota. The names ascomycota, ascomycetes, etc. are based upon the term 'ascus'. Together, the ascomycota and the basidiomycota form the subkingdom dikarya. The more familiar term, ascomycetes, is still loosely used, e.g. at fungal forays it is often said of a fungus, such as *Peziza*, 'It is an ascomycete, not a basidiomycete' in reference to their sexual reproductive mode. The terms are further abbreviated to 'ascos' and 'basidos' which are not officially sanctioned technical names.

Modern classification of ascomycota

There are three subphyla that are described and named:

1. The subphylum pezizomycotina is the largest subphylum and contains all the ascomycota that produce ascocarps (fruiting bodies), except for one genus, *Neolecta*, in the taphrinomycotina. Therefore, it includes virtually all macroscopic 'ascos' such as truffles, ergot, ascolichens, cup fungi (discomycetes), pyrenomycetes, lorchels and caterpillar fungus, as well as many microscopic fungi, e.g. powdery mildews, ring worm fungi, chalkbrood fungus, laboulbeniales and most black moulds around sinks and tubs. The older named taxon euascomycetes is roughly equivalent.

2. The subphylum saccharomycotina comprises most of the 'true' yeasts, such as baker's yeast and *Candida* which are in general single-celled or short chains of cells, and reproduce vegetatively by budding rather than by the production of hyphae. As a result, most were classified in a vaguely defined taxon with the older name hemiascomycetes.

3. The subphylum taphrinomycotina includes a disparate group of ascomycota and were only recognised as a distinctive group after the advent of molecular (DNA) analyses. The group is basal to the other subphyla and hence is considered to be more primitive. Consequently the taxon was originally named archiascomycetes alternatively spelled archaeascomycetes. It includes both hyphal fungi (*Neolecta*, *Taphrina*), and fission yeasts *Schizosaccharomyces* and the peculiar mammalian lung parasite, *Pneumocystis* that was originally believed to be a protozoan.

Evidence from ribosomal RNA gene sequencing of soil indicates that there is likely a fourth, previously unknown subphylum of ascomycota (loosely termed Soil Clone Group I-SCGI), that has never been described via cultures or fruitbodies. SCGI organisms are only known from DNA sequences but have been shown to occur in soils worldwide by Schadt and Porter. Placement of this group based on rRNA gene sequencing indicates that they may fall between the taphriomycotina and the saccharomycotina, however, phenotypic characteristics and environmental roles and significance remain unknown.

Physical make-up

The adjective which describes these fungi is 'ascomycetous'. The majority of ascomycetous fungi grow as a thallus, called a mycelium, consisting of many hyphae which are microscopic multi-branched filaments. If the hyphae of some typical mycelia were laid end to end, they could reach a length of several kilometres. Ascomycota typically produce great numbers of asci at any one time, and these may be contained in a multicellular, often readily visible structure called an 'ascocarp' (also called an 'ascoma', the fruiting body of ascomycetes). Many exceptions to the structure described above occur, for example in one extreme these fungi are single celled yeasts, and there is no mycelium, no fruitbody, and the entire cell is converted into an ascus in such ascomycetous yeasts such as baker's yeast (*Saccharomyces cerevisiae*).

In the case of lichenised species, the thallus of the fungus defines the shape of the symbiotic colony. Other ascomycota are dimorphic, which can mean that they can appear either in single or multi-cellular form. Other species are pleomorphic, exhibiting multiple asexual forms (i.e. anamorphs) as well as a sexual form (a teleomorph). The ascoma come in multiple forms: cup-shaped, club-shaped, potato-like, spongy, seed-like, oozing and pimple-like, coral-like, nit-like, golf-ball-shaped, perforated tennis ball-like, cushion-shaped, plated and feathered in miniature (Laboulbeniales), microscopic classic Greek shield-shaped, stalked or sessile, solitary or clustered, etc. They can be fleshy or carbonaceous (like charcoal), leathery, rubbery, gelatinous, slimy, powdery, or cob-web-like, etc. They come in multiple colours such as red, orange, yellow, and rarely green or blue, although brown or black are more common.

Except for lichens, the mycelium (if produced) is usually inconspicuous because it is subterranean or embedded in the substrate, and only the ascoma is seen in season. But spectacular, bizarre or otherwise noteworthy exceptions occur. Many ascomatous fungi have melanised hyphal walls (referred to as dematiaceous walls) and therefore are black or brown. Black spots on bathroom caulking are often colonies of ascomycota, e.g. *Cladosporium*. Many moulds that grow on spoiled foods are ascomycota, and therefore the pellicles or skins that develop on jams, juices and other foods in containers at home are in fact the thalli of ascomycota (occasionally mucoromycotina and almost never basidiomycota). Sooty moulds that develop on plants, especially in the tropics are the thalli of many species.

Sometimes it is the mass of asci or ascus-like cells or conidia or yeast cells that are the conspicuous elements. Pneumocystis species fill lung cavities causing a form of pneumonia (visible in X-rays). Ascosphaera cysts (asci) fill honey bee larvae and pupae making them appear mummified and chalk-like, hence the name 'chalkbrood'. Free living yeasts form yeast colonies. Excessive *Candida* yeast growth in the mouth or vagina is called 'thrush' or candidiasis.

The cell walls of these fungi are almost always formed of Chitin and β-Glucans; individual cells are formed from divisions of the hyphae called 'septa'. These give stability to the hyphae and prevent a great loss of cytoplasm in the event that the cell membrane should be locally damaged. Mostly the cell divisions are centrally perforated, so they have a small opening in the middle, through which cytoplasm and also nuclei can move more or less freely throughout the system of hyphae. Often hyphae have only one nucleus per cell, and are therefore described as *uninucleate*, but some ascomycetous fungi can also be multinucleate at times.

Metabolism

Like most fungi the ascomycota principally digest living or dead biomass. To achieve this, they secrete into their surroundings powerful digestive enzymes which break down organic substances into small molecules, which are then absorbed through the cell wall. Many species live on dead plant material such as fallen leaves, twigs or logs. Others attack plants, animals or other fungi as parasites and derive their metabolic energy, as well as all the nutrients they need, from the cell tissue of their hosts. Especially in this group extreme specialisation appears; for instance certain species of laboulbeniales attack only one particular leg of one particular insect species. The ascomycota also often take up symbiotic relationships—for instance some combine with green algae or cyanobacteria, from which they obtain photosynthetic nutrients, to form lichens; others form symbioses with tree roots as mycorrhizal fungi. There are also carnivorous fungi, which have developed hyphal traps in which they can catch small protists such as amoebae, as well as roundworms (*Nematoda*), rotifers, tardigrades and small arthropods such as springtails (*Collembola*).

Through their long evolutionary history the ascomycota have developed the capability to break down almost every organic substance. Unlike most organisms they are able to use their own enzymes to digest plant cellulose and the lignin contained in wood. Collagen, an abundant structural protein in animals and keratin (which hair is made of), can also serve as food sources. Exotic examples are given by the ascomycete *Aureobasidium pullulans*, which metabolises wall paint, and the kerosene fungus *Amorphotheca resinae*, which (to the misfortune of the airline industry) feeds on aircraft fue, and in tropical regions sometimes blocks fuel pipes. Others resist osmotic stress to grow on salted fish, and a few live in water.

Distribution and living environment

The ascomycota are present in all land ecosystems worldwide — they even occur in Antarctica — and their spores and hyphal fragments are distributed through the atmosphere and freshwater environments, as well as ocean beaches and tidal zones. The distribution of individual species is very variable: some are found on all continents, while for example the white truffle tuber magnatum, which is much sought after for culinary purposes, only appears in isolated locations in Italy and France. Plant parasitic species are often restricted by their host distributions. *Cyttaria* is only found on *Nothofagus* (Southern Beech) in the Southern Hemisphere.

Reproduction

Asexual reproduction

Asexual reproduction is the dominant form of propagation in the ascomycota and is responsible for the rapid expansion of these fungi into areas which were previously not colonised. It occurs through reproductive structures, the 'conidia', which are genetically identical to the parent and mostly have just one nucleus. They are also called 'mitospores' due to the way they are generated through the cellular process of mitosis. They are generally formed on the ends of specialised hyphae, the 'conidiophores'. Depending on the species they may be dispersed by wind or water, or also by animals.

Asexual spores

In order to further classify the ascomycota in the asexual stages, it is important to consider the spores, which can be distinguished by colour, form and the way they are separated into cells. The most frequent types are the single-celled spores which are designated *amerospores*. If the spore is divided into two by a cross-wall (septum), it is a *didymospore*.

Heterocaryosis and parasexuality

A significant number of ascomycota species either have no sexual stage or none is known. In spite of this, there are two ways in which they can conserve their genetic diversity: Heterocaryosis and parasexuality.

The former happens simply through the merging of two hyphae belonging to different individuals, a process known as anastomosis. As a result there are more cell nuclei than normal in the mycelium and they come from genetically different parent organisms.

Parasexuality, on the other hand, refers to a phenomenon where two cell nuclei merge without any sexual process and the chromosome count is doubled. This involves a complex form of the type of cell division called mitosis, where there is crossing over or recombination, i.e. an exchange of genetic material between corresponding pairs of chromosomes. In sexual reproduction, in contrast, crossing over occurs only during meiosis. Finally the chromosome count will be restored to normal by haploidisation, whereby the nucleus splits into two parts each having a single set of chromosomes, with each daughter genetically different from the original parents.

Sexual reproduction

Sexual reproduction in the ascomycota is marked by a characteristic structure, the *ascus*, which distinguishes these fungi from all others. An ascus is a tube-shaped vessel, a *meiosporangium*, which contains the sexual spores produced by meiosis. The latter are called *ascospores* in contrast to the asexual *conidiospores*.

Apart from exceptions such as baker's yeast (*Saccharomyces cerevisiae*), almost all fungi of the ascomycota are haploid, so their nuclei only contain one set of chromosomes. During sexual reproduction there is a diploid phase (with two sets of chromosomes), which as a rule is very short. Then meiosis occurs, generally very soon, so that the haploid state is re-established.

The sexual part of the life cycle commences when two suitable hyphae meet each other. These come from the same web of hyphae which can also generate asexual spores. The first deciding factor as to whether conjugation—that is, sexual merging—will occur, is whether the hyphae belong to the same organism, or whether they come from different individual fungi. Whilst many species are thoroughly capable of self-propagation, i.e. they are homothallic, others need non-identical partners and so are heterothallic. Besides this, the two hyphae in question must also belong to the same mating type. Mating types are a peculiarity of the fungi and correspond roughly to the sexes in plants and animals; however one species may have more than two mating types.

In the case of compatibility, gametangia form on the hyphae; these are the generative cells for the gametes, in which numerous nuclei gather. A very fine hypha, called the trichogyne, which grows out of one gametangium, now termed the ascogonium, makes a passage to a gametangium of the other individual, which is then the antheridium. Nuclei then pass from the antheridium (playing a 'male' role) to the ascogonium (playing a 'female' role).

Unlike the process in animals and plants, after the union of the cytoplasms of the two gametangia (plasmogamy), the merging of the nuclei (karyogamy) does not usually occur immediately. Instead, the nuclei which have migrated in from the antheridium pair up with the nuclei of the ascogonium, but remain separate next to their partners. With this the dikaryophase of the life cycle begins; during this time the pairs of nuclei repeatedly synchronously divide, so that a great number are produced. In all probability the dikaryophase is an evolutionary adaptation which serves to exploit the potential of sexual reproduction to the full in circumstances where it is a rare event for different individuals to meet each other. After the genetic raw material has been increased by repeated division, recombination will take place independently in each pair during meiosis, so that the greatest possible quantity of genetically different spores will arise. In the red algae (Rhodophyta) a similar solution to the corresponding problem evolved independently.

Next millions of new dinucleate hyphae, into each of which two nuclei migrate, emerge from the fertilised ascogonium. They are also called ascogenous or fertile. They are fed by ordinary uni- or mononucleate hyphae (with only one nucleus), which are also called *sterile*. The tissue of sterile and fertile hyphae now grows in many cases into a macroscopically visible fruiting body, the ascocarp, which may contain millions of fertile hyphae.

In the actual fruiting layer, the hymenium, the asci now appear. At one end of an ascogenous hypha, there develops a U-shaped hook, which points back opposite to the general growth direction. The two nuclei contained in the terminal cell then divide in such a way that the threads of their mitotic spindles run parallel, and thus two pairs of genetically different daughter nuclei arise, with one daughter of each pair near the point of the hook, and the other in the base part of the hypha. Then two parallel cross-walls appear, dividing the hypha into three sections: that at the point of the hook with one nucleus, that at the base of the original hypha with one nucleus, and the middle U-shaped part with two nuclei.

If the positioning in the fruiting layer is right, the karyogamic fusion of the nuclei finally takes place in the U-shaped cell, creating the diploid zygote. It lengthens to form an elongated tube-shaped or cylinder-shaped capsule, the actual ascus. Then meiosis occurs, giving rise to four haploid nuclei. This is almost always followed by a further mitotic division, so that the ascus ultimately has eight daughter nuclei. These become enclosed, together with some of the cell plasma, each by their own membranes, and generally with a hard cell wall. Thus the dissemination cells (the ascospores) develop, lying initially like peas in a pod inside the ascus. Later, when an appropriate opportunity presents itself, they are liberated.

Not having flagella, ascospores are disseminated in various other ways: some are spread by wind and with others the ripe ascus breaks open on contact with water to set free the spores. Certain species have evolved regular 'spore cannons' which can eject them up to 30 cm away. When the spores reach a suitable substrate, they germinate, form new hyphae, and so restart their life cycle, which has come full circle.

The form of the ascus is important for classification and is divided into four basic types: unitunicate-operculate, unitunicate-inoperculate, bitunicate or prototunicate.

Ecology

The ascomycota fulfil a central role in most land-based ecosystems. They are important decomposers which break down such organic materials as dead leaves, twigs, fallen trees, etc. and help the detritivores (animals which live off this decomposing material) to obtain their nutrients. By processing substances like cellulose or lignin, which are otherwise difficult to exploit, they take on an important place in the natural nitrogen cycle and the carbon cycle.

Inversely the fruiting bodies of the ascomycota provide food for a very diverse set of animals from insects and slugs and snails (*Gastropoda*) to rodents and larger mammals such as deer and wild boars.

Fungi of the ascomycota are also known for their numerous symbiotic relationships with other organisms.

Lichens

Probably since early in their evolutionary history the ascomycota have 'domesticated' green algae (*Chlorophyta*), as well as occasionally other types of algae and cyanobacteria. Together they form the mutualistic associations known as lichens, which can survive in the least hospitable terrestrial regions of the earth, including the Arctic, the Antarctic, deserts and mountaintops, and can withstand temperature extremes from −40° to +80°C. While the photoautotrophic algal partner creates metabolic energy through photosynthesis, the fungus offers a stable supportive framework and protects from radiation and drying out. Around 42 per cent of the ascomycota (numerically about 18,000 species) form lichens, and almost all the fungal partners of lichens belong to the ascomycota the proportion of basidiomycota is probably only two to three per cent.

Mycorrhizal fungi and endophytes

Members of the ascomycota make two particularly important types of relationship with plants: as mycorrhizal fungi and as endophytes. The former make symbiotic associations with the root systems of the plants, which for some trees, especially conifers, can be of vital importance, enabling the uptake of mineral salts from the soil. The fungal partner is in a much better position to absorb minerals due to its finely divided mycelium, whilst the plant provides it with metabolic energy in the form of photosynthetic products. Cases are even known where mycorrhizal fungi can transport nutrients from one plant to another, stabilising the recipient. It is likely that mycorrhizal associations enabled the conquest of the land by plants—in any case the earliest known fossils of land plants have mycorrhizae.

Endophytes on the other hand live inside plants, especially in the stem and leaves, but generally do not damage their hosts. The exact nature of the relationship between endophytic fungus and host is not yet well understood, but it seems that this form of colonisation can bestow a higher resistance against insects, roundworms (nematodes) and bacteria; also it can enable or augment the production of poisonous alkaloids, chemicals which can affect the health of plant-eating mammals.

Symbiotic relationships with animals

A series of ascomycota species from the genus *Xylaria* are found in the nests of leafcutter ants and other fungus-growing ants of the tribe attini and in the fungal gardens of termites (isoptera). Since they do not generate fruiting bodies until the insects have left the nests, it is suspected that, as confirmed in several cases of Basidiomycota species, they may be cultivated.

On the other hand bark beetles (family Scolytidae) are certainly important symbiotic partners. The female beetles transport the spores to new hosts in characteristic tucks in their skin, the *mycetangia*. There they eat tunnels in the wood, which lead into large chambers in which they lay their eggs. At this time the spores are released and give rise to hyphae which unlike the beetles can digest the wood. The beetle larvae feed on the fungus and after they have metamorphosed into the adult state they again carry spores with them to renew the cycle of infection. A well-known example of this is Dutch elm disease, caused by fungus *Ophiostoma ulmi*, being carried by the European elm bark beetle *Scolytus multistriatus*.

Ascomycetes make many contributions to the good of humanity, and also have many ill effects. One of their most harmful roles is as the agent of many plant diseases.

Basidiomycota

Basidiomycota is one of two large phyla that, together with the ascomycota, comprise the subkingdom Dikarya (often referred to as the 'higher fungi') within the Kingdom Fungi. More specifically the Basidiomycota include mushrooms, puffballs, stinkhorns, bracket fungi, other polypores, jelly fungi, boletes, chanterelles, earth stars, smuts, bunts, rusts, mirror yeasts, and the human pathogenic yeast, *Cryptococcus*. Basically, basidiomycota are filamentous fungi composed of hyphae (except for those forming yeasts) and reproducing sexually via the formation of specialised club-shaped end cells called basidia that normally bear external meiospores (usually four). These specialised spores are called basidiospores. However, some basidiomycota reproduce asexually, and may or may not also reproduce sexually. Asexually reproducing basidiomycota can be recognised as members of this phylum by gross similarity to others, by the formation of a distinctive anatomical feature, cell wall components, and definitively by phylogenetic molecular analysis of DNA sequence data.

In basidiomycetes, the zygote emerges to form a club-shaped cell, the basidium; at the same time, the diploid nucleus undergoes meiosis. The subsequent course of events is strikingly different from that which occurs in an ascus. No spores are formed within the basidium; instead, a slender projection known as a sterigma develops at its upper end, and a nucleus migrates into this sterigma formed near the based of the sterigma, the cell thus cut off being a basidiospore. The same process is repeated for the remaining three nuclei in the basidium, so that a mature basidium bears on its surface four basidiospores (Fig. 1.2). Basidiospore discharge is a remarkable phenomenon. After the basidiospore has matured, a minute droplet of liquid appears at the point of its attachment to the basidium. This droplet grows rapidly until it is about one-fifth the size of the spore, and then, quite suddenly, both spore and droplet are shot away from the basidium.

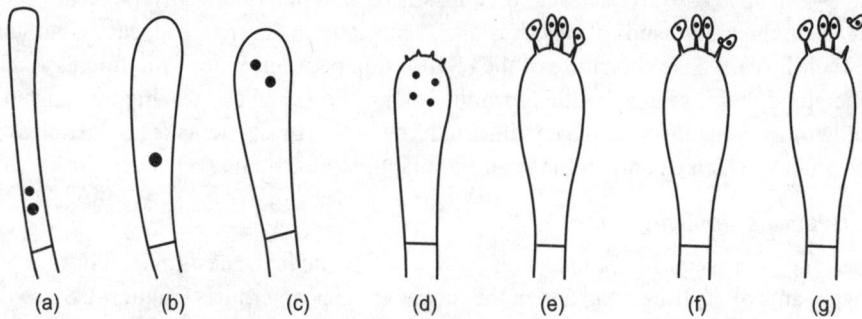

Fig. 1.2. Successive stages in basidium formation and basidiospore discharge: (a) binucleate cell, (b) nuclear fusion, (c), (d) nuclear division, (e) formation of basidiospores, (f), and (g) basidiospore discharge.

Classification

The most recent classification adopted by a coalition of 67 mycologists recognises 3 subphyla (pucciniomycotina, ustilaginomycotina, agaricomycotina) and 2 other class level taxa (wallemiomycetes, entorrhizomycetes) outside of these, among the basidiomycota. As now classified, the subphyla join and also cut across various obsolete taxonomic groups previously commonly used to describe various basidiomycota.

The basidiomycota had traditionally been divided into 2 obsolete classes, the homobasidiomycetes (including true mushrooms); and the heterobasidiomycetes. Previously the entire basidiomycota were called basidiomycetes, an invalid class level name coined in 1959 as a counterpart to the ascomycetes, when neither of these taxa were recognised as phyla. The terms basidiomycetes and ascomycetes are frequently used loosely to refer to basidiomycota and ascomycota. They are often abbreviated to 'basidios' and 'ascos' as mycological slang.

The agaricomycotina includes what had previously been called the hymenomycetes (an obsolete morphological based class of basidiomycota that formed hymenial layers on their fruitbodies), the gasteromycetes (another obsolete class that included species mostly lacking hymenia and mostly forming spores in enclosed fruitbodies), as well as most of the jelly fungi. The ustilaginomycotina are most (but not all) of the former smut fungi and along with the exobasidiales.

The pucciniomycotina includes the rust fungi, the insect parasitic/symbiotic genus *Septobasidium*, a former group of smut fungi (in the microbotryomycetes, which includes mirror yeasts), and a mixture of odd, infrequently seen or seldom recognised fungi, often parasitic on plants.

Two classes, wallemiomycetes and entorrhizomycetes cannot at present be placed in a subphylum.

Typical life cycle

Unlike higher animals and plants which have readily recognisable male and female counterparts, basidiomycota [except for the rust (pucciniales)] tend to have mutually indistinguishable, compatible haploids which are usually mycelia being composed of filamentous hyphae. Typically haploid basidiomycota mycelia fuse via plasmogamy and then the compatible nuclei migrate into each other's mycelia and pair up with the resident nuclei. Karyogamy is delayed, so that the compatible nuclei remain in pairs, called a dikaryon. The hyphae are then said to be dikaryotic. Conversely, the haploid mycelia are called monokaryons. Often, the dikaryotic mycelium is more vigorous than the individual monokaryotic mycelia, and proceeds to take over the substrate in which they are growing. The dikaryons can be long-lived, lasting years, decades or centuries. The monokaryons are neither male nor female. They have either a bipolar (unifactorial) or a tetrapolar (bifactorial) mating system. This results in the fact that following meiosis, the resulting haploid basidiospores and resultant monokaryons, have nuclei that are compatible with 50 per cent (if bipolar) or 25 per cent (if tetrapolar) of their sister basidiospores (and their resultant monokaryons) because the mating genes must differ for them to be compatible. However, there are many variations of these genes in the population, and therefore, over 90 per cent of monokaryons are compatible with each other. It is as if there were multiple sexes.

The maintenance of the dikaryotic status in dikaryons in many basidiomycota is facilitated by the formation of clamp connections that physically appear to help coordinate and re-establish pairs of compatible nuclei following synchronous mitotic nuclear divisions. Variations are frequent and multiple. In a typical basidiomycota life cycle the long lasting dikaryons periodically (seasonally or occasionally) produce basidia, the specialised usually club-shaped end cells, in which a pair of compatible nuclei fuse (karyogamy) to form a diploid cell. Meiosis follows shortly with the production of 4 haploid nuclei that migrate into 4 external, usually apical basidiospores. Variations occur, however. Typically the basidiospores are ballistic, hence they are sometimes also called ballistospores. In most species, the basidiospores disperse and each can start a new haploid mycelium, continuing the life cycle. Basidia are microscopic but they are often produced on or in multicelled large fructifications called basidiocarps (or basidiomes or fruitbodies), variously called mushrooms, puffballs, etc. Ballistic basidiospores are formed on sterigmata which are tapered spine-like projections on basidia and are typically curved, like the horns of a bull. In some basidiomycota the spores are not ballistic, and the sterigmata may be straight, reduced to stubbs or absent. The basidiospores of these non-ballistosporic basidia may either bud off or be released via dissolution or disintegration of the basidia.

Schematic of a typical basidiocarp, the dipoid reproductive structure of a basidiomycete, showing fruiting body, hymenium and basidia.

In summary, meiosis takes place in a diploid basidium. Each one of the four haploid nuclei migrates into its own basidiospore. The basidiospores are ballistically discharged and start new haploid mycelia called monokaryons. There are no males or females, rather there are compatible thalli with multiple compatibility factors. Plasmogamy between compatible individuals leads to delayed karyogamy leading to establishment of a dikaryon. The dikaryon is long lasting but ultimately gives rise to either fruitbodies with basidia or directly to basidia without fruitbodies. The paired dikaryon in the basidium fuse (i.e. karyogamy takes place). The diploid basidium begins the cycle again.

Variations in life cycles

Many variations occur. Some are self-compatible and spontaneously form dikaryons without a separate compatible thallus being involved. These fungi are said to be *homothallic*, versus the normal *heterothallic* species with mating types. Others are secondarily homothallic, in that two compatible nuclei following meiosis migrate into each basidiospore, which is then dispersed as a pre-existing dikaryon. Often such species form only two spores per basidium, but that too varies. Following meiosis, mitotic divisions can occur in the basidium. Multiple numbers of basidiospores can result, including odd numbers via degeneration of nuclei, or pairing up of nuclei, or lack of migration of nuclei.

For example, the chanterelle genus *Craterellus* often has 6-spored basidia, while some corticioid *Sistotrema* species can have 2-, 4-, 6- or 8-spored basidia, and the cultivated button mushroom, *Agaricus bisporus* can have 1-, 2-, 3- or 4-spored basidia under some circumstances. Occasionally monokaryons of some taxa can form morphologically fully formed basidiomes and anatomically correct basidia and ballistic basidiospores in the absence of dikaryon formation, diploid nuclei and meiosis. A rare few number of taxa have extended diploid life cycles, but can be common species. Examples exist in the mushroom genera *Armillaria* and *Xerula*, both in the physalacriaceae. Occasionally basidiospores are not formed and parts of the 'basidia' act as the dispersal agents, e.g. the peculiar mycoparasitic jelly fungus, *Tetragoniomyces* or the entire 'basidium' acts as a 'spore', e.g. in some false puffballs (*Scleroderma*).

Deuteromycotina

Form-class deuteromycetes

Form-class deuteromycetes is an artificial assemblage of those fungi which reproduce by asexual spores. Since all these fungi apparently lack a sexual phase (perfect stage), they are commonly called 'imperfect fungi' or technically 'fungi imperfecti'. In some deuteromycetes sexual stages have been discovered in nature and in cultures and most of these are known to belong to ascomycetes and a few to basidiomycetes. In view of these discoveries, deuteromycetes are considered as conidial stages of ascomycetes or rarely basidiomycetes whose sexual stages have not been discovered or do not exist.

According to Hawksworth there are over 17,000 form-species included in the subdivision deuteromycotina. Majority of these species are terrestrial and a good number have been reported from marine and freshwater habitats. Nutritionally, majority of the deuteromycetes are either saprobes or weak parasites of plants. A few are mycoparasites and some even trap nematodes and consume them. In addition, some are parasites of animals and human beings, lichen symbionts, endophytes of angiosperms and gymnosperms and even mycorrhiza formers. Many species of this group produce a variety of mycotoxins in foods and feeds which have been shown to be carcinogenic to animals including human beings. In contrast to this, members of deuteromycetes also have a positive role in agriculture, forestry and medicines. They decompose organic matter and thus bring about recycling of nutrients in nature. Some of them are used in the commercial production of antibiotics, enzymes and many other chemicals of medicinal importance. Their use in fermentation industry is great. Many genera are even utilised in processing and flavouring foods.

Deuteromycetes typically produce well developed, septate, branched mycelium. The cells are usually multinucleate and the septa are perforated, permitting the streaming of cytoplasm and the migration of nuclei from one cell to another. With few exceptions, deuteromycetes mostly reproduce by means of special spores known as conidia (sing. *conidium*). A conidium is a nonmotile, asexual spore formed at the tip or side of a conidiogenous cell. These may be produced singly or in chains or in a droplet of mucus. The conidiophores may occur singly (*mononematous*) or they may be aggregated to form specialised structures such as sporodochia and synnemata or produced in definite fructifications known as pycnidia or acervuli. When the conidiophores are united or closely appressed at the base and separated at the top, they are called synnematous and the fructification is known as synnema (pl. synnemata) or *coremium* (pl. *coremia*). Conidia may be formed at the apex of the synnema (Fig. 1.3b) or along its length. In a sporodochium, the conidiophores arise from a cushion of loosely interwoven mycelia (Fig. 1.3a). An acervulus (pl. *acervuli*) is typically a flat or saucer-shaped, bed of short conidiophores growing side by side and arising from a more or less stromatic mass of hyphae. A *pycnidium* (pl. *pycnidia*) may be globose or flask shaped, hollow fructification lined on the inside with conidiophores bearing conidia. The pycnidia vary from ostiolate to completely closed and may be provided with a small papilla or a long neck.

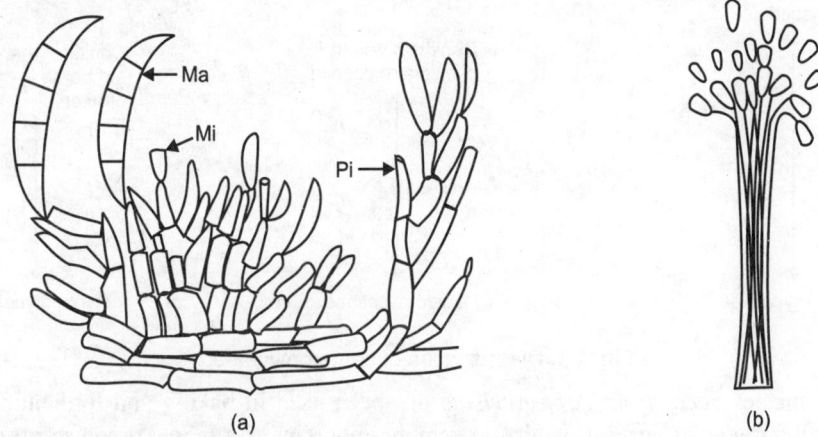

(a)   (b)

Fig. 1.3. Types of asexual fructification: (a) Sporoduchium of *Fusarium* composed of loosely interwoven mycelium bearing phialides (Pi), macroconidia (Ma) and microconidia (Mi), and (b) synnema of *Graphium*.

Conidia of deuteromycetes may be unicellular, bicellular or multicellular. The multicellular conidia may be divided by septa in one to three planes. The shape of the conidia may be varied, for example, globose, elliptical, ovoid, cylindrical, clavate, muriform, sigmoid, reniform, pyriform, filiform, etc. The colour of the conidia may be hyaline (colourless) or brightly coloured (blue, green, pink, grey, brick red) or dark due to the presence of melanins. The colour of the condia and conidiophores form important taxonomical features.

Some of the deuteromycetes derive many of the benefits of sexuality through parasexuality. This is a process in which plasmogamy, karyogamy and haploidisation takes place, but not at specified points in the thallus or the life cycle. Parasexuality was first observed in *Aspergillus nidulans*, the imperfect state of *Emericella nidulans* by Pontecorvo and Roper in 1952. Since then, parasexuality has been found to exist in several imperfect fungi that possess no sexual stage.

Traditionally, the fungi included in the subdivision deuteromycotina have been placed in the single large form-class deuteromycetes. Alexopoulos and Mims classified the deuteromycetes into three subclasses as shown in Fig. 1.4.

Yeast

Yeasts are eukaryotic micro-organisms classified in the kingdom fungi, with about 1500 species currently described; they dominate fungal diversity in the oceans. Most reproduce asexually by budding, although a few do so by binary fission. Yeasts are unicellular, although some species with yeast forms may become multicellular through the formation of a string of connected budding cells known as *pseudohyphae*, or *false hyphae* as seen in most moulds. Yeast size can vary greatly depending on the species, typically measuring 3–4 μm in diameter, although some yeasts can reach over 40 μm.

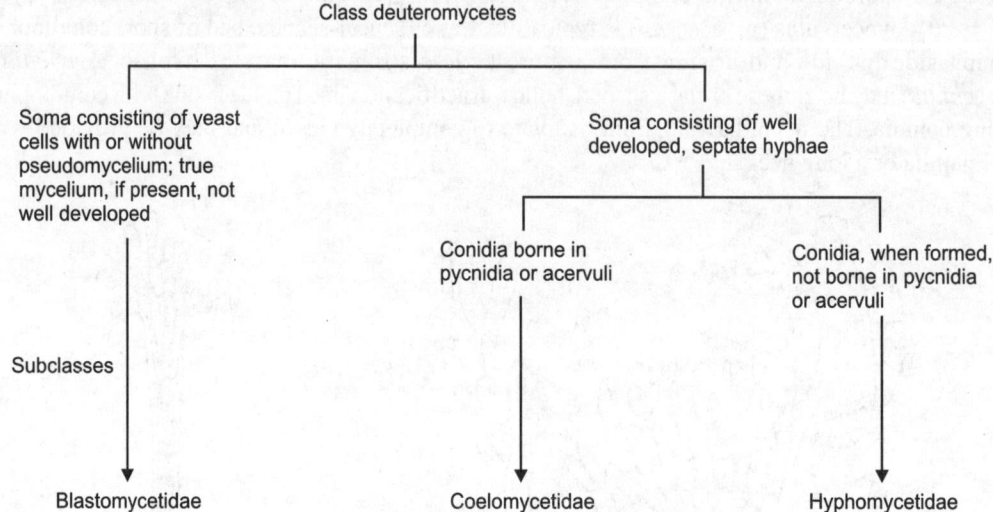

Fig. 1.4. Classification of deuteromycetes.

The yeast species *Saccharomyces cerevisiae* has been used in baking and fermenting alcoholic beverages for thousands of years. It is also extremely important as a model organism in modern cell biology research, and is the most thoroughly researched eukaryotic micro-organism. Researchers have used it to gather information into the biology of the eukaryotic cell and ultimately human biology. Other species of yeast, such as *Candida albicans*, are opportunistic pathogens and can cause infection in humans. Yeasts have recently been used to generate electricity in microbial fuel cells, and produce ethanol for the biofuel industry.

Yeasts do not form a specific taxonomic or phylogenetic grouping. At present it is estimated that only 1 per cent of all yeast species have been described. The term 'yeast' is often taken as a synonym for *S. cerevisiae*, but the phylogenetic diversity of yeasts is shown by their placement in both divisions ascomycota and basidiomycota. The budding yeasts 'true yeasts' are classified in the order saccharomycetales.

Cyanobacteria

Cyanobacteria, also known as blue-green algae, blue-green bacteria or cyanophyta, is a phylum of bacteria that obtain their energy through photosynthesis. The name 'cyanobacteria' comes from the colour of the bacteria. They are a significant component of the marine nitrogen cycle and an important primary producer in many areas of the ocean, but are also found in habitats other than the marine environment; in particular cyanobacteria are known to occur in both freshwater, hypersaline inland lakes and in arid areas where they are a major component of biological soil crusts.

Stromatolites of fossilised oxygen-producing cyanobacteria have been found from 2.8 billion years ago. The ability of cyanobacteria to perform oxygenic photosynthesis is thought to have converted the early reducing atmosphere into an oxidising one, which dramatically changed the composition of life forms on Earth by provoking an explosion of biodiversity and leading to the near-extinction of oxygen-intolerant organisms. Chloroplasts in plants and eukaryotic algae have evolved from cyanobacteria via endosymbiosis.

Forms of cyanobacteria

Cyanobacteria are found in almost every conceivable environment, from oceans to freshwater to bare rock to soil. They can occur as planktonic cells or form phototrophic biofilms in freshwater and marine environments, they occur in damp soil, or even temporarily moistened rocks in deserts. A few are endosymbionts in lichens, plants, various protists, or sponges and provide energy for the host. Some live in the fur of sloths, providing a form of camouflage.

Cyanobacteria include unicellular and colonial species. Colonies may form filaments, sheets or even hollow balls. Some filamentous colonies show the ability to differentiate into several different cell types: vegetative cells, the normal, photosynthetic cells that are formed under favourable growing conditions; akinetes, the climate-resistant spores that may form when environmental conditions become harsh; and thick-walled heterocysts, which contain the enzyme nitrogenase, vital for nitrogen fixation. Heterocysts may also form under the appropriate environmental conditions (anoxic) wherever nitrogen is necessary. Heterocyst-forming species are specialised for nitrogen fixation and are able to fix nitrogen gas, which cannot be used by plants, into ammonia (NH_3), nitrites (NO_2^-) or nitrates (NO_3^-), which can be absorbed by plants and converted to protein and nucleic acids. The rice paddies of Asia, which produce about 75 per cent of the world's rice, could not do so were it not for healthy populations of nitrogen-fixing cyanobacteria in the rice paddy fertiliser.

Many cyanobacteria also form motile filaments, called hormogonia, that travel away from the main biomass to bud and form new colonies elsewhere. The cells in a hormogonium are often thinner than in the vegetative state, and the cells on either end of the motile chain may be tapered. In order to break away from the parent colony, a hormogonium often must tear apart a weaker cell in a filament, called a necridium. Each individual cell of a cyanobacterium typically has a thick, gelatinous cell wall. They differ from other gram-negative bacteria in that the quorum sensing molecules autoinducer-2 and acyl-homoserine lactones are absent. They lack flagella, but hormogonia and some unicellular species may move about by gliding along surfaces. In water columns some cyanobacteria float by forming gas vesicles, like in archaea.

Some of these organisms contribute significantly to global ecology and the oxygen cycle. The tiny marine cyanobacterium *Prochlorococcus* was discovered in 1986 and accounts for more than half of the photosynthesis of the open ocean. Many cyanobacteria even display the circadian rhythms that were once thought to exist only in eukaryotic cells.

Bacteria

The bacteria are a large group of unicellular micro-organisms. Typically a few micrometres in length, bacteria have a wide range of shapes, ranging from spheres to rods and spirals. Bacteria are ubiquitous in every habitat on earth, growing in soil, acidic hot springs, radioactive waste, water, and deep in the earth's crust, as well as in organic matter and the live bodies of plants and animals. There are typically 40 million bacterial cells in a gram of soil and a million bacterial cells in a millilitre of freshwater; in all, there are approximately five nonillion (5×10^{30}) bacteria on earth, forming much of the world's biomass. Bacteria are vital in recycling nutrients, with many steps in nutrient cycles depending on these organisms, such as the fixation of nitrogen from the atmosphere and putrefaction. However, most bacteria have not been characterised, and only about half of the phyla of bacteria have species that can be grown in the laboratory. The study of bacteria is known as bacteriology, a branch of microbiology.

There are approximately ten times as many bacterial cells in the human flora of bacteria as there are human cells in the body, with large numbers of bacteria on the skin and as gut flora. The vast majority of the bacteria in the body are rendered harmless by the protective effects of the immune system, and a few are beneficial. However, a few species of bacteria are pathogenic and cause infectious diseases, including cholera, syphilis, anthrax, leprosy and bubonic plague. The most common fatal bacterial diseases are respiratory infections, with tuberculosis alone killing about 2 million people a year, mostly in sub-Saharan Africa. In developed countries, antibiotics are used to treat bacterial infections and in agriculture, so antibiotic resistance is becoming common. In industry, bacteria are important in sewage treatment, the production of cheese and yoghurt through fermentation, as well as in biotechnology, and the manufacture of antibiotics and other chemicals.

Once regarded as plants constituting the class schizomycetes, bacteria are now classified as prokaryotes. Unlike cells of animals and other eukaryotes, bacterial cells do not contain a nucleus and rarely harbour membrane-bound organelles. Although the term bacteria traditionally included all prokaryotes, the scientific classification changed after the discovery in the 1990s that prokaryotes consist of two very different groups of organisms that evolved independently from an ancient common ancestor. These evolutionary domains are called bacteria and archaea.

Actinobacteria

They include some of the most common soil life, playing an important role in decomposition of organic materials, such as cellulose and chitin and thereby playing a vital part in organic matter turnover and carbon cycle. This replenishes the supply of nutrients in the soil and is an important part of humus formation. Other actinobacteria inhabit plants and animals, including a few pathogens, such as *Mycobacterium*, *Corynebacterium*, *Nocardia*, *Rhodococcus* and a few species of *Streptomyces*.

Actinobacteria are well known as secondary metabolite producers and hence of high pharmacological and commercial interest. In 1940 Selman Waksman discovered that the soil bacteria he was studying made actinomycin, a discovery which granted him a Nobel Prize. Since then hundreds of naturally occurring antibiotics have been discovered in these terrestrial micro-organisms, especially from the genus *Streptomyces*. Some Actinobacteria form branching filaments, which somewhat resemble the mycelia of the unrelated fungi, among which they were originally classified under the older name actinomycetes. Most members are aerobic, but a few, such as *Actinomyces israelii*, can grow under anaerobic conditions. Unlike the Firmicutes, the other main group of Gram-positive bacteria, they have DNA with a high GC-content and some actinomycetes species produce external spores. Some types of Actinobacteria are responsible for the peculiar odour emanating from the soil after rain, mainly on warmer climates. Most actinobacteria of medical or economic significance are in subclass actinobacteridae. While many of these cause disease in humans, streptomyces is notable as a source of antibiotics.

Lactic Acid Bacteria

The lactic acid bacteria (LAB) comprise a clade of Gram-positive, low-GC, acid-tolerant, generally non-sporulating, non-respiring rod or cocci that are associated by their common metabolic and physiological characteristics. These bacteria, usually found in decomposing plants and lactic products, produce lactic acid as the major metabolic end-product of carbohydrate fermentation. This trait has, throughout history, linked LAB with food fermentations, as acidification inhibits the growth of spoilage agents. Proteinaceous bacteriocins are produced by several LAB strains and provide an additional hurdle for spoilage and pathogenic micro-organisms. Furthermore, lactic acid and other metabolic products contribute to the organoleptic and textural profile of a food item. The industrial importance of the LAB is further evidenced by their reputed safe (GRAS) status, due to their ubiquitous appearance in food and their contribution to the healthy microflora of human mucosal surfaces. The genera that comprise the LAB are at its core *Lactobacillus, Leuconostoc, Pediococcus, Lactococcus* and *Streptococcus* as well as the more peripheral *Aerococcus, Carnobacterium, Enterococcus, Oenococcus, Sporolactobacillus, Teragenococcus, Vagococcus* and *Weisella*; these belong to the order Lactobacillales.

Characteristics

The Lactic Acid Bacteria (LAB) are rod-shaped bacilli or coccus. LAB are characterised by an increased tolerance to a lower pH range. This aspect partially enables LAB to outcompete other bacteria in a natural fermentation, as they can withstand the increased acidity from organic acid production (e.g. lactic acid). Laboratory media used for LAB typically includes a carbohydrate source as most species are incapable of respiration. LAB are catalase negative.

LAB metabolism

There are two main hexose fermentation pathways that are used to classify LAB genera. Under conditions of excess glucose and limited oxygen, homolactic LAB catabolise one mole of glucose in the Embden-Meyerhof-Parnas (EMP) pathway to yield two moles of pyruvate. Intracellular redox balance is maintained through the oxidation of NADH, concomitant with pyruvate reduction to lactic acid. This process yields two moles ATP per glucose consumed. Representative homolactic LAB genera include *Lactococcus, Enterococcus, Streptococcus, Pediococcus* and group I lactobacilli. Heterofermentative LAB use the pentose phosphate pathway, alternatively referred to as the pentose phosphoketolase pathway.

One mole Glucose-6-phosphate is initially dehydrogenated to 6-phosphogluconate and subsequently decarboxylated to yield one mole of CO_2. The resulting pentose-5-phosphate is cleaved into one mole glyceraldehyde phosphate (GAP) and one mole acetyl phosphate. GAP is further metabolised to lactate as in homofermentation, with the acetyl phosphate reduced to ethanol via acetyl-CoA and acetaldehyde intermediates. In theory, end-products (including ATP) are produced in equimolar quantities from the catabolism of one mole of glucose. Obligate heterofermentative LAB include *Leuconostoc, Oenococcus, Weissella* and group III lactobacilli.

Algae

Algae (Latin seaweeds, singular Alga) are a large and diverse group of simple, typically autotrophic organisms, ranging from unicellular to multicellular forms. The largest and most complex marine forms are called seaweeds. They are photosynthetic, like plants, and 'simple' because they lack the many distinct organs found in land plants. For that reason they are currently excluded from being considered plants. Though the prokaryotic *Cyanobacteria* (commonly referred to as blue-green algae) were traditionally included as 'algae' in older textbooks, many modern sources regard this as outdated and restrict the term algae to eukaryotic organisms.

All true algae therefore have a nucleus enclosed within a membrane and chloroplasts bound in one or more membranes. Algae constitute a paraphyletic and polyphyletic group, as they do not include all the descendants of the last universal ancestor nor do they all descend from a common algal ancestor, although their chloroplasts seem to have a single origin.

Algae lack the various structures that characterise land plants, such as phyllids and rhizoids in nonvascular plants, or leaves, roots, and other organs that are found in tracheophytes. Many are photoautotrophic, although some groups contain members that are mixotrophic, deriving energy both from photosynthesis and uptake of organic carbon either by osmotrophy, myzotrophy or phagotrophy. Some unicellular species rely entirely on external energy sources and have limited or no photosynthetic apparatus. Nearly all algae have photosynthetic machinery ultimately derived from the cyanobacteria, and so produce oxygen as a by-product of photosynthesis, unlike other photosynthetic bacteria such as purple and green sulphur bacteria.

METABOLISM

Metabolism is the set of chemical reactions that occur in living organisms in order to maintain life. These processes allow organisms to grow and reproduce, maintain their structures, and respond to their environments. Metabolism is usually divided into two categories. Catabolism breaks down organic matter, for example to harvest energy in cellular respiration. Anabolism, on the other hand, uses energy to construct components of cells such as proteins and nucleic acids.

The chemical reactions of metabolism are organised into metabolic pathways, in which one chemical is transformed into another by a sequence of enzymes. Enzymes are crucial to metabolism because they allow organisms to drive desirable but thermodynamically unfavourable reactions by coupling them to favourable ones, and because they act as catalysts to allow these reactions to proceed quickly and efficiently. Enzymes also allow the regulation of metabolic pathways in response to changes in the cell's environment or signals from other cells.

The metabolism of an organism determines which substances it will find nutritious and which it will find poisonous. For example, some prokaryotes use hydrogen sulphide as a nutrient, yet this gas is poisonous to animals. The speed of metabolism, the metabolic rate, also influences how much food an organism will require. A striking feature of metabolism is the similarity of the basic metabolic pathways between even vastly different species. For example, the set of carboxylic acids that are best known as the intermediates in the citric acid cycle are present in all organisms, being found in species as diverse as the unicellular bacteria *Escherichia coli* and huge multicellular organisms like elephants. These striking similarities in metabolism are most likely the result of the high efficiency of these pathways, and of their early appearance in evolutionary history.

GENETICS

Genetics (from Ancient Greek *genetikos*), 'genitive' and that from *genesis*, 'origin', a discipline of biology, is the science of heredity and variation in living organisms. The fact that living things inherit traits from their parents has been used since prehistoric times to improve crop plants and animals through selective breeding. However, the modern science of genetics, which seeks to understand the process of inheritance, only began with the work of Gregor Mendel in the mid-nineteenth century. Although he did not know the physical basis for heredity, Mendel observed that organisms inherit traits in a discrete manner — these basic units of inheritance are now called genes.

Genes correspond to regions within DNA, a molecule composed of a chain of four different types of nucleotides — the sequence of these nucleotides is the genetic information organisms inherit. DNA naturally occurs in a double stranded form, with nucleotides on each strand complementary to each other. Each strand can act as a template for creating a new partner strand — this is the physical method for making copies of genes that can be inherited.

The sequence of nucleotides in a gene is translated by cells to produce a chain of amino acids, creating proteins—the order of amino acids in a protein corresponds to the order of nucleotides in the gene. This is known as the genetic code. The amino acids in a protein determine how it folds into a three-dimensional shape; this structure is, in turn, responsible for the protein's function. Proteins carry out almost all the functions needed for cells to live. A change to the DNA in a gene can change a protein's amino acids, changing its shape and function: this can have a dramatic effect in the cell and on the organism as a whole.

Although genetics plays a large role in the appearance and behaviour of organisms, it is the combination of genetics with what an organism experiences that determines the ultimate outcome. For example, while genes play a role in determining a person's height, the nutrition and health that person experiences in childhood also have a large effect.

Genetic engineering, recombinant DNA technology, genetic modification/manipulation (GM) and gene splicing are terms that apply to the direct manipulation of an organism's genes. Genetic engineering is different from traditional breeding, where the organism's genes are manipulated indirectly. Genetic engineering uses the techniques of molecular cloning and transformation to alter the structure and characteristics of genes directly. Genetic engineering techniques have found some successes in numerous applications. Some examples are in improving crop technology, the manufacture of synthetic human insulin through the use of modified bacteria, the manufacture of erythroprotein in hamster ovary cells, and the production of new types of experimental mice such as the oncomouse (cancer mouse) for research.

The term 'genetic engineering' was coined in Jack Williamson's science fiction novel Dragon's Island, published in 1951, two years before James Watson and Francis Crick showed that DNA could be the medium of transmission of genetic information.

There are a number of ways through which genetic engineering is accomplished. Essentially, the process has five main steps:

1. Isolation of the genes of interest.
2. Insertion of the genes into a transfer vector.
3. Transfer of the vector to the organism to be modified.
4. Transformation of the cells of the organism.
5. Selection of the genetically modified organism (GMO) from those that have not been successfully modified.

Isolation is achieved by identifying the gene of interest that the scientist wishes to insert into the organism, usually using existing knowledge of the various functions of genes. DNA information can be obtained from cDNA or gDNA libraries, and amplified using PCR techniques. If necessary, i.e. for insertion of eukaryotic genomic DNA into prokaryotes, further modification may be carried out such as removal of introns or ligating prokaryotic promoters.

Insertion of a gene into a vector such as a plasmid can be done once the gene of interest is isolated. Other vectors can also be used, such as viral vectors, bacterial conjugation, liposomes or even direct insertion using a gene gun. Restriction enzymes and ligases are of great use in this crucial step if it is being inserted into prokaryotic or viral vectors.

Once the vector is obtained, it can be used to transform the target organism. Depending on the vector used, it can be complex or simple. For example, using raw DNA with gene guns is a fairly straightforward process but with low success rates, where the DNA is coated with molecules such as gold and fired directly into a cell. Other more complex methods, such as bacterial transformation or using viruses as vectors have higher success rates.

After transformation, the GMO can be selected from those that have failed to take up the vector in various ways. One method is screening with DNA probes that can stick to the gene of interest that was supposed to have been transplanted. Another is to package genes conferring resistance to certain chemicals such as antibiotics or herbicides into the vector. This chemical is then applied ensuring that only those cells that have taken up the vector will survive.

Applications

One of the best-known applications of genetic engineering is the creation of genetically modified organisms (GMOs) such as foods and vegetables that resist pest and bacteria infection and have longer freshness than otherwise.

Genetic engineering and research

Although there has been a revolution in the biological sciences in the past twenty years, there is still a great deal that remains to be discovered. The completion of the sequencing of the human genome, as well as the genomes of most agriculturally and scientifically important animals and plants, has increased the possibilities of genetic research immeasurably. Expedient and inexpensive access to comprehensive genetic data has become a reality with billions of sequenced nucleotides already online and annotated.

1. Loss of function experiments, such as in a gene knockout experiment, in which an organism is engineered to lack the activity of one or more genes.
2. Gain of function experiments, the logical counterpart of knockouts.
3. Tracking experiments, which seek to gain information about the localisation and interaction of the desired protein.
4. Expression studies aim to discover where and when specific proteins are produced. In these experiments, the DNA sequence before the DNA that codes for a protein, known as a gene's promoter, is reintroduced into an organism with the protein coding region replaced by a reporter gene such as GFP or an enzyme that catalyses the production of a dye.

Human genetic engineering

Human genetic engineering can be used to treat genetic disease, but there is a difference between treating the disease in an individual and changing the genome that gets passed down to that person's descendants (germ-line genetic engineering).

Human genetic engineering is already being used on a small scale to allow infertile women with genetic defects in their mitochondria to have children. Healthy human eggs from a second mother are used. The child produced this way has genetic information from two mothers and one father. The changes made are germ line changes and will probably be passed down from generation to generation, and, thus, are a permanent change to the human genome.

Human genetic engineering has the potential to change human beings' appearance, adaptability, intelligence, character and behaviour. It may potentially be used in creating more dramatic changes in humans. There are many unresolved ethical issues and concerns surrounding this technology, and it remains a controversial topic. Genetic engineering can either transfer genes between organisms that are unrelated (transgenesis) and could therefore not occur naturally or between organisms that are related (*cis*-genesis) and so could occur naturally.

Chapter 2

Yeasts

INTRODUCTION

Yeasts are eukaryotic micro-organisms classified in the kingdom Fungi, with about 1500 species currently described; they dominate fungal diversity in the oceans. Most reproduce asexually by budding, although a few do so by binary fission. Yeasts are unicellular, although some species with yeast forms may become multicellular through the formation of a string of connected budding cells known as pseudohyphae, or false hyphae as seen in most moulds. Yeast size can vary greatly depending on the species, typically measuring 3–4 μm in diameter, although some yeasts can reach over 40 μm.

The yeast species *Saccharomyces cerevisiae* has been used in baking and fermenting alcoholic beverages for thousands of years. It is also extremely important as a model organism in modern cell biology research, and is the most thoroughly researched eukaryotic micro-organism. Researchers have used it to gather information into the biology of the eukaryotic cell and ultimately human biology. Other species of yeast, such as Candida albicans, are opportunistic pathogens and can cause infection in humans. Yeasts have recently been used to generate electricity in microbial fuel cells, and produce ethanol for the biofuel industry.

Yeasts do not form a specific taxonomic or phylogenetic grouping. The term 'yeast' is often taken as a synonym for *S. cerevisiae*, but the phylogenetic diversity of yeasts is shown by their placement in both divisions Ascomycota and Basidiomycota. The budding yeasts (true yeasts) are classified in the order *Saccharomycetales*.

PROPERTIES OF YEAST

Yeast lack chlorophyll and are unable to manufacture by photosynthesis from inorganic substrates the organic compounds are required for growth, as do higher plants, algae and even some bacteria. Taxonomic consideration of the yeasts relies heavily on morphological characteristics for genera.

Cellular Asexual Reproduction and Morphology

Asexual reproduction is reproduction which does not involve meiosis, ploidy reduction or fertilisation. Only one parent is involved in asexual reproduction. A more stringent definition is agamogenesis which refers to reproduction without the fusion of gametes. Asexual reproduction is the primary form of reproduction for single-celled organisms such as the archaea, bacteria and protists. Many plants and fungi reproduce asexually as well. While all prokaryotes reproduce asexually (without the formation and fusion of gametes), mechanisms for lateral gene transfer such as conjugation, transformation and transduction are sometimes likened to sexual reproduction. A lack of sexual reproduction is relatively rare among multicellular organisms, for reasons that are not completely understood. Current hypotheses suggest that, while asexual reproduction may have short-term benefits when rapid population growth is important or in stable environments, sexual reproduction offers a net advantage by allowing more rapid generation of genetic diversity, allowing adaptation to changing environments.

Because asexual reproduction does not require the formation of gametes (often in separate individuals) and bringing them together for fertilisation, it occurs much faster than sexual reproduction and requires less energy. Asexual lineages can increase their numbers rapidly because all members can reproduce viable offspring. In sexual populations with two genders, some of the individuals are male and cannot themselves produce offspring. This means that an asexual lineage will have roughly double the rate of population growth under ideal conditions when compared with a sexual population half composed of males. This is known as the two-fold cost of sex. Other advantages include the ability to reproduce without a partner in situations where the population density is low (such as for some desert lizards), reducing the chance of finding a mate, or during colonisation of isolated habitats such as oceanic islands, where a single (female) member of the species is enough to start a population.

A consequence of asexual reproduction, which may have both benefits and costs, is that offspring are typically genetically similar to their parent, with as broad a range as that individual receives from one parent. The lack of genetic recombination results in fewer genetic alternatives than with sexual reproduction. Many forms of asexual reproduction, for example budding or fragmentation, produce an exact replica of the parent. This genetic similarity may be beneficial if the genotype is well-suited to a stable environment, but disadvantageous if the environment is changing. For example, if a new predator or pathogen appears and a genotype is particularly defenseless against it, an asexual lineage is more likely to be completely wiped out by it. In contrast, a lineage that reproduces sexually has a higher probability of having more members survive due to the genetic recombination that produces a novel genotype in each individual. Similar arguments apply to changes in the physical environment. From an evolutionary standpoint, one could thus argue that asexual reproduction is inferior because it stifles the potential for change. However, there is also a significantly reduced chance of mutation or other complications that can result from the mixing of genes.

Budding

Some cells split via budding (for example baker's yeast), resulting in a 'mother' and 'daughter' cell. The offspring organism is smaller than the parent. Budding is also known on a multicellular level; an animal example is the hydra, which reproduces by budding. The buds grow into fully matured individuals which eventually break away from the parent organism. Budding represents the most common method of vegetative reproduction.

Budding is a form of asexual reproduction. The new organism is naturally genetically identical to the primary one (a clone). When yeast buds, one cell becomes two cells. When a sponge buds, a part of the parent sponge falls off and starts to grow into a new sponge. These are examples of asexual reproduction.

Pseudomycelia

Similar to chain formation, a pseudomycelium (false mycelium) may be formed when, instead of the bud breaking away from the mother cell at maturity, it elongates and continues to bud breaking away from the mother cell at maturity, it elongates and continues to bud in turn. In this manner chains of cells are formed, which in appearance resemble true mycelium (where cells are separated by a cross-wall or septum) but differ in the manner in which new cells arise (budding). Pseudomycelia vary in their complexity from very primitive, in which the number of cells are limited and where there is little or no differentiation among these cells, to other forms where cells comprising the main chain are rather elongated and the buds arise in clusters on the shoulder of these elongated stem cells. The side buds in turn may remain spherical, ovoidal, or may also elongate giving rise to further branching and complexity of form. While a particular yeast species may produce a characteristic pseudomycelial form, it is more commonly observed that several types of pseudomycelia are found within a single species. Consequently, while the type of pseudomycelium formed by yeast is of little value in classification, the ability or inability to form a pseudomycelium is used.

Fission

Vegetative reproduction by fission is characteristic of 2 genera, *Endomyces* and *Schizosaccharomyces*. In these yeasts, reproduction is carried out by the formation of a cross-wall (septum) without a constriction of the original cell wall. When the process is complete, the new cell wall divides into 2 individual walls and the newly formed vegetative cells separate from each other.

Bud-fission

There are a few yeasts in which asexual reproduction is intermediate between typical budding and fission. This so-called 'bud-fission' results from a type of budding in which the base of the bud is very broad, somewhat like a bowling pin. Separation of the daughter cell from the mother is by the formation of a septum across the broad neck. *Saccharomycodes* and *Nadsonia* are genera exhibiting this type of reproduction. Fundamentally, bud-fission differs from typical budding only in the size of the septum. In budding it is so small that it appears that the bud is 'prinched off' rather than distinctly separated by a septum.

Budding and fission

Some yeasts reproduce vegetatively by both budding and fission. Species of *Trichosporon* usually grow as mycelial strands (hyphae) by cross-wall formation. The strands can undergo disarticulation into individual vegetative cells called arthrospores, which, upon germination again, produce mycelium. Budding cells may also arise on the mycelial strands.

Clamp connections

A special types of mycelium is formed by some of the basidiomycetous yeasts (*Leucosporidium*, *Rhodosporidium* and *Sporidiobolus*) in which clamp connections are formed between adjoining cells during the dikaryotic stage of their special life cycle.

Cell Morphology

Lodder describes the cells of *S. cerevisiae* as being spheroidal, subglobose, ovoid, ellipsoidal or cylindrical to elongate, occurring singly, in pairs, occasionally in short chains or clusters.

Cells may be grouped into three classes on the basis of size. A large type, 4.5–10.5×7.0–21.0 μm (microns); a small-cell type falling within the range 2.5–7.0×4.5–11 μm and an intermediate group with cells measuring 3.5–$8.0 \times$ range 5.0–11.0 μm. Some yeasts may form filaments which may be up to 30 m (in length). Brewing yeast cells fit into any of these categories; however, they tend to be quite large cells, a consequence of polyploidy. Vágvölgyi demonstrated the effect of ploidy on yeast cell size, thus, the mean diameters of haploid, diploid and triploid *S. cerevisiae* cells being 4.2, 5.2 and 5.9 μm, respectively. The relationship between volume and surface are for an ellipsoidal yeast cell (e.g. *S. cerevisiae*) has been given as 45 and 71 μm^2 for haploid and diploid cells with volumes of 25 and 55 μm^3, respectively.

The mean cell size of a particular yeast strain is not a constant but varies according to the stage in the growth cycle, the growth conditions and the age of the individual cell. Changes in cell size associated with age were described by Woldringh and others using a centrifugal elutriation system which allowed the collection of new-born daughter cells. These authors reported that the volume of these increased from a mean value of 17 μm^3 to 34 μm^3 after five generations and 81 μm^3 at 15 generations. Hartwell and Unger concluded that the increase in cell volume occurred during the phase in the cell cycle when budding has finished. In fact, the mean cell volume decreases by approximately a third during the budding phase. Apart from volume changes, predictably, there are also cell cycle-associated oscillations in cell mass. Baldwin and Kubitschek demonstrated that the cellular density reached a peak during the mid-growth cycle and this was attributed to a loss of water with a concomitant increase in dry mass. Such observation serve to illustrate the fact that caution should be exercised interpreting experimental data, expressed as percentage dry mass, regarding fluctuation in the concentrations of individual cellular components during growth.

The growth conditions also influence cell size. Robinow and Johnson reviewed the effects of incubation temperature on cell size and reported a variable response depending on the yeast. Thus, most yeast types, probably including *Saccharomyces*, showed a temperature dependent increase in cell size. However, *Schizosaccharomyces pombé* cell increased in size at temperatures higher and lower than the optimum. Brewing yeast cells growing fermentatively on maltose are significantly bigger than the same cells growing oxidatively on ethanol.

Short-term perturbations in cell size may also occur, presumably as a result of osmatic effects, when yeast is transferred between different media. For example, the effects of pitching yeast suspended in barm ale into wort. Thus, Quain observed that in the first 4 hours after pitching yeast, at laboratory scale, into wort there as a transient increase in cell size. The mean cell volume increased from approximately 170 μm^3 to 200 μm^3. The volume changes occurred before the onset of budding and cell proliferation and were independent of cell dry weight. These results suggest that the degree of turgor of the plasma membrane exerts an influence on cell size and that the cell wall is sufficiently flexible to accommodate such short-term fluctuations.

Changes in cell size over longer periods have also been recorded. Cahill reported that application of image analytical techniques as a method for improving the control of pitching rate. The apparatus was used to monitor cell size of stored pitching yeast. It was observed that for both ale and lager yeast the mean cell volume reduced by 19 per cent (302 to 244 μm^3) and 7 per cent (208 to 194 μm^3), respectively during storage over a period of 14 days at 4°C. The changes in mean cell volume were correlated with glycogen content, the latter being utilised for maintenance energy during storage.

Types of Asexual Reproduction

Binary fission

Many single-celled organisms (unicellular), such as archaea, bacteria and protists, reproduce asexually through binary fission. An exception to the rule are unicellular fungi such as fission yeast, unicellular algae such as *Chlamydomonas*, and ciliates and some other protists, which reproduce both sexually and asexually. Some single-celled organisms (unicellular) rely on one or more host organisms in order to reproduce, but most literally divide into two organisms.

Binary fission is the form of asexual reproduction and cell division used by all prokaryotic and some eukaryotic organisms. This process results in the reproduction of a living prokaryotic cell by division into two parts which each have the potential to grow to the size of the original cell.

Mitosis and cytokinesis are not the same as binary fission. The ability of some multicellular animals, such as echinoderms and flatworms, to regenerate two whole organisms after having been cut in half, is also not the same as binary fission. Neither is vegetative reproduction of plants.

Process

Binary fission begins with DNA replication. DNA replication starts from an origin of replication, which opens up into a replication bubble (note: prokaryotic DNA replication usually has only 1 origin of replication, whereas eukaryotes have multiple origins of replication). The replication bubble separates the DNA double strand, each strand acts as template for synthesis of a daughter strand by semiconservative replication, until the entire prokaryotic DNA is duplicated.

Each circular DNA strand then attaches to the cell membrane. The cell elongates, causing the two chromosomes to separate.

Cell division in bacteria is controlled by the septal ring, a collection of about a dozen proteins that collect around the site of division. There, they direct assembly of the division septum. The cell wall and plasma membrane starts growing transversely from near the middle of the dividing cell. This separates the parent cell into two nearly equal daughter cells, each having a nuclear body.

The cell membrane then invaginates (grows inwards) and splits the cell into two daughter cells, separated by a newly grown cell plate.

Use by eukaryotic organelles

Eukaryotic organelles such as mitochondria, chloroplasts and peroxisomes also reproduce within the eukaryotic cell by binary fission. How they are allotted to one descendant cell or the other during mitosis and cytokinesis is not yet clear.

Virology

Budding is the process by which enveloped viruses acquire their external envelope, often as fragment of the host cell membrane, which bulges outwards and takes the virion inside. Some viruses hijack the host cell proteins normally involved in endocytosis to facilitate this process.

Embryology

The term budding is also applied to the process of embryo differentiation in which old structures are formed in outgrowth from pre-existing parts.

Vegetative reproduction

Vegetative reproduction is a type of asexual reproduction found in plants where new independent individuals are formed without the production of seeds or spores. Examples for vegetative reproduction include the formation of plantlets on specialised leaves (for example in kalanchoe), the growth of new plants out of rhizomes or stolons (for example in strawberry), or the formation of new bulbs (for example in tulips). The resulting plants form a clonal colony.

Fragmentation

Fragmentation is a form of asexual reproduction where a new organism grows from a fragment of the parent. Each fragment develops into a mature, fully grown individual. Fragmentation is seen in many organisms such as animals (some annelid worms and sea stars), fungi and plants. Some plants have specialised structures for reproduction via fragmentation, such as *gemmae* in liverworts. Most lichens, which are a symbiotic union of a fungus and photosynthetic algae or bacteria, reproduce through fragmentation to ensure that new individuals contain both symbionts. These fragments can take the form of *soredia*, dust-like particles consisting of fungal hyphae wrapped around photobiont cells.

Parthenogenesis

Parthenogenesis is a form of agamogenesis in which an unfertilised egg develops into a new individual. Parthenogenesis occurs naturally in many plants, invertebrates (e.g. water fleas, aphids, stick insects, some ants, bees and parasitic wasps) and vertebrates (e.g. some reptiles, amphibians, fish, very rarely birds). In plants, apomixis may or may not involve parthenogenesis.

Agamogenesis

Agamogenesis is any form of reproduction that does not involve a male gamete. Examples are parthenogenesis and apomixis.

Anatomy

Under high magnification, spores can be categorised as either monolete spores or trilete spores. In monolete spores, there is a single line on the spore indicating the axis on which the mother spore was split into four along a vertical axis.

In trilete spores, all four spores share a common origin and are in contact with each other, so when they separate, each spore shows three lines radiating from a centre pole.

Vascular plant spores are always haploid. Vascular plants are either *homosporous* (or *isosporous*) or *heterosporous*. Plants that are *homosporous* produce spores of the same size and type. *Heterosporous* plants, such as spikemosses, quillworts and some aquatic ferns produce spores of two different sizes: the larger spore in effect functioning as a 'female' spore and the smaller functioning as a 'male'.

Trilete spores

Trilete spores, formed by the dissociation of a spore tetrad, are taken as the earliest evidence of life on land, dating to the mid-Ordovician (early Llanvirn, ~470 million years ago).

Dispersal

In fungi, both asexual and sexual spores or sporangiospores of many fungal species are actively dispersed by forcible ejection from their reproductive structures. This ejection ensures exit of the spores from the reproductive structures as well as travelling through the air over long distances. Many fungi thereby possess specialised mechanical and physiological mechanisms as well as spore-surface structures, such as hydrophobins, for spore ejection. These mechanisms include, for example, forcible discharge of ascospores enabled by the structure of the ascus and accumulation of osmolytes in the fluids of the ascus that lead to explosive discharge of the ascospores into the air. The forcible discharge of single spores termed *ballistospores* involves formation of a small drop of water (Buller's drop), which upon contact with the spore leads to its projectile release with an initial acceleration of more than 10,000 g.

Other fungi rely on alternative mechanisms for spore release, such as external mechanical forces, exemplified by puffballs. Attracting insects, such as flies, to fruiting structures, by virtue of their having lively colours and a putrid odour, for dispersal of fungal spores is yet another strategy, most prominently used by the stinkhorns.

In the case of spore-shedding vascular plants such as ferns, wind distribution of very light spores provides great capacity for dispersal. Also, spores are less subject to animal predation than seeds because they contain almost no food reserve; however they are more subject to fungal and bacterial predation. Their chief advantage is that, of all forms of progeny, spores require the least energy and materials to produce. In the spikemoss *Selaginella lepidophylla*, dispersal is achieved in part by an unusual type of diaspore, a tumbleweed.

Alternation between Sexual and Asexual Reproduction

Some species alternate between the sexual and asexual strategies, an ability known as heterogamy, depending on conditions. For example, the freshwater crustacean *Daphnia* reproduces by parthenogenesis in the spring to rapidly populate ponds, then switches to sexual reproduction as the intensity of competition and predation increases. Many protists and fungi alternate between sexual and asexual reproduction. For example, the slime mould *Dictyostelium* undergoes binary fission as single-celled amoebae under favourable conditions. However, when conditions turn unfavourable, the cells aggregate and switch to sexual reproduction leading to the formation of spores. The hyphae of the common mould (*Rhizopus*) are capable of producing both mitotic as well as meiotic spores. Many algae similarly switch between sexual and asexual reproduction. Asexual reproduction is far less complicated than sexual reproduction. In sexual reproduction one must find a mate.

Structure and Function of Cellular Compounds

The following section discusses specific information know about the structure and function of cellular components. These include the cell wall, nucleus, mitochondria, vacules, reticulum and mitochondrion.

Cell wall

A cell wall is a tough, flexible and sometimes fairly rigid layer that surrounds some types of cells. It is located outside the cell membrane and provides these cells with structural support and protection, and also acts as a filtering mechanism. A major function of the cell wall is to act as a pressure vessel, preventing over-expansion when water enters the cell. They are found in plants, bacteria, fungi, algae and some archaea. Animals and protozoa do not have cell walls. The materials in a cell wall vary between species, and in plants and fungi also differ between cell types and developmental stages. In plants, the strongest component of the complex cell wall is a carbohydrate called cellulose, which is a polymer of glucose. In bacteria, peptidoglycan forms the cell wall. Archaean cell walls have various compositions, and may be formed of glycoprotein S-layers, pseudopeptidoglycan, or polysaccharides. Fungi possess cell walls made of the glucosamine polymer chitin and algae typically possess walls made of glycoproteins and polysaccharides. Unusually, diatoms have a cell wall composed of silicic acid. Often, other accessory molecules are found anchored to the cell wall.

Properties

The cell wall serves a similar purpose in those organisms that possess them. The wall gives cells rigidity and strength, offering protection against mechanical stress. In multicellular organisms, it permits the organism to build and hold its shape (morphogenesis). The cell wall also limits the entry of large molecules that may be toxic to the cell. It further permits the creation of a stable osmotic environment by preventing osmotic lysis and helping to retain water. The composition, properties and form of the cell wall may change during the cell cycle and depend on growth conditions.

Rigidity

The rigidity of cell walls is often overestimated. In most cells, the cell wall is flexible, meaning that it will bend rather than holding a fixed shape, but has considerable tensile strength. The apparent rigidity of primary plant tissues is a function of hydraulic turgor pressure of the cells and not due to rigid cell walls. This flexibility is seen when plants wilt, so that the stems and leaves begin to droop, or in seaweeds that bend in water currents. The rigidity of healthy plants results from a combination of the wall construction and turgor pressure.

In plants, a secondary cell wall is a thicker additional layer of cellulose which increases wall rigidity. Additional layers may be formed containing lignin in xylem cell walls, or containing suberin in cork cell walls. These compounds are rigid and waterproof, making the secondary wall stiff. Both wood and bark cells of trees have secondary walls. Other parts of plants such as the leaf stalk may acquire similar reinforcement to resist the strain of physical forces. Certain single-cell protists and algae also produce a rigid wall. Diatoms build a frustule from silica extracted from the surrounding water; radiolarians also produce a test from minerals. Many green algae, such as the Dasycladales encase their cells in a secreted skeleton of calcium carbonate. In each case, the wall is rigid and essentially inorganic.

Permeability

The primary cell wall of most plant cells is semi-permeable and permit the passage of small molecules and small proteins, with size exclusion estimated to be 30-60 kDa. Key nutrients, especially water and carbon dioxide, are distributed throughout the plant from cell wall to cell wall in apoplastic flow.

Plant cell walls

Composition

The major carbohydrates making up the primary (growing) plant cell wall are cellulose, hemicellulose and pectin. The cellulose microfibrils are linked via hemicellulosic ethers to form the cellulose-hemicellulose network, which is embedded in the pectin matrix. The most common hemicellulose in the primary cell wall is xyloglucan. In grass cell walls, xyloglucan and pectin are reduced in abundance and partially replaced by glucuronarabinoxylan, a hemicellulose. Primary cell walls characteristically extend (grow) by a mechanism called acid growth, which involves turgor-driven movement of the strong cellulose microfibrils within the weaker hemicellulose/pectin matrix, catalysed by expansin proteins. The outer part of the primary cell wall of the plant epidermis is usually impregnated with cutin and wax, forming a permeability barrier known as the plant cuticle.

Secondary cell walls contain a wide range of additional compounds that modify their mechanical properties and permeability. The major polymers that make up wood (largely secondary cell walls) include cellulose (35 to 50 per cent), xylan, a type of hemicellulose (20 to 35 per cent) and a complex phenolic polymer called lignin (10 to 25 per cent). Lignin penetrates the spaces in the cell wall between cellulose, hemicellulose and pectin components, driving out water and strengthening the wall. The walls of cork cells in the bark of trees are impregnated with suberin, and suberin also forms the permeability barrier in primary roots known as the Casparian strip. Secondary walls—especially in grasses—may also contain microscopic silica crystals, which may strengthen the wall and protect it from herbivores.

Plant cells walls also contain numerous enzymes, such as hydrolases, esterases, peroxidases and transglycosylases, that cut, trim and cross link wall polymers. Small amounts (1–5 per cent) of structural proteins are found in most plant cell walls; they are classified as hydroxyproline-rich glycoproteins (HRGP), arabinogalactan proteins (AGP), glycine-rich proteins (GRPs), and proline-rich proteins (PRPs). Each class of glycoprotein is defined by a characteristic, highly repetitive protein sequence. Most are glycosylated, contain hydroxyproline (Hyp) and become cross-linked in the cell wall. These proteins are often concentrated in specialised cells and in cell corners. Cell walls of the epidermis and endodermis may also contain suberin or cutin, two polyester-like polymers that protect the cell from herbivores. The relative composition of carbohydrates, secondary compounds and protein varies between plants and between the cell type and age.

Up to three strata or layers may be found in plant cell walls:

1. The middle lamella, a layer rich in pectins. This outermost layer forming the interface between adjacent plant cells and glues them together.
2. The primary cell wall, generally a thin, flexible and extensible layer formed while the cell is growing.
3. The secondary cell wall, a thick layer formed inside the primary cell wall after the cell is fully grown. It is not found in all cell types. In some cells, such as found xylem, the secondary wall contains lignin, which strengthens and waterproofs the wall.
4. Cell walls in some plant tissues also function as storage depots for carbohydrates that can be broken down and resorbed to supply the metabolic and growth needs of the plant. For example, endosperm cell walls in the seeds of cereal grasses, nasturtium, and other species, are rich in glucans and other polysaccharides that are readily digested by enzymes during seed germination to form simple sugars that nourish the growing embryo. Cellulose microfibrils are not readily digested by plants, however.

Formation

The middle lamella is laid down first, formed from the cell plate during cytokinesis, and the primary cell wall is then deposited inside the middle lamella. The actual structure of the cell wall is not clearly defined and several models exist—the covalently linked cross model, the ether model, the diffuse layer model and the stratified layer model. However, the primary cell wall, can be defined as composed of cellulose microfibrils aligned at all angles. Microfibrils are held together by hydrogen bonds to provide a high tensile strength.

The cells are held together and share the gelatinous membrane called the middle lamella, which contains magnesium and calcium pectates (salts of pectic acid). Cells interact though plasmodesma(ta), which are inter-connecting channels of cytoplasm that connect to the protoplasts of adjacent cells across the cell wall.

In some plants and cell types, after a maximum size or point in development has been reached, a secondary wall is constructed between the plant cell and primary wall. Unlike the primary wall, the microfibrils are aligned mostly in the same direction, and with each additional layer the orientation changes slightly. Cells with secondary cell walls are rigid.

Cell to cell communication is possible through pits in the secondary cell wall that allow plasmodesma to connect cells through the secondary cell walls.

Algal cell walls

Like plants, algae have cell walls. Algal cell walls contain cellulose and a variety of glycoproteins. The inclusion of additional polysaccharides in algal cells walls is used as a feature for algal taxonomy.

1. Manosyl form microfibrils in the cell walls of a number of marine green algae including those from the genera, *Codium*, *Dasycladus* and *Acetabularia* as well as in the walls of some red algae, like *Porphyra* and *Bangia*.
2. Xylanes.
3. Alginic acid is a common polysaccharide in the cell walls of brown algae.
4. Sulphonated polysaccharides occur in the cell walls of most algae; those common in red algae include agarose, carrageenan, porphyran, furcelleran and funoran.

Other compounds that may accumulate in algal cell walls include sporopollenin and calcium ions.

The group of algae known as the diatoms synthesise their cell walls (also known as frustules or valves) from silicic acid (specifically orthosilicic acid, H_4SiO_4). The acid is polymerised intra-cellularly, then the wall is extruded to protect the cell. Significantly, relative to the organic cell walls produced by other groups, silica frustules require less energy to synthesise (approximately 8 per cent), potentially a major saving on the overall cell energy budget and possibly an explanation for higher growth rates in diatoms.

Fungal cell walls

There are several groups of organisms that may be called 'fungi'. Some of these groups have been transferred out of the Kingdom Fungi, in part because of fundamental biochemical differences in the composition of the cell wall. Most true fungi have a cell wall consisting largely of chitin and other polysaccharides. True fungi do not have cellulose in their cell walls, but some fungus-like organisms do.

True fungi

Not all species of fungi have cell walls but in those that do, the plasma membrane is followed by three layers of cell wall material. From inside out these are:

1. A chitin layer (polymer consisting mainly of unbranched chains of N-acetyl-D-glucosamine).
2. A layer of β-1,3-glucan.
3. A layer of mannoproteins (mannose-containing glycoproteins) which are heavily glycosylated at the outside of the cell.

Fungus-like protists

The group Oomycetes, also known as water moulds, are saprotrophic plant pathogens like fungi. Until recently they were widely believed to be fungi, but structural and molecular evidence has led to their reclassification as heterokonts, related to autotrophic brown algae and diatoms. Unlike fungi, oomycetes typically possess cell walls of cellulose and glucans rather than chitin, although some genera (such as *Achlya* and *Saprolegnia*) do have chitin in their walls. The fraction of cellulose in the walls is no more than 4 to 20 per cent, far less than the fraction comprised by glucans. Oomycete cell walls also contain the amino acid hydroxyproline, which is not found in fungal cell walls. The dictyostelids are another group formerly classified among the fungi. They are slime moulds that feed as unicellular amoebae, but aggregate into a reproductive stalk and sporangium under certain conditions. Cells of the reproductive stalk, as well as the spores formed at the apex, possess a cellulose wall. The spore wall has been shown to possess three layers, the middle of which is composed primarily of cellulose, and the innermost is sensitive to cellulase and pronase.

Prokaryotic cell walls

Bacterial cell walls

Around the outside of the cell membrane is the bacterial cell wall. Bacterial cell walls are made of peptidoglycan (also called murein), which is made from polysaccharide chains cross-linked by unusual peptides containing D-amino acids. Bacterial cell walls are different from the cell walls of plants and fungi which are made of cellulose and chitin, respectively. The cell wall of bacteria is also distinct from that of Archaea, which do not contain peptidoglycan. The cell wall is essential to the survival of many bacteria, although L-form bacteria can be produced in the laboratory that lack a cell wall. The antibiotic penicillin is able to kill bacteria by inhibiting a step in the synthesis of peptidoglycan.

There are broadly speaking two different types of cell wall in bacteria, called Gram-positive and Gram-negative. The names originate from the reaction of cells to the Gram stain, a test long-employed for the classification of bacterial species.

Gram-positive bacteria possess a thick cell wall containing many layers of peptidoglycan and teichoic acids. In contrast, Gram-negative bacteria have a relatively thin cell wall consisting of a few layers of peptidoglycan surrounded by a second lipid membrane containing lipopolysaccharides and lipoproteins. Most bacteria have the Gram-negative cell wall and only the Firmicutes and Actinobacteria (previously known as the low G+C and high G+C Gram-positive bacteria, respectively) have the alternative Gram-positive arrangement. These differences in structure can produce differences in antibiotic susceptibility, for instance vancomycin can kill only Gram-positive bacteria and is ineffective against Gram-negative pathogens, such as *Haemophilus influenzae* or *Pseudomonas aeruginosa*.

Archaeal cell walls

Although not truly unique, the cell walls of Archaea are unusual. Whereas peptidoglycan is a standard component of all bacterial cell walls, all archaeal cell walls lack peptidoglycan, with the exception of one group of methanogens. In that group, the peptidoglycan is a modified form very different from the kind found in bacteria. There are four types of cell wall currently known among the Archaea.

One type of archaeal cell wall is that composed of pseudopeptidoglycan (also called pseudomurein). This type of wall is found in some methanogens, such as *Methanobacterium* and *Methanothermus*. While the overall structure of archaeal pseudopeptidoglycan superficially resembles that of bacterial peptidoglycan, there are a number of significant chemical differences. Like the peptidoglycan found in bacterial cell walls, pseudopeptidoglycan consists of polymer chains of glycan cross-linked by short peptide connections. However, unlike peptidoglycan, the sugar N-acetylmuramic acid is replaced by N-acetyltalosaminuronic acid, and the two sugars are bonded with a β,1-3 glycosidic linkage instead of β,1-4. Additionally, the cross-linking peptides are L-amino acids rather than D-amino acids as they are in bacteria.

A second type of archaeal cell wall is found in *Methanosarcina* and *Halococcus*. This type of cell wall is composed entirely of a thick layer of polysaccharides, which may be sulphated in the case of *Halococcus*. Structure in this type of wall is complex and as yet is not fully investigated.

A third type of wall among the Archaea consists of glycoprotein, and occurs in the hyperthermophiles, *Halobacterium* and some methanogens. In *Halobacterium*, the proteins in the wall have a high content of acidic amino acids, giving the wall an overall negative charge. The result is an unstable structure that is stabilised by the presence of large quantities of positive sodium ions that neutralise the charge. Consequently, *Halobacterium* thrives only under conditions with high salinity.

In other Archaea, such as *Methanomicrobium* and *Desulphurococcus*, the wall may be composed only of surface-layer proteins, known as an *S-layer*. S-layers are common in bacteria, where they serve as either the sole cell-wall component or an outer layer in conjunction with polysaccharides. Most Archaea are gram-negative, though at least one gram-positive member is known.

Capsular materials

Capsular materials, while not strictly a component of the cell wall, are produced extracellularly by representatives of several yeast genera. Capsular materials are generally classified as phosphomannas, β-linked mannans, heteropolysaccharides (contain more than one type of sugar), and finally a number of hydrophobic substances belonging to the sphingolipid type compounds.

Plasmalemma (Cytoplasmic membrane)

This membrane is between the cell wall layers and the cytoplasm and functions in the selective transport of nutrients from the medium into the cell and conversely protects the cell from the loss of low molecular weight compounds from the cytoplasm. During the growth of the cell it also represents the structure upon which the cell wall components are deposited. Physically the plasmalemma shows numerous deep invaginations. The outer surface is composed of particles which contain mannan-protein, and these particles may be involved in the formation of the mannan-protein complex of the cell wall.

Cytoplasmic matrix

The ground substance or matrix in which various yeast structures such as the nucleus, vacuoles, etc. are located also contains large quantities of polyphosphates, glycolytic enzymes, ribosomes, reserve glycogen, and, in some yeasts, the reserve sugar trehalose. Some of the polyphosphates are highly polymerised and are a reservoir of high-energy phosphate utilisable in various metabolic processes such as sugar transport, synthesis of cell wall polysaccharides, etc. Glycogen, one of the main carbohydrate storage products, is a highly polymerised glucose molecule which accumulates primarily in a cell's stationary stage of growth when nitrogen is limiting and glucose is still available.

Cell nucleus

HeLa cells stained for DNA with the Blue Hoechst dye. The central and rightmost cell are in interphase, thus their entire nuclei are labelled.

Typical animal cell, contain subcellular components. Organelles: (i) nucleolus, (ii) nucleus, (iii) ribosome, (iv) vesicle, (v) rough endoplasmic reticulum (ER), (vi) golgi apparatus, (vii) cytoskeleton, (viii) smooth ER, (ix) mitochondria, (x) vacuole, (xi) cytoplasm, (xii) lysosome, and (xiii) centrioles.

In cell biology, the nucleus (pl. *nuclei*; from Latin *nucleus* or *nuculeus*, or kernel), also sometimes referred to as the 'control centre', is a membrane-enclosed organelle found in eukaryotic cells. It contains most of the cell's genetic material, organised as multiple long linear DNA molecules in complex with a large variety of proteins, such as histones, to form chromosomes. The genes within these chromosomes are the cell's nuclear genome. The function of the nucleus is to maintain the integrity of these genes and to control the activities of the cell by regulating gene expression—the nucleus is therefore the control centre of the cell. The main structures making up the nucleus are the nuclear envelope, a double membrane that encloses the entire organelle and separates its contents from the cellular cytoplasm, and the nuclear lamina, a meshwork within the nucleus that adds mechanical support, much like the cytoskeleton supports the cell as a whole. Because the nuclear membrane is impermeable to most molecules, nuclear pores are required to allow movement of molecules across the envelope. These pores cross both of the membranes, providing a channel that allows free movement of small molecules and ions. The movement of larger molecules such as proteins is carefully controlled, and requires active transport regulated by carrier proteins. Nuclear transport is crucial to cell function, as movement through the pores is required for both gene expression and chromosomal maintenance. Although the interior of the nucleus does not contain any membrane-bound subcompartments, its contents are not uniform, and a number of subnuclear bodies exist, made up of unique proteins, RNA molecules, and particular parts of the chromosomes. The best known of these is the nucleolus, which is mainly involved in the assembly of ribosomes. After being produced in the nucleolus, ribosomes are exported to the cytoplasm where they translate mRNA.

Vacuole

A vacuole is a membrane organelle which is present in all plant and fungal cells and some protist, animal and bacterial cells. Vacuoles are essentially enclosed compartments which are filled with water containing inorganic and organic molecules including various enzymes in solution, though in certain cases they may contain solids which have been engulfed. Vacuoles are formed by the fusion of multiple membrane vesicles and are effectively just larger forms of these. The organelle has no basic shape or size, its structure varies according to the needs of the cell.

The function and importance of vacuoles varies greatly according to the type of cell in which they are present, having much greater prominence in the cells of plants, fungi and certain protists than those of animals and bacteria. In general, the functions of vacuole include:

1. Isolating materials that might be harmful or a threat to the cell.
2. Containing waste products.
3. Maintaining internal hydrostatic pressure or turgor within the cell.
4. Maintaining an acidic internal pH.
5. Containing small molecules.
6. Exporting unwanted substances from the cell.

Vacuoles also play a major role in autophagy, maintaining a balance between biogenesis (production) and degradation (or turnover), of many substances and cell structures in certain organisms. They also aid in destruction of invading bacteria or of misfolded proteins that have begun to build up within the cell. In protists, vacuoles have the additional function of storing food which has been absorbed by the organism, and assist in the digestive and waste management process for the cell.

Endoplasmic reticulum

The endoplasmic reticulum (ER) is a eukaryotic organelle that forms an interconnected network of tubules, vesicles and cisternae within cells. The lacey membranes of the endoplasmic reticulum were first seen by Keith R. Porter, Albert Claude and Ernest F. Fullam in 1945. These structures are responsible for several specialised functions: protein translation, folding and transport of proteins to be used in the cell membrane (e.g. transmembrane receptors and other integral membrane proteins), or to be secreted (exocytosed) from the cell (e.g. digestive enzymes); sequestration of calcium; and production and storage of glycogen, steroids and other macromolecules. The endoplasmic reticulum is part of the endomembrane system. The basic structure and composition of the ER membrane is similar to the plasma membrane.

Function

The endoplasmic reticulum serves many general functions, including the facilitation of protein folding and the transport of synthesised proteins in sacs called cisternae.

Correct folding of newly-made proteins is made possible by several endoplasmic reticulum chaperone proteins, including protein disulphide isomerase (PDI), ERp29, the Hsp70 family member Grp78, calnexin, calreticulin and the peptidylpropyl isomerase family. Only properly-folded proteins are transported from the rough ER to the Golgi complex.

Transport of proteins

Secretory proteins, mostly glycoproteins, are moved across the endoplasmic reticulum membrane. Proteins that are transported by the endoplasmic reticulum and from there throughout the cell are marked with an address tag called a signal sequence. The N-terminus (one end) of a polypeptide chain (i.e. a protein) contains a few amino acids that work as an address tag, which are removed when the polypeptide reaches its destination. Proteins that are destined for places outside the endoplasmic reticulum are packed into transport vesicles and moved along the cytoskeleton toward their destination.

The endoplasmic reticulum is also part of a protein sorting pathway. It is, in essence, the transportation system of the eukaryotic cell. The majority of endoplasmic reticulum resident proteins are retained in the endoplasmic reticulum through a retention motif. This motif is composed of four amino acids at the end of the protein sequence. The most common retention sequence is KDEL (*lys-asp-glu-leu*). However, variation on KDEL does occur and other sequences can also give rise to endoplasmic reticulum retention. It is not known if such variation can lead to sub-endoplasmic reticulum localisations. There are three KDEL receptors in mammalian cells, and they have a very high degree of sequence identity. The functional differences between these receptors remain to be established.

Other functions

1. Insertion of proteins into the endoplasmic reticulum membrane: Integral membrane proteins are inserted into the endoplasmic reticulum membrane as they are being synthesised (co-translational translocation). Insertion into the endoplasmic reticulum membrane requires the correct topogenic signal sequences in the protein.
2. Glycosylation: Glycosylation involves the attachment of oligosaccharides.
3. Disulphide bond formation and rearrangement: Disulphide bonds stabilise the tertiary and quaternary structure of many proteins.
4. Drug metabolism: The smooth ER is the site at which some drugs are modified by microsomal enzymes which include the cytochrome P450 enzymes.

Mitochondrion

In cell biology, a mitochondrion (plural mitochondria) is a membrane-enclosed organelle found in most eukaryotic cells. These organelles range from 0.5–10 micrometers (μm) in diameter. Mitochondria are sometimes described as 'cellular power plants' because they generate most of the cell's supply of adenosine triphosphate (ATP), used as a source of chemical energy. In addition to supplying cellular energy, mitochondria are involved in a range of other processes, such as signalling, cellular differentiation, cell death, as well as the control of the cell cycle and cell growth. Mitochondria have been implicated in several human diseases, including mitochondrial disorders and cardiac dysfunction, and may play a role in the ageing process.

Several characteristics make mitochondria unique. The number of mitochondria in a cell varies widely by organism and tissue type. Many cells have only a single mitochondrion, whereas others can contain several thousand mitochondria. The organelle is composed of compartments that carry out specialised functions. These compartments or regions include the outer membrane, the intermembrane space, the inner membrane and the cristae and matrix. Mitochondrial proteins vary depending on the tissues and species. In human, 615 distinct types of proteins were identified from cardiac mitochondria; whereas in murinae (rats), 940 proteins encoded by distinct genes were reported. The mitochondrial proteome is thought to be dynamically regulated. Although most of a cell's DNA is contained in the cell nucleus, the mitochondrion has its own independent genome. Further, its DNA shows substantial similarity to bacterial genomes.

Lipid globules

Yeasts have globules of lipid material stainable with Sudan Black or Sudan Red. While most yeast cells contain a small amount of these lipid materials, some yeasts, particularly when grown in a medium with a limiting nitrogen supply, can accumulate up to 50 per cent of the dry weight as lipids. *Lipomyces starkeyi, Metschnikowia pulcherrima* and *Rhodotorula glutinis* are notable fat-producing yeasts.

Sexual Reproduction

Sexual reproduction is characterised by processes that pass a combination of genetic material to offspring, resulting in diversity. The main two processes are: meiosis, involving the halving of the number of chromosomes; and fertilisation, involving the fusion of two gametes and the restoration of the original number of chromosomes. During meiosis, the chromosomes of each pair usually cross over to achieve genetic recombination.

The evolution of sexual reproduction is a major puzzle. The first fossilised evidence of sexually reproducing organisms is from eukaryotes of the Stenian period, about 1 to 1.2 billion years ago. Sexual reproduction is the primary method of reproduction for the vast majority of macroscopic organisms, including almost all animals and plants. Bacterial conjugation, the transfer of DNA between two bacteria, is often mistakenly confused with sexual reproduction, because the mechanics are similar.

A major question is why sexual reproduction persists when parthenogenesis appears in some ways to be a superior form of reproduction. Contemporary evolutionary thought proposes some explanations. It may be due to selection pressure on the clade itself—the ability for a population to radiate more rapidly in response to a changing environment through sexual recombination than parthenogenesis allows. Alternatively, sexual reproduction may allow for the 'ratcheting' of evolutionary speed as one clade competes with another for a limited resource.

Spores

The term spore derives from the ancient Greek word (spora), meaning a seed. In biology, a spore is a reproductive structure that is adapted for dispersal and surviving for extended periods of time in unfavourable conditions. Spores form part of the life cycles of many plants, algae, fungi and some protozoans. A chief difference between spores and seeds as dispersal units is that spores have very little stored food resources compared with seeds.

Spores are usually haploid and unicellular and are produced by meiosis in the sporangium by the sporophyte. Once conditions are favourable, the spore can develop into a new organism using mitotic division, producing a multicellular gametophyte, which eventually goes on to produce gametes.

Two gametes fuse to create a new sporophyte. This cycle is known as alternation of generations, but a better term is 'biological life cycle', as there may be more than one phase and so it cannot be a direct alternation. Haploid spores produced by mitosis (known as mitospores) are used by many fungi for asexual reproduction.

Many ferns, especially those adapted to dry conditions, produce diploid spores. This form of asexual reproduction is called apogamy. It is a form of apomixis.

Spores are the units of asexual reproduction, because a single spore develops into a new organism. By contrast, gametes are the units of sexual reproduction, as two gametes need to fuse to create a new organism. In common parlance, the difference between a 'spore' and a 'gamete' (both together called gonites) is that a spore will germinate and develop into a sporeling, while a gamete needs to combine with another gamete before developing further. However, the terms are somewhat interchangeable when referring to gametes. A chief difference between spores and seeds as dispersal units is that spores have little food storage compared with seeds, and thus require more favourable conditions in order to successfully germinate. (This is not without its exceptions, however: many orchid seeds, although multicellular, are microscopic and lack endosperm, and spores of some fungi in the Glomeromycota commonly exceed 300 μm in diameter.) Seeds, therefore, are more resistant to harsh conditions and require less energy to start mitosis. Spores are produced in large numbers to increase the chance of a spore surviving in a number of notable examples.

Classification

Spores can be classified in several ways such as:

By spore-producing structure

In contrast, in many seed plants and heterosporous ferns, only a single product of meiosis will become a megaspore (macrospore), with the rest degenerating.

In fungi and fungus-like organisms, spores are often classified by the structure in which meiosis and spore production occurs. Since fungi are often classified according to their spore-producing structures, these spores are often characteristic of a particular taxon of the fungi.

1. Sporangiospores: spores produced by a sporangium in many fungi such as zygomycetes.
2. Zygospores: spores produced by a zygosporangium, characteristic of zygomycetes.
3. Ascospores: spores produced by an ascus, characteristic of ascomycetes.
4. Basidiospores: spores produced by a basidium, characteristic of basidiomycetes.
5. Aeciospores: spores produced by a aecium in some fungi such as rusts or smuts.
6. Urediospores: spores produced by a uredinium in some fungi such as rusts or smuts.
7. Teliospores: spores produced by a telium in some fungi such as rusts or smuts.
8. Oospores: spores produced by a oogonium, characteristic of oomycetes.
9. Carpospores: spores produced by a carposporophyte, characteristic of red algae.
10. Tetraspores: spores produced by a tetrasporophyte, characteristic of red algae.

By function

1. Chlamydospores: thick-walled resting spores of fungi produced to survive unfavourable conditions.
2. Parasitic fungal spores may be classified into internal spores, which germinate within the host, and external spores, also called environmental spores, released by the host to infest other hosts.

By origin during life cycle

1. Meiospores: spores produced by meiosis; they are thus haploid, and give rise to a haploid daughter cell(s) or a haploid individual. Examples are the precursor cells of gametophytes of seed plants found in flowers (angiosperms) or cones (gymnosperms).
2. Microspores: meiospores that give rise to a male gametophyte (pollen in seed plants).

3. Megaspores (or macrospores): meiospores that give rise to a female gametophyte (an ovule in seed plants).
4. Mitospores (or conidia, conidiospores): spores produced by mitosis; they are characteristic of Ascomycetes. Fungi in which only mitospores are found are called 'mitosporic fungi' or 'anamorphic fungi', and are previously classified under the taxon Deuteromycota.

By motility

Spores can be differentiated by whether they can move or not.
1. Zoospores: mobile spores that move by means of one or more flagella, and can be found in some algae and fungi.
2. Aplanospores: immobile spores that may nevertheless potentially grow flagella.
3. Autospores: immobile spores that cannot develop flagella.
4. Ballistospores: spores that are actively discharged from the body of the fungal fruiting body. Most basidiospores are also ballistospores, and another notable example is spores of *Pilobolus*.
5. Statismospores: spores that are not actively discharged from the fungal fruiting body. Examples are puffballs.

Spore formation

Many multicellular organisms form spores during their biological life cycle in a process called sporogenesis. Exceptions are animals and some protists, who undergo gametic meiosis immediately followed by fertilisation. Plants and many algae on the other hand undergo sporic meiosis where meiosis leads to the formation of haploid spores rather than gametes. These spores grow into multicellular individuals (called gametophytes in the case of plants) without a fertilisation event. These haploid individuals give rise to gametes through mitosis. Meiosis and gamete formation therefore occur in separate generations or 'phases' of the life cycle, referred to as alternation of generations. Since sexual reproduction is often more narrowly defined as the fusion of gametes (fertilisation), spore formation in plant sporophytes and algae might be considered a form of asexual reproduction (agamogenesis) despite being the result of meiosis and undergoing a reduction in ploidy. However, both events (spore formation and fertilisation) are necessary to complete sexual reproduction in the plant life cycle.

Fungi and some algae can also utilise true asexual spore formation, which involves mitosis giving rise to reproductive cells called mitospores that develop into a new organism after dispersal. This method of reproduction is found for example in conidial fungi and the red alga Polysiphonia, and involves sporogenesis without meiosis. Thus, the chromosome number of the spore cell is the same as that of the parent producing the spores. However, mitotic sporogenesis is an exception and most spores, such as those of plants, most Basidiomycota and many algae, are produced by meiosis.

Yeast Sexuality

Various yeast species depending upon the strain, are found to exhibit homothallism, heterothallism and parasexuality.

Homothallism

Homothallism occurs in fungi in the form of sexual incompatibility. Gametes produced by one type of thallus are compatible only with gametes produced by the other type. Such fungi are said to be heterothallic. Many fungi, however, are homothallic, i.e. sex organs produced by a single thallus are self-compatible, and a second thallus is unnecessary for sexual reproduction.

Heterothallism

Four mechanisms of heterothallism are known at the present time the simplest being the biallelic, bipolar, sexual compatibility system in which species require mating type of sexual conjugation; the determinant for sex is located at 1 locus on a chromosome.

It actually occurs quite commonly among the various groups of yeasts and its importance cannot be overemphasised. Due in part to the classic method of isolation for obtaining pure cultures, where one selects single well isolated colonies on an isolation medium, many species have been described as lacking a sexual phase when in fact the isolation has been of only 1 matting type. Thus, the recognition of heterothallism has aided in the proper taxonomic designation of many of these organisms when the isolate has been mixed with compatible strains of a known species and the matting results in sporulation.

Parasexuality

Studies by various investigators have shown cases where yeasts and other fungi alternate between the haploid and diploid phases without the formation of sexual spores. This process, observed to occur in *Aspergillus nidulans* by Pontecorvo is know as parasexuality. Subsequent to that time, similar observations have been made in other fungi, including some yeast species. This alternation of haploid and diploid phases is of particular interest since it is functional not in fungi without known sexual stages, but also in yeasts where a sexual stage has been established.

Yeast Life Cycle

There are two forms in which yeast cells can survive and grow: haploid and diploid. The haploid cells undergo a simple life cycle of mitosis and growth, and under conditions of high stress will generally simply die. The diploid cells (the preferential 'form' of yeast) similarly undergo a simple life cycle of mitosis and growth, but under conditions of stress can undergo sporulation, entering meiosis and producing a variety of haploid spores, which can go on to mate.

Yeasts secrete enzymes that break down carbohydrates (through fermentation) to yield carbon dioxide and alcohol. The source of carbohydrates are either living hosts or non-living hosts such as rotting vegetation, or the moist body cavities of animals. Yeasts are considered by some scientists to be closely related to the algae, lacking only in photosynthetic capability—perhaps as a result of an evolutionary trend toward a lifestyle dependent upon host nutrition. Ecologically yeasts are decomposers that secrete enzymes which dismantle the complex carbon compounds of plant cell walls and animal tissues, which they convert to sugars for their own growth and sustenance. Yeast reproduction may involve sexual spore production or asexual budding, dependent upon surrounding conditions. Though yeasts are highly tolerant of environmental variations in temperature and acidity, they thrive in warm and moist places high in oxygen and low in carbon dioxide. Whether or not they reproduce through asexual budding depends on the favourability of surrounding conditions: when times are good, yeast clones are produced by budding. In times of environmental stress, yeasts produce spores which are capable of withstanding periods of environmental hardship—perhaps even to lie dormant, until conditions improve and the mingling of genes can take place with the spore of another yeast. This rare version of yeast reproduction provides for genetic.

Ascosporogenous yeasts

Ascosporogenous yeasts can be broadly subdivided into two classes, those in which the vegetative phase exists in the haploid condition and those in which the diplophase predominates. In the haploid class, such as the subgenus *Zygosaccharomyces*, the nucleus of the vegetative cell contains only a single set of chromosomes (1n). Thus, there must be a fusion of 2 nuclei to establish the diploid (2n) condition before reduction division can begin and subsequent sporulation can take place. In those yeasts which exist vegetatively primarily as diploid cells, such as *Saccharomyces cerevisiae*, the ascus can develop directly from the vegetative cell by reduction division of the diploid nucleus followed by spore formation.

Haploid vegetative phase

In ascosporogenous yeasts which characteristically exist as haploids in the vegetative phase, the diploid generation is usually limited to the zygote formed after fusion of 2 haploid cells and their nuclei. These yeasts normally have 1 of 3 types of life cylces.

Conjugation tube

Connecting that allows two individuals to fuse together temporarily in order to exchange micronuclear material. A conjugation tube; a hollow hair-like appendage of a donor *Escherichia coli* cell that acts as a bridge for transmission of donor DNA to the recipient cell during conjugation.

Some bacteria have şex pili which are responsible for bacteria recognising one another and the consequent formation of a conjugation tube which allows the transfer of DNA from a 'male' cell to a 'female' cell.

Meiosis bud

In order to discuss meiosis bud first of all let us define meiosis. In biology, meiosis is a process of reductional division in which the number of chromosomes per cell is halved. In animals, meiosis always results in the formation of gametes, while in other organisms it can give rise to spores. As with mitosis, before meiosis begins, the DNA in the original cell is replicated during S-phase of the cell cycle. Two cell divisions separate the replicated chromosomes into four haploid gametes or spores.

Meiosis is essential for sexual reproduction and therefore occurs in all eukaryotes (including single-celled organisms) that reproduce sexually. A few eukaryotes, notably the Bdelloid rotifers, have lost the ability to carry out meiosis and have acquired the ability to reproduce by parthenogenesis. Meiosis does not occur in archaea or bacteria, which reproduce via asexual processes such as binary fission.

During meiosis, the genome of a diploid germ cell, which is composed of long segments of DNA packaged into chromosomes, undergoes DNA replication followed by two rounds of division, resulting in four haploid cells. Each of these cells contain one complete set of chromosomes, or half of the genetic content of the original cell. If meiosis produces gametes, these cells must fuse during fertilisation to create a new diploid cell, or zygote before any new growth can occur. Thus, the division mechanism of meiosis is a reciprocal process to the joining of two genomes that occurs at fertilisation. Because the chromosomes of each parent undergo genetic recombination during meiosis, each gamete, and thus each zygote, will have a unique genetic *blueprint* encoded in its DNA. Together, meiosis and fertilisation constitute sexuality in the eukaryotes, and generate genetically distinct individuals in populations.

In all plants, and in many protists, meiosis results in the formation of haploid cells that can divide vegetatively without undergoing fertilisation, referred to as spores. In these groups, gametes are produced by mitosis. Meiosis uses many of the same biochemical mechanisms employed during mitosis to accomplish the redistribution of chromosomes. There are several features unique to meiosis, most importantly the pairing and genetic recombination between homologous chromosomes. Meiosis comes from the root-meio, meaningless.

Meiosis bud is the second type of life cycle exhibited by some haploid yeasts varies from the first in that the haploid vegetative cell produces a bud which, instead of separating in a normal fashion, stays attached to the mother cell, retaining a rather large connective opening. Nuclear division occurs (mitosis) and the 2 daughter nuclei move into the bud structure where karyogamy occurs. Meiosis also occurs in the bud resulting in 2 or 4 haploid nuclei. Because meiosis does occur in this bud-like structure, it has been termed the 'meiosis bud'.

Cell fusion

Cell fusion is an important cellular process that occurs during differentiation of muscle, bone and trophoblast cells, during embryogenesis and during morphogenesis. Cell fusion is a necessary event in the maturation of cells so that they maintain their specific functions throughout growth.

Diploid vegetative phase

Diploid cells have two homologous copies of each chromosome, usually one from the mother and one from the father. The exact number of chromosomes may be one or two different from the 2 number yet the cell may still be classified as diploid (although with aneuploidy). Nearly all mammals are diploid organisms (the Plains Viscacha Rat is an exception), although all individuals have some small fraction of cells that display polyploidy. Human diploid cells have 46 chromosomes and human haploid gametes (egg and sperm) have 23 chromosomes.

Retroviruses that contain two copies of their RNA genome in each viral particle are also said to be diploid. Examples include human foamy virus, human T-lymphotropic virus and HIV. In diploid vegetative phase ascosporogenous yeasts which spend their vegetative days in the diploid condition procure their spores within the vegetative cells, which become the asci. For these yeasts there are 4 means known by which the diploid condition in the vegetative cell can arise from the haploid ascospore.

Basidiomycetous yeasts

Life cycles of the basidiomycetous yeasts also show variations but, in general, after fusion of 2 haploid (1n) yeast cells, there is a stage not found in the ascomycetous yeasts. This is the development of a dikaryotic conditions (1n plus 1n) where the 2 nuclei after plasmogamy do not fuse in the zygote but rather are incorporated in pairs into the cells of mycelium by a clamp connection. The clamp connection mechanism assures that 2 compatible nuclei are duplicated and propagated in subsequent cells of the mycelium. At the time of sporulation either thick-walled teliospores or thin-walled basidia are formed on the mycelium. The sexual spores (sporidia) are not forceably discharged for the promycelium or basidia of these yeasts. They are formed by budding and further vegetative reproduction is also by this means.

Nutritional requirements

All strains of *Saccharomyces cerevisiae* can grow aerobically on glucose, maltose and trehalose and fail to grow on lactose and cellobiose. However, growth on other sugars is variable. It was shown that galactose and fructose were two of the best fermenting sugars. The ability of yeasts to use different sugars can differ depending on whether they are grown aerobically or anaerobically. Some strains cannot grow anaerobically on sucrose and trehalose.

All strains can utilise ammonia and urea as the sole nitrogen source, but cannot utilise nitrate since they lack the ability to reduce them to ammonium ions. They can also utilise most amino acids, small peptides and nitrogen bases as a nitrogen source. Histidine, glycine, cystine and lysine are however, not readily utilised. *S. cerevisiae* does not excrete proteases so extracellular protein cannot be metabolised.

Yeasts also have a requirement for phosphorus, which is assimilated as a dihydrogen phosphate ion, and sulphur, which can be assimilated as a sulphate ion or as organic sulphur compounds like methionine and cystine. Some metals like magnesium, iron, calcium, zinc also are required for good growth of the yeast.

Sporulation

The determination of a yeast isolate's ability to form asco- or basidiospores is of prime importance in determining its identification. This determination can be complicated by the fact that some yeasts can grow in a vegetative state for an indefinite number of generations and that very specific conditions must be met before the sexual cycle can be induced. Further, in heterothallic species, fertile matings and successful completion of the sexual cycle depend upon the mixing of compatible strains. Early workers were of the opinion that yeasts would sporulate only when conditions for growth became unfavourable. Today it is known that this is not necessarily true. Many yeasts freshly isolated from nature often sporulate very heavily on the relatively rich media commonly used for isolation. Further, yeasts cultured in a laboratory are propagated on much richer media than would normally be available to them in their natural habitat. However, many so-called domestic cultivated yeasts, for example, bakers' and brewers' yeasts, as well as many species commonly isolated from spoiled beverages and other food products, often sporulate poorly or not at all on media rich in nutrients. Some yeast species have a tendency to lose their ability to form sexual spores while others are not affected when they are held in laboratory culture for a period of years.

Innumerable media and various techniques have been used over the years for the purpose of inducing ascospore formation or to increase the percentage of sporulating cells. Yeast ascospores are somewhat more resistant to adverse conditions such as freezing, drying and exposure to high temperatures and to harmful chemicals than are the vegetative cells. The heat resistance of the ascospore is only a few degrees (6°–12°C) greater than the vegetative cells under the same conditions. Thus, by heating a cell suspension for a short time at mildly elevated temperatures, such as 55°–60°C, vegetative cells can be killed but spores that might be present would still be viable.

Experience has shown that success in obtaining sporulation is best when the culture is well nourished and relatively young. In species of *Saccharomyces* it was found that young daughter cells which have not produced buds sporulate—either very poorly or not at all. However, after producing one or more buds, sporulation occurs normally.

Fermentative (anaerobic) conditions do not promote sporulation. In *Saccharomyces cerevisiae* sporulation is enhanced when the vegetative cells are adapted for aerobic growth. However, it has been found that with some species of *Hanseniaspora* which produce 1 to 2 spheroidal spores, a reduced oxygen tension stimulates spore formation. When part of the vegetative cell inoculum is covered by a sterile cover slip, large numbers of asci may develop under the cover slip near the outer edge, but are infrequently found in the uncovered portion of the growth or far under the cover slip.

In the laboratory most yeasts will sporulate at room temperature (18°–25°C) although reduced temperatures (12°–15°C) are beneficial to some species of *Nadsonia* and *Metschnikowia*.

As one might expect from the diversity of the many yeast species, there is no one medium capable of inducing sporulation for all of the yeasts. Most media are adjusted so that the pH is in the neutral to slightly acid range (pH 5.8–7.0). Certain media have been found to be better for some species than others. For example, acetate agar is commonly used for achieving sporulation with species of *Saccharomyces*, although potato extract glucose agar (PDA) works better for some haploid species of this genus. Gorodkowa agar works well for most species of *Debaryomyces*; YM agar (yeast extract malt extract maltose agar) induces sporulation of many species of *Pichia* and *Hansenula* and other yeasts. A medium based on vegetable juices (V-8), with or without added bakers' yeast, is also an excellent sporulation medium for species of a number of genera. In certain special cases a medium composed of the substrate from which the yeast was isolated may be used.

Since heterothallic yeasts require compatible mating types, cultures in which sporulation cannot be induced and which would be classified in the so-called imperfect genera should be mixed with similar cultures in various combinations, or, when the mating types for a species are known, mixed with the same mating types and reobserved for sporulation. Many yeast isolates formerly believed to be asporogenous are properly classified into their perfect generally these techniques.

Yeasts being observed for ability to sporulate should be checked frequently over a period of several weeks because the time required to sporulate as well as the number of asci formed varies a great deal among the yeast species and even within strains of the same species. Some can produce spores in 1–2 days, whereas other yeasts may not form asci for a week or two or longer. Frequent examination is necessary because with many yeasts the spores formed can also germinate on the same medium, and if observation were delayed or infrequent, one might not observe that sporulation had taken place.

Thus, although the ability or inability to produce sexual spores is not always easy to determine, the type of sexual spore formed is the primary criterion used by the taxonomist to place a yeast into 1 of 3 subdivisions of shape, size, surface markings and colour. Generally, most of these features are quite constant for a given species. For some genera, all species have a similar morphology, although in other genera, spore morphology differs among the species. Sporulation among the yeasts also has made possible genetic studies. However, from the standpoint of the yeast itself, it is the, most important biological event in its life cycle and it governs to a large extent the evolutionary development of the various groups of the yeasts. Therefore, inspite of the time spent and difficulties encountered in determining a yeast's ability to sporulate, the importance is justified.

FERMENTATION

Man has used the ability of certain yeasts to carry out an alcoholic fermentation long before the responsible agent was recognised as a living thing. The everyday use of alcoholic beverages and panary products has also made large quantities of yeasts available, facilitating the work of the investigators elucidating the basic metabolic processes of living cells.

Yeast cells will use oxygen if it is present, and break down sugars all the way to CO_2 and H_2O. In the absence of oxygen, yeast will switch to an alternative pathway that does not require oxygen. The end products of this pathway are CO_2 and ethanol. The first pathway yields a lot more energy per sugar molecule consumed, and so it is the 'preferred' pathway if oxygen is present. So, the first thing you need to do is set up a yeast culture that can grow anaerobically, i.e. in the absence of oxygen.

A low-tech way of doing this is to use a plastic soft drink bottle. Fill it with warm, 'not hot' (which will kill the yeast) water and dissolve a few tablespoons of sucrose (table sugar) in it. Dump in a packet of baker's yeast and mix. Fill the bottle right up to the top of the neck with water, and fit a deflated balloon over the neck.

Incubate the culture in a warm place; even room temperature will work. (If you have ever made bread, you will know that it's possible to overheat the yeast and kill the culture.) Within a day you should see the balloon start to puff up with the CO_2 that is expelled as a waste product from the yeast. You won't get tons of gas, since the resistance of the balloon prevents it from expanding to a large size, but you will get carbon dioxide.

For a more elegant collection method, replace the balloon with a stopper that has a short piece of tubing inserted through it. Attach a couple of feet of flexible tubing to the tube on the stopper. Now the CO_2 will be expelled out the tubing. How to capture it.... Fill a test tube or similar item 'full' of water, put your finger on top to seal it, and insert it upside down into a beaker or glass that is half full of water. You now have a setup that is similar to the waterers found on bird cages, for example. Run the flexible tubing so that the end of it is located underneath the end of the test tube, in the water. As gases escape from the tubing, they will bubble up into the test tube, and displace the water in the test tube. Once sufficient gas has collected, you can remove the test tube and test for CO_2 by seeing if the gas in the test tube will support combustion. The hardest part about the second setup is just getting everything clamped to stay in place.

During the primary fermentation, the fermentable sugars, mainly maltose and glucose are converted to ethanol and carbon dioxide. This action is performed by the brewing yeast, which during the brewing process also produces many of the characteristic aroma compounds found in beer. At the end of the primary fermentation, the yeast cells flocculate and sediment at the bottom of the fermenter and can be cropped and used for a new fermentation. Not all yeast cells sediment; some will remain in suspension, and these cells are responsible for maturation of the beer. During this process the off-flavour, diacetyl is degraded to below the taste threshold. The fermentation characteristics of brewer's yeast are strain-dependent and are genetically inherited. Much of the genetics of *Saccharomyces* yeasts has been elucidated, and the knowledge gained, forms the basis for breeding of brewing yeast. Thus, new types of beer with altered aromas can be produced with yeast strains selected through breeding.

Three basic rules regarding yeasts' capabilities to ferment were formulated many years ago by Kluyver. The first rule is that if a yeast is unable to ferment D-glucose, it cannot ferment any other sugar. The second rule states that if a yeast can ferment D-glucose, then D-fructose and D-mannose will also be fermented. The third rule is that if a yeast can ferment maltose, it cannot ferment lactose, and *vice versa*. Exceptions are known for the third rule in that there are a few yeasts capable of fermenting both maltose and lactose. *Brettanomyces claussenii* is an example of a yeast able to ferment both disaccharides.

Respiration

Aerobic metabolism is affected by the level of oxygen present and also concentration of the sugars. For example, both with *Saccharomyces cerevisiae* and with *Candida utilis* the Embden-Meyerhof pathway accounts for approximately 90 per cent of the glycolytic metabolism. Under aerobic conditions, however, the hexose monophosphate pathway is responsible for 6 to 30 per cent glycolysis in *Saccharomyces cerevisiae* and for 3 to 50 per cent in strains of *Candida utilis*. In contrast, species of *Rhodotorula* which are unable to ferment metabolise 60 to 80 per cent of the glucose taken from the medium through the hexose monophosphate pathway.

The effect of substrate concentration can be illustrated fur *S. cerevisiae* as follows. In media with glucose concentrations in excess of 5 per cent, there is a total inhibition of synthesis of respiratory enzymes so that the yeast continues to ferment even though the medium is aerated. This phenomenon is known as the 'glucose effect' or 'Crabtree effect'. Not all yeasts exhibit the Crabtree effect, e.g. species of *Kluyveromyces* and some haploid *Saccharomyces*. In contrast, a yeast (such as *Saccharomyces cerevisiae*) growing in low concentrations of glucose (0.1 per cent) can shift from fermentation to respiration upon aeration of the medium. The decrease in fermentative ability upon aeration was first demonstrated by Pasteur (Pasteur effect) and industrially utilised by producers of bakers' yeast and of feed yeasts. As the level of the sugar decreases in an aerated growth medium, there is a corresponding increase in the activity of the enzymes of the tricarboxylic acid cycle (TCA) and increased activity of enzymes involved in the glyoxylate cycle and in the electron-transport system. Since the enzymes for the TCA and glyoxylate cycles are located in the mitochondrial fraction of the yeast, the observation that the presence of sugar inhibits mitochondrial formation is not unexpected.

The TCA cycle starts with pyruvate's being oxidised to acetyl coenzyme A instead of decarboxylation to acetaldehyde, which occurs during alcoholic fermentation. The β-oxidation of fatty acids also results in acetyl CoA. Acetyl CoA then condenses with oxaloacetate, giving rise to citrate. Subsequent reactions of the TCA cycle release 2 molecules of CO_2 per cycle and generate ATP by oxidative phosphorylation. Several of the intermediate compounds also may be used in the synthesis of amino acids and other cellular constituents. The glyoxylate cycle or bypass has been more recently elucidated and was found to function for the replenishment of TCA cycle intermediates — especially L-malate and succinate removed from the cycle due to the synthesis of cellular constituents. The glyoxylate cycle also serves as the mechanism by which yeast can grow on 2-carbon molecules such as ethanol and acetate. A biotin-dependent reaction producing oxaloacetate from pyruvate and CO_2 serves to supply additional oxaloacetate for incorporation into the TCA cycle.

The hexose monophosphate shunt pathway, also known as the pentose, cycle, starts with glucose-6-phosphate which is oxidised to 6-phosphogluconate. This reaction is dependent, upon the reduction or NADP to $NADPH_2$. Subsequently, 1 molecule of CO_2 is released and additional molecule of $NADPH_2$ is formed. Aerobically, the cycle can result in the complete oxidation of glucose to 6 CO_2 and the formation of 12 molecules of $NADPH_2$. While the hexose monophosphate shunt does not generate high energy phosphate in the form of ATP, a portion of the $NADPH_2$ formed is oxidised in other metabolic pathways and in this way does contribute to ATP formation. The $NADPH_2$ is utilised in large part in synthetic reactions requiring reductions, such as the formation of lipids. The hexose monophosphate pathway also serves as a mechanism by which yeasts respire pentoses and methyl pentose sugars if the yeasts have the proper pentose kinases and other enzymes that will convert the substrates into intermediates of the pentose cycle.

GROWTH REQUIREMENTS

Carbohydrates

In order to grow, yeasts require oxygen, proper temperature and pH, utilisable organic carbon and nitrogen sources, and various minerals; and some require vitamins and other growth factors. All yeasts are able to utilise D-glucose, D-fructose and D-mannose, although a particular yeast may utilise other carbon sources more efficiently. Besides these 3 hexoses, another hexose, D-galactose, may be fermented, but this requires enzymatic adaptation by yeasts can possessing the potential to ferment the sugar. Other monosaccharides and all L-sugars are unfermentable although a particular yeast maybe able to utilise them by respiration.

In the fermentation of di-, tri-, or polysaccharides, the fermentation always goes through the hexose stage after enzymatic hydrolysis either at the cell surface of internally, depending upon the location of the specific enzymes. Consequently, if the particular hexose sugar is not fermented by the particular yeast, the di- or oligosaccharides are not fermented either. Enzymes for the hydrolysis of sucrose, raffinose, melibiose, starch and inulin apparently are situated outside of the cell membrane (plasmalemma) although their precise location has still to be determined. Enzymes for the hydrolysis of other sugars such as maltose, lactose, cellobiose and melezitose are located internally; the sugars are transported by specific permeases across the membrane and hydrolysed within the cell. Fermentation of polysaccharides such as starch, and inulin (a fructose-containing polysaccharide) is possible by relatively few yeasts, and then generally a reduced rates of fermentation. The ability to ferment pentose sugars of methyl pentoses is not found in any yeast, although it is not unusual for these compounds to be utilised by respiration. Thus, among the yeasts which are able to ferment, glucose (fructose, mannose), galactose, sucrose, maltose, raffinose, melibiose, lactose, and trehalose are the most commonly utilised sugars.

In brief, the breakdown of a sugar and its transformation to ethanol and carbon dioxide proceed in the following manner: D-glucose, D-fructose and D-mannose are all transported across the cell membrane by a common transport system termed 'facilitated diffusion'. In addition, these 3 hexoses are all phosphorylated by the same enzyme, yeast hexokinase, to the corresponding hexose-6-phosphates. Both the rate of transportation and the rate of phosphorylation of these sugars vary depending upon the sugar and also on the species, in fact, even on the strain of yeast. Glucose-6- and mannose-6-phosphate are subsequently transformed to fructose-6-phosphate. The other fermentable hexose, D-galactose, when utilised by a yeast, is transported by a separate, induced transport system, and once in the cell it is phosphorylated by a specific enzyme and transformed by 3 additional enzymes before it can enter the glycolytic cycle.

Hydrolysis to hexose components is obviously required before di-, trio and oligosaccharides may be fermented. After the hexoses are phosphorylated to the hexose-6-phosphate, a reaction requiring adenosine triphosphate (ATP) and other enzymes converts fructose-6-phosphate into fructose-1,6-diphosphate using another molecule of ATP. The fructose-1,6-diphosphate is converted to pyruvic acid via the Embden-Meyerhof pathway of glycolysis. The net results are 2 molecules of pyruvate and the generation of 4 molecules of ATP, a net gain of 2 molecules of ATP. The 2 pyruvate molecules are subsequently decarboxylated yielding 2 molecules of CO_2 and 2 molecules of acetaldehyde. Finally, the 2 molecules of acetaldehyde are reduced to ethanol by alcohol dehydrogenase and the reduced form of the coenzyme nicotinic acid adenine dinucleotide (NAD). It had been formed during one of the intermediate steps of the Embden-Meyerhof pathway. The 2 molecules of ATP formed during the transformation of 1 molecule of hexose to 2 molecules of CO_2 and 2 of ethanol are used as a supply of energy required for cell growth and for synthesis of storage reserve products (glycogen and trehalose).

It should be noted that under conditions of no growth, for example, in a medium containing glucose but no nitrogen source, the yeast cells will still convert about 70 per cent of the glucose to ethanol and CO_2 with the remainder going to reserve carbohydrates. When the glucose of the medium is depleted, it is felt that these reserve carbohydrates furnish the energy necessary for maintenance of the cell in replacement of the proteins and ribonucleic acids which are being constantly 'recycled'.

The concentration of ethanol produced depends not only on the conditions of fermentation, but perhaps even moreso upon the species and particular strain of a species. Suitable strains of *Saccharomyces cerevisiae*, for example, strains of wine yeast or distillers' yeast, can attain an ethanol concentration of 12 to 14 per cent by volume with relative ease if a sufficient supply of fermentable sugar is supplied. As the ethanol concentration increases above this level, the rate of fermentation is greatly reduced and will eventually cease. Ethanol levels of 18 to 20 per cent by volume have been achieved with select strains and specific fermentation conditions. In contrast, species of *Hanseniaspora* (and the asporogenous forms in the genus *Kloeckera*), which frequently are predominant yeasts in the early stages of natural fruit fermentations, are relatively sensitive to the presence of alcohol (about 3.5 to 6.0 per cent alcohol).

Of industrial interest is the ability of some yeasts to ferment L-malic acid to ethanol and carbon dioxide. Some wine yeasts (strains of *Saccharomyces cerevisiae*) have this ability, but species of *Schizosaccharomyces* (*S. pombe* and *S. malidevorans*) are more efficient. This property is especially of interest in the fermentation of grape and fruit musts of low sugar content and high levels of malic acid.

Other Organic Carbon Sources

Yeasts can respire all sugars that they are capable of fermenting and in addition may respire a wide array of other organic compounds. In addition to pentoses and methyl pentose sugars, compounds which yeasts can respire include organic acids, sugar alcohols, methanol and ethanol, as well as some aromatic compounds and hydrocarbons. Only a limited number of yeasts can utilise the last 2 classes of compounds and then only a few of these. Hydrocarbons used are primarily limited to the *n*-alkanes, particularly those with 12 to 18 carbon skeletons.

Nitrogen

Inorganic sources

The ability of yeasts to assimilate various compounds as a source of nitrogen also varies greatly among the yeasts. Among the inorganic sources of nitrogen, ammonium sulphate is utilisable by virtually all yeasts. In fact, most ammonium salts can supply nitrogen for the growth of yeasts, although some salts are more suitable than others. The ability to use nitrate is much more restricted and is, in fact, a criterion used in yeast classification. *Candida utilis* is an example of an industrially important yeast which utilises nitrate. Bakers' and brewers' yeast (*Saccharomyces cerevisiae* strains) are unable to grow on nitrate. Nitrite is utilised by all of the yeasts which can use nitrate, although the toxicity of the nitrite ion varies among these yeasts, and caution must be used to assure that too high a concentration is not used.

Amino acid

In chemistry, an amino acid is a molecule containing both amine and carboxyl functional groups. These molecules are particularly important in biochemistry, where this term refers to α-amino acids with the general formula $H_2NCHRCOOH$, where, R is an organic substituent. Amino acids also serve as a source of nitrogen for yeasts. While it was previously thought that yeasts could incorporate assimilated amino acids directly into proteins, it has more recently been shown that the utilisation of a particular amino acid depends upon the ability of the particular yeast to deaminate the amino acid and to incorporate that nitrogen into other constituents of the cell. Glutamic and aspartic acids and their amines are easily deaminated or transaminated by most yeasts and serve as good sources of nitrogen. In general, yeasts take up on the L-form of the amino acid, although certain D-isomers can be assimilated.

Other organic sources

Of other compounds which can act as a source of nitrogen, urea has been found to be utilised by virtually all yeasts and is as good a source as is ammonium sulphate. It was found, however, far a yeast to grow well, the medium must also contain ample biotin. The ability to utilise purine and pyrimidine bases varies greatly among the yeasts, as does the growth response to the various bases. Bakers' and brewers' yeasts in general utilise very few whereas *Candida utilis* can assimilate a greater number of these nitrogen-containing compounds. It has been shown for a number of yeasts that, during fermentation and growth, the yeasts actually excrete nitrogenous compounds into the medium. In many instances, these nitrogen-containing compounds are reabsorbed by the cell. Excreted compounds include amino acids, oligopeptides and nucleotides, components also to be found in the intracellular pool of nitrogenous compounds.

Vitamins

The requirement of yeasts for an exogenous source of vitamins varies widely, as some yeasts can synthesise all of their required vitamins, whereas other yeasts have multiple requirements. In recognition of requirement variability only the ability or inability to grow in a medium lacking vitamins is presently used in classification. With the exception of meso-inositol, the vitamins serve catalytic functions, normally as part of a particular coenzyme. Meso-inositol serves a structural function in membrane synthesis where it is incorporated into the phospholipids. The requirement for a particular vitamin in the medium is often qualified as to whether it is an absolute requirement, in which case the yeasts cannot grow if the vitamin is not regularly supplied, regardless of time or condition of growth, or whether it is a relative requirement, meaning that the yeasts can grow very slowly by synthesising the vitamin at a very reduced rate, but that the yeasts will grow much more vigorously if the vitamin is supplied in the medium. Yeasts having absolute requirements for a particular growth factor find use as a biological assay tool.

Biotin is the most commonly required vitamin to be supplemented in the medium whereas riboflavin and folic acid are apparently synthesised in sufficient quantities by all yeasts. Vitamin B_{12} is not known to be required or even synthesise. Adding high levels of vitamins, or in some cases their precursors, can 'enrich' yeasts by taking advantage of their ability to concentrate vitamins, particularly the B complex, from a medium into the yeast cell.

Minerals

Analysis of the minerals found in yeast cells show about 50 elements to be present, most in extremely minute amounts. Trace and small amounts of elements such as iron, copper, zinc, cobalt, calcium and magnesium are added to the medium as they are required by yeasts as enzyme activators, structural stabilisers, and components of proteins , pigments, etc. Some yeasts can utilise the amino acid, methionine, or the tripeptide, glutathione, as sources of sulphur but most yeasts cannot use cystine or cysteine. Sulphite can be used, but a number of yeasts are sensitive to bisulphite and to sulphurous acid. This sensitivity is used industrially for inhibiting 'wild yeasts' in certain fermentations, notably wine.

pH and Temperature

Besides adequately supplying a yeast's nutritional needs, attention to proper pH values and temperature of incubation are essential for desired activities and growth of the yeast. Actually most yeasts are relatively tolerant of a wide range of pH values; most will grow at pH 2.8–3.0 if hydrochloric acid is used to adjust the pH of the medium. Lactic and acetic acids at low pH values are often inhibitory due to the high concentrations of the undissociated acid form which can pass through the cell membrane into the cytoplasm. Most yeasts will also grow well at neutrality and in slightly alkaline conditions (pH 8–8.5). Optimum pH for growth varies from 4.5 to 6.5 for most species. Temperature ranges for growth vary from relatively narrow, particularly for a few yeasts found associated with warm-blooded animals, to relatively broad ranges. Many yeasts can grow at 0°C or slightly below but the rate of growth is extremely slow; some have a maximum of 18°–20°C, whereas others can grow at 46°–47°C. Most species encountered grow from about 5°C to 30°–37°C with an optimum approximating 25°C.

While optimum conditions are known for many yeasts, manipulation of nutrient concentrations, pH, temperature, and oxygen tension are used in industrial fermentations to best meet the desired purposes as economically as possible. Industrial fermenters further improve their processes by careful selection of yeast strains. Strain improvement by genetic selection or mutation often results in strains performing many-fold better than the original wild type.

Killer Yeasts

Killer yeasts are yeasts, such as *Saccharomyces cerevisiae*, which can carry a double-stranded RNA virus, causing them to secrete a number of toxic proteins which are lethal to receptive cells. These yeast cells are immune to the toxic effects of the protein due to an intrinsic immunity. Killer yeast strains can be a problem in commercial processing because they kill desirable strains.

RNA virus

The virus, L-A, is an icosahedral virus of *S. cerevisiae* comprising a 4.6 kb genomic segment and several satellite double-stranded RNA sequences, which are called M dsRNAs. The genomic segment encodes for the viral coat protein and a protein which replicates the viral genomes. The M dsRNAs encode the toxin, of which there are at least three variants in *S. cerevisiae*, and many more variants across all species.

L-A is not released into the environment. It spreads between cells during yeast mating.

Saccharomyces pastorianus

Saccharomyces pastorianus is a yeast, used industrially for the production of lager beer. It is a synonym of the yeast species *Saccharomyces carlsbergensis*, which was originally described in 1883 by Emil Christian Hansen, who was working for the Danish brewery Carlsberg.

Saccharomyces uvarum

Saccharomyces uvarum is a species of yeast that is believed to have originated as a hybrid of *S. cerevisiae* and *S. monacensis*, because of its allopolyploid genome. It is a bottom-fermenting yeast, so-called because it does not form the foam on top of the wort that top-fermenting yeast does.

Saccharomyces cerevisiae

Saccharomyces cerevisiae is a species of budding yeast. It is perhaps the most useful yeast owing to its use since ancient times in baking and brewing. It is believed that it was originally isolated from the skins of grapes (one can see the yeast as a component of the thin white film on the skins of some dark-coloured fruits such as plums; it exists among the waxes of the cuticle). It is one of the most intensively studied eukaryotic model organisms in molecular and cell biology, much like *Escherichia coli* as the model prokaryote. It is the micro-organism behind the most common type of fermentation. *Saccharomyces cerevisiae* cells are round to ovoid, 5–10 micrometers in diameter. It reproduces by a division process known as budding.

Many proteins important in human biology were first discovered by studying their homologs in yeast; these proteins include cell cycle proteins, signalling proteins and protein-processing enzymes. The petite mutation in *S. cerevisiae* is of particular interest.

'*Saccharomyces*' derives from Greek, and means 'sugar mould' or 'sugar fungi'. *Saccharo-* being 'of sugar' and *Myco-* being 'of fungi', '*cerevisiae*' comes from Latin, and means 'of beer'.

Other names for the organism are:

1. *S. cerevisiae* short form of the scientific name.
2. Brewer's yeast (the apostrophe may be after the *s* or missing), though other species are also used in brewing.
3. Ale yeast.
4. Top-fermenting yeast.
5. Baker's yeast (the apostrophe may be after the *s* or missing).
6. Budding yeast.

This species is also the main source of nutritional yeast and yeast extract.

Genomics

As *S. pastorianus* is a hybrid of *Saccharomyces bayanus* and *Saccharomyces cerevisiae* it is not surprising that there is a degree of phenotypic and genomic similarity between the two species. The hybrid nature of *S. pastorianus* also explains the genome size, which is up to 60 per cent larger than that of *S. cerevisiae* as it includes large parts of the two genomes. However, there is growing evidence that *S. pastorianus* has inherited most of its genetic material from *S. bayanus*. Indeed the mitochondrial DNA and ribosomal DNA of *S. pastorianus* appear to be derived from *S. bayanus* rather than *S. cerevisiae*.

The genomic difference between *S. pastorianus* and *S. cerevisiae* is responsible for a number of phenotypic traits which *S. pastorianus* share with *S. bayanus*, but not *S. cerevisiae*. The ability of *S. pastorianus* to break down melibiose is dependent on up to ten MEL genes, which are exclusive to strains metabolising melibiose such as *S. bayanus*. *S. pastorianus* never grows above 34°C, whereas *S. cerevisiae* will grow at 37°C. *S. pastorianus* exhibits a higher growth rate than *S. cerevisiae* at 6° to 12°C. It has been suggested that *S. pastorianus* may be a hybrid of *S. cerevisiae* and *Saccharomyces monacensis*, as the LEU2, MET2 and ACB1 genes of *S. pastorianus* had been reported to have a high level of similarity or be identical to the *S. monacensis* homologues. However, subtelomeric sequence hybridisation has suggested that *S. monacensis* is likely to be a closely related hybrid to *S. pastorianus*, rather than an ancestor.

Ale strains are genetically more diverse than lager strains, as lager strains are thought to derive from a hybrid gene pool. It is thought that the lager strains in use are derived from only one or two primary strains; Tuborg and Carlsberg.

Chapter 3

Pure Culture Methods

INTRODUCTION

Micro-organisms necessary in food fermentation may be added as pure cultures or mixed cultures, or, in some instances, no cultures may be added if the desired micro-organisms are known to be present in sufficient numbers in the original raw material. In the food fermentations for the manufacture of sauerkraut, fermented pickles and green olives and in the processing of cocoa, coffee, poi and citron, the original raw product carries enough of the desired organisms, which will act in proper succession if favourable environmental conditions are provided and maintained. Therefore, the addition of pure or mixed cultures of the organisms responsible for the fermentations has not been found necessary, although in some of the fermentations, e.g. pickles and green olives, it is advantageous. On the other hand, controlled 'starter' cultures, pure or mixed, usually are employed in the manufacture of certain dairy products, such as fermented milks, some kinds of butter and most types of cheese, and in most of the other food fermentations, e.g. bread, malt beverages, wines, distilled liquors and vinegar.

GENERAL PRINCIPLES OF CULTURE MAINTENANCE AND PREPARATION

Selection of Cultures

Cultures for food fermentations are selected primarily on the basis of their stability and their ability to produce desired products or changes efficiently. These cultures may be established ones obtained from other laboratories or may be selected after the testing of numerous strains. Stability is an important characteristic; yields and rates of changes must not be erratic. Some cultures may be improved by breeding, e.g. the sporogenous yeasts, but selection is the most commonly used method for the improvement of strains. Selection of cultures with desirable traits can be made from new strains isolated from the environment, from existing strains, or following mutation of strains by various means.

Refinement of plasmid transfer systems in the lactic acid bacteria will allow for gene cloning or gene amplification of a highly desirable trait such as lactic acid production. Since the gene responsible for lactose fermentation in some lactic streptococci is located on plasmids, the trait can be easily lost. Stabilising these industrially important traits has been demonstrated to be possible. McKay and coworkers have cloned the lac$^+$ genes of S. lactis and incorporated them into S. sanguis. The lac$^+$ genes, via a vector plasmid and transformation, were integrated into the chromosome of the host cell. As an integrated part of the chromosome, the lac$^+$ gene is much more stable than it is when it is plasmid-borne.

Maintenance of Activity of Cultures

Once a satisfactory culture has been obtained, it must be kept pure and active. Usually this objective is attained by periodic transfer of the culture into the proper culture medium, incubation until the culture reaches the maximal stationary phase of growth, and then storage at temperatures low enough to prevent further growth. Too frequent transfer of an unstable culture may lead to undesirable changes in its characteristics.

Stock cultures should be prepared for storage of cultures over long periods without transfer. Such cultures tend to remain stable and serve as a source of culture if the active culture deteriorates or is lost. Lyophilisation (freeze drying) and freezing in liquid nitrogen (–196°C) are now frequently used to prepare stock cultures, although some use still is made of a paraffin oil seal over ordinary tube cultures. Bacterial cultures have been preserved for months to years at room temperature on slants of agar in which 1 per cent NaCl had been incorporated. A dry spore stock on sterilised soil can be used to preserve spores of bacteria or moulds for long periods.

Maintenance of Purity of Cultures

To ensure the purity of cultures, they should be obtained periodically from a culture laboratory or be checked regularly for purity. Methods for testing a culture for purity vary with the type of culture being tested. Microscopic examination will indicate contamination only if the contaminant differs from the desired organism in appearance and is high in numbers. Another method is to plate the culture with an agar medium that will grow contaminants but not the desired organism. Tests may be made for the presence of substances not produced by the desired organism, e.g. for catalase in a culture of catalase-negative lactic acid bacteria as indicative of the presence of catalase-positive contaminants.

Preparation of Cultures

Mother culture is usually prepared daily from a previous mother culture and originally from the stock culture. These mother cultures can be used to inoculate a larger quantity of culture medium to produce the mass or bulk culture to be used in the fermentation process. Often, however, the fermentation is on such a large scale that several intermediate cultures of increasing size must be built up between the mother culture and the final bulk or mass culture. Culture makers attempt to produce and maintain a culture that: (i) contains only the desired micro-organism(s), (ii) is uniform in microbial numbers, proportions (if a mixed culture), and activity from day-to-day, (iii) is active in producing the products desired, and (iv) has adequate resistance to unfavorable conditions if necessary, e.g. heat resistance, if it has to take heating in a cheese curd. They try to maintain uniformity by standardising methods of preparation and sterilisation of the culture medium, inoculation and incubation temperature and time. The stage of growth to which they will grow the culture depends on the purpose for which it is to be used. If they wish prompt and rapid growth, they use a culture that is late in its logarithmic phase of growth. If they want more resistance to heat or other unfavourable conditions, they use a culture that has just entered the maximal stationary phase. The temperature of incubation usually is somewhere near the optimal temperature for the organism, although there are exceptions. Temperature and time of incubation often are adjusted so that the culture will be ready at the time it is needed. Otherwise, it may have to be cooled to stop further development.

Activity of Culture

The activity of a culture is judged by its rate of growth and production of products. It should be good if the mother or the intermediate culture is satisfactory and culture medium, incubation time, and temperature are optimal. Deterioration of cultures may result from improper handling and cultivation, frequent transfer over long periods in an inadequate culture medium, selection, variation or mutation, or attack of bacteria by a bacteriophage.

Mixed Cultures

Known mixtures of pure cultures sometimes are prepared, being grown together continuously or grown separately and mixed at the time of use. The so-called of butter or lactic, culture used in the dairy industry is an example of a mixture of several species of bacteria growing together and sometimes several strains of individual species. When different strains of the same species or different species are grown together, these organisms must be compatible, i.e. grow well together without any causing the elimination of others. The maintenance of the desired balance of kinds of organisms within these mixed cultures is difficult.

Unknown mixtures of organisms are present in starters used in some food products. Examples are the dough carried over from one lot of special French bread to a succeeding lot and the mixture of yeasts and bacteria carried from the surface smear of one Limburger cheese to the surface of another.

MICROBIOLOGICAL CULTURE

A microbiological culture or microbial culture, is a method of multiplying microbial organisms by letting them reproduce in predetermined culture media under controlled laboratory conditions. Microbial cultures are used to determine the type of organism, its abundance in the sample being tested, or both. It is one of the primary diagnostic methods of microbiology and used as a tool to determine the cause of infectious disease by letting the agent multiply in a predetermined media. For example, a throat culture is taken by scraping the lining of tissue in the back of the throat and blotting the sample into a media to be able to screen for harmful micro-organisms, such as, streptococcus pyogenes, the caustive agent of strep throat. Furthermore, the term culture is more generally used informally to refer to 'selectively growing' a specific kind of micro-organism in the laboratory.

Microbial cultures are foundational and basic diagnostic methods used extensively as a research tool in molecular biology. It is often essential to isolate a pure culture of micro-organisms. A pure (or *axenic*) culture is a population of cells or multicellular organisms growing in the absence of other species or types. A pure culture may originate from a single cell or single organism, in which case the cells are genetic clones of one another. For the purpose of gelling the microbial culture, the medium of agarose gel (Agar) is used. Agar is a gelatinous substance derived from seaweed. A cheap substitute for agar is 'guar gum', which can be used for the isolation and maintenance of thermophiles.

Bacterial Cultures

Microbiological cultures utilise petri dishes of differing sizes that have a thin layer of agar based growth medium in them. Once the growth medium in the petri dish is inoculated with the desired bacteria, the plates are incubated in an oven usually set at 37 degrees Celsius. Another method of bacterial culture is liquid culture, in which case desired bacteria are suspended in liquid broth, a nutrient medium. These are ideal for preparation of an antimicrobial assay. The experimenter would inoculate liquid broth with a bacteria and let it grow overnight in a shaker for uniform growth, then take aliquots of the sample to test for the antimicrobial activity of a specific drug or protein (antimicrobial peptides).

Most of the bacterial cultures employed as starters for dairy products, sausage, and bread are pure or mixed cultures of lactic acid bacteria, exceptions being the propionic acid bacteria added to

Swiss cheese. Acetic acid bacteria are used in vinegar making, and various bacteria are used for the manufacture of certain enzymes.

Virus and phage culture

Virus or phage cultures require host cells for the virus or phage to multiply in. For bacteriophages, cultures are grown by infecting bacterial cells. The phage can then be isolated from the resulting plaques in a lawn of bacteria on a plate. Virus cultures are obtained from their appropriate eukaryotic host cells.

Eukaryotic cell culture

The term culture can also apply to eukaryotic micro-organisms such as yeast and be used as a synonym for tissue culture, which involves the growth of cells or tissues explanted from a multi-cellular organism.

Lactic acid cultures

Although a few dairy plants still maintain their own cultures that they have carried successfully for years, most operators obtain new cultures periodically or use frozen, concentrated cultures prepared by commercial culture laboratories. The majority of commercially available cultures are now liquid-nitrogen frozen culture concentrates prepared by growing the cultures in a suitable medium followed by harvesting and concentrating by centrifugation. The harvested cell pastes are standardised for activity and then packaged in pull-top cans and rapidly frozen in liquid nitrogen. Shipping, distribution and storage of the frozen culture concentrates are feasible, and numerous advantages are evident. Acquiring such cultures eliminates the need for the maintenance and routine transfers involved in a company maintained culture collection. Problems with contamination of the cultures during transfer and routine maintenance are eliminated. The use of the various strains of commercially available cultures can be rotated to provide a broader protection against bacteriophage infection. The numbers of cells are so high in many of these culture concentrate products that a 16-oz can (containing 11 oz of concentrate) can be used for direct inoculation of a cheese vat containing up to 5000 lb of milk. This procedure would eliminate the older practice of preparing increasingly larger bulk-starter inocula over a succession of days. Preparation of enough bulk starter for a large cheese vat used to require several days of transferring to larger and larger volumes, all of which would have originated from the stock culture.

The most common dairy starter is the lactic starter, which ordinarily consists of a mixture of strains of *Streptococcus lactis* subsp. *lactis*, and *S. mesenteroides* subsp. *cremoris* for the production of lactic acid and *Leuconostoc cremoris* or *Streptococcus lactis* subsp. *diacetlactis* for the production of flavour and aroma. Several strains of lactic streptococci of different sensitivities to bacteriophage usually are included in the same culture concentrate as an insurance against trouble with phage.

Generally the lactic culture is incubated at 21.1° to 22.2°C, although 23.9° to 26.7°C has been employed in making starters for cheese. A culture is ripened to the desirable titratable acidity to suit the purpose for which the culture is to be used.

A mixed lactic culture is used in the manufacture of cultured buttermilk, yogurt and several types of cheese. The aroma bacteria are especially important in flavour production in cultured buttermilk. The typical yogurt starter is a mixture of *Streptococcus thermophilus* and *Lactobacillus delbrueckii* subsp. *bulgaricus*. The transfer and handling of mixed cultures must take into account the temperature and length of incubation which will best maintain the desired mixed population and thereby prevent domination by one strain or species over another. The use of frozen concentrated cultures eliminates many of these concerns. In addition, cultures from commercial culture laboratories provide the benefit of purchasing previously determined and tested compatible strains.

As already mentioned the 'sour' used by the makers of rye bread is a mixture of various lactic acid bacteria ordinarily grown in mixed and impure culture in flour paste, dough or other medium. It is claimed that *L. delbrueckii* subsp. *bulgaricus* must grow if enough acid is to be produced and that heterofermentative lactics are desirable from the standpoint of flavour production. Some breadmakers use pure cultures of *Streptococcus lactis* subsp. *lactis*, *Leuconostoc* spp., *Lactobacillus plantarum*, *L. casei*, *L. brevis*, *L. delbrueckii* subsp. *bulgaricus* and *Streptococcus thermophilus* to inoculate bread. Other breadmakers also add yeasts. Lactobacilli and *Pediococcus acidilactici* or *P. pentosaceus* cultures may be used as starters for summer, Thuringer and similar fermented sausages. Broth cultures, dried cultures and frozen culture concentrates have been prepared.

Propionic culture

Spray-dried or lypohilised cultures of *Propionibacterium freudenreichii* are added to milk used in the manufacture of Swiss cheese to improve the flavour and assist eye formation.

Cheese smear organisms

Most cheese makers inoculate the surfaces of smear-ripened cheese from previous cheeses, shelves, cloths, brine tank, hands and other sources in the plant. The micrococci, *Brevibacterium linens* and film yeasts important in the smear have been isolated and used in pure or mixed cultures to wash cheese surfaces, thereby inoculating them.

Acetic acid bacteria

Pure cultures of *Gluconobacter* or *Acetobacter* are not efficient in the production of acetic acid. Therefore, in vinegar making, impure mixed cultures are allowed to develop naturally, are added by means of raw vinegar from a previous run, or are transferred from a vinegar cask or generator.

YEAST CULTURES

Most yeasts of industrial importance are of the genus *Saccharomyces* and mostly of the species *S. cerevisiae*. These ascospore forming yeasts are readily bred for desired characteristics. A yeast for a given purpose may be improved for that use but must also be guarded against possible undesirable changes.

Bakers Yeast

Strains of *S. cerevisiae* used to manufacture bakers' yeast are usually single cell isolates that have been selected especially for the purpose. They should give a good yield of cells in the mash or medium chosen for their cultivation, should be stable, should remain viable in the cake or dried form for a reasonably long period, and should produce carbon dioxide rapidly in the bread dough when used for leavening. Like other cultures used on a large scale, this culture is built up from the original mother culture through several intermediate cultures of increasing size to the final 'seed' culture. The cells from the seed-culture tank are concentrated into a 'cream' by centrifugation, and this heavy suspension is added to the large volume of mash in which the yeast is to be grown, so that about 3 to 5 lb of yeast is added per 100 gal of medium.

The most commonly used medium for the buildup of cultures and the production of bakers' yeast is a cane or beet molasses—mineral-salts mash that contains molasses, nitrogen foods in the form of ammonium salts, urea, malt sprouts, etc. inorganic salts as phosphates and other mineral salts and accessory growth substances in the form of extracts of vegetables, grain or yeast, or small quantities of vitamin precursors or vitamins. The pH is adjusted to about 4.3 to 4.5, and the incubation temperature is around 30°C. During growth of the yeast the medium is aerated at a rapid rate and molasses is added gradually to maintain the sugar level at about 0.5 to 1.5 per cent. After four or five budding cycles, the yeast is centrifuged out in the form of a 'cream', which is put through a filter press to remove excess liquid. The mass of yeasts is made into cakes of different sizes after incorporation of small amounts of vegetable oils.

Active dry yeast now is made by drying the yeast cells to less than 8 per cent moisture. Cells so dried are grown especially for the purpose and are dried fully at low temperatures so that most of the cells will survive and will retain for some months their ability to actively leaven dough.

Bakers' yeast also can be prepared from grain mashes, waste sulphite liquor from paper mills, wood hydrolyzate and other materials.

Yeasts for Malt Beverages

Yeasts for malt beverages may be carried in pure culture in brewery laboratories or obtained when needed from specialised laboratories. The strain selected is one intended for the product to be made, a special bottom yeast for beer, usually a top yeast for ale but sometimes a bottom yeast, and a top yeast for stout and porter. The top yeasts used are strains of *Saccharomyces cerevisiae*, and the bottom yeast used is *S. uvarum* (*carlsbergensis*). When the yeast is started from a pure culture, it must be built up in wort from a laboratory culture to a final large seed or 'pitching' culture. In practice, however, the pitching yeast is nearly always yeast recovered from a previous fermentation. The recovered yeast is concentrated and may or may not be washed. It is obvious that such a yeast culture will always be contaminated with other organisms, which ordinarily include bacteria and wild yeasts that build up during successive fermentations and recoveries. Fortunately, most of the contaminants, although able to grow in the yeast culture, are inhibited by the hops and low pH in the wort and do not damage the malt beverage appreciably. It is possible, however, for organisms causing 'beer diseases' to build up in the pitching yeast.

Wine Yeasts

For wine making, a special strain of *Saccharomyces cerevisiae* var. *ellipsoideus*, adapted to the making of the specific type of wine, is selected. Famous types are the Burgundy, Tokay, and champagne cultures so widely used. The cultures are grown and built up in volume in must (juice of the grape or other fruit) like that to be used in the main fermentation.

Distillers' Yeast

Distillers' yeast ordinarily is a high-alcohol-yielding strain of *S. cerevisiae* var. *ellipsoideus*, usually one adapted to growing in the medium or mash to be employed. The medium or mash would be malted grain, usually corn or rye for whiskey, molasses for rum, or juices or mashes of fruits for brandy. The liquors are distillates of the fermented mashes.

MOULD CULTURES

Stock cultures of moulds usually are carried on slants of a suitable agar medium, e.g. malt-extract agar, and may be preserved in the spore state for long periods by lyophilisation (freeze drying) or as soil stocks. There are a number of different ways of preparing spore or mycelial cultures for use on a plant scale. These include: (i) surface growth on a liquid or agar medium in a flask or similar container,

(ii) surface growth on media in shallow layers in trays, (iii) growth on loose, moistened wheat bran which may be acidified or may have liquid nutrient added, e.g. corn-steep liquor, (iv) growth on previously sterilised and moistened bread or crackers, and (v) growth by the submerged method in an aerated liquid medium, usually resulting in pellets composed of mycelium, with or without spores. The mould spores are recovered in different ways, depending on the method of production. They may be washed or drawn from dry surfaces, may be left in dry material that is ground up or powdered, or for convenience in use may be incorporated in some dry powder, e.g. flour. The pellets, of course, are used as such.

Spores of *Penicillium roqueforti* for blue cheeses, Roquefort, Stilton, Gorgonzola, etc. usually are grown on cubes of sterilised, moistened and usually acidified bread; whole wheat or bread of a special formula may be employed. After the sporulation of the mould is complete, bread and culture are dried, powdered and packaged, commonly in cans.

P. camemberti spores are prepared by growing the mould on moistened sterile crackers. A spore suspension is prepared for the surface inoculation of the Camembert, Brie, or similar cheese.

Mould starters used as inoculum in industrial submerged fermentations usually are prepared in the form of pellets or masses of mycelium that are produced during submerged growth while the culture is being actively shaken. When surface growth is desired on liquid or agar medium or on bran, mould spores, produced by the methods listed previously, ordinarily serve as the inoculum.

The koji, or starter, for soya sauce, usually is a mixed culture carried over from a previous lot, although pure cultures of *Aspergillus oryzae*, together with a yeast and *Lactobacillus delbrueckii*, have been used. The mould culture is grown on cooked, sterilised rice.

PURE CULTURE TECHNIQUE

Micro-organisms are ubiquitous, so the preparation of a pure culture involves not only the isolation of a given micro-organism from a mixed natural microbial population, but also the maintenance of the isolated individual and its progeny in an artificial environment to which the access of other micro-organisms is prevented. Micro-organisms do not require much space for development; hence an artificial environment can be created within the confines of a test tube, a flask, or a petri dish, the three kinds of containers most commonly used to cultivate micro-organisms. The culture vessel must be rendered initially sterile (free of any living micro-organism) and, after the introduction of the desired type of micro-organism, it must be protected from subsequent external contamination. The primary source of external contamination is the atmosphere, which always contains floating micro-organisms. The form of a petri dish, with its overlapping lid, is specifically designed to prevent atmospheric contamination. Contamination of tubes and flasks is prevented by closure of their orifices with an appropriate stopper. This has traditionally been a plug of cotton wool, although metal caps or plastic screw caps are now often employed, particularly for test tubes. The external surface of a culture vessel is, of course, subject to contamination, and the interior of a flask or tube can become contaminated when it is opened to introduce or withdraw material. This danger is minimised by passing the orifice through a flame, immediately after the stopper has been removed and again just before it is replaced.

The *inoculum* (i.e. the microbial material used to seed or inoculate a culture vessel) is commonly introduced on a metal wire or loop, which is rapidly sterilised just before its use by heating in a flame. Transfers of liquid cultures can also be made by pipette. For this purpose, the mouth end of the pipette may be plugged with cotton wool, and the pipette is sterilised in a paper wrapping or in a glass or metal container, which keeps both inner and outer surfaces free of contamination until the time of use.

The risks of accidental contamination may be further reduced by performing transfers in a hood or in a small closed room, the air of which has been specially treated to reduce its microbial content. Special hoods and other precautions may also be necessary to prevent accidental release of the organism if it causes disease, or if it has been constructed using recombinant DNA techniques.

Isolation of Pure Cultures

For single-celled eukaryotes, such as yeast, the isolation of pure cultures uses the same techniques as for bacterial cultures. Pure cultures of multicellular organisms are often more easily isolated by simply picking out a single individual to initiate a culture. This is a useful technique for pure culture of fungi, multicellular algae and small metazoa, for example.

Developing pure culture techniques is crucial to the observation of the specimen in question. The most common method to isolate individual cells and produce a pure culture, is to prepare a streak plate. The streak plate method is a way to physically separate the microbial population, and is done by spreading the inoculate back and forth with an inoculating loop over the solid agar plate. Upon incubation, colonies will arise and, hopefully, single cells will have been isolated from the biomass.

Isolation of Pure Cultures by Plating Methods

Pure cultures of micro-organisms that form discrete colonies on solid media (e.g. yeasts, most bacteria, many fungi and unicellular algae) may be most simply obtained by one of the modifications of the plating method. This method involves the separation and immobilisation of individual organisms on or in a nutrient medium solidified with agar or some other appropriate gelling agent. Each viable organism gives rise, through growth, to a colony from which transfers can be readily made.

The streaked plate is in general the most useful plating method. A sterilised bent wire is dipped into a suitable diluted suspension of organisms and is then used to make a series of parallel, non-overlapping streaks on the surface of an already solidified agar plate. The inoculum is progressively diluted with each successive streak, so that even if the initial streaks yield confluent growth, well-isolated colonies develop along the lines of later streaks (Fig. 3.1). Alternatively, isolations can be made with poured plates: successive dilutions of the inoculum are placed in sterile petri dishes and mixed with the cooled but still molten agar medium, which is then allowed to solidify. Colonies subsequently develop embedded in the agar.

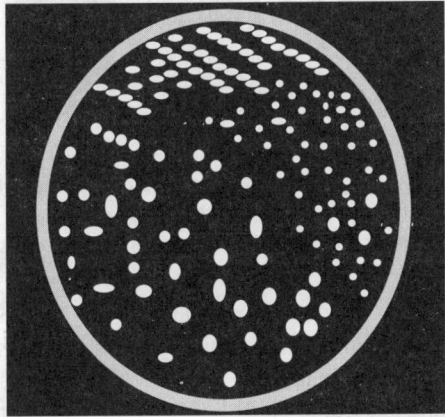

Fig. 3.1. Isolation of a pure culture by the streak method. A petri dish containing nutrient agar was streaked with a suspension of bacterial cells. As a result of subsequent growth, each cell has given rise to a macroscopically visible colony.

The isolation of anaerobic bacteria by plating methods poses special problems. Provided that the desired organisms are not rapidly killed by exposure to oxygen, plates may be prepared in the usual manner and then incubated in closed containers, from which the oxygen is removed either by chemical absorption or evacuation. For more oxygen-sensitive anaerobes, a modification of the pour plate method, known as the dilution shake culture, is preferred. A tube of melted and cooled agar medium is inoculated and mixed, and approximately one-tenth of its contents is transferred to a second tube, which is then mixed and used to inoculate a third tube in a similar fashion. After 6 to 10 successive dilutions have been prepared, the tubes are rapidly cooled and sealed, by pouring a layer of sterile petroleum jelly and paraffin on the surface, thus preventing access of air to the agar column. In shake culture the colonies develop deep in the agar column (Fig. 3.2), and are thus not easily accessible for transfer. To make a transfer, the petroleum jelly-paraffin seal is removed with a sterile needle, and the agar column is extruded from the tube into a sterile petri dish by gently blowing a stream of gas through a capillary pipette inserted between the tube wall and the agar. The column is sectioned into discs with a sterile knife to permit examination and transfer of colonies.

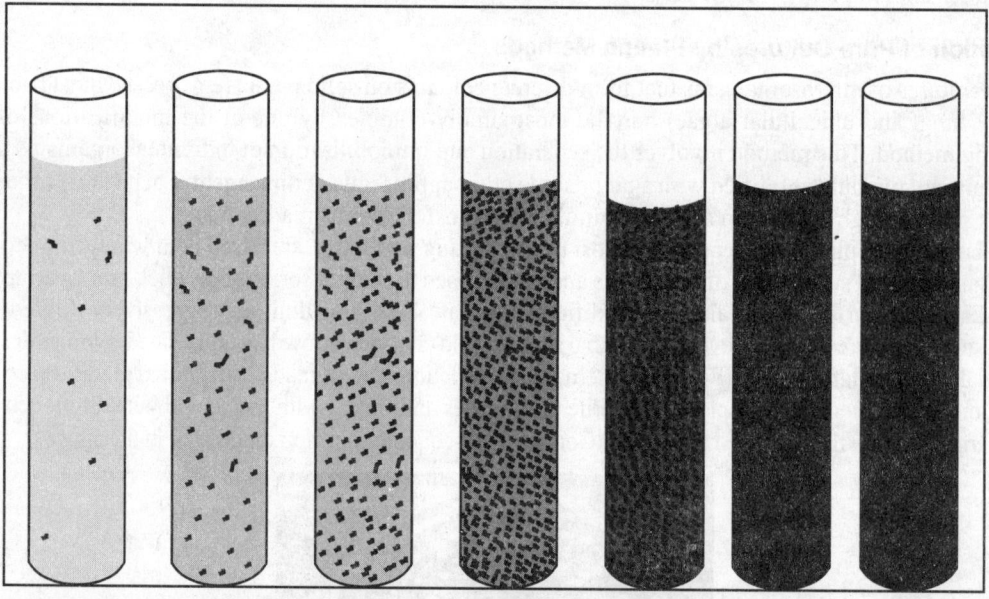

Fig. 3.2. Isolation of a pure culture of anaerobic bacteria by the dilution shake method. A complete series of dilution shakes is shown. Note the confluent growth in the more densely seeded tubes (at right), and the well-isolated colonies in the two final tubes of the series (at left). After the agar had solidified, each tube was sealed with a mixture of sterile vaseline and paraffin to prevent the access of atmospheric oxygen, which inhibits the growth of anaerobic bacteria.

Many bacteria are killed by even momentary exposure to air; thus, successful cultivation of these strict anaerobes, as they are called, requires extraordinary measures to exclude at all times even traces of oxygen. Two principal techniques are currently used to culture bacteria in the complete absence of oxygen; they are the roll tube, and anaerobic glove box techniques. The roll tube procedure, developed by Hungate, is used to obtain pure cultures of strict anaerobes by distributing cells in a thin layer of agar on the walls of a test tube, where they develop into isolated colonies. The test tube contains a few millilitres of molten agar medium that has been reduced chemically to remove dissolved oxygen and is tightly stoppered with a butyl rubber bung (small but lethal quantities of oxygen diffuse through ordinary rubber). The molten agar is inoculated with appropriate dilutions of the source of bacteria by inserting them through the rubber stoppers with a sterile syringe. The tubes are then laid on their sides in ice and rolled until the agar solidifies in a thin layer on the wall of the tube. After a period of incubation when colonies become visible, the bung is removed and isolated colonies picked from the agar with a needle or capillary tube. Whenever a tube is unstoppered, entry of air is prevented by continuously passing a stream of O_2 free gas (normally CO_2 or N_2) into the tube. To ensure that some entry of air has not inadvertently occurred, it is usual to include in the medium the redox dye *resazurine*, which changes from colourless to red at a midpoint E_h of -0.042 V (E_h is the effective reduction potential of a medium reduced forms of all redox-active compounds. In the construction of media for the culture of strict anaerobes, it is lowered by the inclusion of strong reducing agents).

Strict anaerobes may also be isolated using conventional streak plate techniques if all procedures are done within a glove box (a glove box is a sealed chamber in which objects are manipulated with hands inserted into rubber gloves that are attached to the front of the unit, a transparent panel allows the manipulations to be viewed from the outside) that encloses a reducing atmosphere.

In isolating from a mixed natural population it is often possible, provided one's technique is good, to prepare a first plate, or dilution shake or roll tube series, in which many of the colonies that develop are well separated from one another. Can one then pick material from such a colony, transfer it to an appropriate medium, and call it a pure culture? Although this is often done, a culture so isolated may be far from pure. There is a significant probability that any particular colony was initiated by two similar micro-organisms seeded together on the plate to produce a mixed colony. Furthermore, because micro-organisms vary greatly in their nutritional requirements, no single medium and set of growth conditions will permit the growth of all the micro-organisms present in a natural population. Indeed, it is probable that only a very small fraction of the micro-organisms initially present will be able to form colonies on any given medium. Hence, for every visible colony on a first plate, there may be thousands of other micro-organisms that were also deposited on the agar surface but that failed to give macroscopically visible growth, although they may still be viable. The probability is high that some of these organisms will be picked up and carried over when a transfer is made. One should never pick from a first plate for the preparation of a pure culture. Instead, a second plate should be streaked from a cell suspension prepared from a well-isolated colony. If all the colonies on this second plate appear identical, a well-isolated colony can be used to establish a pure culture.

Not all micro-organisms able to grow on solid media necessarily give rise to well-isolated colonies. Certain motile flagellated bacteria (Proteus, Pseudomonas, for example) can rapidly spread over the slightly moist surface of a freshly poured plate. This can be prevented by the use of plates with well-dried surfaces, on which the cells are immobilised. Spirochetes and organisms that show gliding movement (e.g. myxobacteria, many cyanobacteria) can move over or through an agar gel, even when its surface is well dried. In such cases, the movement of the organisms in question may be an aid to their purification, since they can move away from other kinds of micro-organisms immobilised on the agar. Thus, purification can often be achieved by allowing migration to occur and transferring repeatedly to fresh plates from the advancing edge of the migrating population.

The incorporation into the medium of selectively inhibitory substances is also sometimes helpful in making isolations from nature. Because of their biological specificity, certain antibiotics are particularly useful in this respect. Bacteria vary greatly in their sensitivity to the antibiotic penicillin, which can consequently be used at low concentrations to prevent the development of sensitive bacteria in the initial population. At higher concentrations penicillin is generally toxic for procaryotic organisms but not for eucaryotic ones. It is thus a very useful agent for the purification of protozoa, fungi, and eucaryotic algae that are contaminated by bacteria. Conversely, procaryotic organisms are insensitive to polyene antibiotics such as nystatin, which are generally toxic for eucaryotic organisms. The incorporation of this kind of antibiotic into the isolation medium can sometimes be used to advantage in the purification of bacteria heavily contaminated by fungi or amebae. Many other variations on the theme of selective toxicity can be used to facilitate isolations by the plating method.

Isolation of Pure Cultures in Liquid Media

Plating methods are in general satisfactory for the isolation of bacteria and fungi because the great majority of the representatives of these groups can grow well on solid media. However, some of the larger-celled bacteria have not yet been successfully cultivated on solid media, and many protozoa and algae are also cultivable only in a liquid medium. Although plating methods for the isolation of viruses have been greatly extended in recent years, many of these organisms are most easily isolated by the use of liquid media. In the case of viruses, of course, a pure culture is never obtainable, since these organisms are obligate intracellular parasites; a two-membered culture, consisting of a specific virus and its biological host, represents the goal of purification for this microbial group.

The simplest procedure of isolation in liquid media is the dilution method. The inoculum is subjected to serial dilution in a sterile medium, and a large number of tubes of medium are inoculated with aliquots of each successive dilution. The goal of this operation is to inoculate a series of tubes with a microbial suspension so dilute that the probability of introducing even one individual into a given tube is very small: a probability of the order of 0.05. When a large number of tubes is seeded with an inoculum of this size, it can be calculated from probability theory that the fraction of tubes receiving one organism is 0.048; the fraction receiving two organisms is 0.0012; the fraction receiving three organisms is 0.00002. As a result, (a tube shows any subsequent growth, there is a very high probability that this growth has resulted from the introduction of a single organism. The probability that growth has originated from a single organism declines very rapidly as the mean number of organisms in the inoculum increases. It is, therefore, essential to isolate from a series of tubes the great majority of which show no growth.

The dilution method has, however, one major disadvantage: it can be used only to isolate the numerically predominant member of a mixed microbial population. It can almost never be effectively used for the isolation of larger micro-organisms that are incapable of developing on solid media (e.g. protozoa, algae), because in nature these micro-organisms are, as a rule, greatly outnumbered by bacteria. Hence, the usefulness of the dilution method is limited.

When neither plating nor dilution methods can be applied, the only alternative is to resort to the microscopically controlled isolation of a single-cell or organism from the mixed population, a technique known by the name of single-cell isolation. The technical difficulty of single-cell isolation is inversely related to the size of the organism which one wishes to isolate: it is relatively easy to use with large-celled micro-organisms, such as algae and protozoa, but becomes much harder with bacteria.

In the case of large micro-organisms, purification involves the capture of a single individual in a fine capillary pipette and the subsequent transfer of this individual through several washings in relatively large volumes of sterile medium to eliminate microbial contaminants of smaller size. The successive operations can be performed manually, with control by direct microscopic observation at a relatively low magnification, such as that provided by a dissecting microscope.

The technique of the capillary pipette can no longer be applied if the organism that one wishes to isolate is so small that it cannot be readily observed at a magnification of 100 times or less, because one cannot achieve the necessary fineness of control to manipulate a capillary pipette directly at higher magnifications. In this event, a mechanical device known as a micromanipulator must be used in conjunction with specially prepared, very fine glass operating instruments. The essential purpose of a micromanipulator is to gear down manual control, so that very slight and precisely controlled movements of the operating instruments can be effected in a small operating area (a microdrop) under continuous microscopic observation at high magnifications (500 to 1000 ×).

Two-Membered Cultures

The goal of isolation is normally to obtain a pure culture. However, there are certain situations where this cannot be achieved or where achievement is so difficult as to be impractical. Under such circumstances, the alternative is to obtain the next best degree of purification, in the shape of a two-membered culture, which contains only two kinds of micro-organisms. As already mentioned, a two- membered culture is in principle the only possible way to maintain viruses, since these organisms are all obligate intracellular parasites of cellular organisms. Obligate intracellular parasitism is also characteristic of several groups of cellular micro-organisms. In all these instances a two-membered culture represents the nearest approach to cultivation under controlled laboratory conditions that can be achieved.

Many of the protozoa, which feed in nature on smaller micro-organisms, are also most easily maintained in the laboratory as two-membered cultures in association with their smaller microbial prey. This is true, for example, of ciliates, amebaes and slime moulds. In such instances the association is probably never an obligate one, since careful nutritional studies on a few representatives of these groups have shown that they can be grown in pure culture; however, the nutritional requirements of protozoa are often extremely complex, so that the preparation of media for the maintenance of pure cultures is both difficult and laborious. For purposes of routine maintenance, and also for many experimental purposes, two-membered cultures are satisfactory.

The establishment of a two-membered culture is an operation that is conducted in two phases. First, it is necessary to establish a pure culture of the food organism (the host in the cases of obligate intracellular parasites, the prey in the case of protozoa). Once this has been achieved, the parasite or predator can be isolated by anyone of a variety of methods (plating on solid media in the presence of the food organism, dilution in a liquid medium, single-cell isolation) and introduced into the pure culture of the food organism.

The successful maintenance of two-membered cultures requires considerable art because a reasonably stable biological balance between the two components is essential. The medium must be one that permits sufficient growth of the food organism to meet the needs of the parasite or predator but should not be so rich that the food organism can outgrow its associate or produce metabolic products that are deleterious to it.

Construction of Culture Media

In constructing a culture medium for any micro-organism, the primary goal is to provide a balanced mixture of the required nutrients, at concentrations that will permit good growth. It might seem at first sight reasonable to make the medium as rich as possible, by providing all nutrients in great excess. However, this approach is not a wise one. In the first place, many nutrients become growth inhibitory or toxic as the concentration is raised. This is true of many organic substrates, such as salts of fatty acids (e.g. acetate) and even of sugars, if the concentration is high enough. Some inorganic constituents may also become inhibitory if provided in excess; many algae are very sensitive to the concentration of inorganic phosphate. Second, even if growth can occur in a concentrated medium, the metabolic activities of the growing microbial population will eventually change the nature of the environment to the point where it becomes highly unfavourable and the population becomes physiologically abnormal or dies. This may be brought about by a drastic change in the hydrogen ion concentration (pH), by the accumulation of toxic organic metabolites, or in the case of strict aerobes, by the depletion of oxygen. Since the usual goal of the microbiologist is to study the properties and behaviour of healthy micro-organisms, it is wise to limit the total growth of cultures by providing a limiting quantity of one nutrient; in the case of chemoheterotrophs, the principal carbon source is usually selected for this purpose. Examples of the appropriate concentrations of nutrients will be provided in the various media described below.

The rational point of departure for the preparation of media is to compound a mineral base, which provides all those nutrients that can be supplied to any organism in inorganic form. This base can then be supplemented, as required, with a carbon source, an energy source, a nitrogen source, and any required growth factors; these supplements will, of course, vary with the nutritional properties of the particular organism that one wishes to grow. A medium composed entirely of chemically defined nutrients is termed a synthetic medium. One that contains ingredients of unknown chemical composition is termed a complex medium.

Suitable chemical adjustments may be required to accommodate the osmotic conditions and hydrogen ion concentration to the needs of some micro-organisms for which these media are satisfactory with respect to their content of nutrients.

Control of pH

Although a given medium may be suitable for the initiation of growth, the subsequent development of a bacterial population may be severely limited by chemical changes that are brought about by the growth and metabolism of the organisms themselves. For example, in glucose-containing media, organic acids that may be produced as a result of fermentation may become inhibitory to growth.

In contrast, the microbial decomposition or utilisation of anionic components of a medium tends to make the medium more alkaline. For example, the oxidation of a molecule of sodium succinate liberates two sodium ions in the form of the very alkaline salt, sodium carbonate. The decomposition of proteins and amino acids may also make a medium alkaline as a result of ammonia production.

To prevent excessive changes in hydrogen ion concentration either buffers or insoluble carbonates are often added to the medium.

In some instances neither buffers nor insoluble carbonates can be used to maintain a relatively constant pH in a culture medium. Special problems arise, for example, when very large amounts of acid are formed in media in which the presence of calcium carbonate is not desired. Even more serious difficulties are encountered in controlling the pH of slightly alkaline media in which basic substances are produced as a result of bacterial growth. This is due to the fact that phosphate buffers are not effective in the pH range 7.2 to 8.5, and few suitable buffers in this range are available. In certain cases, therefore, it is necessary to adjust the pH of the culture, either periodically or continuously, by the aseptic addition of strong acids or bases. In some laboratories and in industrial plants elaborate mechanical devices are used for this purpose. With their aid, a continuous titration of the medium is feasible and the pH is kept nearly constant.

Many organisms prefer neutral or slightly acidic conditions, which can be achieved by the use of appropriate buffers.

Avoidance of mineral precipitates: chelating agents

A troublesome problem often encountered in the preparation of synthetic media is the formation of a precipitate upon sterilisation, particularly if the medium has a relatively high phosphate concentration. This results from the formation of insoluble complexes between phosphates and certain cations, particularly calcium and iron. Although it usually does not affect the nutrient value of the medium, it may make the observation or quantitation of microbial growth difficult. The problem can be avoided by sterilising separately the calcium and iron salts in concentrated solution and adding them to the sterilised and cooled medium. Alternatively, one can incorporate in the medium a small amount of a chelating agent, which will form a soluble complex with these metals and thus prevent them from forming an insoluble complex with phosphates. The chelating agent most commonly used for this purpose is ethylenediaminetetraacetic acid (EDTA), at a concentration of approximately 0.01 per cent.

Control of oxygen concentration

Oxygen is an essential nutrient for the obligately aerobic bacteria. Aerobic micro-organisms can be grown easily on the surface of agar plates and in shallow layers of liquid medium. In unshaken liquid cultures, growth usually occurs at the surface. Below the surface, however, conditions become anaerobic, and growth is impossible. To obtain large populations in liquid cultures, it is, therefore, necessary to aerate the medium. Various types of shaking machines that constantly agitate, and thus aerate, the medium are available for laboratory use. Another method of aeration is the continuous passage of a stream of sterile air through a culture. To ensure a large surface of contact between gas and liquid, the air may be introduced through a porous 'sparger', which delivers it in the form of very fine bubbles. However, even vigorous aeration is often insufficient to maintain an adequate concentration of dissolved oxygen, because the rate of O_2 utilisation by the culture may exceed the rate of its diffusion into the culture medium.

These methods all have as their goal the maintenance of O_2 concentrations at the saturation point with respect to the partial pressure of O_2 in air. Maintaining constant dissolved O_2 concentrations less than saturation requires continuous adjustment of the rate of aeration in response to the dissolved oxygen concentrations sensed by an oxygen electrode; or alternatively, that the culture be aerated with a gas mixture in which the partial pressure of O_2 is less than that of air.

Techniques for cultivation of obligate anaerobes

Many of the more sensitive, strictly anaerobic micro-organisms are rapidly killed by contact with molecular oxygen. The exposure of cultures to air should accordingly be minimised or avoided completely.

Liquid cultures of strict anaerobes are usually prepared in tubes or flasks completely filled with medium and closed by rubber stoppers or plastic screw caps. Isolation in solid media can be undertaken by several methods. Organisms able to tolerate a transient exposure to air can be isolated in shake tubes, or on streaked plates, which are placed after inoculation in sealed anaerobic jars. The atmosphere of the jars is then rendered O_2 free by evacuation and refilling with an inert gas (e.g. N_2); by chemical destruction of oxygen; or by a combination of both methods. Organisms unable to tolerate even momentary exposure to air are often isolated using roll tubes.

Although roll tubes allow the convenient isolation and subculturing of the most strict anaerobes, they are not well suited to growth of cultures for genetic or physiological study. Consequently, glove boxes containing a reducing atmosphere at slightly higher pressure than the surrounding air (to ensure that gas will not leak in through undetected holes) are being used increasingly. Within such a glove box the full range of microbiological and biochemical techniques may be performed.

Provision of carbon dioxide

A problem frequently encountered in the cultivation of photoautotrophs and chemoautotrophs is the provision of CO_2 in sufficient amounts. Although the diffusion of CO_2 from the atmosphere into the culture medium will permit growth to occur, the CO_2 concentration in the atmosphere is very low (0.03 per cent in the open atmosphere, somewhat higher inside a building), and the growth rates of autotrophs are often limited by the availability of CO_2 under these conditions. The solution is to gas the cultures with air that has been artificially enriched with CO_2 and contains from 1 to 5 per cent of this gas. The control of pH becomes a problem, for and if this solution is adopted, care must be taken to modify the buffer composition of the medium. In the case of autotrophs that can be grown under anaerobic conditions in stoppered bottles (e.g. the purple and green sulphur bacteria) the requirement for CO_2 can be met by the incorporation of $NaHCO_3$ in the medium. Soluble carbonates cannot be used in media exposed to air because the rapid loss of CO_2 to the atmosphere causes the medium to become extremely alkaline.

Provision of light

For the cultivation of phototrophic micro-organisms (algae, photosynthetic bacteria), light is a requirement. The provision of adequate illumination combined with control of temperature is not a simple matter. In the cultivation of non-photosynthetic organisms, temperature control is provided by the use of incubators, maintained by a thermostatic device at the desired value; however, most commercially available models are not designed with a system of internal illumination and cannot be used for the cultivation of phototrophic organisms.

A relatively uncontrolled and discontinuous illumination may be obtained by the exposure of cultures to daylight. Direct exposure to sunlight should be avoided, because the intensity may be too high, and the temperature may rise to a point where growth is prevented. Many phototrophic micro-organisms can tolerate continuous illumination, and their growth is much more rapid under these conditions, so artificial light sources are advantageous. The emission spectrum of the lamp employed is important. Fluorescent light sources have the practical advantage of producing relatively little heat, so maintenance of a suitable temperature is not difficult. However, their emission spectra are deficient, compared to sunlight, in the longer wavelengths of the visible spectrum and the near infrared region. They are satisfactory for the cultivation algae and cyanobacteria, which perform photosynthesis with light of wavelengths shorter than 700 nm, but provide little or no photosynthetically effective light for purple and green bacteria, which use wavelengths in the range 750 to 1000 nm. The only suitable artificial light sources for the latter photosynthetic bacteria are incandescent lamps; however, if high intensities are used, the dissipation of heat becomes a problem. The easiest solution to immerse culture vessels in a glass or plastic water bath that can be subjected to lateral illumination and maintained at the desired temperature by the circulation of water. The other solution is to construct a light cabinet with internal incandescent illumination, in which the temperature can be controlled by ventilation or refrigeration.

Selective Media

It is clear that no single medium or set of conditions will support the growth of all the different types of organisms that occur in nature. Conversely, any medium that is suitable for the growth of a specific organism is, to some extent, selective for it. In a medium inoculated with a variety of organisms, only those that can grow in it will reproduce, and all, others will be suppressed. Further, if the growth requirements of an organism are known, it is possible to devise a set of conditions that will specifically favour the development of this particular organism, thus permitting its isolation from a mixed natural population, even when the organism in question is a minor component of the total population. Micro-organisms can be selectively obtained from natural habitats (e.g. soil or water) either by direct isolation or by enrichment.

Direct isolation

If a mixed microbial population is spread over the surface of a selective medium solidified with agar (or some other gelling agent), every cell in the inoculum capable of development will grow and eventually form a colony. The spatial dispersion of the microbial population on a solid medium considerably reduces the competition for nutrients: under these circumstances, even organisms that grow relatively slowly will be able to produce colonies. Direct plating on a selective medium is the technique of choice when one wishes to isolate a considerable diversity of micro-organisms, all able to grow under the conditions of culture employed.

Enrichment

If a mixed microbial population is introduced into a liquid selective medium, there is a direct competition for nutrients among the members of developing population. Liquid enrichment media therefore tend to select the micro-organism of highest growth rate among all the members of introduced population that are able to grow under the conditions provided.

The selectivity of an enrichment culture is not determined solely by the chemical composition of the medium used. The outcome of enrichment in a given medium can be significantly modified by variation of such other factors as temperature, pH, ionic strength, illumination, aeration or source of inoculum.

Temperature selection can also be used with great effectiveness for the isolation of cyanobacteria, which closely resemble many algae in nutritional and metabolic respects. Both algae and cyanobacteria can grow in a simple mineral medium, incubated in the light at 25°C. However, development of algae can be almost wholly prevented by incubation at a temperature of 35°C, since algae in general have lower temperature maxima than cyanobacteria.

An enrichment medium that is not initially highly selective may acquire greatly increased selectivity for a particular type of micro-organism as result of chemical changes produced by this organism during its development. Thus, fermentative bacteria and yeast are typically more tolerant than other organisms of the organic end-products that they themselves produce from carbohydrates; in a carbohydrate-rich medium their development will, therefore, tend to suppress competing micrco-organisms

In the isolation of endospore-forming bacteria (genera *Bacillus* and *Clostridium*), competition from nonsporulating bacteria can be largely eliminated by a pretreatment of the inoculum. Pasteurisation of the inoculum, involving brief exposure to a high temperature (two to five minutes at 80°C) will destroy most vegetative cells, leaving the much more heat-resistant spores relatively unaffected.

Chapter 4

Introduction to Food Microbiology

INTRODUCTION

Micro-organisms have been used for centuries to modify food stuffs and fermented foods and beverages, and thus constitute a major and extremely positive role in food industry. They can be consumed as foods in themselves as in edible fungi mycoprotein and algae. They can also effect desirable transformations in a food, changing its properties in a way that is beneficial.

Historically, of course, the micro-organisms employed in these fermentation processes were adventitious. Even then, however, it was realised that the addition of a part of the previous process stream to the new batch could serve to 'kick off' the process. In some businesses, this was called 'back slopping'. We now know that what the ancients were doing was seeding the process with a hefty dose of the preferred organism(s). Only relatively recently have the relevant microbes been added in a purified and enriched form to knowingly seed fermentation processes.

The two key components of a fermentation system are the organism and its feedstock. For some products, such as wine and beer, there is a radical modification of the properties of the feedstock, rendering them more palatable (especially in the case of beer: the grain extracts prefermentation are most unpleasant in flavour; by contrast, grape juice is much more acceptable). For other products, the organism is less central, albeit still important. One thinks, for instance, of bread, where not all styles involve yeast in their production.

For products such as cheese, the end product is quite distinct from the raw materials as a result of a series of unit operations. For products such as beer, wine and vinegar, our product is actually the spent growth medium—the excreta of living organisms if one had to put it crudely. Only occasionally is the product the actual micro-organism itself—for example, the surplus yeast generated in a brewery fermentation or that generated in a 'single-cell protein' operation such as mycoprotein.

Organisms employed in food fermentations are many and diverse. The key players are lactic acid bacteria, in dairy products for instance, and yeast, in the production of alcoholic beverages and bread. Lactic acid bacteria, to illustrate, may also have a positive role to play in the production of certain types of wines and beers, but equally they represent major spoilage organisms for such products. It truly is a case of the organism being in the right niche for the product in question.

MICRO-ORGANISMS

Table 4.1 lists some of the organisms used in food fermentation. Some of the relevant fungi are unicellular, for example, Saccharomyces. However, the major class of fungi, namely the filamentous fungi with their hyphae (moulds), are of significance for a number of the foodstuffs, notably those Asian products involving solid-state fermentations, for example, sake and miso, as well as the only successful and sustained single-cell protein operation.

Table 4.1. Some micro-organisms involved in food fermentation processes.

Bacteria		Fungi	
Gram negative	Gram positive	Filamentous	Yeasts and non-filamentous fungi
Acetobacter	Arthrobacter	Aspergillus	Brettanomyces
Acinetobacter	Bacillus	Aureobasidium	Candida
Alcaligenes	Bifidobacterium	Fusarium	Cryptococcus
Escherichia	Cellulomonas	Mucor	Debaromyces
Flavobacterium	Corynebacter	Neurospora	Endomycopsis
	Lactobacillus	Penicillium	Geotrichum
Gluconobacter	Lactococcus	Rhizomucor	Hanseniaspora (Kloeckera)
Klebsiella	Leuconostoc	Rhizopus	Hansenula
Methylococcus	Micrococcus	Trichoderma	Kluyveromyces
Methylomonas	Mycoderma		Monascus
Propionibacter	Staphylococcus		Pichia
Pseudomonas	Streptococcus		Rhodotorula
Thermoanaerobium	Streptomyces		Saccharomyces
Xanthomonas			Saccharomycopsis
Zymomonas			Schizosaccharomyces
			Torulopsis
			Trichosporon
			Yarrowia
			Zygosaccharomyces

Microbial Metabolism

In order to grow, any living organism needs a supply of nutrients that will feature as, or go on to form, the building blocks from which that organism is made. These nutrients must also provide the energy that will be needed by the organism to perform the functions of accumulating and assimilating those nutrients, to facilitate moving around, etc.

The microbial kingdom comprises a huge diversity of organisms that are quite different in their nutritional demands. Some organisms (*phototrophs*) can grow using light as a source of energy and carbon dioxide as a source of carbon, the latter being the key element in organic systems. Others can get their energy solely from the oxidation of inorganic materials (*lithotrophs*).

All of the organisms considered are *chemotrophs*, insofar as their energy is obtained by the oxidation of chemical species. Furthermore, unlike the *autotrophs*, which can obtain all their carbon from carbon dioxide, the organisms that are at the heart of fermentation processes for making foodstuffs are *organotrophs* (or *heterotrophs*) in that they oxidise organic molecules, of which the most common class is the sugars.

Nutritional needs

The four elements required by organisms in the largest quantity (gram amounts) are carbon, hydrogen, oxygen and nitrogen. This is because these are the elemental constituents of the key cellular components of carbohydrates (Fig. 4.1), lipids (Fig. 4.2), proteins (Fig. 4.3) and nucleic acids (Fig. 4.4). Phosphorus and sulphur are also important in this regard. Calcium, magnesium, potassium, sodium and iron are demanded at the milligram level, while microgram amounts of copper, cobalt, zinc, manganese, molybdenum, selenium and nickel are needed. Finally, organisms need a preformed supply of any material that is essential to their well-being, but that they cannot themselves synthesise, namely vitamins (Table 4.2). Micro-organisms differ greatly in their ability to make these complex molecules. In all instances, vitamins form a part of coenzymes and prosthetic groups that are involved in the functioning of the enzymes catalysing the metabolism of the organism.

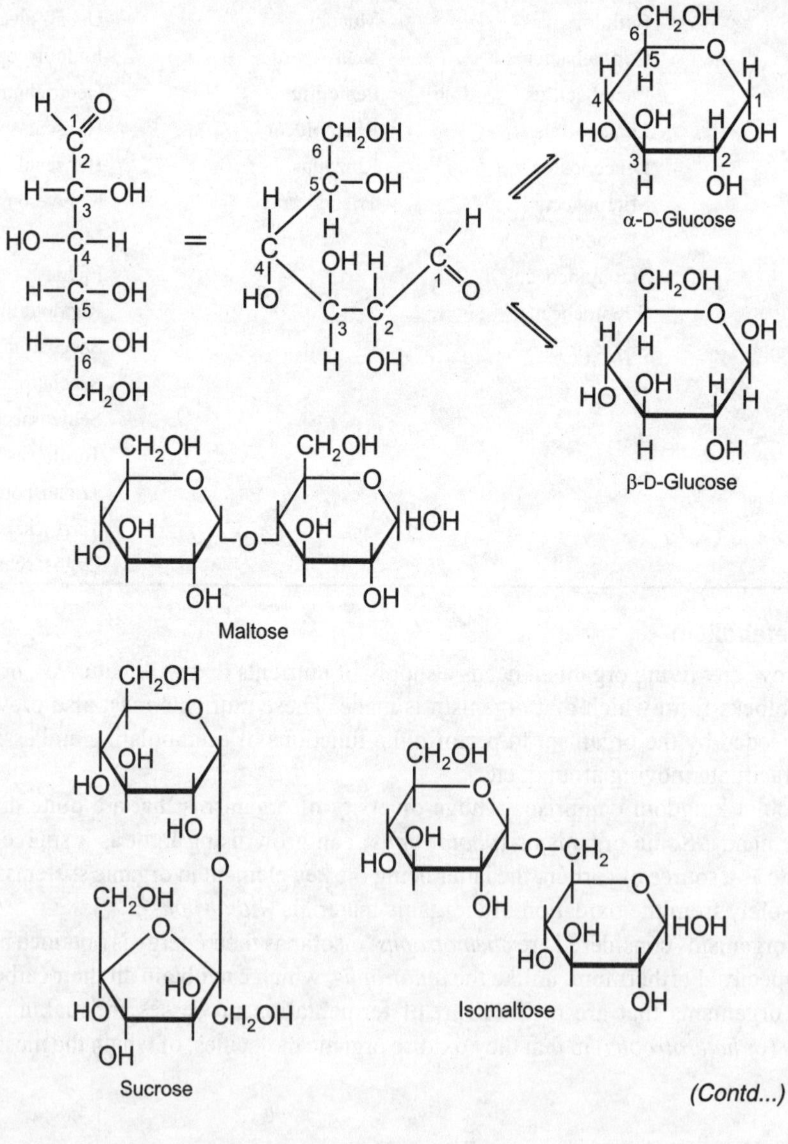

α-D-Glucose

β-D-Glucose

Maltose

Sucrose

Isomaltose

(Contd...)

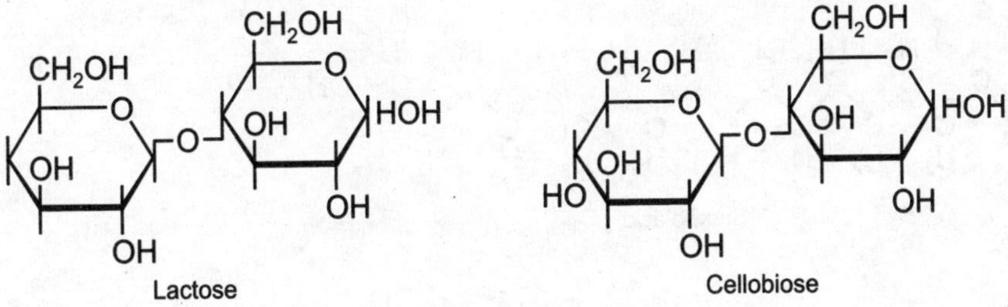

Fig. 4.1. Carbohydrate. (a) Hexoses (sugars with six carbons), such as glucose, exist in linear and cyclic forms in equilibria (top). The numbering of the carbon atoms is indicated. In the cyclic form, if the OH at C_1 is lowermost, the configuration is α. If the OH is uppermost, then the configuration is p. At C_1 in the linear form is an aldehyde grouping, which is a reducing group. Adjacent monomeric sugars (monosaccharides, in this case glucose) can link (condense) by the elimination of water to form disaccharides. Thus, maltose comprises two glucose moieties linked between C_1 and C_4, with the OH contributed by the C_1 of the first glucosyl residue being in the α configuration. Thus, the bond is $\alpha 1 \longrightarrow 4$. For isomaltose, the link is $\alpha 1 \longrightarrow 6$. For cellobiose, the link is $\beta 1 \longrightarrow 4$. Sucrose is a disaccharide in which glucose is linked $\beta 1 \longrightarrow 4$ to a different hexose sugar, fructose. Similarly, lactose is a disaccharide in which galactose (note the different conformation at its C_4) is linked $\beta 1 \longrightarrow 4$ to glucose. (b) Successive condensation of sugar units yields oligosaccharides. This is a depiction of part of the amylopectin fraction of starch, which includes chains of $\alpha 1 \longrightarrow 4$ glucosyls linked by $\alpha 1 \longrightarrow 6$ bonds. The second illustration shows that there is only one glucosyl (marked by) that retains a free C_1 reducing group, all the others (o) being bound up in glycosidic linkages.

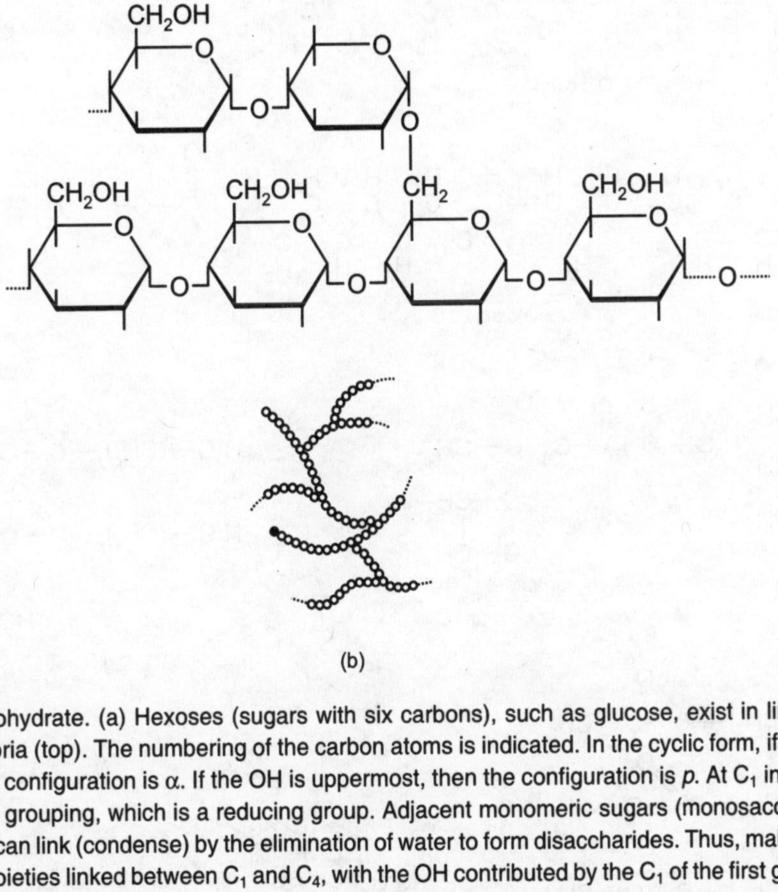

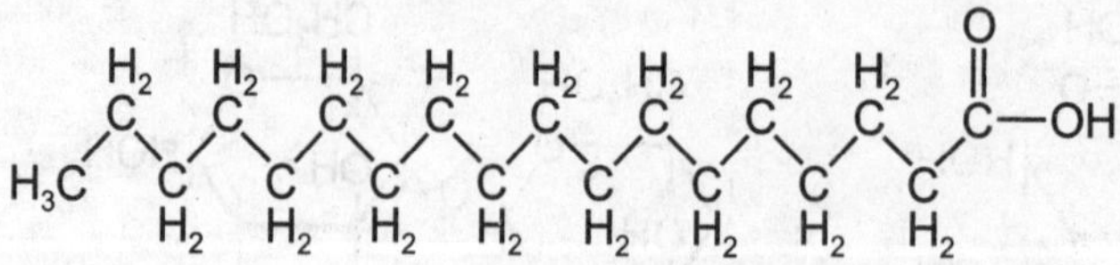

Stearic acid $C_{18:0}$

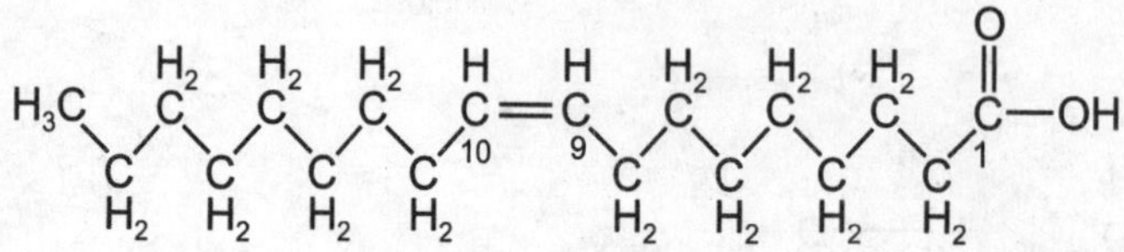

Oleic acid $C_{18:1}$

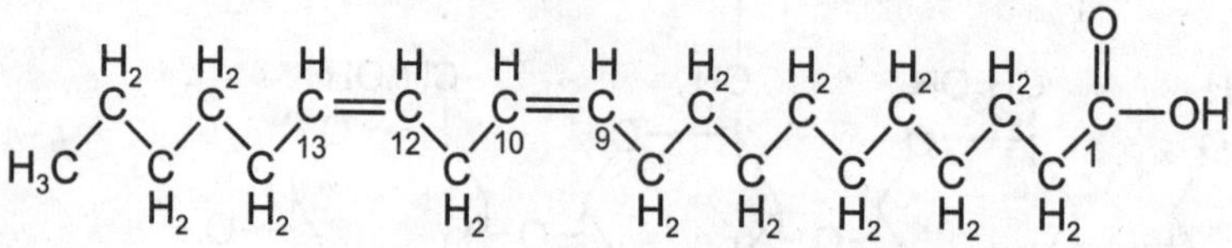

Linoleic acid $C_{18:2}$

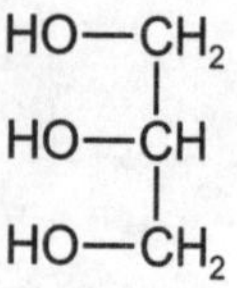

Glycerol 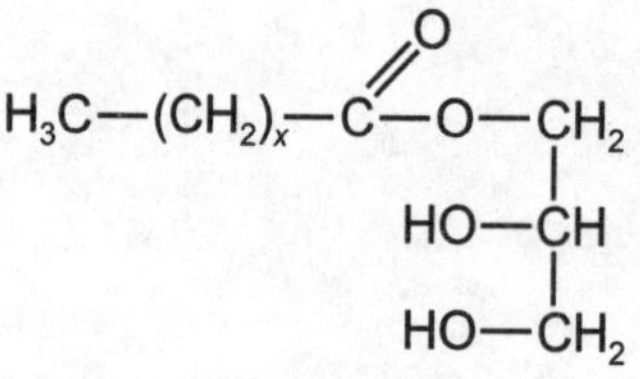   Monoglyceride

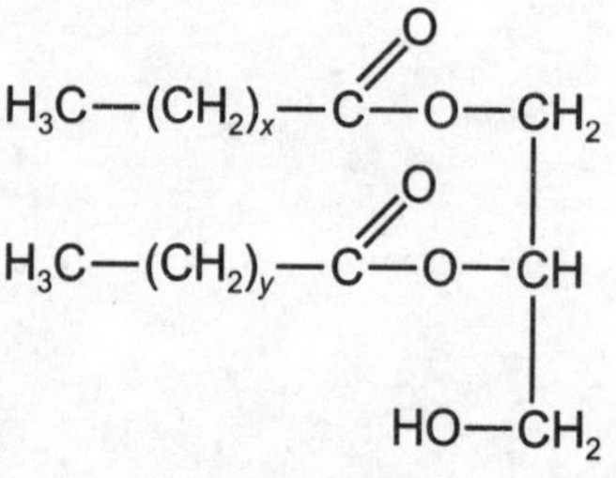

Diglyceride

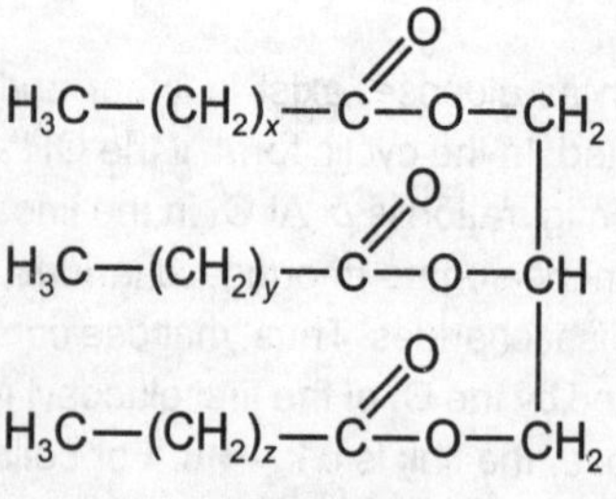

Triglyceride 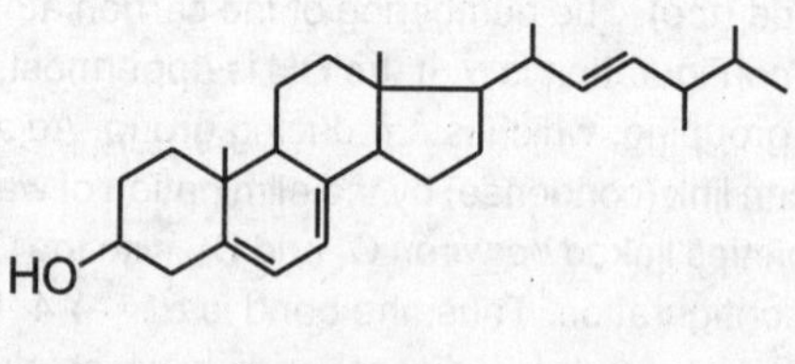   Ergosterol

Fig. 4.2. Lipids fatty acids comprise hydrophobic hydrocarbon chains varying in length, with a single polar carboxyl group at C_1. Three different fatty acids with 18 carbons (hence C_{18}) are shown. They are the 'saturated' fatty acid stearic acid (so-called because all of its carbon atoms are linked either to another carbon or to hydrogen with no double bonds) and the unsaturated fatty acids, oleic acid (one double bond, hence $C_{18:1}$) and linoleic acid (two double bonds, $C_{18:2}$). Fatty acids may be in the free form or attached through ester linkages to glycerol, as glycerides.

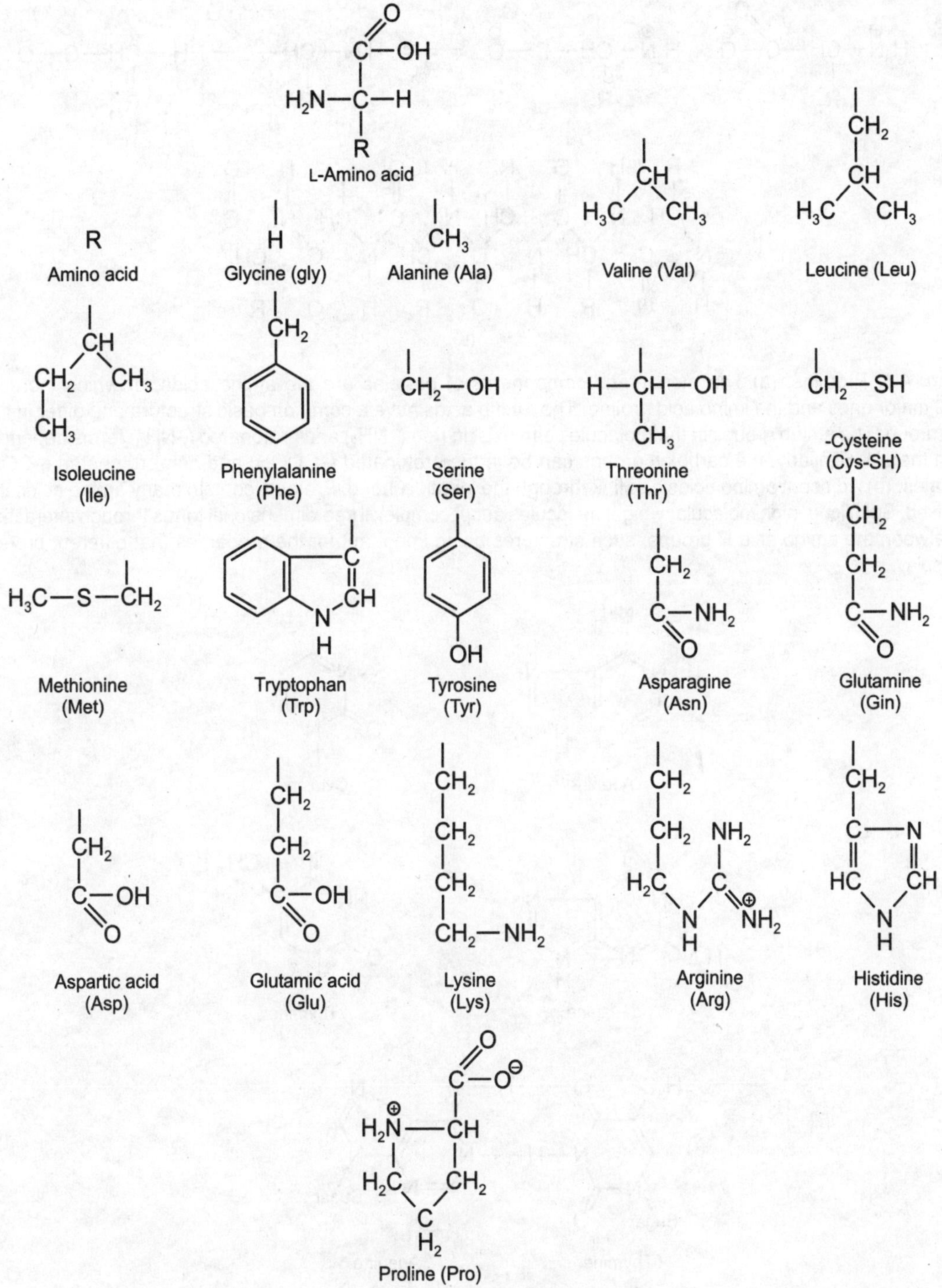

$$
\begin{array}{c}
O \\
\parallel \\
C-OH \\
| \\
H_2N-C-H \\
| \\
R
\end{array}
$$

L-Amino acid

R
Amino acid

Glycine (gly)

Alanine (Ala)

Valine (Val)

Leucine (Leu)

Isoleucine
(Ile)

Phenylalanine
(Phe)

-Serine
(Ser)

Threonine
(Thr)

-Cysteine
(Cys-SH)

Methionine
(Met)

Tryptophan
(Trp)

Tyrosine
(Tyr)

Asparagine
(Asn)

Glutamine
(Gln)

Aspartic acid
(Asp)

Glutamic acid
(Glu)

Lysine
(Lys)

Arginine
(Arg)

Histidine
(His)

Proline (Pro)

(a)

(Contd...)

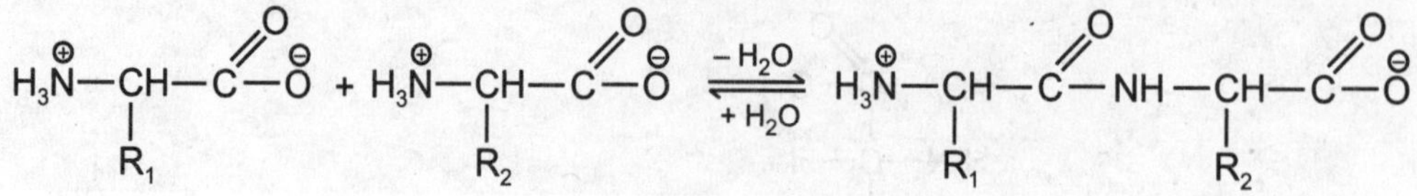

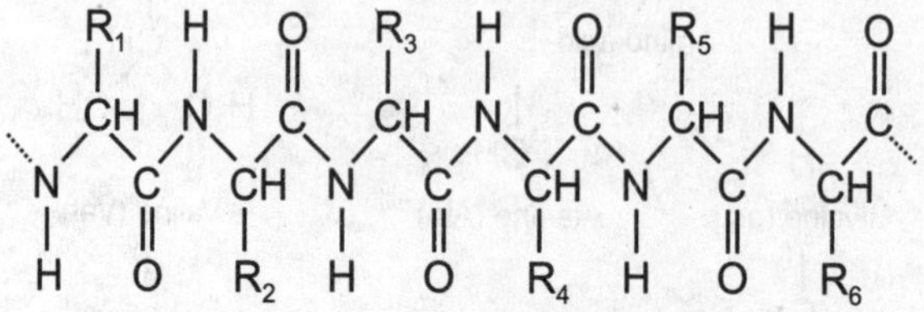

(b)

Fig. 4.3. Proteins. (a) The monomeric components of proteins are the amino acids, of which there are 19 major ones and the imino acid proline. The amino acids have a common basic structure and differ in their R group. The amino groups in the molecules can exist in free (–NH$_2$) and protonated (–NH$_3^+$) forms depending on the pH. Similarly, the carboxyl groups can be in the protonated (–COOH) and non-protonated (–COO$^-$) states. (b) Adjacent amino acids can link through the 'peptide' bond. Proteins contain many amino acids thus linked. Such long, high molecular weight molecules adopt complex three-dimensional forms through interactions between the amino acid R groups, such structures being important for the properties that different proteins display.

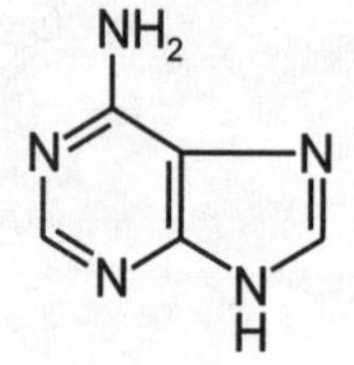

Adenine

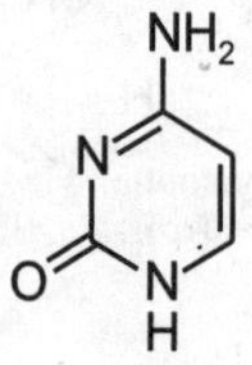

Cytosine

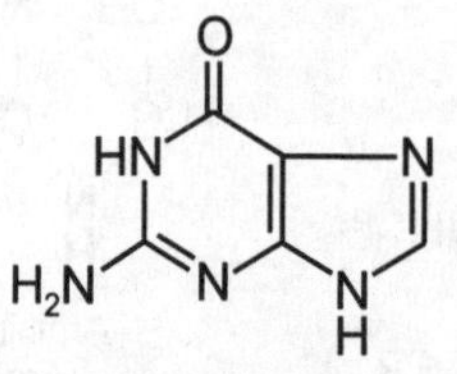

Guanine

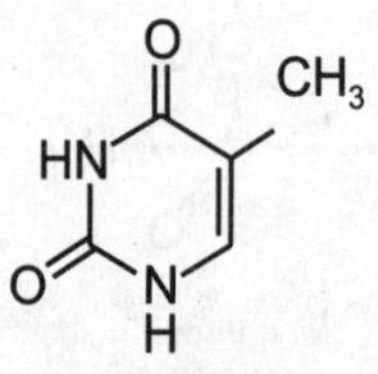

Thymine

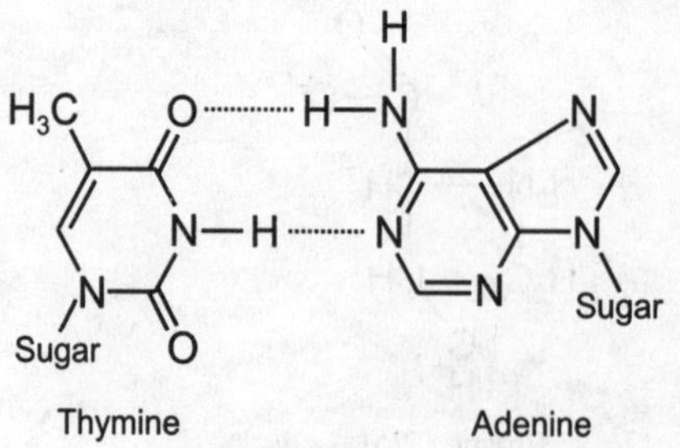

Thymine   Adenine

(Contd...)

Cytosine　　　　Guanine

(a)

(Contd...)

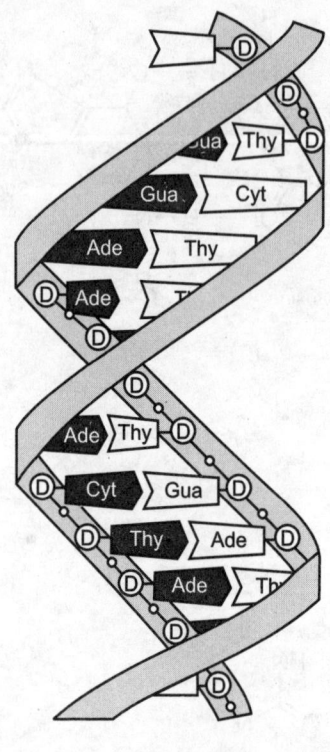

(b)

Fig. 4.4. Nucleic acids. (a) Nucleic acids comprise three building blocks: bases, pentose (sugars with five carbon atoms) and phosphate. There are four bases in DNA: the purines adenine (A) and guanine (G) and the pyrimidines thymine (T) and cytosine (C). A and T or G and C can interact through hydrogen bonds and this binding affords the linking between adjacent chains in DNA. The bases are linked to the sugar-phosphate backbone. (b) In the famous double-helix form of DNA, adjacent strands of deoxyribose (D)–phosphate (o) are linked through the bases. The sequence of bases represents the genetic code that determines the properties of any living organism. In ribonucleic acid (RNA), there is only one strand: thymine is replaced by another pyrimidine (uracil) and the sugar is ribose, whose C_2 has an –OH group rather than two H atoms.

Table 4.2. Role of vitamins in micro-organisms.

Vitamin	Coenzyme it forms part of
Thiamine (vitamin B_1)	Thiamine pyrophosphate
Riboflavin (B_2)	Flavin adenine dinucleotide, flavin mononucleotide
Niacin	Nicotinamide adenine dinucleotide
Pyridoxine (B_6)	Pyridoxal phosphate
Pantothenate	Coenzyme A
Biotin	Prosthetic group in carboxylases
Folate	Tetrahydrofolate
Cobalamin (B_{12})	Cobamides

As the skeleton of all the major cellular molecules (other than water) comprises carbon atoms, there is a major demand for carbon. Hydrogen and oxygen originate from substrates such as sugars, but of course also come from water.

The oxygen molecule, O_2, is essential for organisms growing by aerobic respiration. Although fermentation is a term that has been most widely applied to an anaerobic process in which organisms do not use molecular oxygen in respiration, even those organisms that perform metabolism in this way generally do require a source of this element. To illustrate, a little oxygen is introduced into a brewer's fermentation so that the yeast can use it in reactions that are involved in the synthesis of the unsaturated fatty acids and sterols that are essential for it to have healthy membranes. Aerobic metabolism, too, is necessary for the production of some of the foodstuffs, for example, in the production of vinegar. All growth media for micro-organisms must incorporate a source of nitrogen, typically at $1-2$ g l^{-1}. Most cells are about 15 per cent protein by weight, and nitrogen is a fundamental component of protein (and nucleic acids).

As well as being physically present in the growth medium, it is equally essential that the nutrient should be capable of entering into the cell. This transport is frequently the rate-limiting step. Few nutrients enter the cell by passive diffusion and those that do tend to be lipid-soluble. Passive diffusion is not an efficient strategy for a cell to employ as it is very concentration-dependent. The rate and extent of transfer depend on the relative concentrations of the substance inside and outside the cell. For this reason, facilitated transportation is a major mechanism for transporting materials (especially water-soluble ones) into the cell, with proteins known as permeases selectively and specifically catalysing the movement. These permeases are only synthesised as and when the cell requires them. In some instances, energy is expended in driving a substance into the cell if a thermodynamic hurdle has to be overcome, for example, a higher concentration of the molecule inside than outside. This is known as 'active transport'.

An additional challenge is encountered with high molecular weight nutrients. Whereas some organisms, for example, the protozoa, can assimilate these materials by engulfing them (*phagocytosis*), micro-organisms secrete extracellular enzymes to hydrolyse the macromolecule outside the organism, with the resultant lower molecular weight products then being assimilated. These extracellular enzymes are nowadays produced commercially in fermentation processes that involve subsequent recovery of the spent growth medium containing the enzyme and various degrees of ensuing purification. A list of such enzymes and their current applications is given in Table 4.3.

Table 4.3. Exogenous enzymes.

Enzyme	Major sources	Application in foods
α-Amylase	Aspergillus, Bacillus	Syrup production, baking, brewing
β-Amylase	Bacillus, Streptomyces, Rhizopus	Production of high maltose syrups, brewing
Glucoamylase	Aspergillus, Rhizopus	Production of glucose syrups, baking, brewing, wine making
Glucose isomerase	Arthrobacter, Streptomyces	Production of high fructose syrups
Pullulanase	Klebsiella, Bacillus	Starch (amylopectin) degradation
Invertase	Kluyveromyces, Saccharomyces	Production of invert sugar, production of soft-centred chocolates

(Contd...)

Enzyme	Major sources	Application in foods
Glucose oxidase (coupled with catalase)	Aspergillus, Penicillium	Removal of oxygen in various foodstuffs
Pectinase	Aspergillus, Penicillium	Fruit juice and wine production, coffee bean fermentation
β-Glucanases	Bacillus, Penicillium, Trichoderma	Browing fruit juices, olive processing
Pentosanases	Cryptococcus, Trichosporon	Baking, brewing
proteinases	Aspergillus, Bacillus, Rhizomucor, Lactococcus, recombinant Kluyveromyces, Papaya	Baking, brewing, meat tenderisation, cheese
Catalase	Micrococcus, Corynebacterium, Aspergillus	Cheese (see also glucose oxidase above)
Lipases	Aspergillus, Bacillus, Rhizopus, Rhodotorula	Dairy and meat products
Urease	Lactobacillus	Wine
Tannase	Aspergillus	Brewing
β-Galactosidase	Aspergillus, Bacillus, Escherichia, Kluyveromyces	Removal of lactose
Acetolactate decarboxylase	Thermoanaerobium	Accelerated maturation of beer

Environmental impacts

A range of physical, chemical and physico-chemical parameters impact the growth of micro-organisms, of which we may consider temperature, pH, water activity, oxygen, radiation, pressure and 'static' agents.

Temperature

The rate of a chemical reaction was shown by Svante Arrhenius to increase two to three-fold for every 10°C rise in temperature. However, cellular macromolecules, especially the enzymes, are prone to denaturation by heat, and this accordingly limits the temperatures that can be tolerated. Although there are organisms that can thrive at relatively high temperatures (*thermophiles*), most of the organisms discussed here do not fall into that class. Neither do they tend to be *psychrophiles*, which are organisms capable of growth at very low temperatures. They have a minimum temperature at which growth can occur, below which the lipids in the membranes are insufficiently fluid. It should be noted that many organisms can survive (if not grow) at lower temperatures and advantage is taken of this in the storage of pure cultures of defined organisms (discussed later). Organisms which prefer the less-extreme temperature brackets, say 10°–40°C, are referred to as *mesophiles*.

pH

Most organisms have a relatively narrow range of pH within which they grow best. This tends to be lower for fungi than it is for bacteria. The optimum pH of the medium reflects the best compromise position in respect of:

1. The impact on the surface charge of the cells (and the influence that this has on behaviours such as flocculation and adhesion.
2. On the ability of the cells to maintain a desirable intracellular pH and, in concert with this, the charge status of macromolecules (notably the enzymes) and the impact that this has on their ability to perform.

Water activity

The majority of microbes comprise between 70 per cent and 80 per cent water. Maintaining this level is a challenge when an organism is exposed variously to environments that contain too little water (dehydrating or hypertonic locales) or excess water (hypotonic).

The water that is available to an organism is quantifiable by the concept of water activity (A_w). Water activity is defined as the ratio of the vapour pressure of water in the solution surrounding the micro-organism to the vapour pressure of pure water. Thus, pure water itself has an A_w of 1 while an absolutely dry, water-free entity would have an A_w of 0. Micro-organisms differ greatly in the extent to which they will tolerate changes in A_w. Most bacteria will not grow below A_w of 0.9, so drying is a valuable means for protecting against spoilage by these organisms. By contrast, many of the fungi that can spoil grain ($A_w = 0.7$) can grow at relatively low moisture levels and are said to be *xerotolerant*. Truly *osmotolerant* organisms will grow at an A_w of 0.6.

Oxygen

Microbes differ substantially in their requirements for oxygen. *Obligate aerobes* must have oxygen as the terminal electron acceptor for aerobic growth (Fig. 4.5). *Facultative anaerobes* can use oxygen as terminal electron acceptor, but they can function in its absence. Microaerophiles need relatively small proportions of oxygen in order to perform certain cellula activities, but the oxygen exposure should not exceed 2–10 per cent v/v (cf. the atmospheric level of 21 per cent v/v). *Aerotolerant anaerobes* do not use molecular oxygen in their metabolism but are tolerant of it. *Obligate anaerobes* are killed by oxygen.

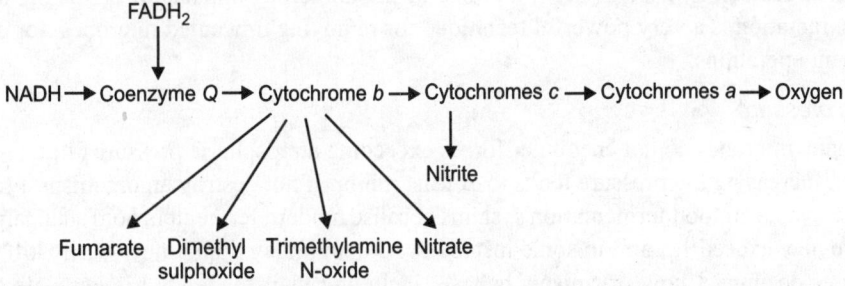

Fig. 4.5. Electron transport chains. Reducing power captured as NADH or FADH₂ is transferred successively through a range of carriers until ultimately reducing a terminal electron acceptor. In aerobic organisms, this acceptor is oxygen, but other acceptors found in many microbial systems are illustrated. This can impact parameters such as food flavour—for example, reduction of trimethylamine N-oxide affords trimethylamine (fishy flavour) while reduction of dimethyl sulphoxide (DMSO) yields dimethyl sulphide (DMS), which is important in the flavour of many foodstuffs.

Clearly these differences have an impact on the susceptibility of foodstuffs to spoilage. Most foods when sealed are (or rapidly become) relatively anaerobic, thus obviating the risk from the first three categories of organism.

Irrespective of which class an organism falls into, oxygen is still a potentially damaging molecule when it becomes partially reduced and converted into radical forms (Fig. 4.6). Organisms that can tolerate oxygen have developed a range of enzymes that scavenge radicals, amongst them superoxide dismutase, catalase and glutathione peroxidase.

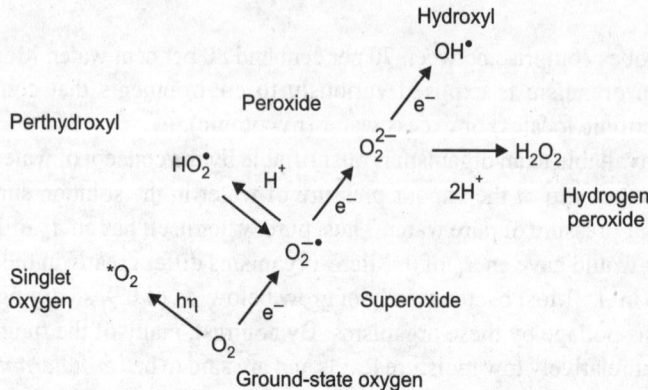

Fig. 4.6. Activation of oxygen. Ground-state oxygen is relatively unreactive. By acquiring electrons, it become successively more reactive—superoxide, peroxide, hydroxyl. Superoxide exists in charged and protonated forms, the latter (perhydroxyl) being the more reactive. Exposure to light converts oxygen to another reactive form, singlet oxygen.

Radiation

One of the radical forms of oxygen, singlet oxygen, is produced by exposure to visible light. An even more damaging segment of the radiation spectrum is the ultraviolet light, exposure to which can lead to damage of DNA. Ionising radiation, such as gamma rays, causes the production of an especially reactive oxygen derived radical, hydroxyl (OH·), and one of the numerous impacts of this is the breakage of DNA. Thus, radiation is a very powerful technique for removing unwanted microbes, for example, in food treatment operations.

Hydrostatic pressure

In nature, many microbes do not encounter forces exceeding atmospheric pressure (1 atm = 101.3 kPa = 1.013 bar). Increasing the pressure tends to at least inhibit if not destroy an organism. Pressure is of increasing relevance in food fermentation systems because modern fermenters hold such large volumes that pressure may exceed 1.5 atm in some instances. Although they do not necessarily kill organisms, high pressures do impact how organisms behave, including their tendency to aggregate and certain elements of their metabolism. The latter is at least in part due to the accumulation of carbon dioxide that occurs when pressure is increased.

Controlling or inhibiting growth of micro-organisms

It is important to regulate those organisms that are present during the making of fermentation products and also those that are able to grow and survive in the finished product. On the one hand, we have nowadays the deliberate seeding of the desired organism(s), which therefore gain a selective advantage in outgrowing other organisms. Conversely, there are physical or chemical '-cidal' treatments or sterilisation procedures that are employed to achieve the depletion or total kill of organisms.

Relevant factors are:

1. How many organisms are present.
2. The types of organism that are present.
3. The concentration of antimicrobial agents that are present or the intensity of the physical treatment.

4. The prevailing conditions of temperature, pH and viscosity.
5. The period of exposure.
6. The concentration of organic matter.

Fermentation by itself comprises a procedure that originally emerged as a means for preserving the nutritive value of foodstuffs. Through fermentation there was either the lowering of levels of substances that contaminating organisms would need to support their growth or the development of materials or conditions that would prevent organisms from developing, for example, a lowering of pH. In the case of a product like beer, there is the deliberate introduction of antiseptic agents, in this case, the bitter acids from hops.

Heating

Moist heat is used for sterilising a greater diversity of materials than dry heat. Moist heat employs steam under pressure and is very effective for the sterilisation of production vessels and pipe work. Dry heat is less efficient and requires a higher temperature (e.g. 160°C as opposed to 120°C); it is used in systems like glassware and for moisture-sensitive materials.

The microbial content of finished food products is frequently lowered by heat treatment. Ultra-high temperature (UHT) treatments are used where especially high kills are necessary. Pasteurisation is a milder process, one in which the temperature and the time of exposure are regulated to achieve a sufficient kill of spoilage organisms without deleteriously impacting the other properties of the foodstuff. In batch pasteurisation, filled containers (e.g. bottles of beer) are held at, say, 62°C for 10 minutes in chambers through which the product slowly passes on a conveyor (tunnel pasteurisation). In flash pasteurisation, the liquid is heated as it flows through heat exchangers en route to the packaging operation. Residence times are much shorter so temperatures are higher (e.g. 72°C for 15 secs). In the specific example of beer, this might be the way in which beer destined for kegs is processed. One pasteurisation unit (PU) is defined as exposure to 60°C for 1 minute. As the temperature is increased, the shorter exposure time equates to 1 PU. The more organisms, the more extensive is the heat treatment, so the onus is on the operator to minimise the populations by good hygienic practice.

Cooling

The ability of organisms to grow is curtailed as the temperature is lowered (refrigeration, freezing).

Drying

As organisms usually require significant amounts of water (discussed earlier), drying affords preservation. Thus, for example, starting materials for fermentation (such as grains and fruits) may be subjected to some degree of drying if they are to be stored successfully prior to use. The other way in which water activity can be lowered is by adding solutes such as salt or sugar.

Irradiation

The use of irradiation to eliminate spoilage organisms is charged with emotion. Critics hit on the tendency of the technique to reduce the food value, for example, by damaging vitamins. However, the procedure really should be considered on a case-by-case basis, and only if there is some definite negative impact on the quality of a product should it necessarily be avoided. Thus, to take beer as our example again, there is evidence for the increased production of hydrogen sulphide when beer is irradiated.

Filtration

Undesirable organisms can be removed by physically filtering them from the product. Depth filters operate by trapping and adsorbing the cells in a fibrous or granular matrix. Membrane filters possess defined pore sizes through which organisms of greater dimensions cannot pass. Typically these pore sizes may be 0.45 μm or, for especially rigorous 'clean-up', 0.2 μm. Practical systems may employ successive filters—for example, a depth filter followed by membranes of different sizes. The approach may be most valuable for heat-sensitive products.

Chemical agents

Modern food production facilities are designed so that they are readily cleanable between production runs by chemical treatment regimes, often called 'cleaning in place' or CIP. This demands fabrication with resilient material, for example, stainless steel, as well as design that ensures that the agent reaches all nooks and crannies. CIP protocols generally involve an initial water rinse to remove loose soil, followed by a 'detergent' wash. This is not so much a detergent proper as sodium hydroxide or nitric acid and it is targeted at tougher adhering materials. Next is another water rinse to eliminate the detergent, followed by a sterilant. Various chemical sterilants are available, the most commonly used being chlorine, chlorine dioxide and peracetic acid.

Some foodstuffs are formulated so that they contain preservatives (Table 4.4). In other foodstuffs there are natural antimicrobial compounds present, for example, polyphenols and the hop iso-α-acids in beer. And, of course, the end products of some fermentations are historically the basis of protection for fermented foodstuffs, for example, low pH, organic acids, alcohol, carbon dioxide. Of especial interest here is nisin (Fig. 4.7) that is a natural product from lactic acid bacteria, capable of countering the invasion of other bacteria.

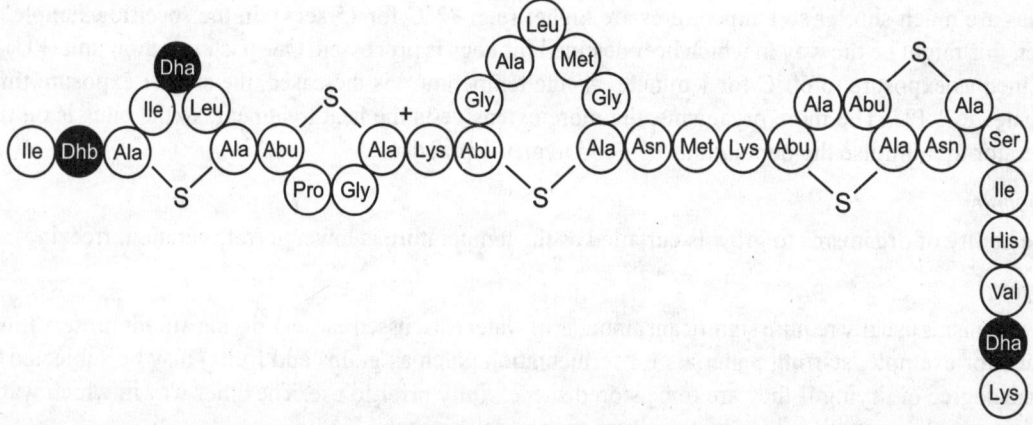

Fig. 4.7. Nisin. This antimicrobial destroy Gram-positive organisms by making pores in their membranes. It includes some unusual amino acids, including dehydrated serine (Dha), dehydrated threonine (Dhb), lanthionine (Ala–S–Ala) and β-methyllanthionine (Abu–S–Ala). The last two originate from the coupling of cysteine with dehydrated serine or threonine, respectively.

An essential aspect of the long-term success of lactic acid bacteria as a protective agent within the fermentation industries is the multiplicity of ways in which it counters the growth of competing organisms. Apart from nisin and other bacteriocins, we might draw attention to the production of:

1. Organic acids, such as lactic, acetic and propionic acids, with acetic acid being especially valuable in countering bacteria, yeasts and moulds.

2. Hydrogen peroxide, which, as we have seen is an activated (and therefore potentially damaging) derivative of oxygen.

3. Diacetyl and acetaldehyde, although some argue that the levels developed are not of practical significance as antimicrobial agents.

Table 4.4. Food grade antimicrobial agents.

Preservative
Acetic acid and its sodium, potassium and calcium salts
Benzoic acid and its sodium, potassium and calcium salts
Biphenyl
Formic acid and its sodium and calcium salts
Hydrogen peroxide
p-Hydroxybenzoate, ethyl, methyl and propyl variants and their sodium salts
Lactic acid
Nisin
Nitrate and nitrite, and its sodium and potassium salts
o-Phenylphenol
Propionic acid and its sodium, potassium and calcium salts
Sorbic acid and its sodium, potassium and calcium salts
Sulphur dioxide, sodium and potassium sulphites, sodium and potassium bisulphites, sodium and potassium metabisulphites (disulphites)
Thiabendazole

Metabolic events

Catabolism

Catabolism refers to the metabolic events whereby a foodstuff is broken down so as to extract energy in the form of adenosine triphosphate (ATP), as well as reducing power (customarily generated primarily in the form of nicotinamide adenine dinucleotide (NADH, reduced form) but utilised as nicotinamide adenine dinucleotide phosphate (NADPH, reduced form) to fuel the reactions (anabolism) wherein cellular constituents are fabricated (Fig. 4.8).

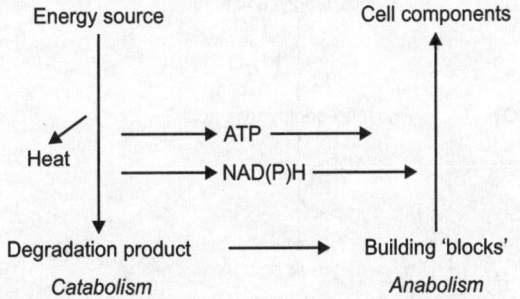

Fig. 4.8. Energy sources (e.g. sugars) are successively broken down in catabolic reactions, resulting in the capture of energy in the form of ATP and reducing power (as reduced NADH). Building blocks are transformed into the polymers from which cells are comprised (Figs 4.1 to 4.4) in anabolic reactions that draw on energy (ATP) and reducing power (many of the anabolic processes use the phosphorylated form of NADH, i.e. NADPH).

In focusing on the organotrophs, and in turn even more narrowly (for the most part) on those that use sugars as the main source of carbon and energy, we must first consider the Embden–Meyerhof–Parnas (EMP) pathway (Fig. 4.9).

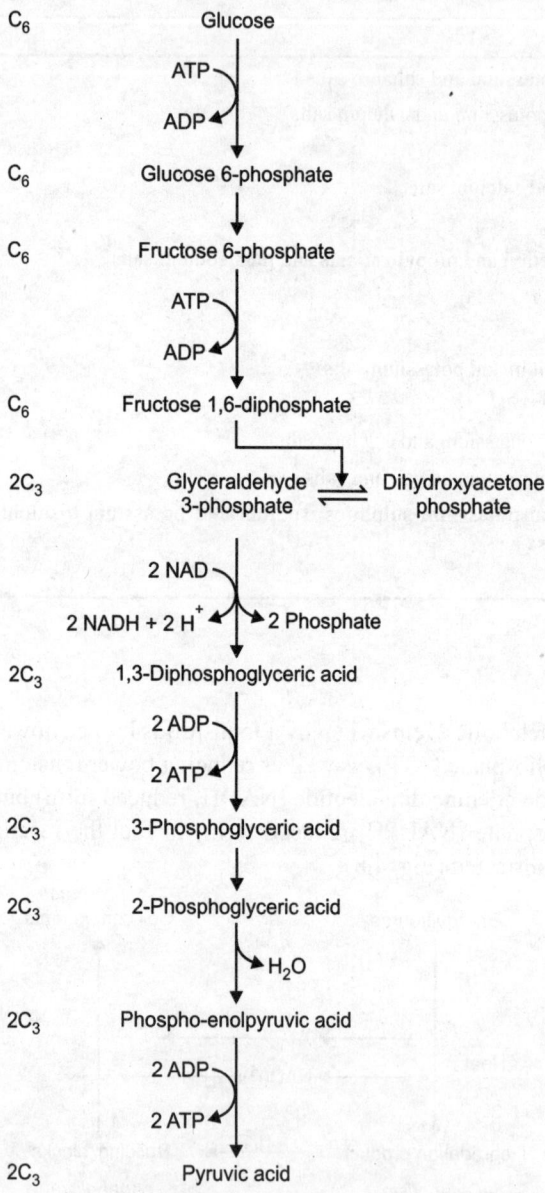

Fig. 4.9. The EMP pathway.

This is the most common route by which sugars are converted into a key component of cellular metabolism, pyruvic acid. This pathway, for example, is central to the route by which alcoholic fermentations are performed by yeast. In this pathway, the sugar is 'activated' to a more reactive phosphorylated state by the addition of two phosphates from ATP. There follows a splitting of the diphosphate to two three-carbon units that are in equilibrium. It is the glyceraldehyde 3-phosphate that is metabolised further, but as it is used up, the equilibrium is strained and dihydroxyacetone phosphate is converted to it. Hence we are in reality dealing with two identical units proceeding from the fructose diphosphate. The first step is oxidation, the reducing equivalents (electrons, hydrogen) being captured by NAD. En route to pyruvate are two stages at which ATP is produced by the splitting off of phosphate this is called *substrate-level phosphorylation*. As there are two three-carbon (C_3) fragments moving down the pathway, this therefore means that four ATPs are being produced per sugar molecule. As two ATPs were consumed in activating the sugar, there is a net ATP gain of two.

Anabolism

The above-named pathways are examples of how cells deal with sugars, thereby obtaining carbon, hydrogen and oxygen. As observed earlier, cells must also secure a supply of other elements from the medium. Nitrogen may be provided as amino acids (e.g. in the case of brewing yeast), urea or inorganic nitrogen forms, primarily as ammonium salts (often used in wine fermentations).

Sulphur can variously be supplied in organic or inorganic forms. Brewing yeast, for example, can assimilate sulphate, but will also take up sulphur-containing amino acids (Fig. 4.10).

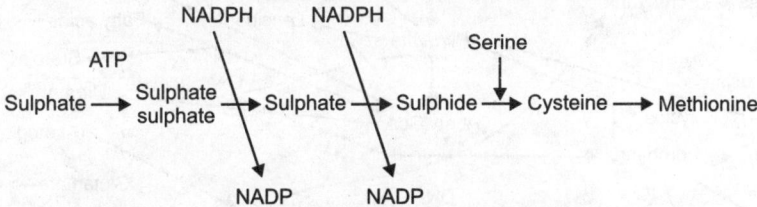

Fig. 4.10. The assimilation of sulphur.

The major structural and functional molecules in cells are polymeric and include the following:

1. Polysaccharides—notably the storage molecules such as glycogen in yeast, which has a structure closely similar to the amylopectin fraction of starch (see later), and the structural components of cell walls, for example, the mannans and glucans in yeast and the complex polysaccharides in bacterial cell walls.
2. Proteins—notably the enzymes and the permeases.
3. Lipids—notably the components at the heart of membrane structure.
4. Nucleic acids—DNA and RNA.

A greatly simplified summary of cellular metabolism, incorporating the essential features of anabolic reactions is given in Fig. 4.11. It is sufficient in the present discussion to state that pyruvate is at the heart of the metabolic pathways. There are clearly various draws on it, both catabolic and anabolic. Of particular note is the draw off from the tricarboxylic acid cycle to satisfy biosynthetic needs, meaning that there is a failure to regenerate the oxaloacetate needed to collect a new acetyl-CoA residue emerging from pyruvate. Thus, cells have so-called anaplerotic pathways by which they can replenish necessary intermediates such as oxaloacetate. The best-known such pathway is the glyoxylate cycle (Fig. 4.12).

It is essential that the multiplicity of reactions, which as a whole constitute cellular metabolism, are controlled so that the whole is in balance to achieve the appropriate needs of the cell under the prevailing conditions within which it finds itself. It is outside the scope of this chapter to dwell on these regulatory mechanisms, but they include coarse controls on the synthesis of the necessary permeases and enzymes (the general rule being that a protein is only synthesised as and when it is needed) and fine controls on the rate at which the enzymes are able to act. Examples of the impact of these control strategies will be encountered in this chapter, for example, whether brewing yeast degrades sugars by respiration or fermentation.

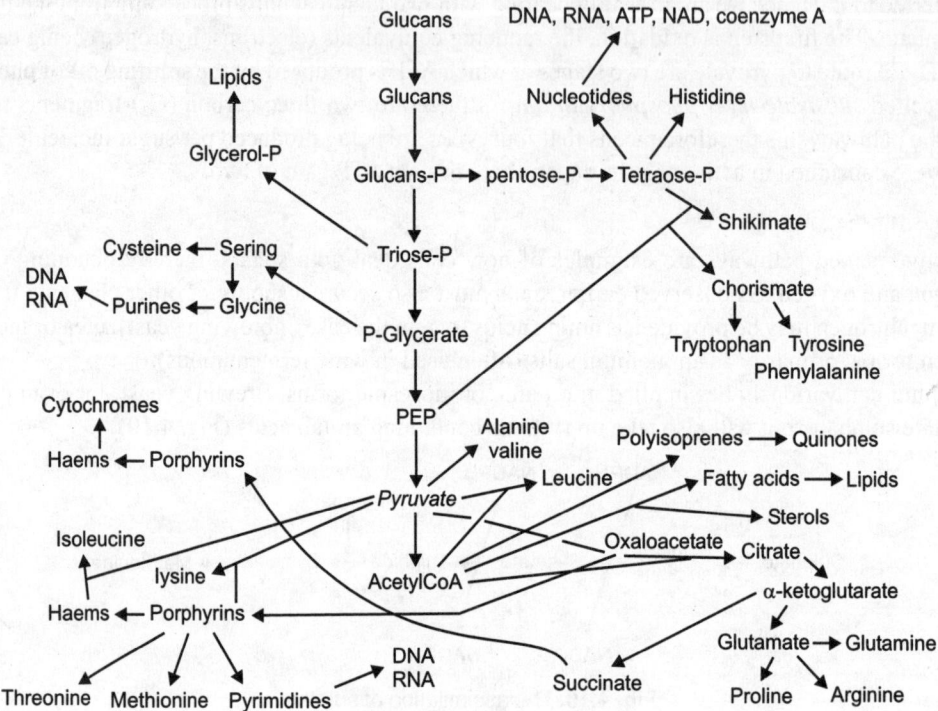

Fig. 4.11. A simplified overview of intermediary metabolism.

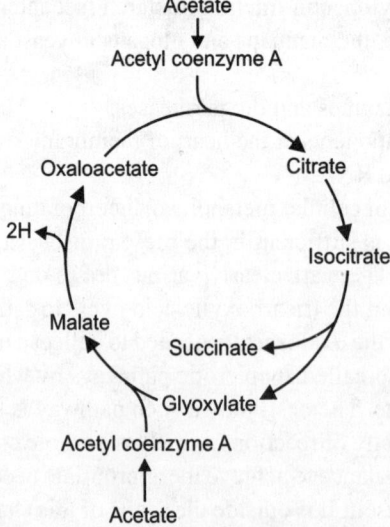

Fig. 4.12. The glyoxylate cycle.

Origins of the organisms employed in food fermentations

For the longest time, the foodstuffs described in this chapter were prepared using endogenous microflora. Increasingly, however, and starting first with the isolation of pure strains of brewing yeast by Emil Christian Hansen in 1883, many of the products employ starter cultures in their production. The organisms conform to the criterion of being Generally Recognised as Safe (GRAS). They are selected for their advantageous properties in terms of process performance and impact on final product quality.

Many companies and academic laboratories are seeking newer, improved cultures. This can be achieved in what may be called 'serendipity mode' by screening a broad swathe of samples taken from multitudinous habitats, the screening employing growth media and cultivation conditions that are best suited to an organism with the desired characteristics. Alternatively, some narrowing of odds can be achieved by specifically looking in locales where certain types of organisms are known to thrive—for example, yeasts are plentiful on the surface of fruit. One extreme example of this approach might most reasonably be described as 'theft', with the pure culture of one company finding its way, through whatever mechanism, into the clutches of another corporation.

A more honest approach is by purchasing samples of pure organisms of the desired character from culture collection. Nowadays the cultures are likely to be in the form of vials frozen in liquid nitrogen (–196°C) or they may be lyophilised. For some industries, notably bread making and wine making, companies do not produce their own yeast but rather bring it into the production facility on a regular basis from a supplier company. This might be supplied frozen or merely refrigerated with cryoprotectants such as sucrose, glycerol or trehalose. The latest technology here is active dried yeast, with the organism cultured optimally to ensure its ability to survive drying in a state that will allow it to perform vigorously and representatively when rehydrated. In other industries, notably beer brewing, companies tend to maintain their own strains of yeast and propagate these themselves. This is probably on account of the fact that beer-making is essentially the only industry described in this chapter where the surplus organism that grows in the process is reused.

There are various opportunities for enhancing the properties of the organisms that are already employed in food companies. Mutagenesis to eliminate undesirable traits has been employed. However, this is a challenge for eukaryotes as such cells tend to have multiple copies of each gene (polyploidy), and it is a formidable challenge to eliminate all the alleles of the undesirable gene. Classic recombination techniques (conjugation, transduction and transformation) have been pursued, but there is always the risk that an undesirable trait will be introduced as an accompaniment to the trait of interest. Much more selectivity is afforded by modern genetic modification strategies. However, as noted earlier, this attracts far more emotion for organisms used in food production than it does in the production of, say, fuels or pharmaceuticals.

Some of the Major Micro-organisms

The organisms that one encounters most widely in these processes are undoubtedly the yeasts, notably Saccharomyces, and lactic acid bacteria. It is important to note in passing that if these organisms 'stray' from where they are supposed to be, then they are spoilage organisms with a ruinous nature. For example, lactic acid bacteria have a multiplicity of values in the production of many foodstuffs, including cheese, sourdough bread, some wines and a very few beers. However, their development in the majority of beers is very much the primary source of spoilage.

Yeast

In most instances, use of the word yeast in a food context is synonymous with *S. cerevisiae*, namely, brewer's yeast or baker's yeast. However, as we shall discover, there are other yeasts involved in fermentation processes.

Yeasts are heterotrophic organisms whose natural habitats are the surfaces of plant tissues, including flowers and fruit. They are mostly obligate aerobes, although some (such as brewing yeast) are facultative anaerobes. They are fairly simple in their nutritional demands, requiring a reduced carbon source, various minerals and a supply of nitrogen and vitamins. Ammonium salts are readily used, but equally a range of organic nitrogen compounds, notably the amino acids and urea, can be used. The key vitamin requirements are biotin, pantothenic acid and thiamine.

Focusing on brewing yeast, and following the most recent taxonomic findings, the term *S. cerevisiae* is properly applied only to ale yeasts. Lager yeasts are properly termed *Saccharomyces pastorianus*, representing as they do organisms with a 50 per cent larger genome and tracing their pedigree to a coupling of *S. cerevisiae* with *Saccharomyces bayanus*.

Saccharomyces is spherical or ellipsoidal. Whereas laboratory strains are haploid (one copy of each of the 16 linear chromosomes), industrial strains are polyploid (i.e. they have multiple copies of each chromosome) or aneuploid (varying numbers of each chromosome). Some 6000 genes have been identified in yeast and indeed the entire genome has now been sequenced.

Brewing yeast does have a sex life, but reproduces in production conditions primarily by budding. A single cell may bud up to 20 times, each time leaving a scar, the counting of which indicating how senile the cell has become.

The surface of the wall surrounding the yeast cell is negatively charged due to the presence of phosphate groups attached to the mannan polysaccharides that are located in the wall. This impacts the extent to which adjacent cells can interact, and the presence of calcium ions serves to bridge cells through ionic bonding. Coupled with other interactions between lectins in the surface, there are varying degrees of association between different strains, resulting in differing extents of flocculation, advantage of which is taken in the separation of cells from the liquid at the end of fermentation.

The underlying plasma membrane (as well as the other membranes in the cellular organelles) is comprised primarily of sterols (notably ergosterol), unsaturated fatty acids and proteins, notably the permeases (discussed earlier) (Fig. 4.13). As oxygen is needed for the desaturation reactions involved in the synthesis of the lipids, relatively small quantities of oxygen must be supplied to the yeast, even when it is growing anaerobically by fermentation.

The control mechanisms that drive the mode of metabolism in the yeast cell (i.e. by aerobic respiration or by fermentation) are based on the concentration of sugar that the yeast is exposed to. At high concentrations of sugar, the cell is switched into the fermentative mode, and the pyruvate is metabolised via acetaldehyde to ethanol. At low sugar concentrations, the pyruvate shunts into acetyl-CoA and the respiratory chain. This is the so-called Crabtree effect. The rationale is that when sugar concentrations are high, the cell does not need to generate as many ATP molecules per sugar molecule, whereas if the sugar supply is limited, the yeast must maximise the efficiency with which it utilises that sugar (ATP yield via fermentation and respiration are 2 molecules and 32 molecules, respectively). The significance of this in commercial fermentation processes is clear. In brewing, where the primary requirement is a high yield of alcohol, the sugar content in the feedstock (wort) is high, whereas in the production of baker's yeast, where the requirement is a high cell yield, the sugar concentration is always kept low, but the sugar is continuously passed into the fermenter (fed batch).

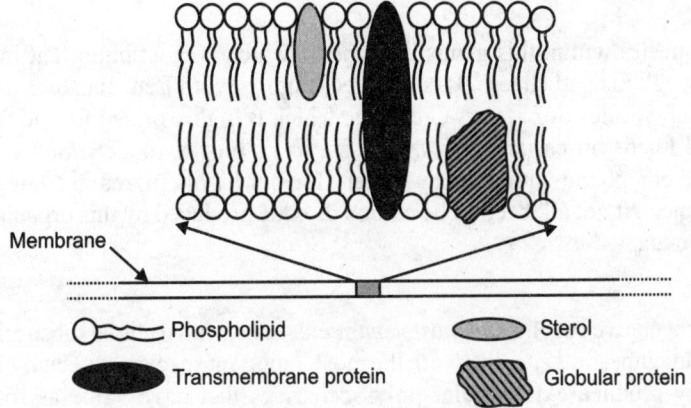

Membrane

○⌇⌇ Phospholipid   Sterol

▬ Transmembrane protein   Globular protein

Fig. 4.13. Membrane structure.

Lactic acid bacteria

Throughout the centuries it has been the practice in various fermentation based processes to add back a proportion of the previously produced food to the new batch, so-called back slopping. What of course this did was to seed the fermentation with the preferred micro-organism, and for many foodstuffs this organism is a lactic acid bacterium. Such bacteria are only weakly proteolytic and lipolytic, which means that they are quite 'mild' with respect to their tendency to produce pungent flavours. They are also naturally present in the intestine and the reproductive tract, so it is no surprise that nowadays we talk of probiotics and prebiotics in the context of enriching the level of lactic acid bacteria in the gut. Probiotics are organisms, notably lactobacilli and bifidobacteria, which are added to the diet to boost the flora in the large intestine. For example, they are added to yoghurt. Prebiotics are nutrients that boost the growth of these organisms.

Like the brewing and baking yeasts, lactic acid bacteria tend to be GRAS, although some strains are pathogenic. Joseph Lister isolated the first lactic acid bacterium. This organism that we now refer to as *Lactococcus lactis* is a species of great significance in the fermentation of milk products.

There are 16 genera of lactic acid bacteria, some 12 of which are active in a food context. They are Gram-positive organisms, are either rod-shaped, cocci (spherical) or coccobacilli. For the most part they are mesophilic, but some can grow at refrigerator temperatures (4°C) and as high as 45°C. Generally they prefer a pH in the range 4.0–4.5, but certain strains can tolerate and grow at pHs above 9.0 or as low as 3.2. They need preformed purines, pyrimidines, amino acids and B vitamins. Lactic acid bacteria do not possess a functional tricarboxylic acid cycle or haem-linked electron transport systems, so they use substrate level phosphorylation to gain their energy.

As we saw previously, their metabolism can be classified as either homofermentative, where lactic acid represents 95 per cent of the total end products, or heterofermentative, in which acetic acid, ethanol and carbon dioxide are produced alongside lactic acid.

Lactic acid bacteria produce antimicrobial substances known as bacteriocins. For the most part, these are cationic amphipathic peptides that insert into the membranes of closely related bacteria, causing pore formation, leakage and an inability to sustain metabolism, ergo death. The best known of these agents is nisin (discussed earlier), which has been used substantially as a 'natural' antimicrobial agent. Lactic acid bacteria also produce acids and hydrogen peroxide as antimicrobials.

Lactococcus

The most notable species within this genus is *L. lactis*, which is most important in the production of foodstuffs such as yoghurts and cheese. It is often co-cultured with Leuconostoc.

There are two sub-species of *L. lactis* Cremoris, which is highly prized for the flavour it affords to certain cheese, and Lactis, in particular *L. lactis* ssp. *lactis* biovar, *diacetyllactis*, which can convert citrate to diacetyl, a compound with a strong buttery flavour highly prized in some dairy products but definitely taboo in most, if not all, beers. The carbon dioxide produced by this organism is important for eye formation in Gouda.

Leuconostoc

These are heterofermentative cocci. *Leuconostoc mesenteroides*, with its three subspecies: mesenteroides, cremoris and dextranicum, and *Leuc. lactis* are the most important species, especially in the fermentation of vegetables. They produce extracellular polysaccharides that have value as food thickeners and stabilisers. These organisms also contribute to the CO_2 production in Gouda. *Oenococcus oeni* (formerly *Leuc. oenos*) plays an important role in malolactic fermentations in wine.

Streptococcus

These are mostly pathogens; however, *Streptococcus thermophilus* is a food organism, featuring alongside *Lactobacillus delbrueckii* ssp. *bulgaricus* in the production of yoghurt. Furthermore, it is used in starter cultures for certain cheeses, notably Parmesan.

Lactobacillus

There are some 60 species of such rod-shaped bacteria that inhabit the mucous membranes of the human, ergo the oral cavity, the intestines and the vagina. However, they are equally plentiful in foodstuffs, such as plants, meats and milk products.

Lb. delbrueckii ssp. *bulgaricus* is a key starter organism for yoghurts and some cheeses. However, lactobacilli have involvement in other fermentations, such as sourdough and fermented sausages, for example, salami. Conversely, they can spoil beer and either fresh or cooked meats, etc.

Pediococci

Pediococcus halophilus (now *Tetragenococcus*) is extremely tolerant of salt (>18 per cent) and as such is important in the production of soya sauce. *Pediococci* also function in the fermentation of vegetables, meat and fish. On the other hand, *Pediococcus damnosus* growth results in ropiness in beer and the production of diacetyl as an off-flavour.

Enterococcus

These faecal organisms have been isolated from various indigenous fermented foods; however, no positive contribution has been unequivocally demonstrated and their presence is debatably indicative of poor hygiene.

Providing the Growth Medium for the Organisms

The microflora is of course one of the two key inputs to food fermentation. The other is the substrate that the organism(s) converts. With the possible exception of mycoproteins, the substrates that we encounter in this chapter are very traditional and well-defined insofar as the end product is what it is as much because of that substrate as through the action of the microbe that deals with it. Thus, for beers, the final product, whether it is an ale, lager or stout, a wheat beer or a lambic has clear characteristics that are afforded by the raw materials (malt, adjunct and hops) used to make the wort that the yeast ferments. The same applies for the cereal used to make bread, the milk going to cheese and yoghurt, the meat destined for salami, the cabbage en route to sauerkraut.

In all instances there are defined preparatory steps that must be undertaken to render the substrate in the state that is ready for the microbial fermentative activity. For some foodstuffs (e.g. yoghurt), there is relatively little processing of the milk. However, for a product like beer, there is prolonged initial processing, notably the malting of grain and its subsequent extraction in the brewery.

The growth substrate must always include sources of carbon, nitrogen, water and, usually, oxygen, as well as the trace elements. These nutritional considerations have already been discussed.

Fermenters

Most food fermentations are generally classified as being 'non-aseptic' to distinguish them from microbial processes where rigorous hygiene must be ensured, for example, production of antibiotics and vaccines. This is not to say that those practising food fermentations are less than hygienic.

A diversity of fermenter types is employed ranging from the relatively sophisticated cylindroconical vessels in modern brewery operations through to the relatively crude set-ups used in some of the indigenous fermentation operations, not the least the fermentation of cocoa. Key issues in all instances are the ability to maintain the required degree of cleanliness, the ability to mix, the ability to regulate temperature and change temperature smoothly and efficiently, the access of oxygen (aeration or oxygenation) and the ability to monitor and control.

Downstream Processing

For many of the foodstuffs that we address, some form of post-fermentation clarification is necessary to remove surplus microbial cells and various other types of insoluble particles. Cells may be harvested by sedimentation (perhaps encouraged by agents such as isinglass or egg white), centrifugation or filtration. Additionally, there may be other downstream treatments, such as the adsorption of materials that might (if not removed) fall out of solution and ruin the appearance of a product, for example, polyphenols and proteins in beer. Many products have their microbial populations depleted either by pasteurisation or filtration through depth and/or membrane filters. Finally, of course, they receive varying degrees of primary and secondary packaging.

Some General Issues for a Number of Foodstuffs

Non-enzymatic browning

These are chemical reactions that lead to a brown colour when food is heated. The relevant chemistry is known as the Maillard reaction, which actually comprises a sequence of reactions that occurs when reducing sugars are heated with compounds that contain a free amino group, for example, amino acids, proteins and amines (Fig. 4.14, Table 4.5). In reflection of the complexity of the chemistry, there are many reaction intermediates and products. As well as colour, Maillard reaction products have an impact on flavour and may act as antioxidants. These antioxidants are mostly produced at higher pHs and when the ratio of amino acid to sugar is high. It must also be stressed that some of the Maillard reaction products can promote oxidative reactions. Other Maillard-type reactions occur between amino compounds and substances other than sugars that have a free carbonyl group. These include ascorbic acid and molecules produced during the oxidation of lipids.

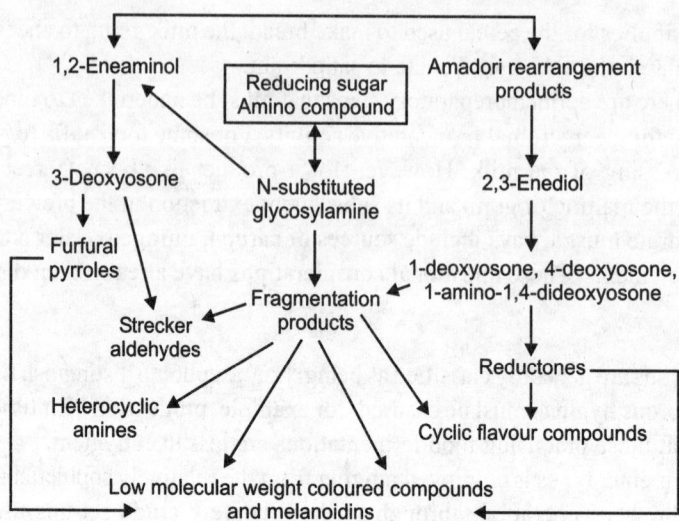

Fig. 4.14. The Maillard reaction.

Table 4.5. Some products of the Maillard reaction.

Type of compound	Example	Flavour descriptors
Products derived from interactions of sugars and amino acids		
Pyrolle	2-Acetyl-1-pyrroline	Newly baked crust of wheat bread
Pyridine	2-Acetyl-1,4,5,6-tetrahydropyridine	Cream crackers
Pyrazine	Methylpyrazine	Nut
Oxazole	Trimethyloxazole	Green, nutty, sweet
Thiophene	2-Acetylthiphene	Onion, mustard
Products derived from the sugar		
Furan	Furaneol	Caramel, strawberry
Carbonyl	Diacetyl	Butterscotch
Products derived from the amino acid		
Cyclic polysulphur	5-Methyl-5-pentyl-1,2,4-trithiolane	Fried chicken
Sulphur-container	Methional	Mashed potato
Thiazole	2-Acetylthiazole	Popcorn

The maillard reaction should not be confused with caramelisation, which is the discolouration of sugars as a result of heating in the absence of amino compounds.

In the primary Maillard reaction, the amino compound reacts with the reducing sugar to form an N-substituted glycosylamine that rearranges to 1-amino-1-deoxy-2-ketose (the so-called Amadori rearrangement product). This goes forward in a cascade of reactions in various ways depending on the pH. At the pH of most foods (4–6), the primary route involves melanoidin formation by further reaction with amino acids. Other products are Strecker aldehydes, pyrazines, pyrolles and furfurals. The substances produced in these reactions have flavours that are typical of roasted coffee and nuts, bread and cereals. The pyrolle derivatives afford bitter tastes. The Maillard reaction may also lead to aged or cooked characters in products such as processed orange juice and dried milk products.

The early products in the Maillard reaction are colourless, but when they get progressively larger, they become coloured and responsible for the hue of a wide range of foods. Some of these coloured compounds have low molecular weights, but others are much larger and may include complexes produced by heat-induced reactions of the smaller compounds and proteins.

The exact events in any Maillard-based process depend on the proportion of the various precursors, the temperature, pH, water activity and time available. Metals, oxygen and inhibitors such as sulphite also impact. The flavour developed differs depending on the time and intensity of heating for instance — high temperature for a short time gives a different result when compared with low temperature for a long time. Pentose sugars react faster than do hexoses, which in turn react more rapidly than disaccharides such as maltose and lactose. With regard to the amino compounds, lysine and glycine are much more reactive than is cysteine, for instance, but more than that, for the flavour also depends on the amino acid. Cysteine affords meaty character; methionine gives potato, while proline gives bready.

As water is produced in the Maillard reaction, it occurs less readily in foods where the water activity is high. The Maillard reaction is especially favoured at A_w 0.5–0.8. Finally sulphite, by combining with reducing sugars and other carbonyl compounds, inhibits the reaction.

Enzymatic browning

This arises by the oxidation of polyphenols to o-quinones by enzymes such as polyphenol oxidase (PPO) and peroxidase (Fig. 4.15). A day-to-day example would be the browning of sliced apple. In other foods, the reaction is wanted, for example, in the readying of prunes, dates and tea for the marketplace.

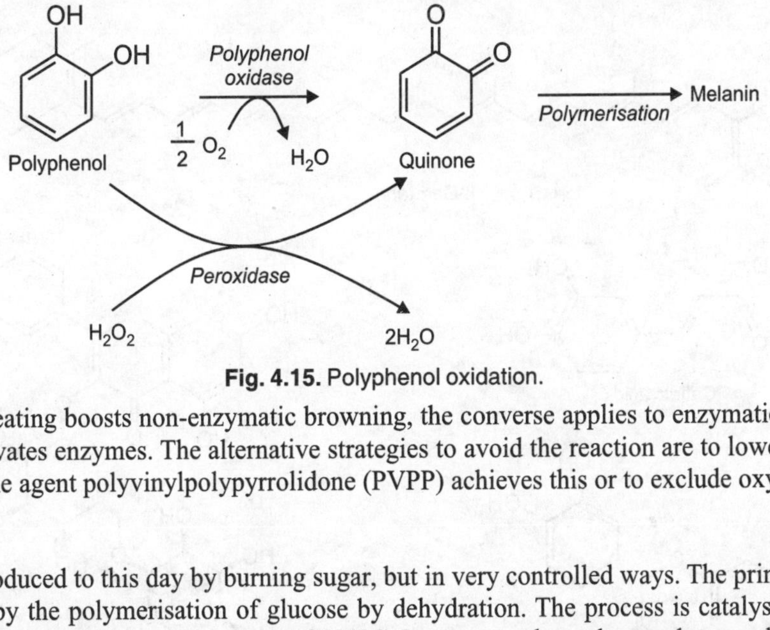

Fig. 4.15. Polyphenol oxidation.

Whereas heating boosts non-enzymatic browning, the converse applies to enzymatic browning, as the heat inactivates enzymes. The alternative strategies to avoid the reaction are to lower the levels of polyphenols the agent polyvinylpolypyrrolidone (PVPP) achieves this or to exclude oxygen.

Caramel

This is still produced to this day by burning sugar, but in very controlled ways. The principal products are produced by the polymerisation of glucose by dehydration. The process is catalysed by acids or bases and requires temperatures in excess of 120°C. In some markets, the word caramel is retained for materials that are produced in the absence of nitrogen-containing compounds and these products are used for flavouring value. Where N is present, then 'sugar colours' are produced and these are used for colouring purposes. Caramel is polymeric in nature, but also contains several volatile and nonvolatile lower molecular weight components that afford the characteristic flavour compounds, such as maltol and isomaltol (Fig. 4.16).

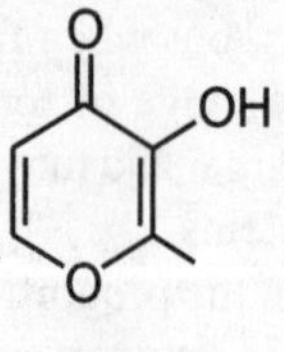

Maltol 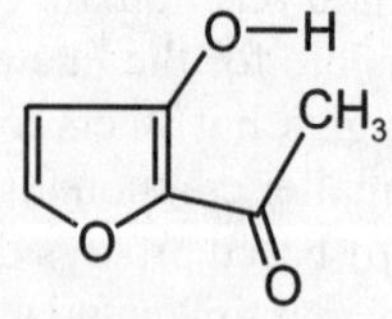   Isomaltol

Fig. 4.16. Some flavour compounds produced in caramelisation reactions.

Antioxidants

There is much interest in antioxidants from the perspective of protecting foodstuffs from flavour decay, but increasingly for their potential value in countering afflictions such as cancer, rheumatoid arthritis and inflammatory bowel diseases. Figure 4.17 presents a range of these antioxidants. Many are phenolics and act either by scavenging or by neutralising (reduction) the radicals that effect deterioration or by chelating the metal ions that cause the production of these radicals.

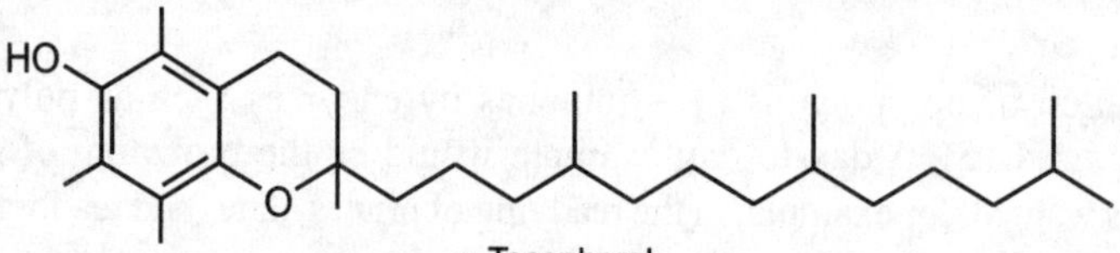

α-Tocopherol

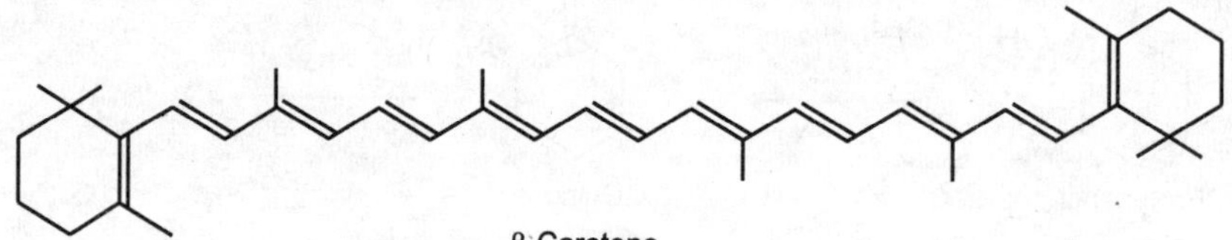

β-Carotene

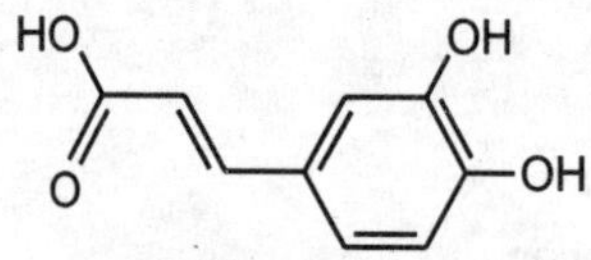

Caffeic acid

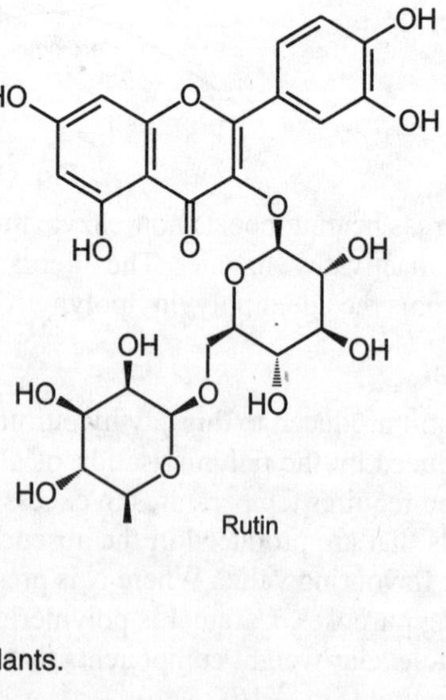

Rutin

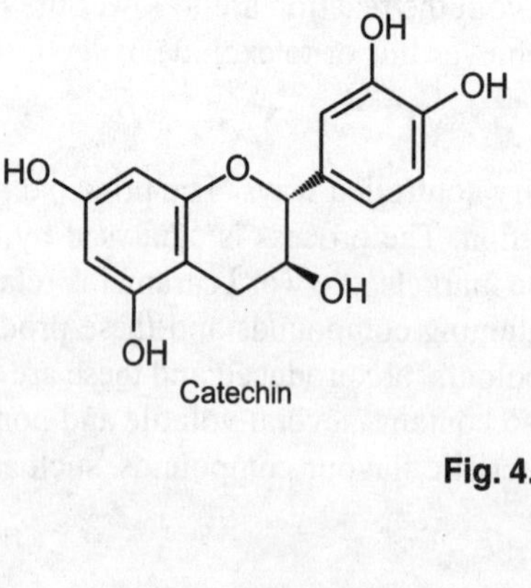

Catechin

Fig. 4.17. Some antioxidants.

The tocopherols are fat soluble and are found in vegetable oils and the fatty regions of cereals, for example, the germ. The carotenoids (e.g. lycopene) are water soluble and are found in fruits and vegetables. The flavonoids are water-soluble polyphenols found in fruits, vegetables, leaves and flowers. Such molecules have particular significance for some of the products discussed in various chapters of the book notably wine, beer and tea. The phenolic acids, for example, caffeic and ferulic acids and their esters, are abundant in cereal grains such as wheat and barley.

Chapter 5

Chemical Changes Caused by Micro-organisms

INTRODUCTION

A product is fit for food if a discriminating consumer, knowing the story of its production and seeing the material itself, will eat it, and, conversely the same product is spoiled when such an examiner refuses it as food. According to this definition, the fitness of the food will depend on the person judging it, for what one person will eat another will not. The buried fish, titmuck, eaten by the Eskimos is a malodorous, semiliquid product that most of us would consider inedible. Starving people might eat food they would not consume under normal conditions.

Despite differences between individuals in their judgement of fitness of food, they would agree on certain criteria for assurance of fitness:

1. The desired stage of development or maturity: Fruits should be at a certain but differing stage of ripeness; sweet corn should be young enough to be tender and milky; poultry preferably is from birds that are fairly young.

2. Freedom from pollution at any stage in production or handling: Vegetables should not be consumed raw if they had been fertilised with sewage; oysters from waters contaminated with sewage should be rejected; food handled by dirty or diseased workers should be spurned; food contaminated by flies or rodents should be suspected.

3. Freedom from objectionable change resulting from microbial attack or action of enzyme of the food: Sometimes it is difficult to draw a line between spoilage by micro-organisms and harmless growth; or the same type of change may be considered undesirable in one food and desirable in another. Thus the homemaker says that sour milk has spoiled, but the cultured buttermilk made by a lactic acid fermentation is good. Putrefaction in meat means definite spoilage, but putrefactive changes in Limburger cheese are normal to the ripening process. Some changes termed spoilage may be only changes in appearance or physical characteristics, as in wilted lettuce or flabby carrots, although the product probably has undergone no microbial spoilage and there has been little loss in nutritive value. Yet each one of us has his or her own idea about whether a food is spoiled and usually can come to a decision about its edibility without much difficulty.

CAUSES OF SPOILAGE

Decay or decomposition of an undesirable nature usually is implied when the term 'spoiled' is applied to food, while food unfit to eat for sanitary reasons usually is not called spoiled.

Spoilage may be due to one or more of the following:

1. Growth and activity of micro-organisms (or higher forms occasionally). Often a succession of organisms is involved.
2. Insects.
3. Action of the enzymes of the plant or animal food.
4. Purely chemical reactions, i.e. those not catalysed by enzymes of the tissues or of micro-organisms.
5. Physical changes, such as those caused by freezing, burning, drying, pressure, etc.

The discussion to follow will be devoted chiefly to spoilage caused by micro-organisms.

CLASSIFICATION OF FOODS BY EASE OF SPOILAGE

On the basis of ease of spoilage, foods can be placed in three groups:

1. Stable or nonperishable foods: These foods, which do not spoil unless handled carelessly, include such products as sugar, flour and dry beans.
2. Semiperishable foods: If these foods are properly handled and stored, they will remain unspoiled for a fairly long period, e.g. potatoes, some varieties of apples, waxed rutabagas and nutmeats.
3. Perishable foods: This group includes most important daily foods that spoil readily unless special preservative methods are used. Meats, fish, poultry, most fruits and vegetables, eggs and milk belong in this classification.

Most foods fall into one of these three groups, but some are near enough to the borderline to be difficult to place.

FACTORS AFFECTING KINDS AND NUMBERS OF MICRO-ORGANISMS IN FOOD

The kind of spoilage of foods by micro-organisms and enzymes will depend on the kinds and numbers of these agents present and on the environment about them. Most raw foods contain a variety of bacteria, yeasts, and moulds and may contain plant or animal enzymes as the case may be. Because of the particular environmental conditions, only a small proportion of the kinds of micro-organisms present will be able to grow rapidly and cause spoilage — usually a single kind of organism but sometimes two or three types — and these may not have been predominant in the original food. If spoilage by the first organism or organisms is allowed to proceed, one or more other kinds of organisms are likely to produce secondary spoilage, or a further succession of organisms and changes may be involved.

The kinds and numbers of micro-organisms that will be present on or in food will be influenced by the kind and extent of contamination, previous opportunities for the growth of certain kinds, and pretreatments which the food has received.

Contamination may increase numbers of micro-organisms in the food and may even introduce new kinds. Thus wash water may incorporate surface-taint bacteria in butter; plant equipment may add spoilage organisms to foods during processing; washing machines may add them to eggs; and dirty boats may add them to fish. The increased 'bioburden' of micro-organisms, especially those which cause spoilage, makes preservation more difficult, i.e. spoilage is more likely and more rapid and perhaps takes a different form from that which would have appeared without the contamination.

Growth of micro-organisms in or on the food obviously will increase numbers or the bioburden of micro-organisms and presumably in most foods will bring about the greatest increase in the organisms most likely to be involved in spoilage. The heavier bioburden will add to the difficulty of preventing spoilage of the food and may influence the kind of spoilage to be anticipated.

Pretreatments of foods may remove or destroy some kinds of micro-organisms, add organisms, or change the proportions of those present or inactivate part or all of the food enzymes and thus limit the number of spoilage agents and hence the possible types of spoilage. Washing, for example, may remove organisms from the surface or may add some from the wash water. If washing is by means of an antiseptic or germicidal solution, numbers of organisms may be greatly reduced and some kinds may be eliminated. Treatment with rays, ozone, sulphur dioxide, or germicidal vapours will reduce numbers and be selective of kinds. High temperatures will kill more and more organisms and leave fewer and fewer kinds as the heat treatment is increased. Storage under various conditions may either increase or decrease kinds and numbers. Any of these methods, as well as other treatments not mentioned, will influence the numbers, kinds, proportions, and health of the micro-organisms.

FACTORS AFFECTING THE GROWTH OF MICRO-ORGANISMS IN FOOD

Associative Growth

Associations of micro-organisms with each other are involved in spoilage or fermentations of most kinds of food. Competition between the different kinds of bacteria, yeasts, and moulds in a food ordinarily determines which one will outgrow the others and cause its characteristic type of spoilage. If conditions are favourable for all, bacteria usually grow faster than yeasts, and yeasts faster than moulds. Therefore, yeasts outgrow bacteria only when they are predominant in the first place or when conditions are such as to slow the bacteria. Moulds can predominate only when conditions are better for them than for yeasts or bacteria. The different kinds of bacteria present compete among themselves, with one kind usually outstripping the others. Likewise, if yeasts are favoured, one kind usually will outgrow others; and among the moulds one kind will find conditions more favourable than will other kinds. Micro-organisms are not always antagonistic, or antibiotic, to each other, however, and may sometimes be symbiotic, i.e. mutually helpful, or they may grow simultaneously without seeming to aid or hinder each other. Two kinds of micro-organisms may be synergistic, i.e. when growing together they may be able to bring about changes, such as fermentations, that neither could produce alone. *Pseudomonas syncyanea* growing alone in milk produces only a light-brownish tinge, and *Streptococcus lactis* causes no colour change in milk; however, when the two organisms grow together, a bright blue colour develops, resulting from a pH effect on the brown pigment produced by *P. syncyanea*.

A most important effect of a micro-organism on another is the metabiotic one, which occurs when one organism makes conditions favourable for growth of the second. Both organisms may be growing at the same time, but more commonly one succeeds the other. Most natural fermentations or decompositions of raw foods illustrate metabiosis. Raw milk at room temperature normally first supports an acid fermentation by *Streptococcus lactis* and coliform bacteria until the bacteria are inhibited by the acid they have produced. Next the acid-tolerant lactobacilli increase the acidity further until they are stopped. Then film yeasts and moulds grow over the top, finally reducing the acidity so that proteolytic bacteria can become active. The normal succession of organisms is first, miscellaneous bacteria, chiefly coliform; second, *Leuconostoc mesenteroides*; third, *Lactobacillus plantarum*; and last, *Lactobacillus brevis*.

Effect of Environmental Conditions

The environment determines which of the different kinds of micro-organisms present in a food will outgrow the others and cause its characteristic type of change or spoilage. The factors that make up this environment are interrelated and in combination determine the organisms that will grow and the effects to be produced. Chief among these factors are the physical and chemical properties of the food, the availability of oxygen, and the temperature.

Physical state and structure of the food

The physical state of the food, its colloidal nature, and whether it has been frozen, heated, moistened or dried, together with its biological structure, may have an important influence on whether a food will spoil and the type of spoilage.

The water in food, its location, and its availability constitute one of the most important factors influencing microbial growth. Water may be considered both as a chemical compound necessary for growth and as part of the physical structure of the food.

It has been emphasised that all micro-organisms require moisture for growth and that all grow best in the presence of a plentiful supply. This moisture must be available to the organisms, i.e. not tied up in any way, such as by solutes or by a hydrophilic colloid such as agar. Solutes such as salt and sugar dissolved in the water cause an osmotic pressure that tends to draw water from the cells if the concentration of dissolved materials is greater outside the cells than inside. It should be recalled that when the relative humidity of the air about the food corresponds to the available moisture or the water activity a_w of the food, the food and air about it will be in equilibrium in regard to moisture.

A dry food such as bread is most likely to be spoiled by moulds; sirups and honey, with their fairly high sugar content and hence lowered a_w favour the growth of osmophilic yeasts; and moist, neutral foods such as milk, meats, fish and eggs ordinarily are spoiled by bacteria. However, environmental factors other than moisture should be kept in mind in predicting the type of micro-organism apt to cause spoilage. Grape juice, for example, may favour yeasts because of its fairly high sugar content and low pH but will support the growth of bacteria if incubation temperatures are too high or too low for fermentative yeasts. Refrigerated foods may mould in the presence of air but undergo bacterial spoilage in its absence. Honey, although its sugar content is too high for most yeasts but not for some of the moulds, rarely is spoiled by moulds because of fungistatic substances present.

An a_w as low as 0.70 makes unlikely any spoilage by micro-organisms of a food held at room temperature. This is approximately the level of available moisture in dry milk at 8 per cent total moisture, dried whole egg at 10 to 11 per cent, flour at 13 to 15 per cent, nonfat dry milk at 15 per cent, dehydrated fat-free meat at 15 per cent, seeds of leguminous crops at 15 per cent, dehydrated vegetables at 14 to 20 per cent, dehydrated fruits at 18 to 25 per cent, and starch at 18 per cent.

It is possible for micro-organisms growing in food to change the level of available moisture by release of metabolic water or by changing the substrate so as to free water. In the production of ropiness in bread, for example, it is supposed that *Bacillus subtilis* causes the release of moisture as a result of the decomposition of starch and in this way makes conditions more favourable for its own growth. Destruction of moisture-holding tissues, as in fruits by moulds, may make water available to yeasts or bacteria.

Freezing not only prevents microbial growth if the temperature is sufficiently low but also is likely to damage tissues, so that juices released on thawing favour microbial growth. Freezing also increases the concentration of solutes in the unfrozen portion as the temperature is lowered, slowing and finally stopping the growth of organisms able to grow at temperatures below 0°C. Freezing also effects the removal of water from hydrophilic colloids that is not wholly reabsorbed on thawing.

Heat processing may change not only the chemical composition of the food but also its structure by softening tissues; releasing or tying up moisture; destroying or forming colloidal suspensions, gels or emulsions; and changing the penetrability of the food to moisture and oxygen. Protein may become denatured and therefore more available to some organisms than it was in the native state. Starch or protein may become gelated, releasing moisture and becoming more easily decomposed. For the reasons indicated, cooked food usually is more easily decomposed than is the original fresh food.

Changes in the colloidal constituents of foods may be caused by agencies other than the freezing or heating processes, e.g. by sound waves, but the results are similar. Emulsions of fat and water are more likely to spoil, and the spoilage will spread more rapidly when water is the continuous phase and fat the discontinuous one, as in French dressing, compared with butter, where the reverse is true.

Chemical properties of the food

The chemical composition of a food determines how satisfactory it will be as a culture medium for micro-organisms. Each organism has its own characteristic ability to utilise certain substances as a source of energy, a carbon source and/or a source of nitrogen.

Properties of a food dictating the numbers and type of organisms that will grow in and possibly spoil a food have been discussed already and include: (i) pH, or hydrogen-ion concentration, (ii) nutrient content, (iii) moisture availability, (iv) O-R potential, and (v) possible presence of inhibitory substances.

Temperature

Any nonsterile food is likely to spoil in time if it is moist enough and unfrozen. There is likelihood of spoilage at any temperature between –5°C and 70°C. Since micro-organisms differ so widely in their optimal, minimal and maximal temperatures for growth, it is obvious that the temperature at which a food is held will have a great influence on the kind, rate and amount of microbially induced change that will take place. Even a small change in temperature may favour an entirely different kind of organism and result in a different type of spoilage. Moulds and yeasts, for the most part, do not grow well above 35° to 37°C and therefore would not be important in foods held at high temperatures. On the other hand, moulds and yeasts grow well at ordinary room temperatures, and many of them grow fairly well at low temperatures, some even at freezing or slightly below. Although most bacteria grow best at ordinary temperatures, some (thermophiles) grow well at high temperatures and others (psychrophiles and psychrotrophs) at chilling temperatures. Therefore, moulds often grow on refrigerated foods, and thermophilic bacteria grow in the hot pea blanchers. Raw milk held at different temperatures supports the initial growth of different bacteria. At temperatures near freezing, cold-tolerant bacteria, e.g. species of *Pseudomonas* and *Alcaligenes*, are favoured; at room temperatures *Streptococcus lactis* and coliform bacteria usually predominate; at 40° to 45°C thermoduric species, e.g. *S. thermophilus* and *S. faecalis*, grow first; and at 55° to 60°C thermophilic bacteria such as *Lactobacillus thermophilus* will grow.

It should be kept in mind that the temperature at which a raw food is stored may affect its self-decomposition and therefore its susceptibility to microbial spoilage. As discussed, wrong storage temperatures for fruits weaken them and may make them more likely to spoil.

Temperatures commonly used in handling and storing foods, especially in the market and in the home, are very different in different countries. In some countries, refrigeration of most perishable foods is the rule and keeping such foods at atmospheric temperatures for very long is the exception, but the reverse is true in many foreign lands. Therefore, the most commonly occurring type of spoilage of a food may be entirely different in different countries. In the United States, concern with spoilage of most perishable foods mostly concerns changes at chilling temperatures, and psychrotrophic strains of *Pseudomonas*, *Flavobacterium*, *Alcaligenes* and other genera and certain yeasts and moulds would be important. Where foods are not refrigerated customarily, the prevailing atmospheric temperatures of the area would be significant, and differences during the seasons of the year would have to be considered. During seasons or at times when the climate is temperate, ordinary mesophilic bacteria, yeasts and moulds would assume importance. During hot weather, 26.7° to 43°C and above, organisms favoured by these temperatures would be important, such as coliform bacteria and species of *Bacillus*, *Clostridium*, *Streptococcus*, *Lactobacillus* and other genera. Tropical temperatures would be unfavourable to most yeasts and moulds. Under exceptional conditions, foods, especially canned varieties, sometimes are held at temperatures favouring thermophiles, as was often true during World War II, when canned foods were stored under tarpaulins in the tropics.

The combination of all of the factors just discussed and the kinds, numbers and proportions of micro-organisms present and their environment as controlled by physical and chemical properties of the food, oxygen tension and oxidation-reduction potential, and temperature will determine the kinds of micro-organisms most likely to grow in a food and hence the changes to be produced. All these factors should be considered in making predictions regarding the stability of shelf life. Table 5.1 summarises frequently employed processing modifications and their effect on the resulting keeping quality and on the microbial flora of major foods.

Sometimes a change in only one of the factors mentioned will be enough to limit the change to be expected, but more often several factors exert a combined effect.

Thus, a combination of low moisture, refrigerator temperature, high acidity and high sugar would make mould growth more likely than growth of yeasts or bacteria. But increasing the moisture content and the temperature would change conditions to favour yeasts, and decreasing the acidity and sugar content would encourage bacteria.

CHEMICAL CHANGES CAUSED BY MICRO-ORGANISMS

Because of the great variety of organic compounds in foods and the numerous kinds of micro-organisms that can decompose them, many different chemical changes are possible and many kinds of products can result. The following discussion is concerned only with the important types of decomposition of main constituents of foods and the chief products produced.

Changes in Nitrogenous Organic Compounds

Most of the nitrogen in foods is in the form of proteins which must be hydrolysed by enzymes of the micro-organisms or of the food to polypeptides, simpler peptides, or amino acids before they can serve as nitrogenous food for most organisms. Proteinases catalyse the hydrolysis of proteins to peptides, which may give a bitter taste to foods. Peptidases catalyse the hydrolysis of polypeptides to simpler peptides and finally to amino acids. The latter give flavours, desirable or undesirable, to some foods; e.g. amino acids contribute to the flavour of ripened cheeses.

For the most part these hydrolyses do not result in particularly objectionable products. Anaerobic decomposition of proteins, peptides or amino acids, however, may result in the production of obnoxious odours and is then called putrefaction. It results in foul-smelling, sulphur-containing products, such as hydrogen, methyl and ethyl sulphides and mercaptans, plus ammonia, amines (e.g. histamine, tyramine, piperidine, putrescine and cadaverine), indole, skatole and fatty acids.

Table 5.1. Classification of the major foods in order of increasing microbiological keeping quality.

Class	'Processing' including heat treatment, compositional modification, and packing	Stability characteristic		Examples	Predominant microbial flora at retail
		Temp., °C	Time of spoilage-free storage		
1	None of functional nature	<10	10–40 hr	Fresh meat, milk, fish, poultry, eggs, vegetables	Psychrotrophic, nonfermentative gram-negative rods
2	Pasteurisation, followed by hermetic packing	<10	3 days to 2 weeks	Dairy products, sliced cured meat products	Sporing rods and Lancefield group D streptococci
3	Reduction of water activity to ca. 0.95, pH reduction and addition of preservatives, in combination with hermetic packing	<10	A few weeks	'Gaffelbitter' and similar semipreserved fish products	Lactobacilli, streptococci, yeasts and moulds
4	Reduction of water activity to ca. 0.85, pH/a_w/lactic acid combinations of equivalent microbistatic effect, pasteurisation	25	Many weeks	Condensed milk, mayonnaise, margarine, smoked sausage	Yeasts, moulds
5	Reduction of water activity to ca. 0.80 sometimes in combination with pH reduction	25	Unlimited, i.e. until chemical reactions interfere	Shelf-stable products such as salami, stockfish, sauces	Moulds
6	Reduction of water activity, to <0.60	35	Unlimited	Dehydrated foods	Bacilli, group D streptococci, mould spores
7	Appertisation	35	Unlimited	Canned cured meat products and fruits	An occasional spore, i.e. counts of <10^2/g
8	Sterilisation	Any	Unlimited	Canned milk, soups, meat, vegetables, and fish	None

When micro-organisms act on amino acids, they may deaminate them, decarboxylate them or both, resulting in the products listed in Table 5.2. *Escherichia coli*, for example, produces glyoxylic acid, acetic acid and ammonia from glycine; *Pseudomonas* also produces methylamine and carbon dioxide; and clostridia give acetic acid ammonia, and methane. From alanine these three organisms produce: (i) an α-keto acid, ammonia and carbon dioxide, (ii) acetic acid, ammonia, and carbon dioxide and (iii) propionic acid, acetic acid, ammonia, and carbon dioxide, respectively. From serine, *E. coli* produces pyruvic acid and ammonia, and species of *Clostridium* give propionic acid, formic acid and ammonia. As stated previously, the sulphur in sulphur-bearing amino acids may be reduced to foul-smelling sulphides or mercaptans. *Desulphotomaculum nigrificans* (formerly *C. nigrificans*), an obligate anaerobe, can reduce sulphate to sulphide and produces hydrogen sulphide from cystine.

Table 5.2. Products from the microbial decomposition of amino acids.

Chemical process	Products
Oxidative deamination	Keto acid + NH_3
Hydrolytic deamination	Hydroxy acid + NH_3
Reductive deamination	Saturated fatty acid + NH_3
Desaturation deamination (at α and β positions)	Unsaturated fatty acid + NH_3
Mutual O-R between pairs of amino acids	Keto acid + fatty acid + NH_3
Decarboxylation	Amine + CO_2
Hydrolytic deamination + decarboxylation	Primary alcohol + NH_3 + CO_2
Reductive deamination + decarboxylation	Hydrocarbon + NH_3 + CO_2
Oxidative deamination + decarboxylation	Fatty acid + NH_3 + CO_2

Other nitrogenous compounds decomposed include: (i) amides, imides and urea, from which ammonia is the principal product, (ii) guanidine and creatine, which yield urea and ammonia, and (iii) amines, purines, and pyrimidines, which may yield ammonia, carbon dioxide and organic acids (chiefly lactic or acetic).

Changes in Non-nitrogenous Organic Compounds

The main non-nitrogenous foods for micro-organisms, mostly used to obtain energy but possibly serving as sources of carbon, include carbohydrates, organic acids, aldehydes and ketones, alcohols, glycosides, cyclic compounds and lipids.

Carbohydrates

Carbohydrates, if available, usually are preferred by micro-organisms to other energy-yielding foods. Complex di-, trio or polysaccharides usually are hydrolysed to simple sugars before utilisation. A monosaccharide, such as glucose, aerobically would be oxidised to carbon dioxide and water and anaerobically would undergo decomposition involving any of six main types of fermentation: (i) an alcoholic fermentation, as by yeasts, with ethanol and carbon dioxide as the principal products, (ii) a simple lactic fermentation, as by homofermentative lactic acid bacteria, with lactic acid as the main product, (iii) a mixed lactic fermentation, as by heterofermentative lactic acid bacteria, with lactic and acetic acids, ethanol, glycerol and carbon dioxide as the chief products, (iv) the coliform type of fermentation, as by coliform bacteria, with lactic, acetic and formic acids, ethanol, carbon dioxide, hydrogen, and perhaps acetoin and butanediol as likely products, (v) the propionic fermentation, by propionibacteria, producing propionic, acetic, and succinic acids and carbon dioxide, and (vi) the butyric-butyl-isopropyl fermentations, by anaerobic bacteria, yielding butyric and acetic acids, carbon dioxide, hydrogen, and in some instances acetone, butylene glycol, butanol, and 2-propanol. A variety of other products are possible from sugars when different micro-organisms are active, including higher fatty acids, other organic acids, aldehydes, and ketones.

Organic acids

Many of the organic acids usually occurring in foods as salts are oxidised by organisms to carbonates, causing the medium to become more alkaline. Aerobically the organic acids may be oxidised completely to carbon dioxide and water, as is done by film yeasts. Acids may be oxidised to other, simpler acids or to other products similar to those from sugars. Saturated fatty acids or lower ketonic derivatives are degraded to acetic acid, two carbons at a time, aided by coenzyme A. Unsaturated or hydroxy fatty acids may be degraded partially in a similar manner but must be converted to a saturated acid (or ketonic derivative) for complete beta oxidation.

Other compounds

Alcohols usually are oxidised to the corresponding organic acid, e.g. ethanol to acetic acid. Glycerol may be dissimilated to products similar to those from glucose. Glycosides, after hydrolysis to release the sugar, will have the sugar dissimilated characteristically. Acetaldehyde may be oxidised to acetic acid or reduced to ethanol. Cyclic compounds are not readily attacked.

Lipids

Fats are hydrolysed by microbial lipase to glycerol and fatty acids, which are then dissimilated as outlined previously. Micro-organisms may be involved in the oxidation of fats, but auto-oxidation is more common. Phospholipids may be degraded to their constituent phosphate, glycerol, fatty acids, and nitrogenous base, e.g. choline. Lipoproteins are made up of proteins, cholesterol esters and phospholipids.

Pectic substances

Protopectin, the water-insoluble parent pectic substance in plants, is converted to pectin, a water-soluble polymer of galacturonic acid which contains methyl ester linkages and varying degrees of neutralisation by various cations. It gels with sugar and acid. Pectinesterase causes hydrolysis of the methyl ester linkage of pectin to yield pectic acid and methanol. Polygalacturonases destroy the linkage between galacturonic acid units of pectin or pectic acid to yield smaller chains and ultimately free D-galacturonic acid, which may be degraded to simple sugars.

Chapter 6

Milk and Dairy Products

INTRODUCTION

Dairy milk is an opaque white liquid produced by the mammary glands of mammals (including monotremes). It provides the primary source of nutrition for newborn mammals before they are able to digest other types of food. The early lactation milk is known as colostrum, and carries the mother's antibodies to the baby. It can reduce the risk of many diseases in the baby. The exact components of raw milk varies by species, but it contains significant amounts of saturated fat, protein and calcium as well as vitamin C. Cow's milk has a pH ranging from 6.4 to 6.8, making it slightly acidic.

The specific gravity of milk ranges from 1.029 to 1.039. The specific gravity of milk decreases with the increasing fat content and increases with increasing amounts of proteins, sugar and salts. The freezing point of milk is almost a constant value at 0.53°–0.55°C and is suitable indicator for detection of dairy cheese and yoghurt are +0.05 and –0.15 V respectively.

OTHER ANIMAL SOURCES

In addition to cows, the following animals provide milk used by humans for dairy products: (i) buffalo, (ii) camels, (iii) donkeys, (iv) goats, (v) horses, (vi) reindeer, (vii) sheep, (viii) water buffalo, and (ix) yaks.

In Russia and Sweden, small moose dairies also exist.

Human milk is not produced or distributed industrially or commercially; however, milk banks exist that allow for the collection of donated human milk and its redistribution to infants who may benefit from human milk for various reasons (premature neonates, babies with allergies or metabolic diseases, etc.). All other female mammals do produce milk, but are rarely or never used to produce dairy products for human consumption.

PHYSICAL AND CHEMICAL STRUCTURE

Milk is an emulsion or colloid of butterfat globules within a water-based fluid. Each fat globule is surrounded by a membrane consisting of phospholipids and proteins; these emulsifiers keep the individual globules from joining together into noticeable grains of butterfat and also protect the globules from the fat-digesting activity of enzymes found in the fluid portion of the milk. In unhomogenised cow milk, the fat globules average about four micrometers across. The fat-soluble vitamins A, D, E and K are found within the milkfat portion of the milk.

The largest structures in the fluid portion of the milk are casein protein micelles: aggregates of several thousand protein molecules, bonded with the help of nanometer-scale particles of calcium phosphate. Each micelle is roughly spherical and about a tenth of a micrometer across. There are four different types of casein proteins, and collectively they make up around 80 per cent of the protein in milk, by weight. Most of the casein proteins are bound into the micelles. There are several competing theories regarding the precise structure of the micelles, but they share one important feature: the outermost layer consists of strands of one type of protein, kappa-casein, reaching out from the body of the micelle into the surrounding fluid. These kappa-casein molecules all have a negative electrical charge and therefore repel each other, keeping the micelles separated under normal conditions and in a stable colloidal suspension in the water-based surrounding fluid.

Both the fat globules and the smaller casein micelles, which are just large enough to deflect light, contribute to the opaque white colour of milk. Skimmed milk, however, appears slightly blue because casein micelles scatter the shorter wavelengths (blue compared to red).

The fat globules contain some yellow-orange carotene, enough in some breeds—Guernsey and Jersey cows, for instance to impart a golden or 'creamy' hue to a glass of milk. The riboflavin in the whey portion of milk has a greenish colour, which can sometimes be discerned in skim milk or whey products. Fat-free skim milk has only the casein micelles to scatter light, and they tend to scatter shorter wavelength blue light more than they do red, giving skim milk a bluish tint.

Milk contains dozens of other types of proteins besides the caseins. They are more water-soluble than the caseins and do not form larger structures. Because these proteins remain suspended in the whey left behind when the caseins coagulate into curds, they are collectively known as whey proteins. Whey proteins make up around twenty per cent of the protein in milk, by weight. Lactoglobulin is the most common whey protein by a large margin.

The carbohydrate lactose gives milk its sweet taste and contributes about 40 per cent of whole cow milk's calories. Lactose is a composite of two simple sugars, glucose and galactose. In nature, lactose is found only in milk and a small number of plants. Other components found in raw cow milk are living white blood cells. Mammary-gland cells, various bacteria and a large number of active enzymes are some other components in milk.

NATURAL COMPONENTS IN MILK

Lactoferrin, lactoperoxidase and xanthine oxidase are naturally present in milk and have some specific properties that have been found to be beneficial for the shelf life and quality of dairy products. These compounds are nonimmune antimicrobial proteins that have been investigated by several researchers.

Lactoferrin

Lactoferrin is an iron-binding glycoprotein in milk that inhibits the growth of pathogenic bacteria by its high affinity with iron. The antimicrobial mechanism of lactoferrin is more complex than simple binding of iron. Lactoferrin also disrupts bacterial cell membranes by binding bacterial lipopolysaccharide and modifies membrane permeability by binding porin molecules in the outer membrane. This interaction with the cell membranes facilitates the bactericidal properties of lactoferrin. When the antimicrobial effects of lactoferrin on *Escherichia coli*, *Salmonella typhimurium*, *Shigella dysenteriae* and *Listera monocytogenes* were investigated, lactoferrin was shown to inhibit the growth of these microbes.

Lactoperoxidase

Lactoperoxidase is an antibacterial enzyme naturally present in colostrum and milk. This enzyme catalyses the oxidation of thiocyanate (SCN^-) in the presence of hydrogen peroxide (H_2O_2), producing hypothiocyanite ($OSCN^-$), which is a toxic intermediary oxidation product. This product inhibits bacterial metabolism by oxidation of essential sulphydryl groups in proteins. This reaction produces a severe change in the cytoplasmic membrane of spoilage bacteria. The use of lactoperoxidase is not approved in the United States because its activation requires a thiocyanide compound, which is unsafe for children. The activation of the lactoperoxidase system in refrigerated raw milk retarded the growth of psychrotrophic bacteria for several days. The lactoperoxidase system has been used to extend the shelf life of raw, pasteurised and ultra high temperature (UHT)-treated milk and to preserve cream, cottage cheese, mozzarella cheese and yogurt.

Xanthine Oxidase

Xanthine oxidase is a complex metallo-flavo enzyme present in the fat globule membrane. The enzyme catalyses the reaction to produce bactericide superoxide radicals and hydrogen peroxide in the presence of oxygen. Hydrogen peroxide can also be used to activate the lactoperoxidase system. Xanthine oxidase was studied for its activity in dairy products such as raw, evaporated and powdered milks; ice cream; yogurt; cheese; and butter and creams. Nielsen reported that xanthine oxidase, an oxido-reductase enzyme, catalyses the oxidation of purine bases and reduces nitrate to nitrite. Nitrate inhibits the germination of spore butyric acid bacteria in cheese.

MILK PROCESSING OPERATIONS

The steps in milk processing operations carried out in a dairy plant are: (i) blending, (ii) clarification and cream separation, (iii) heat treatment, primarily pasteurisation, (iv) homogenisation, and (v) bottling. The process steps are shown in the Fig. 6.1.

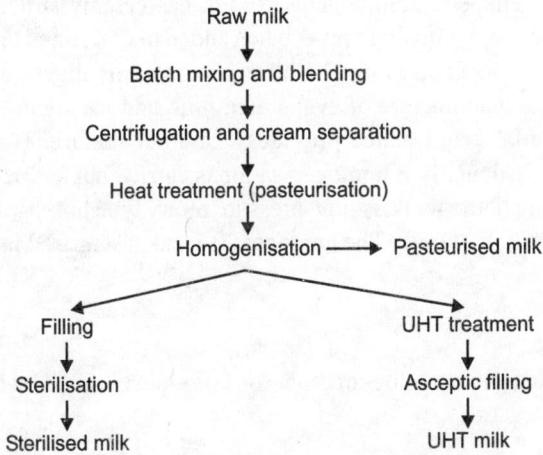

Fig. 6.1. Milk processing operations.

Blending of different batches of milk in cold condition (~5°C) is carried out to obtain a specified fat content. In the second step, the blended milk is clarified by a centrifugal clarifier to remove any sediments, body cells from the cow's udder and some-bacteria. A high speed centrifuge called bactofuge is used for almost complete removal of bacteria. Cream separation is often achieved simultaneously in this step. This operation is carried out at 40°C at 5000–6000 rpm.

The clarified milk is then given appropriate heat treatment depending on the requirement. Pasteurisation is carried out to destroy lipase activity and other milk enzymes and also to destroy pathogenic organisms in batch or harding method by heating the milk at 62°–65°C for at least 30 minutes or by HTST method (high temperature short time method) at 71°–74°C for 15 seconds or in a short time process at 85°C for 2 seconds. Pasteurised milk is not sterile and hence it is quickly cooled to prevent multiplication of souring bacteria. Raw milk contains several enzymes of which alkaline phosphatase is important. This enzyme has heat destruction characteristics that closely approximate the time-temperature exposures of proper pasteurisation and hence its activity is indicative of the effectiveness of pasteurisation. If alkaline phosphatase activity beyond a certain level is found in pasteurised milk, it is indicative of inadequate pasteurisation. The enzyme liberates phenol from phenol phosphoric acid compounds and free phenol gives a deep blue colour with certain organic compounds, which forms the basis for phosphatase test.

Ultra high temperature (UHT) treatment involves indirect heating by coils or plates at 135°–140°C for 6–10 seconds or by direct heating by live stream injection at 140°–150°C for 2–4 seconds followed by aseptic packaging. Milk may also be sterilised in retail packages by heating in autoclaves at 110°–120°C for 15–20 minutes.

Homogenisation may be carried out before or after pasteurisation. This process makes a stable emulsion of milk fat and milk serum by mechanical treatment. Homogenisation is achieved by passing milk or cream through a small aperture under high pressure and velocity. The fat globules of milk with varying sizes in the range of 0.1 to 20 μm in diameter have a tendency to gather into clumps and rise due to their lower density than milk, thereby separating into a cream layer. Homogenisation breaks the fat globules to uniform size of about 2 μm or less which are covered by an adsorbed layer of plasma proteins including casein micelles.

This stabilises the milk emulsion. Homogenised milk has creamy structure, bland flavour and a whiter appearance. It has greater whitening power when added to coffee and tea compared to skim milk. A soft curd is formed from homogenised milk, which is more easily digested than curd obtained from unhomogenised milk. In the manufacture of evaporated milk and ice cream, homogenisation reduces the chance of separation of fat and hence provides smoother texture. Homogenisation, however, accelerates lipase activity, particularly if homogenisation is carried out before pasteurisation leading to rancid flavour. High pressure homogenisers, low pressure rotary type homogenisers and sonic vibrators may be used for homogenisation of milk. The homogenised and pasteurised milk is then cooled, bottled and marketed.

MILK PRODUCTS

Fresh milk is the starting point for a number of other food products, some of which are shown in Fig. 6.2

Microflora of Raw Milk

Its high water activity, moderate pH (6.4–6.6) and ample supply of nutrients make milk an excellent medium for microbial growth. This demands high standards of hygiene in its production and processing; a fact recognised in most countries where milk was the first food to be the focus of modern food hygiene legislation.

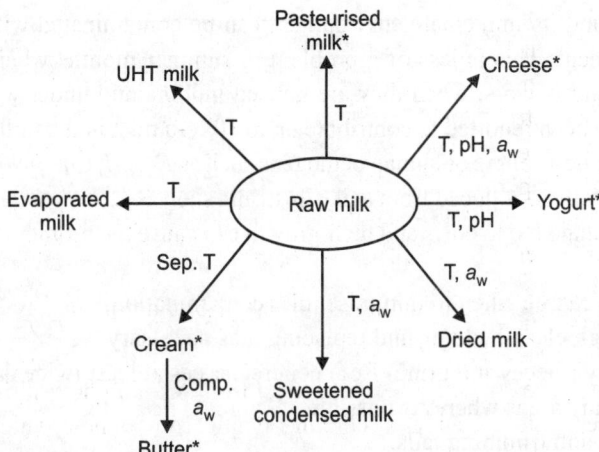

Fig. 6.2. Milk and milk products. T indicates elevated temperature; pH, reduced pH; a_w, reduced a_w; sep., separation, comp., compartmentalisation; and * stored at chill temperatures.

Milk does possess a number of antimicrobial features, present either to protect the udder from infection or to protect the newborn calf. Generally these are present at too low a concentration in cow's milk to have a very marked effect on its keeping quality or safety. In some cases the antimicrobial activity is antagonised by other milk constituents such as the effect of citrate and bicarbonate on lactoferrin activity. Stimulation of lactoperoxidase activity through the addition of exogenous hydrogen peroxide has been investigated as a means of preserving raw milk in developing countries where ambient temperatures are high and refrigeration is not often available. In one trial in Africa, use of this technique increased the proportion of samples passing the 10 minutes resazurin quality test from 26 to 88 per cent.

Three sources contribute to the micro-organisms found in milk: the udder interior, the teat exterior and its immediate surroundings, and the milking and milk-handling equipment.

Bacteria that get on to the outside of the teat may be able to invade the opening and thence the udder interior. Aseptically taken milk from a healthy cow normally contains low numbers of organisms, typically fewer than 10^2–10^3 cfu ml^{-1}, and milk drawn from some quarters may be sterile. The organisms most commonly isolated are micrococci, streptococci and the diptheroid *Corynebacterium bovis*. Counts are frequently higher though due to mastitis, an inflammatory disease of the mammary tissue, which is a major cause of economic loss in the dairy industry.

Many organisms can cause mastitis, the most important being *Staphylococcus aureus*, *Escherichia coli*, *Streptococcus agalactiae*, *Strep. uberis*, *Pseudomonas aeruginosa* and *Corynebacterium pyogenes*. The first three of these are all potential human pathogens and a number of other human pathogens such as *Salmonella*, *Listeria monocytogenes*, *Mycobacterium bovis* and *Mycobacterium tuberculosis* are also occasionally reported.

Infected cows are treated by injection of antibiotics into the udder. Milk from these cows must be withheld from sale for several days following treatment because antibiotic residues can cause problems in sensitive consumers and inhibit starter culture activity in fermented milks. Attempts to control mastitis by good milking hygiene, use of a disinfectant teat dip after milking and an antibiotic infusion at the end of lactation have helped to reduce streptococcal and staphylococcal infections but have had little success in preventing *E. coli* mastitis.

The udder exterior and its immediate environment can be contaminated with organisms from the cow's general environment. This is less of a problem in summer months when cows are allowed to graze in open pasture and is worst when they are housed indoors and under wet conditions. Heavily contaminated teats have been reported to contribute up to 10^5 cfu ml^{-1} in the milk. Contamination from bedding and manure can be a source of human pathogens such as *E. coli*, *Campylobacter* and *Salmonella* and *Bacillus* species may be introduced from soil. Clostridia such as *C. butyricum* and *C. tyrobutyricum* can get into milk from silage fed to cows and their growth can cause the problem known as late blowing in some cheeses.

Following measures can be taken to minimise milk contamination:

1. Providing enough clean bedding and replacing it as necessary.
2. Removing slurry (faeces and urine) from concrete areas at least twice daily.
3. Preventing muddy areas wherever possible.
4. Shaving udders and trimming tails.
5. Washing teats with warm water containing disinfectant and drying individually with paper towels.
6. Keeping the milking parlour floor clean during milking.
7. Thoroughly cleaning teat cups if they fall off during milking and discarding foremilk.

Although such procedures certainly improve the microbiological quality of milk, economic constraints such as increasing size of individual dairy herds and decreased manning levels in milking parlours encouraged their neglect.

Milk-handling equipment such as teat cups, pipework, milk holders and storage tanks, is the principal source of the micro-organisms found in raw milk. As the overall quality of the milk decreases so the proportion of the microflora derived from this source increases. Milk is a nutritious medium and, if equipment is poorly cleaned, milk residues on surfaces that are frequently left wet will act as a focus for microbial growth which can contaminate subsequent batches of milk. Occasional neglect of cleaning and sanitising procedures is usually less serious since, although it may contribute large numbers of micro-organisms to the product, these tend to be fast growing bacteria that are heat sensitive and will be killed by pasteurisation. They are also sensitive to sanitising practices used and will be eliminated once effective cleaning is resumed. If cleaning is persistently neglected though, the hydrophobic, mineral-rich deposit known as milks tone can build up on surfaces, particularly heated ones. This will protect organisms from sanitisers and allow slower growing organisms to develop such as micrococci and enterococci. Many of these are thermoduric and may not be removed by pasteurisation.

In most developed countries milk is chilled almost immediately after it issues from the cow and is held at a low temperature thereafter. It is stored in refrigerated holding tanks before being transported by refrigerated lorry to the dairy where it is kept in chill storage tanks until use. Throughout this time, its temperature remains below 7°C and the only organisms capable of growing will be psychrotrophs. There are many psychrotrophic species, but those most commonly found in raw milk include gram-positive rods of the genera *Pseudomonas*, *Acinetobacter*, *Alcaligenes*, *Flavobacterium*, psychrotrophic coliforms, predominantly, *Aerobacter* spp., and gram-positive *Bacillus* spp.

Types of Milk and Milk Products

A variety of milk and milk products are produced in the dairy depending on consumer requirements. These include the following categories of products.

Vitamin D milk

Vitamin D content in cow's milk depends on the cattle feed and exposure of the cow to sunlight. The diet of most children is deficient in Vitamin D and hence Vitamin D enriched milk is marketed. Vitamin D activity in milk is enhanced by irradiating milk with UV light which converts the milk sterol, 7-dehydrocholesterol into Vitamin D_3. Alternatively, Vitamin D concentrates may be added to milk to bring the potency to about 400 units per quart.

Low sodium milk

Low sodium milk is required by people with high blood pressure or edema. It is prepared by passing milk through an ion-exchange resin that replaces sodium with potassium. Low sodium milk contains 3–10 mg of sodium per 100 ml compared to about 50 mg in ordinary milk.

Concentrated milk

Evaporated milk is whole milk from which most of the water has been evaporated. Raw whole milk is clarified and concentrated in the vacuum pans at a temperature of 74°–77°C. It is then fortified with the Vitamin D, homogenised, and filled into can and sterilised at 118°C for 15 minutes and cooled. This heat treatment gives evaporated milk a light brown colour due to sugar-protein interaction and also its characteristic flavour. Khoa is a semi solid obtained by evaporating milk in open pans and is used in preparing Indian sweetmeats. Malai is made by simmering milk to a thick layer of milk fat and coagulated proteins consumed with or without sugar.

Sweetened condensed milk

This is made from pasteurised milk by concentration and sucrose is added to sweeten the concentrate to the extent of 65 per cent in the final product. Sweetened condensed milk is not sterile but microbial growth is prevented by the added sugar. Kheer is concentrated milk, obtained by evaporating milk to nearly half its original volume, resembling sweetened condensed milk.

Dry milk

Whole milk is dehydrated to the extent of 97 per cent by spray drying or vacuum drying. Skim milk and low-fat milk are also dehydrated to manufacture milk powder. Vitamins A and D are added to enhance the nutritive value. The low-cost dry milk has a long shelf life and can be reconstituted to fluid milk by mixing with the required amount of water. Dried milk is stored in dry air tight containers.

Skim milk

Whole milk from which fat has been removed by centrifugation is called skim milk. It contains all other constituents of milk except fat and fat-soluble Vitamins A and D. These vitamins can be added to skim milk. By varying the amount of fat removed from whole milk, low fat milk (containing 0.5–2 per cent fat) is prepared. Condensed skim milk finds extensive use in baking and confectionery industries.

Cream

Concentrated milk fat is called cream. Cream is formed as a layer of fat globules, which rise to the top in unhomogenised milk. Cream is separated from milk by centrifugation. Table cream (coffee cream) contains about 18 per cent fat while whipping cream contains about 35 per cent fat. Cream, used for butter making, contains about 40 per cent fat. Sour cream, which is extensively used in bakery items as salad dressings, is prepared by pasteurising cream with about 18 per cent fat at 75°C for 30 minutes to kill all bacteria and then inoculating with a controlled culture of lactic acid bacteria to develop the desired acid tang in the finished product.

Yoghurt

Yoghurt (or yogurt) or dahi in India is a fermented milk product with a fine curdled gel like consistency having a sour and aromatic flavour. It is obtained by fermenting homogenised pasteurised milk with about 3 per cent thermophylic lactic acid bacteria (mixed cultures of Streptococcus thermophilus or Lactobacillus bulgaricus) at 42°–45°C for about 3 hours. During fermentation, the curdled gel-like consistency and acid flavour due to formation of carbonyl compounds such as diacetyl and acetaldehyde develop. Sugar and fruit pastes may be added to the final product to achieve distinct fruity flavours.

Sour milk

Sour milk or buttermilk is fermented fluid milk either by spontaneous souring (by *Streptococcus lactis* or *cremoris*) or by fermentation with aroma forming bacteria (*Streptococcus diacetylactis* or *Betacoccus citrovorus*) or by fermentation with pure bacterial cultures to give cultured buttermilk. During fermentation lactose is converted into lactic acid which coagulates casein at pH 4.5–5 to give the final sour tasting curdled buttermilk.

Kefir and kumiss

Kefir and kumiss are sparkling, carbonated alcoholic beverages derived from milk. The microflora such as *Torula* yeast (for alcoholic fermentation) and *Streptococcus lactis* and *Lactobacillus caucasicus* (for lactic acid fermentation) which form clotted milk particles are added to fluid milk to give kefir. Kumiss is made from goat's or mare's milk by fermentation with *Thermobacterium bulgaricus* and yeast Candida.

Taette milk

Milk is fermented with *Streptococcus lactis* var. *hollandicus* to yield a sour viscous thread-like product due to the symbiotic growth of the lactic acid bacteria and yeast. Taette is popular in Sweden, Norway and Finland. Typical milk composition are listed in Table 6.1 and composition of fresh cow's milk are listed in Table 6.2.

Table 6.1. Typical milk composition [% weight (volume) $^{-1}$].

	Fat	Protein	Lactose	Total solids
Human	3.8	1.0	7.0	12.4
Cow	3.7	3.4	4.8	12.7
Jersey	5.1	3.8	5.0	14.5
Ayrshire	4.0	3.5	4.8	13.0
Short-horn	3.6	4.9	4.9	12.6
Sheep	7.4	5.5	4.8	19.3
Goat	4.5	2.9	4.1	13.2
Water buffalo	7.4	3.8	4.8	17.2
Horse	1.9	2.5	6.2	11.2

Table 6.2. Composition of fresh cow's milk.

	Concentration g litre^{-1}	
Lipids	37	
	of which	% w/w
Triglycerides		95–96
Diglycerides		1.3–1.6
Free fatty acids		0.1–0.5
Total phospholipids		0.8–1.0
Proteins	34	
Casein	26	
α_{S1}	11.1	
α_{S2}	1.7	
β	8.2	
γ	1.2	
κ	3.7	
Whey proteins		
α-Lactalbumin	0.7	
β-Lactoglobulin	3.0	
Serum albumin	0.3	
Immunoglobulins	0.6	
Non-protein nitrogen	1.9	
Lactose	48.0	
Citric acid	1.75	
Ash	7.0	
Calcium	1.25	
Phosphorus	0.96	

PROCESSING OF CULTURED DIARY PRODUCTS

The following discussion highlights the unique processing steps that are involved in the production of cultured dairy products. These processing steps contribute to the unique flavour, texture, and overall sensory characteristics of these products.

Cheese

Milk and other dairy foods have been recognised as important foods since ancient times. In Egyptian tombs, dating back to 2300 BC, remains of cheese have been found. With advances in the dairy industry over the years, a wide variety of products derived from milk are available today.

Cheese has all the beneficial attributes of an ideal dairy product. Until the 18th century cheese making was essentially a farmhouse industry, which rapidly progressed, as processes of manufacture and ripening of cheese were refined.

Cheese is a food consisting of proteins and fat from milk, usually the milk of cows, buffalo, goats, or sheep. It is produced by coagulation of the milk protein casein. Typically, the milk is acidified and addition of the rennet causes coagulation. The solids are then separated and pressed into final form. Some cheeses also contain moulds, either on the outer rind or throughout.

Hundreds of types of cheese are produced. Their different styles, textures and flavours depend on the origin of the milk (including the animal's diet), whether it has been pasteurised, butterfat content, the species of bacteria and mould, and the processing including the length of ageing. Herbs, spices or wood smoke may be used as flavouring agents. The yellow to red colour of many cheeses is a result of adding annatto. Cheeses are eaten both on their own and cooked in various dishes; most cheeses melt when heated. For a few cheeses, the milk is curdled by adding acids such as vinegar or lemon juice. Most cheeses are acidified to a lesser degree by bacteria, which turn milk sugars into lactic acid, then the addition of rennet completes the curdling. Vegetarian alternatives to rennet are available; most are produced by fermentation of the fungus *Mucor miehei*, but others have been extracted from various species of the Cynara thistle family.

Cheese has served as a hedge against famine and is a good travel food. It is valuable for its portability, long life, and high content of fat, protein, calcium, and phosphorus. Cheese is more compact and has a longer shelf life than the milk from which it is made. Cheese-makers near a dairy region may benefit from fresher, lower-priced milk and lower shipping costs. The long storage life of cheese allows selling it when markets are more favourable.

Some cheese varieties are made from milk whey solids that remain after the removal of coagulated casein. Some of the well-known names include Cheddar, Camembert, Edam, Romano, Swiss, Roquefort, Trappist, brick and whey cheese. Cheese may also be classified on the basis of texture and kind of ripening. Thus there are hard cheese (Cheddar, Cheshire, Emmental), semi-hard cheese (Edam, Gouda, Molbo, Port Salut, Roquefort, Blue Dorset, Blue Cheese) and soft cheese (Chevre, Brie, Camembert, Limburger, Le Munster) depending on their moisture content. The varieties of cheese may be ripened by bacteria or moulds, or they may be unripened (Quark, Cottage Cheese, Mozzarella, Petit Suisse). The bacteria may produce gas and form 'eyes' in the cheese as in Swiss cheese or they may not produce gas and hence no eyes as in the case of Cheddar cheese. Among the soft and semi-hard cheeses, Limburger is ripened primarily by bacteria and Camembert by a mould while cottage cheese is not ripened. Whey cheese has high lactalbumin content, the second principal protein in milk. Lactalbumin is not coagulated by rennin or the acid and so it remains soluble in whey. However, it is easily coagulated from the whey as curd by the process of heating.

Nutritional value

Fermentation has occupied a place of pride in food preservation practices from time immemorial. It enhances the nutritional value and enriches flavour and texture of the product. Fermented milk products have been reported to have many therapeutic properties. This is accomplished by multifarious biological activities of desirable micro-organisms. As a net result they may add certain vitamins and may enhance the digestion and assimilation of major food constituents, namely, carbohydrates, proteins and fats. Cheese represents a balanced food with concentrated form of energy and good quality protein. It is rich in essential amino acids and binds large amounts of minerals and vitamins. Cheese has high food and nutritive value. In addition to fats, 100 g of cheese has protein (23.7 g), calcium (870 mg), phosphorus (610 mg), vitamin A (1740 IU), vitamin D (13 IU) and riboflavin (0.50 mg). By adjusting the fat content of cheese milk to different values, cheeses of widely different fat and other compositional components are produced. Average fat and protein content of cheeses is given in Table 6.3.

Cheddar cheese, one of the most popular cheeses, contains about 25 per cent protein compared with 20 per cent in meat and 8 per cent in bread, and is usually one of the finest sources of high value protein. One kg of cheddar cheese is approximately equivalent in food value to 10 litres of milk or 30 eggs or 1.5–2.0 kg meat, or 2–3 kg fish or 18–20 kg cabbage. Depending upon the ratio of fat to protein in cheese, the consumption of cheese with other foods, i.e. vegetables and bread or other cereal products may raise the biological value of proteins in diet as a whole, which is a distinct advantage. On the other hand, soft cheese made from skim milk or very low fat milk is among the best of slimming foods.

Table 6.3. Average fat and protein content of cheeses.

Cheese variety	Moisture %	Fat %	FDM %	Protein %
Cheddar	37.0	32.5	50.0	25.5
Swiss	38.5	29.0	47.0	29.0
Mozzarella	54.0	18.0	40.0	22.0
Edam/Gouda	46.0	25.4	45.0	24.0
Parmesan	31.0	26.0	35.0	37.5
Blue	43.0	29.0	50.0	22.5
Feta	63.0	16.0	40.0	18.4
Cottage	80.0	5.0	20.0	10.0

Cheese and cardiovascular health

Coronary heart disease (CHD), the most common and serious form of cardiovascular disease, is the leading cause of death in mainly developed industrialised countries. Many risk factors, both genetic and environmental, contribute to the development of CHD. The three most important modifiable risk factors for CHD are cigarette smoking, high blood pressure and elevated blood cholesterol levels, particularly high low-density lipoprotein (LDL). Other risk factors likely to contribute to CHD risk include Diabetes mellitus, physical inactivity, low blood levels of high-density lipoprotein (HDL), elevated blood triglyceride levels and obesity.

Some dairy food nutrients, namely, saturated fatty acids such as palmitic, myristic and lauric acids, and cholesterol are hypercholesterolemic, whereas others like monounsaturated fatty acids, poly-unsaturated fatty acids, stearic acid and medium chain saturated fatty acids may have a modest hypocholesterolemic effect in comparison with longer chain saturated fatty acids. The effect of any single nutrient on blood lipid levels is highly individualised, mainly because of genetic variability. In addition, the effect of single nutrient may be different when delivered in the complex matrix of food and the overall diet. In studies where various milks or dairy products such as yoghurt and cheese are consumed in moderate amounts, blood lipid levels generally do not increase. Mineral contents in cheeses are given in Table 6.4. Health awareness has prompted many people to be conscious of the quantity of fat in their diet. There are some severe problems associated with high fat consumption. Dietary fat, especially fat containing more saturated fatty acid increases plasma lipid level. A strong correlation has been found between plasma lipid levels, in particular low-density lipoprotein and coronary arterial disease (CAD). Fat is the richest source of energy and excessive calorie consumption from fat may cause obesity. Obesity frequently predisposes an individual to hyperlipidemia, diabetes and hypertension, and thus adversely affects health.

Table 6.4. Mineral contents in cheeses.

Cheese variety	Calcium	Phosphorus	Sodium	Potassium	Magnesium
Parmesan	1300	850	1200	100	44
Cheddar	760	500	640	90	30
Emmental	1080	730	250	90	43
Edam/Gouda	800	600	800	100	40
Mozzarella	400	340	450	100	16
Camembert	350	300	930	150	20
Processed cheese	600	600	135	100	24
Cottage cheese	80	140	380	75	8

There is a strong association between calorie intake, especially that from fat, and the incidence of many common cancers. Low fat cheeses and cottage cheese are, therefore, highly beneficial. Trace element contents in various cheese variety are given in Table 6.5.

Table 6.5. Trace elements content per 100 g of cheese.

Cheese variety	Zn (mg)	Fe (mg)	l (µg)	Mn (µg)	Se (µg)	Cu (µg)	Al (mg)
Cheddar	3.8	0.6	52	40	11	50	0.02
Parmesan	3.6	0.6	40	40	12	200	–
Emmental	5.0	0.5	40	40	11	200	0.2
Edam/Gouda	4.0	0.5	35	40	–	100	0.3
Mozzarella	3.5	0.4	45	30	3	60	–
Processed cheese	3.4	0.35	48	22	10	50	1.4
Cottage cheese	0.5	0.2	20	6	5	17	0.1

Cheese and colon cancer

Colorectal cancer is one of the leading causes of morbidity and mortality in both men and women. Although some dietary factors are suspected of contributing to specific cancers, others may be protective. Several components of dairy foods, especially calcium and vitamin D, bacterial cultures (*Lactobacillus acidophilus*), a class of fatty acids known as conjugated dieonoic derivatives of linoleic acid (CLA), sphingolipids, butyric acid and milk proteins are believed to protect against colon cancer. Further, new clinical findings in human beings indicate that increasing the intake of low fat dairy foods may reduce the risk of colon cancer. Vitamin content in various variety of cheese are given in Table 6.6.

Table 6.6. Vitamin content per 100 g of cheese.

Cheese variety	A (mg)	B_1 (µg)	B_2 (µg)	B_6 (µg)	Folic acid (µg)	B_{12} (µg)	Tocopherol (mg)
Emmental	0.33	35	0.30	105	12	2.7	0.9
Cheddar	3.36	35	0.40	75	25	1.9	0.7
Edam/Gouda	0.21	35	0.35	70	25	1.9	0.7
Blue cheese	0.40	36	0.50	100	45	1.2	0.9
Cottage cheese	0.08	28	0.24	55	15	1.0	0.2
Processed cheese	0.3	23	0.30	55	15	1.0	0.4

New findings from a clinical trial indicate that increasing intake of low-fat dairy foods to reach 1500 mg calcium/day may reduce the risk of colon cancer. There is also suggestive evidence that intake of culture containing dairy foods such as cheese and yoghurt may protect against colon cancer. However, further research is needed to confirm the potential anti carcinogenic role of CLA, sphingolipids and other components in dairy foods.

Cheese and osteoporosis

Osteoporosis (porous bones) is defined as a metabolic bone disease characterised by low bone mass and micro architectural deterioration of bone tissue leading to enhanced bone at fragility and a consequent increase in fracture risk. The cause(s) of osteoporosis, similar to other chronic diseases, is multifactorial, involving both genetic and environmental factors. As more than 99 per cent of the total calcium content of the body is found in the skeleton, it is not surprising that considerable interest lies in the role of calcium and vitamin D (which enhances calcium absorption) in bone health. Scientific evidence indicates that increasing calcium and/or vitamin D intake has a beneficial impact on bone health. Amongst all the milk products cheese is the major source of calcium. Cheese is also rich in other nutrients important to bone health such as vitamin D, protein, phosphorus, magnesium, vitamin A, vitamin B_6 and trace elements such as zinc.

Cheese and oral health

Cheese is a rich source of minerals. The mineral content of cheese varies both within and among various varieties. Cheddar cheese contains 721 mg and cottage cheese 32 mg calcium per 100 g. Generally, cheeses that are high in calcium contain other minerals such as magnesium in appreciable amount. Studies in experimental animals and in human beings have demonstrated that intake of natural and processed cheese reduces the risk of tooth decay. Dental caries and periodontal diseases are the two most prevalent, but preventable oral diseases. The elderly are particularly at high risk of developing these diseases. Food intake has been recognised as a contributing factor to dental caries. Components in cheese such as calcium and phosphorus may inhibit demineralisation and favour the remineralisation of teeth.

Non-cariogenicity of cheese

Human dental pH studies have shown that a number of cheeses such as aged Cheddar, Swiss, Blue, Mozzarella, Gouda, etc. produce little or no plaque acidity. Most of these cheeses have been demonstrated to eliminate sucrose induced decrease in the plaque pH when consumed just prior to or after sucrose intake. Skimmed milk powder has been ranked as the food with the lowest potential cariogenicity. Therefore, consuming cheese before, during, or after a meal may reduce the risk of dental caries. Demineralisation/Remineralisation Cheese and milk consumption have been reported to prevent demineralisation of enamel and favour its remineralisation. Consumption of aged cheddar cheese immediately after sucrose intake dramatically reduces sucrose-induced demineralisation of enamel. Processed cheese also has been shown to prevent demineralisation and enhance remineralisation of enamel and root lesions.

Cheese and lactose intolerance

It has been estimated that about 75 per cent of the world's adult population have a genetically controlled limited ability to digest lactose, the principal carbohydrate in milk and other dairy foods. This condition is called lactose non-persistence. Limited digestion of lactose can lead to unpleasant gastrointestinal symptoms of varying severity, termed lactose intolerance. During the manufacture of cheese, most of the lactose is removed with the whey. In addition, any residual lactose is transformed into lactic acid, which inhibits the growth of undesirable bacteria. Due to their low lactose content, cheeses, especially natural aged or ripened cheeses such as Swiss and Cheddar are suitable foods to individuals who are lactose intolerant. Lactose content of dairy products are given in Table 6.7.

Table 6.7. Lactose content of dairy products.

Product	Lactose (g)
Milk (1 cup)	
Whole	9–12
2% reduce fat	9–13
1% low fat	12–13
Fat free	11–14
Chocolate	10–12
Buttermilk	9–12
Evaporated	24–28
Sweetened condensed	31–50
Lactaid (lactose-reduced low-fat milk)	3
Goat's milk	11–12
Acidophilus, skim	11
Yoghurt, low-fat (1 cup)	4–17
Cheese (1 oz.)	0.7–4
Cottage (1/2 cup)	0.4–0.6
Cheddar, sharp	0.5–1
Swiss Mozzarella, part skim, low moisture	0.08–0.9
American, pasteurised, processed	0.5–4
Ricotta (1/2 cup)	0.3–6
Cream	0.1–0.8
Butter (1 pat)	0.04–0.05
Cream (1 tbsp.)	
Light	0.6
Whipping	0.4–0.5
Sour	0.4–0.5
Ice cream (1/2 cup)	2–6
Ice milk (1/2 cup)	5
Sherbet (1/2 cup)	0.6–2

Probiotical attributes

Cheese is a bio-enriched food the enrichment being brought about by vitamins and micronutrients produced as metabolites of the starter bacteria. A 'probiotic' can be defined as a viable mono- or mixed culture of micro-organisms which, applied to animal or man, beneficially affects the host by improving the properties of the indigenous microflora. The beneficial effects of cheese and fermented milk products as health foods have been clinically established. The most beneficial among the lactic acid bacteria (LAB) are the lactobacilli and the bifidobacteria. Various nutritional, probiotical and physiological benefits of fermented milks including cheeses in the gastrointestinal tract (GIT), for decreasing harmful bacteria, have been well documented. Specific microbial strains could play an important role in colonisation resistance in the intestinal respiratory and progenitor tracts, cholesterol metabolism, inhibiting carcinogenesis and the metabolism of lactose, absorption of calcium and the synthesis of vitamins.

Many formulated foods have today made a major impact on traditional foods and beverages. Popular cheese products include cheese butter spread, flavoured processed cheese in cans, cheese slices, cheese sauces and cheese powder for soups, etc. Pizza is one of the fastest growing segments in the food industry and major ingredient of pizza is Mozzarella cheese.

Natural cheeses

A simplified overview of the steps involved in processing fresh and ripened natural cheeses is presented in Fig. 6.3. Fresh cheeses are consumed immediately after processing and are characterised as having a high moisture content and mild flavour. In most cases, lactic acid produced by the starter cultures cause the precipitation of the caseins.

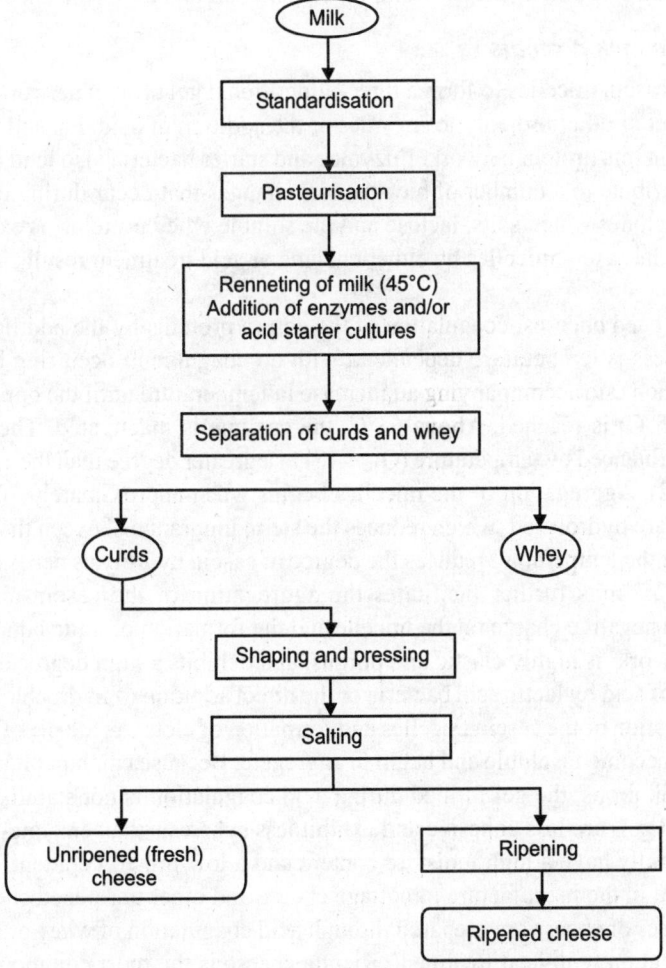

Fig. 6.3. Processing scheme for natural cheeses.

The final pH of the acid-coagulated cheeses in 4.6. Ripened cheeses undergo a ripening period, ranging from 3 weeks to more than 2 years, following processing, which contributes to the development of the flavour and texture of the cheese. The moisture content of these cheeses ranges from 30 to 55 per cent and the pH ranges from 5.0 to 5.3. Rennet is primarily used for the coagulation of the casein proteins and curd formation. Starter cultures are added to produce acid and contribute enzymes for flavour and texture development during ripening.

Standardisation of the milk

The casein and fat content of the milk are standardised to minimise variations in the quality of the cheese due to seasonal effects and variation in the milk supply. The casein-to-fat ratio can be adjusted by the addition of skim milk, cream, milk powder, or evaporated milk or the removal of fat. Calcium chloride (0.1 per cent) may also be added to improve coagulation of the milk by rennet and further processing of the cheese. The actual casein and fat content of the milk will vary for each cheese type and influence the curd formation, cheese yield, fat content and texture of the cheese.

Coagulation of the milk proteins

Aggregation of the casein micelles to form a three-dimensional gel protein network is initiated through the addition of rennet or other proteolytic enzymes or the addition of acid. Fat and water molecules are also entrapped within this protein network. Enzymes and starter bacteria also tend to associate with the curds, and thus contribute to a number of biochemical changes that occur during the ripening process. The whey, which includes water, salts, lactose and the soluble whey proteins, is expelled from the gel. The aggregation of the casein micelles by either enzyme or acid treatment results in gels with different characteristics.

In most natural, aged cheeses, coagulation of the casein proteins by the addition of rennet is most common. This process is temperature dependent, with no coagulation occurring below 10°C, and an increase in coagulation rate accompanying an increase in temperature until the optimal temperature for coagulation (40°–45°C) is reached. Above 65°C, the enzyme is inactivated. The aggregation of the casein micelles is influenced by temperature ($Q_{10} \sim 12$) to a greater degree than the enzymatic hydrolysis of κ-casein ($Q_{10} \sim 2$). Aggregation of the micelles begins when approximately 70–85 per cent of the κ-casein molecules are hydrolysed, which reduces the steric hindrance between the micelles. Reducing the pH or increasing the temperature reduces the degree of casein hydrolysis necessary for coagulation. The presence of Ca^{2+} ions further facilitates the aggregation of the casein micelles through the neutralisation of the negative charge on the micelle and the formation of ionic bonds. The resulting gel has an irregular network, is highly elastic and porous, and exhibits a high degree of syneresis.

The production of acid by lactic acid bacteria or the direct addition of hydrochloric or lactic acid can also result in aggregation of the casein micelles and formation of clots. As the pH of the milk is reduced, the casein micelles become insoluble and begin to aggregate. Because calcium phosphate is solubilised as the pH of the milk drops, the gel formed during acid coagulation is not stabilised by calcium ions. The acid-coagulated gels are less cohesive and exhibit less syneresis than enzyme-coagulated cheeses. These cheeses generally have a high moisture content and a low mineral content. Acid coagulation is most frequently used in the manufacture of cottage cheese and other unripened cheeses.

A few unique types of cheese are prepared through acid coagulation of whey or a blend of whey and skim milk in conjunction with heat treatment. Ricotta cheese is the most common cheese prepared in this manner.

Lactic acid bacteria (LAB) cultures are added to the milk in conjunction with the rennet. Although the LAB cultures do not have a significant role in the coagulation of casein, they contribute to the changes that occur during the ripening process. The different strains of starter cultures differ in such characteristics as growth rate, metabolic rate, phage interactions, proteolytic activity, and flavour promotion. Frequently, mixed-strain cultures, which contain unknown numbers of strains of the same species are used.

Mesophilic L cultures contain *Leuconostoc* species, including *Ln. mesenteroides* spp. *cremoris* and *Ln. lactis*, while the main species in mesophilic D cultures are *Lactococcus lactis* ssp. *cremoris* with lesser amounts of *Lc. lactis* ssp. *lactis*. Mesophilic DL cultures would consist of both lactococci and leuconostocs. The thermophilic cultures consist of *Streptococcus thermophilus* and one of the following: *Lactobacillus helveticus*, *Lb. delbrueckii* ssp. *lactis* or *Lb. delbrueckii* ssp. *bulgaricus*.

Cutting the coagulum

Cutting the coagulum increases the drainage of the whey from the curds and contributes to a sharp decrease in the moisture content of the curds. Acid-coagulated and rennet-coagulated cheeses differ in the pH at which curd formation occurs and, subsequently, the pH at which the coagulum is cut. For acid-coagulated cheeses, curd formation occurs at pH 4.6, the isoelectric point of casein. Curd formation of rennet-coagulated cheeses occurs at higher pH, ranging from pH 6.3 to 6.6. Following the cutting of the coagulum, the curd and whey mixture is heated and agitated in a process called 'scalding'. The agitation is necessary to keep the curds suspended in the whey and to promote drainage of whey from the curds. The temperature during the scalding process is dependent on the type of the cheese and ranges from 20° to 55°C. The temperature affects gel formation and gel viscoelasticity and regulates the growth of the lactic acid bacteria. A high temperature results in greater drainage from the cheese and a firmer cheese.

The conversion of lactose to lactic acid by starter cultures decreases the pH of the curd, which contributes to the loss of whey from the curd and a decrease in moisture content. While the curds are in the whey, diffusion of lactic acid into the whey and lactose into the curds occurs. The rate of acid production is affected by the amount and type of the starter culture, the composition of the milk, and the temperature during acid production.

When the required acidity of the cheese curds is reached, the whey is drained to recover the curds. Following the separation of the curds from the whey, acid production continues at an increased rate, because of the lack of diffusion of the lactic acid from the curd. To minimise excess acid development following the drainage of the whey, some types of cheese include a washing step to reduce the lactose content. The moisture content of the curd is affected by the extent the coagulum is cut, the temperature of the curd after cutting, and agitation of the curd in the whey.

The handling of the curd following the cutting of the coagulum greatly affects the characteristics of the cheese. The cheddaring process, used in the manufacture of Cheddar, Colby, Monterey and mozzarella cheeses, involves piling blocks of curd on top of each other, with regular turning to allow the curds to fuse together. In Colby and Monterey cheeses, vigorous stirring during the drainage of the whey inhibits the development of a curd structure and results in a softer cheese with a higher moisture content. Frequently, the whey may be partially drained off and replaced with water or salt brine to remove lactose and reduce the development of acidity, as is done in the processing of Gouda and Limburger cheeses.

Shaping and pressing

The resulting curds are shaped to form a coherent mass that is easy to handle. The curds are placed in a mould and are often pressed with an external force to cause the curds to deform and fuse. The pressure and time of pressing ranges from a few grams per square centimetre for a few minutes for moist cheeses to 200–500 g/cm^2 for up to 16-48 hours for cooked and hard cheeses. The temperature (20°–27°C) and humidity (95 per cent relative humidity) of the pressing room is controlled to optimise the growth of the lactic acid bacteria and facilitate the deformation and shaping of the curd. Acid production by LAB and additional drainage of whey from the curd continues during the shaping and pressing stage. Deformability is affected by the composition of the cheese, and it increases until the curds reach a pH of 5.2–5.3. Deformability also increases with an increase in moisture content and temperature.

Salting

The salting step reduces the moisture content of the curd, inhibits the growth of starter bacteria and affects the flavour, preservation, texture, and rate of ripening of the cheese. The final salt content of cheese ranges from 0.7 to 4 per cent (2–10 per cent salt in moisture content). The amount of salt, the method of application of the salt and the timing of the salting is dependent on the specific type of cheese. The salt may be incorporated through: (i) mixing with drymilled curd pieces, (ii) rubbing onto the surface of the moulded cheese, and (iii) immersing the cheese in a salt brine. Following the salting step, the salt diffuses into the interior of the cheese, with the subsequent displacement of whey. Depending on the size of the cheese block and the composition of the cheese, it may take from 7 days to over 4 months for the salt to equilibrate within the cheese.

Ripening

Fresh, green cheese has a bland flavour and a smooth, rubbery texture. During the ripening process, the characteristic texture and flavour of the cheese develop through a complex series of biochemical reactions. Ripening starter cultures are selected to develop the texture and flavour characteristics of the specific cheese type. Enzymes released following lysis of the micro-organisms catalyse the degradation of proteins, lipids and lactose in the cheese. As the ripening time increases, the moisture content of the cheese decreases and the intensity of the flavour increases. The resulting quality attributes of the finished cheese depend not only on the initial composition of the milk and the starter cultures used, but also on the water activity of the cheeses and the temperature, time and humidity during the ripening period. Depending on the type of cheese, the ripening period can range from 3 weeks to more than 2 years.

The ripening temperature influences the rate of the microbia growth and enzyme activity during the process and the equilibrium between the biochemical reactions that occurs during ripening. Ripening temperatures generally range from 5° to 20°C, which is well below the optimum temperatures for microbial growth and enzyme activity. Soft cheeses are often ripened at 4°C to slow the biochemical processes. An increase in ripening temperature for hard cheeses reduces the ripening time necessary for flavour development, with a 5°C increase in ripening temperature reducing the ripening time 2 to 3 months. However, caution must be exercised in altering ripening temperatures since not all micro-organisms and enzymes respond to temperature changes in the same manner, resulting in an imbalance in flavour characteristics.

The growth of most of the starter bacteria added to the milk in the initial stages of cheese making is slowed as the pH of the cheese approaches 5.7 and following the addition of salt, but fermentation and the decrease in pH continue. The fermentation of lactose to lactic acid by the starter cultures provides an environment that prevents the growth of undesirable micro-organisms through reduced pH and the formation of an anaerobic environment. The optimal activity for proteases is between pH 5.5 and 6.5 and that for lipases is between pH 6.5 and 7.5.

Protease and lipase activity during the ripening is probably most important to the development of the flavour and texture of the cheese. Enzymes of the starter bacteria, nonstarter lactic acid bacteria, and secondary cultures added during cheese making are most important in the development of the flavour and texture of the cheese during ripening. These enzymes are released by the lysis of the cell wall of the bacteria. Rennet enzymes and endogenous milk enzymes, such as plasmin, also contribute to these hydrolytic reactions during ripening. The extent of these enzymatic reactions depends on the activity and specificity of the enzymes, the concentration of the substrates, pH, water activity, salt concentration and ripening temperature and duration. The degradation of the amino acids and fatty acids, through enzymatic and nonenzymatic reactions, result in the formation of several important volatile flavour compounds, including sulphur-containing compounds, amines, aldehydes, alcohols, esters and lactones. Rennet and plasmin are associated with the primary phase of proteolysis and hydrolyse the caseins to large polypeptides. This proteolysis alters the three-dimensional protein network of the cheese to form a less firm and less elastic cheese. Although these polypeptides do not have a direct impact on flavour, they do function as a substrate for the proteases associated with the starter and nonstarter bacteria. However, if the primary proteolysis is extensive, bitter peptides, with a high percentage of hydrophobic amino acids, predominate. Free amino acids and short-chain peptides contribute sweet, bitter and brothy-like taste characteristics to the cheese. Further degradation and chemical reactions of these peptides and amino acids through the action of decarboxylases, transaminases, or deaminases contribute to the formation of amines, acids, ammonia and thiols, which contribute to cheese flavour.

Lipases break down triglycerides into free fatty acids and mono- and diglycerides. The short-chain free fatty acids contribute to the sharp, pungent flavour characteristics of the cheese. The degree of lipolysis that is acceptable without producing soapy and rancid flavours depends on the type of cheese. Several *Penicillium* strains form methyl ketones, lactones and unsaturated alcohols through their enzymatic systems associated with β-oxidation and decarboxylation, β-oxidation and lactonisation, and lipoxygenase activity. Aliphatic and aromatic esters are synthesised by esterases present in a range of micro-organisms, including mesophilic and thermophilic LAB.

The texture of cheese is attributed to the three-dimensional protein network that entraps fat and whey. This structure is altered through proteolysis during ripening to form a less firm and less elastic cheese.

Carbon dioxide produced by the metabolism of the bacteria and entrapped within the curd results in the formation of eyes in several types of cheeses. The small eyes characteristics of Edam, Gouda and related cheese varieties are formed by carbon dioxide produced from citrate by the *Leuconostoc* ssp. In Swiss type cheeses, *Propionibacterium freudenreichii* ssp. *shermanii* metabolise lactate to form the carbon dioxide responsible for the eye formation. These cheeses are ripened in hot rooms (20°–22°C) to optimise the growth of the propionibacteria and allow eye formation.

Ripening of cheese is a time-intensive process, thus, there is much interest in accelerating the ripening process without an adverse effect on cheese quality. The addition of attenuated starters or a mixture of enzymes has been explored as a possible means to shorten the ripening processing. An important consideration is that increased proteolysis or an imbalance of enzyme activity can result in higher contents of hydrophobic amino acids and peptides that contribute to bitterness.

Processed Cheese

Processed cheeses are produced by blending and heating several natural cheeses with emulsifiers, water, butterfat, whey powder, and/or caseinates to form a homogeneous mixture. The proportion of cheese used in the formulation ranges from 51 per cent for cheese spreads and cheese foods to 98 per cent in processed cheeses. Different types of natural cheeses will produce processed cheeses with different flavour and textural characteristics. The formulation of these ingredients affects the consistency, texture, flavour and melting characteristics of the processed cheese. The heating process inactivates the micro-organisms and denatures enzymes to produce a stable product. The flavour of the processed cheese is generally milder than the natural cheeses, due to the effects of the heat. However, the melting properties of the processed cheese are much improved due to the addition of the emulsifiers. Processed cheeses range in consistency from block cheese to sliced cheese to cheese for spreading.

Butter

Butter is commonly sold in sticks or blocks, and frequently served with the use of a butter knife. Butter is a dairy product made by churning fresh or fermented cream or milk. It is generally used as a spread and a condiment, as well as in cooking applications such as baking, sauce making and frying. Butter consists of butterfat, water and milk proteins.

Most frequently made from cows' milk, butter can also be manufactured from that of other mammals, including sheep, goats, buffalo and yaks. Salt, flavourings and preservatives are sometimes added to butter. Rendering butter produces clarified butter or ghee, which is almost entirely butterfat.

Butter is an emulsion which remains a solid when refrigerated, but softens to a spreadable consistency at room temperature, and melts to a thin liquid consistency at $32°–35°C$ ($90°–95°F$). The density of butter is 911 kg/m^3 (1535.5 lb/yd^3).

It generally has a pale yellow colour, but varies from deep yellow to nearly white. Its colour is dependent on the animal's feed and is commonly manipulated with food colourings in the commercial manufacturing process, most commonly annatto or carotene

In general use, the term 'butter' refers to the spread dairy product when unqualified by other descriptors. The word commonly is used to describe puréed vegetable or nut products such as peanut butter and almond butter. It is often applied to spread fruit products such as apple butter. Fats such as cocoa butter and shea butter that remain solid at room temperature are also known as 'butters'. In addition to the act of applying butter being called 'to butter', non-dairy items that have a dairy butter consistency may use 'butter' to call that consistency to mind, including food items such as maple butter and Witch's butter and non-food items such as baby bottom butter, hyena butter and rock butter.

Flavour and consistency are the most important quality attributes to consider during the processing of butter. The characteristic flavour of butter is a result of the formation of diacetyl by heterofermentative LAB. Off-flavours due to lipolysis, oxidation or other contaminants should be avoided. The butter should be firm enough to hold its shape, yet soft enough to spread easily. Figure 6.4 outlines the process involved for making butter and the by-product buttermilk.

The first step in the processing of butter is skimming the milk to obtain cream with a fat content of at least 35 per cent, in which the fat is dispersed as droplets within the aqueous phase. This step increases the efficiency of the process through increasing the yield of butter, reducing the yield of buttermilk and reducing the size of machinery needed. The function of the pasteurisation step is to kill micro-organisms, inactivate enzymes, and make the butter less susceptible to oxidative degradation. Following pasteurisation, the cream is inoculated with a starter culture mixture (1–2 per cent) of *Lactococcus* ssp.

and *Leuconostoc* ssp., which contributes to the development of the characteristic butler flavour. It is desirable that the starter cultures grow rapidly at low temperatures. During ripening, the cream begins to ferment and the fat begins to crystallise. The formation of lactic acid and diacetyl by the starter cultures contributes to flavour development in the butter and buttermilk.

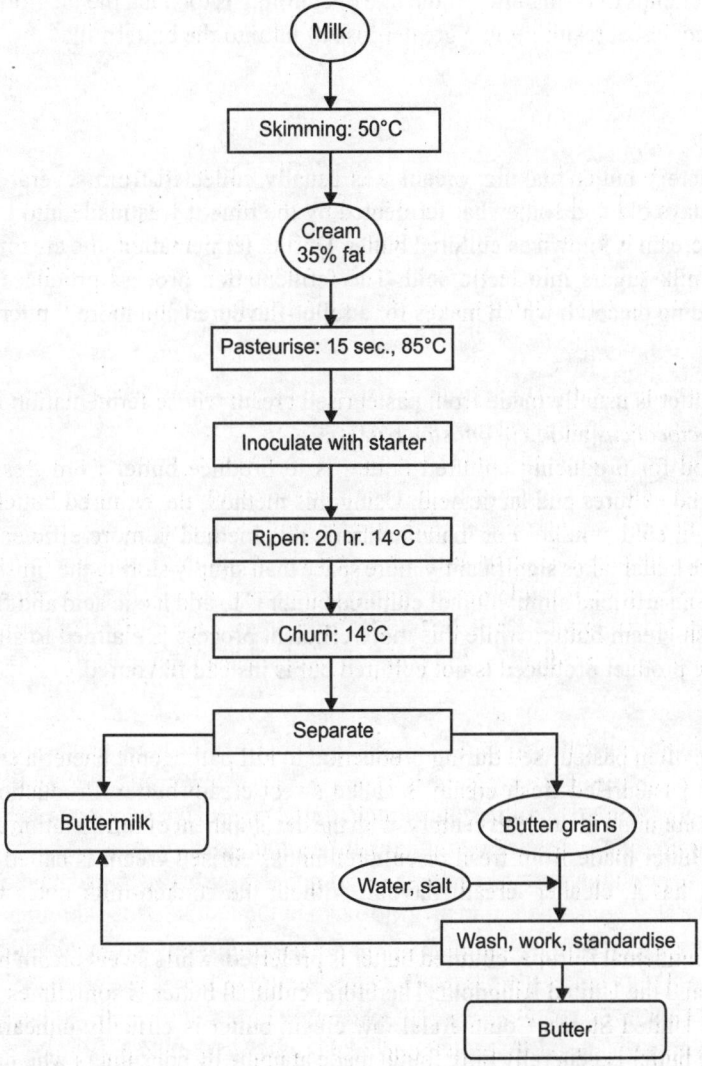

Fig. 6.4. Processing scheme for butter processed from ripened cream.

Crystallisation of the fat is important to maximise the yield of the butter and minimise loss of fat into the buttermilk during the churning process. During the churning process, air is incorporated into the cream using dashboards or rotary agitators, contributing to the aggregation of fat globules to form butter granules. The resulting butter grains may be washed with water to remove nonfat solids, followed by working or kneading the butter grains. During the working step, a water-in-oil emulsion is formed as the small water droplets are dispersed into the fat matrix.

The churning process is probably most critical to the textural quality of the butter. As air is incorporated into the cream, the fat globules surround the air bubbles and coalesce with other fat-coated air bubbles to form clumps. These clumps continue to coalesce during the churning process, and the volume of air bubbles decreases. The proportion of solid fat, which is influenced by temperature, is critical to the aggregation of fat clumps to form butter. If the rate of churning is too fast, the fat globules are less stable and less likely to coalesce, resulting in a greater loss of fat into the buttermilk.

Types of butter

Hand-made butter

Before modern factory butter making, cream was usually collected from several milkings and was therefore several days old and somewhat fermented by the time it was made into butter. Butter made from a fermented cream is known as cultured butter. During fermentation, the cream naturally sours as bacteria convert milk sugars into lactic acid. The fermentation process produces additional aroma compounds, including diacetyl, which makes for a fuller-flavoured and more 'buttery' tasting product.

Cultured butter

Today, cultured butter is usually made from pasteurised cream whose fermentation is produced by the introduction of *Lactococcus* and *Leuconostoc* bacteria.

Another method for producing cultured butter, is to produce butter from fresh cream and then incorporate bacterial cultures and lactic acid. Using this method, the cultured butter flavour grows as the butter is aged in cold storage. For manufacturers, this method is more efficient since ageing the cream used to make butter takes significantly more space than simply storing the finished butter product. A method to make an artificial simulation of cultured butter is to add lactic acid and flavour compounds directly to the fresh-cream butter; while this more efficient process is claimed to simulate the taste of cultured butter, the product produced is not cultured but is instead flavoured.

Sweet butter

Dairy products are often pasteurised during production to kill pathogenic bacteria and other microbes. Butter made from pasteurised fresh cream is called sweet cream butter. Production of sweet cream butter first became common in the 19th century, with the development of refrigeration and the mechanical cream separator. Butter made from fresh or cultured unpasteurised cream is called raw cream butter. Raw cream butter has a 'cleaner' cream flavour, without the cooked-milk notes that pasteurisation introduces.

Throughout Continental Europe, cultured butter is preferred, while sweet cream butter dominates in the United States and the United Kingdom. Therefore, cultured butter is sometimes labelled European style butter in the United States. Commercial raw cream butter is virtually unheard-of in the United States. Raw cream butter is generally only found made at home by consumers who have purchased raw whole milk directly from dairy farmers, skimmed the cream themselves, and made butter with it. It is rare in Europe as well.

Spreadable butter

Several spreadable butters have been developed; these remain softer at colder temperatures and are therefore easier to use directly out of refrigeration. Some modify the make-up of the butter's fat through chemical manipulation of the finished product, some through manipulation of the cattle's feed, and some by incorporating vegetable oils into the butter. Whipped butter, another product designed to be more spreadable, is aerated via the incorporation of nitrogen gas—normal air is not used, because doing so would encourage oxidation and rancidity.

All categories of butter are sold either in salted and unsalted forms. Either granular salt or a strong brine are added to salted butter during processing. In addition to enhanced flavour, the addition of salt acts as a preservative.

The amount of butterfat in the finished product is a vital aspect of production. In the United States, products sold as 'butter' are required to contain a minimum of 80 per cent butterfat; in practice most American butters contain only slightly more than that, averaging around 81 per cent butterfat. European butters generally have a higher ratio, which may extend up to 85 per cent.

Clarified butter

Clarified butter is butter with almost all of its water and milk solids removed, leaving almost-pure butterfat. Clarified butter is made by heating butter to its melting point and then allowing it to cool off; after settling, the remaining components separate by density. At the top, whey proteins form a skin which is removed, and the resulting butterfat is then poured off from the mixture of water and casein proteins that settle to the bottom.

Ghee is clarified butter which is brought to higher temperatures of around 120°C (250°F) once the water has cooked off, allowing the milk solids to brown. This process flavours the ghee, and also produces antioxidants which help protect it longer from rancidity. Because of this, ghee can keep for six to eight months under normal conditions.

Different varieties are found around the world. Smen is a spiced Moroccan clarified butter, buried in the ground and aged for months or years.

Yak butter

Yak butter is important in Tibet; tsampa, barley flour mixed with yak butter, is a staple food. Butter tea is consumed in the Himalayan regions of Tibet, Bhutan, Nepal and India. It consists of tea served with intensely flavoured or 'rancid' yak butter and salt. In African and Asian developing nations, butter is traditionally made from sour milk rather than cream. It can take several hours of churning to produce workable butter grains from fermented.

Storage and cooking

Normal butter softens to a spreadable consistency around 15°C (60°F), well above refrigerator temperatures. The 'butter compartment' found in many refrigerators may be one of the warmer sections inside, but it still leaves butter quite hard. Until recently, many refrigerators sold in New Zealand featured a 'butter conditioner', a compartment kept warmer than the rest of the refrigerator—but still cooler than room temperature—with a small heater. Keeping butter tightly wrapped delays rancidity, which is hastened by exposure to light or air, and also helps prevent it from picking up other odours. Wrapped butter has a shelf life of several months at refrigerator temperatures.

'French butter dishes' or 'Acadian butter dishes' involve a lid with a long interior lip, which sits in a container holding a small amount of water. Usually the dish holds just enough water to submerge the interior lip when the dish is closed. Butter is packed into the lid. The water acts as a seal to keep the butter fresh, and also keeps the butter from overheating in hot temperatures. This allows butter to be safely stored on the counter-top for several days without spoilage.

Once butter is softened, spices, herbs or other flavouring agents can be mixed into it, producing what is called a compound butter or composite butter (sometimes also called composed butter). Compound butters can be used as spreads, or cooled, sliced, and placed onto hot food to melt into a sauce. Sweetened compound butters can be served with desserts; such hard sauces are often flavoured with spirits.

Melted butter plays an important role in the preparation of sauces, most obviously in French cuisine. Beurre noisette (hazel butter) and Beurre noir (black butter) are sauces of melted butter cooked until the milk solids and sugars have turned golden or dark brown; they are often finished with an addition of vinegar or lemon juice. Hollandaise and béarnaise sauces are emulsions of egg yolk and melted butter; they are in essence mayonnaises made with butter instead of oil. Hollandaise and béarnaise sauces are stabilised with the powerful emulsifiers in the egg yolks, but butter itself contains enough emulsifiers— mostly remnants of the fat globule membranes —to form a stable emulsion on its own. Beurre blanc (white butter) is made by whisking butter into reduced vinegar or wine, forming an emulsion with the texture of thick cream. Beurre monté (prepared butter) is melted but still emulsified butter; it lends its name to the practice of 'mounting' a sauce with butter: whisking cold butter into any water-based sauce at the end of cooking, giving the sauce a thicker body and a glossy shine as well as a buttery taste.

In Poland, the butter lamb (Baranek wielkanocny) is a traditional addition to the Easter meal for many Polish Catholics. Butter is shaped into a lamb either by hand or in a lamb-shaped mould.

Butter is used for sautéing and frying, although its milk solids brown and burn above 150°C (250°F) a rather low temperature for most applications. The smoke point of butterfat is around 200°C (400°F), so clarified butter or ghee is better suited to frying. Ghee has always been a common frying medium in India, where many avoid other animal fats for cultural or religious reasons.

Butter fills several roles in baking, where it is used in a similar manner as other solid fats like lard, suet, or shortening, but has a flavour that may better complement sweet baked goods. Many cookie doughs and some cake batters are leavened, at least in part, by creaming butter and sugar together, which introduces air bubbles into the butter. The tiny bubbles locked within the butter expand in the heat of baking and aerate the cookie or cake. Some cookies like shortbread may have no other source of moisture but the water in the butter. Pastries like pie dough incorporate pieces of solid fat into the dough, which become flat layers of fat when the dough is rolled out. During baking, the fat melts away, leaving a flaky texture. Butter, because of its flavour, is a common choice for the fat in such a dough, but it can be more difficult to work with than shortening because of its low melting point. Pastry makers often chill all their ingredients and utensils while working with a butter dough.

Health and nutrition

According to Smith, one tablespoon of butter (14 grams/0.5 ounces) contains 420 kilojoules (100 kcal), all from fat, 11 grams (0.4 oz) of fat, of which 7 grams (0.25 oz) are saturated fat and 30 milligrams (0.46 gram) of cholesterol. In other words, butter consists mostly of saturated fat and is a significant source of dietary cholesterol. For these reasons, butter has been generally considered to be a contributor to health problems, especially heart disease. For many years, vegetable margarine was recommended as a substitute, since it is an unsaturated fat and contains little or no cholesterol. In recent decades, though, it has become accepted that the *trans* fats contained in partially hydrogenated oils used in typical margarines significantly raise undesirable LDL cholesterol levels as well. Trans-fat free margarines have since been developed.

Butter contains only traces of lactose, so moderate consumption of butter is not a problem for the lactose intolerant. People with milk allergies need to avoid butter, which contains enough of the allergy-causing proteins to cause reactions.

Butter can form a useful role in dieting by providing satiety. A small amount added to low fat foods such as vegetables may stave off feelings of hunger. Comparative properties of common cooking fats are listed in Table 6.8.

Table 6.8. Comparative properties of common cooking fats (per 100 g).

	Total fat	Saturated fat	Monounsaturated fat	Polyunsaturated fat	Protein fat
Butter	81g	51 g	21 g	3 g	1 g
Vegetable shortening (hydrogenated)	71 g	23 g	8 g	37 g	0 g
Olive oil	100 g	14 g	73 g	11 g	0 g
Lard	100 g	39 g	45 g	11 g	0 g

Buttermilk

Natural buttermilk is a by-product of butter manufacture (Fig. 6.5) and is categorised as sweet (nonfermented) or acidic (fermented). Sweet and acid buttermilk are obtained from the manufacture of butter from nonfermented, sweet cream and sour or cultured cream, respectively. The fat content of natural buttermilk is approximately 0.4 per cent and consists primarily of the membrane components of the fat globules. Because of the high content of unsaturated fatty acids associated with the membrane lipids, natural buttermilk has a characteristic flavour and is also more susceptible to the development of oxidised off-flavours.

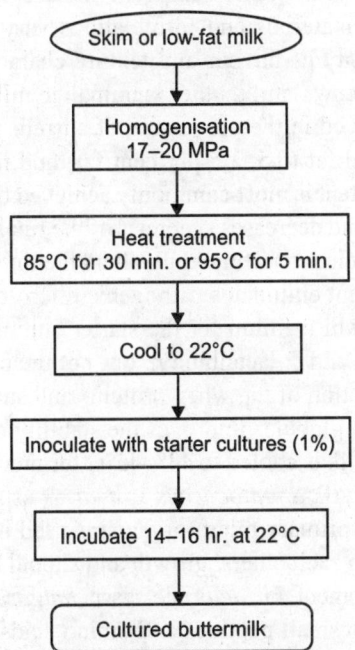

Fig. 6.5. Processing scheme for cultured buttermilk.

Cultured buttermilk and cultured skim milk are more frequently produced as alternatives to the traditional buttermilk (Fig. 6.5). The solids-not-fat and fat content of cultured buttermilk range from

7.4–11.4 per cent and 0.25–1.9 per cent, respectively. The homogenised and pasteurised milk with the desired fat content is inoculated with a 1 per cent starter culture of *Lc. lactis* ssp. *lactis* and *Lc. lactis* biovar. *diacetylactis* and *Ln. mesenteroides* ssp. *cremoris*. These bacteria metabolise citrate to diacetyl to contribute to the development of 'buttery' flavour. Acid is produced by these bacteria at a relatively slow rate.

Sour Cream

Sour cream is produced from pasteurised, homogenised cream (20–30 per cent fat) and has a pleasant acidic taste and buttery aroma (Fig. 6.6). Low-fat sour cream has a fat content ranging from 10 to 12 per cent. Following standardisation of the milk and cream to the desired fat content, the mixture is warmed and homogenised to improve the consistency of the final product. The starter cultures include *Lc. lactis* ssp. *lactis* and *Lc. lactis* biovar. *diacetylactis* and *Ln. mesenteroides* ssp. *cremoris*. As in buttermilk, these cultures contribute to the acid and buttery flavour of the sour cream. The sour cream may be packaged prior to or following fermentation at 20°C until the pH is reduced to 4.5. Packaging prior to fermentation results in a thicker product because the gel is not disturbed. As the pH decreases, the fat clusters aggregate to form a viscous cream. Rennet or thickening agents are sometimes added to increase the firmness of the sour cream.

Yogurt

The tremendous increase in the popularity of yogurt in recent decades has been attributed to its health food image and the wide diversity of flavours, compositions, and viscosities available to consumers. The manufacturing methods, raw materials and formulations vary widely from country to country, resulting in products with a diversity of flavour and texture characteristics. While in many Western societies, yogurt is produced from cows' milk, other mammalian milks can be used to produce yogurt. Figure 6.7 outlines the steps involved in the processing of stirred- and set-style yogurts. The milk is initially standardised to the desired fat (0.5–3.5 per cent fat) and milk solids-not-fat (12.5 per cent) content. Increase in the protein content is most commonly achieved through the addition of nonfat milk powder, which improves the body and decreases syneresis of the final product. In addition to decreasing the size of the fat globule, homogenisation of the milk alters the milk proteins to reduce syneresis and increase firmness. The heat treatment eliminates pathogenic micro-organisms and reduces the oxygen in the milk to provide a good growth medium for the starter cultures. Enzymes and the major whey proteins, including β-lactoglobulin and α-lactalbumin, but not the casein proteins, are also denatured by the heat treatment. The denaturation of the whey proteins and subsequent interactions between the whey proteins and casein and/or fat globules improves the stability of the gel and decreases syneresis.

Following heat treatment, the milk is cooled to 43°–45°C for inoculation of the starter cultures. The fast acid-producing thermophilic LAB *Streptococcus salivarius* ssp. *thermophilus* and *Lactobacillus delbrueckii* ssp. *bulgaricus* are the primary micro-organisms used in the production of yogurt. These bacteria have a synergistic effect on each others' growth and should be present in approximately equal numbers for optimal flavour development. *Lb. delbrueckii* ssp. *bulgaricus* has important protease activity and hydrolyses the milk proteins to small peptides and amino acids. These peptides and amino acids enhance the growth of *S. thermophilus*, which has limited proteolytic activity. *S. thermophilus* metabolises pyruvic acid to formic acid and carbon dioxide, which in turn, stimulates the growth of *Lb. delbrueckii*. Initially, *S. thermophilus* grows faster than *Lb. delbrueckii*; however, at the later stages of the fermentation process, the growth of the *S. thermophilus* is inhibited by the reduced pH of the yogurt. The mutual stimulation of the yogurt cultures through their metabolic activity significantly increases the formation of lactic acid to a rate greater than would be possible by the individual cultures.

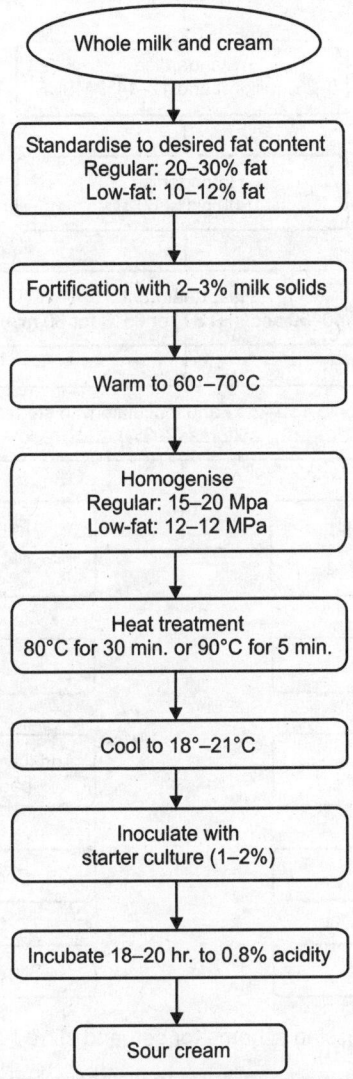

Fig. 6.6. Processing scheme for sour cream.

The acid production by the yogurt cultures results in the aggregation of casein micelles and gel formation. Two types of yogurt, set and stirred, are produced. Set-style yogurt is fermented following packaging, with colour and flavours added to the container prior to the addition of the inoculated milk, resulting in a gel that forms a firm, unbroken coagulum. Stirred yogurt is fermented in a vat prior to packaging, with the gel structure broken following fermentation during the addition of flavours and colours and during the cooling and packaging stages. For both types of yogurt, either a short incubation period at 4°–5°C for 2–3 hours or a long incubation period at 30°C for 16–18 hours may be used to attain a pH of 4.5 or titratable acidity of 0.9 per cent lactic acid prior to cooling.

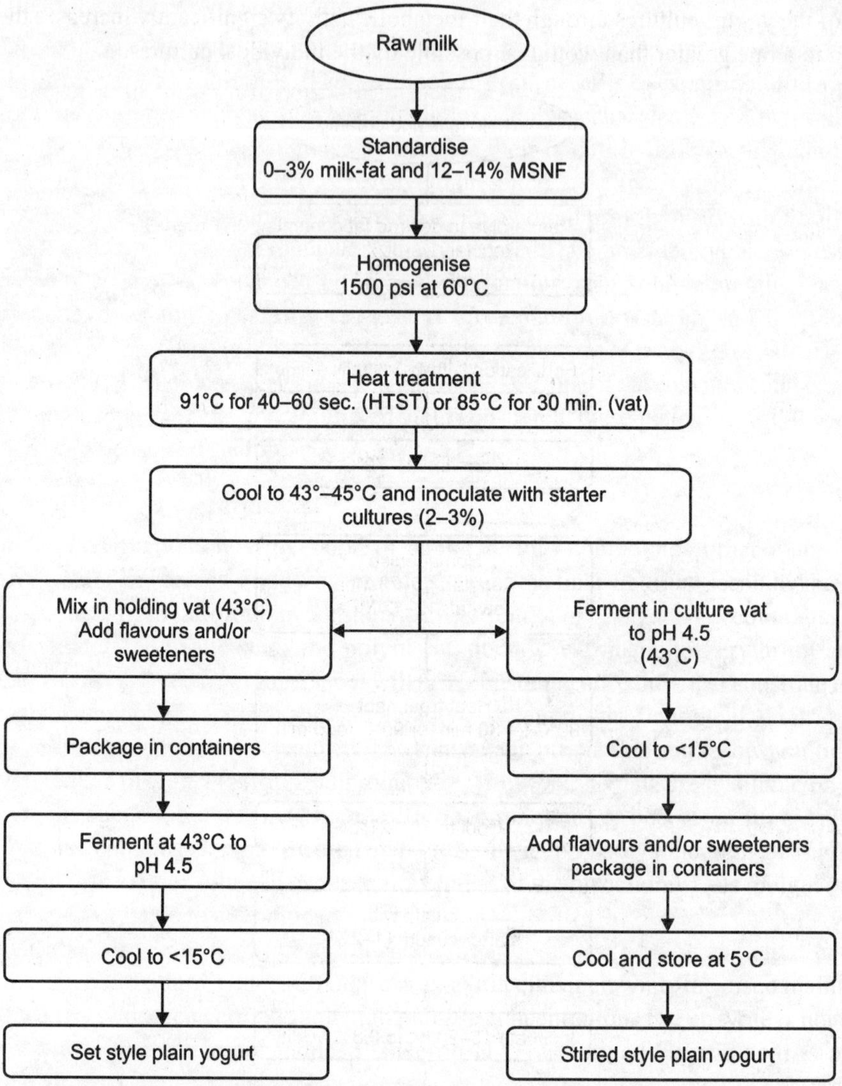

```
                          ┌─────────────┐
                          │  Raw milk   │
                          └─────────────┘
                                 │
                                 ▼
                    ┌──────────────────────────┐
                    │        Standardise        │
                    │ 0–3% milk-fat and 12–14% MSNF │
                    └──────────────────────────┘
                                 │
                                 ▼
                    ┌──────────────────────────┐
                    │        Homogenise         │
                    │     1500 psi at 60°C      │
                    └──────────────────────────┘
                                 │
                                 ▼
              ┌────────────────────────────────────────┐
              │            Heat treatment               │
              │ 91°C for 40–60 sec. (HTST) or 85°C for 30 min. (vat) │
              └────────────────────────────────────────┘
                                 │
                                 ▼
              ┌────────────────────────────────────────┐
              │ Cool to 43°–45°C and inoculate with starter │
              │              cultures (2–3%)             │
              └────────────────────────────────────────┘
```

Mix in holding vat (43°C) Add flavours and/or sweeteners ◄──────► Ferment in culture vat to pH 4.5 (43°C)

Package in containers | Cool to <15°C

Ferment at 43°C to pH 4.5 | Add flavours and/or sweeteners package in containers

Cool to <15°C | Cool and store at 5°C

Set style plain yogurt | Stirred style plain yogurt

Fig. 6.7. Processing scheme for set- and stirred-style yogurts.

The metabolism of the yogurt cultures contributes to the characteristic flavour of yogurt. Both bacteria are heterofermentative and produce lactic acid from glucose, yet are unable to metabolise galactose. Acetaldehyde, a key flavour component of yogurt, is produced by the degradation of threonine to acetaldehyde and glycine by the enzyme threonine aldolase. Although *S. thermophilus* forms a majority of the acetaldehyde produced, the proteolytic activity of *Lb. delbrueckii* ssp. *bulgaricus* generates the precursors for the formation of acetaldehyde.

Syneresis, the expelling of interstitial liquid due to association of the protein molecules and shrinkage of a gel network, is undesirable in yogurt. Syneresis increases with an increase in incubation temperature. In stirred yogurt, extensive syneresis results in a thin product. Therefore, incubation of the yogurt at a lower temperature, such as 32°C, is recommended to maintain the desirable viscosity.

Acidophilus Milk

Acidophilus milk was developed as a fluid milk product that provides therapeutic benefits through the alleviation of intestinal disorders. Following homogenisation and heat treatment of the milk to minimise contamination by other micro-organisms, the milk is cooled to 37°C and inoculated with a 1 per cent culture of *Lactobacillus acidophilus* (Fig. 6.8). The milk is incubated at this temperature for 18–24 hours until the titratable acidity reaches 0.63–0.72 per cent. *Lb. acidophilus* is a thermophilic starter that grows slowly in milk and has a relatively high acid tolerance. To provide the desired therapeutic effects, the milk should contain 5×10^8 cfu/ml at the time of consumption.

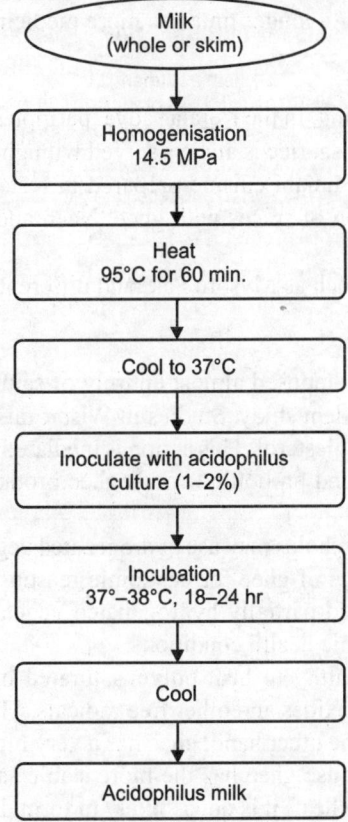

Fig. 6.8. Processing scheme for acidophilus milk.

Ghee

Ghee is made by simmering unsalted butter in a large pot until all water has boiled off and protein has settled to the bottom. The cooked and clarified butter is then spooned off to avoid disturbing the milk solids on the bottom of the pan. Unlike butter, ghee can be stored for extended periods without refrigeration, provided it is kept in an airtight container to prevent oxidation and remains moisture-free. Texture, colour or taste of ghee depends on the source of the milk from which the butter was made and the extent of boiling. In India, ghee is usually made with water buffalo's milk as it tends to be whiter than cow's milk.

Ayurvedic medicine attributes many physical and mental healing qualities to ghee, including the following:

1. Absorption: Ghee is an integral part of the practice of ayurvedic herbal formulation. Since ghee is an oil, it can bond with lipid-soluble nutrients and herbs to penetrate the lipid-based cell membranes of the body. It is stated to increase the potency of certain herbs by carrying the active components to the interior of the cells where they impart the most benefit.
2. Digestion: The ayurvedic texts say that ghee helps balance excess stomach acid, and helps maintain/repair the mucus lining of the stomach.
3. Mild burns: Like aloe, ghee is said to prevent blisters and scarring if applied quickly to affected skin. Also, ghee stored over a longer time has more medicinal value.

Usage in food

Ghee is widely used in Indian cooking. In the Kerala sadya, parippu is eaten with ghee. In many parts of India, especially in Bengal and Orissa, rice is always served with ghee. Ghee is an ingredient as well as used in the preparation of kadhi. Punjabi cuisine prepared in restaurants use large amounts of ghee. Masala is made by the combination of spices with ghee. Naan and roti are brushed with ghee either during preparation or while serving.

Ghee is used in Indian sweets such as Mysore Pak, and different varieties of halva and laddu.

Nutrition aspects

Like any clarified butter, ghee is composed almost entirely of saturated fat. Ghee has been shown to reduce serum cholesterol in one rodent study. Studies in Wistar rats have revealed one mechanism by which ghee reduces plasma LDL cholesterol. This action is mediated by an increased secretion of biliary lipids. The nutrition facts label found on bottled cow's ghee produced in the USA indicates 8 mg of cholesterol per teaspoon.

Indian restaurants and some households may use hydrogenated vegetable oil (also known as vanaspati, Dalda, or 'vegetable ghee') in place of ghee for economic reasons. This 'vegetable ghee' is actually polyunsaturated or monounsaturated partially hydrogenated vegetable oil, a trans fat. Trans fats are increasingly linked to serious chronic health conditions.

When cooking, it can be unhealthy to heat polyunsaturated oils such as vegetable oils to high temperatures. Doing so creates peroxides and other free radicals. These substances lead to a variety of health problems and diseases. On the other hand, ghee has a very high smoke point and doesn't burn or smoke easily during cooking. Because ghee has the more stable saturated bonds (i.e. it lacks double bonds which are easily damaged by heat) it is not as likely to form dangerous free radicals or advanced glycation end products when cooking. Ghee's short chain fatty acids are also metabolised very readily by the body, which would seem to negate concerns of its health effects. However, there is significant controversy between traditional oils and modern industrially processed oils which tends to heavily cloud the facts and issues surrounding oil consumption.

Ice Cream

Ice cream is a frozen dessert usually made from dairy products, such as milk and cream, combined with fruits or other ingredients. Most varieties contain sugar, although some are made with other sweeteners. In some cases, artificial flavourings and colourings are used in addition to (or in replacement of) the natural ingredients. This mixture is stirred slowly while cooling to prevent large ice crystals from forming; the result is a smoothly textured ice cream.

The meaning of the term ice cream varies from one country to another. Terms like frozen custard, frozen yogurt, sorbet, gelato and others are used to distinguish different varieties and styles. In some countries, like the USA, the term ice cream applies only to a specific variety, and their governments regulate the commercial use of all these terms based on quantities of ingredients. In others, like Italy and Argentina, one word is used for all the variants. Alternatives made from soya milk, rice milk and goat milk are available to those who are unable to enjoy traditional ice cream due to lactose intolerance or allergy to dairy protein.

The most common method for producing ice cream at home is to use an ice cream maker, in modern times generally an electrical device that churns the ice cream mixture while cooled inside a household freezer, or using a solution of pre-frozen salt and water, which gradually melts while the ice cream freezes. Some more expensive models have an inbuilt freezing element. A newer method of making home-made ice cream is to add liquid nitrogen to the mixture while stirring it using a spoon or spatula. Some ice cream recipes call for making a custard, folding in whipped cream, and immediately freezing the mixture.

Ice cream can be mass-produced and thus is widely available in developed parts of the world. Ice cream can be purchased in large cartons (vats and squrounds) from supermarkets and grocery stores, in smaller quantities from ice cream shops, convenience stores and milk bars, and in individual servings from small carts or vans at public events. In Turkey and Australia, ice cream is sometimes sold to beach-goers from small powerboats equipped with chest freezers. Some ice cream distributors sell ice cream products from travelling refrigerated vans or carts (commonly referred to in the US as 'ice cream trucks'), sometimes equipped with speakers playing children's music. Traditionally, ice cream vans in the United Kingdom make a music box noise rather than actual music.

ROLE OF CHEMICALS AND CHEMISTRY IN ICE CREAM

Most people are familiar with the appearance, taste and texture of ice cream. But certain ingredients and a time consuming preparation process are required as ice cream is an extremely complex, intricate and delicate substance. The science of ice cream consists of understanding its ingredients, processing, microstructure and texture, and crucially the links between them.

Ice cream is composed primarily of water (from milk and cream), with sweeteners such as corn syrup or sugar, flavourings, emulsifiers, stabilisers, milk solids and milk fat. The fat component adds richness of flavour, contributes to a smooth texture with creamy body and good meltdown, and adds lubrication to the plate as it is consumed. The components in milk solids also contribute to the flavour but more importantly improves the body and texture of the ice cream, offering some chew resistance and enhances the ability of the ice cream to hold its own.

Colour

The colour of ice cream has a significant influence on the consumer's perception of its flavour and quality. Colours are added for several reasons: to give colour to products that would otherwise be virtually colourless, to reinforce colours already present or to ensure uniformity of colours between different batches. Natural colours extracted from plants have been used as colouring agents for many years. Synthetic colours based on petrochemical products were developed in the 20th century. Commonly used natural colours include: anthocyanins which are red-purple, chlorophyulls and chlorophyllins, which are green-yellow and vegetable carbon black, which is black. A number of other compounds such as chocolate, fruits and nuts are also used to add value and interest to the ice cream.

Role of Sugar in Ice Cream

The sugars give the product its characteristic sweetness and palatability and enhance the perception of various fruit flavours. In addition, the sugars, including the lactose from the milk components, contribute to a depressed freezing point so that the ice cream has some unfrozen water associated with it at very low temperatures. Without this unfrozen water, the ice cream would be too hard to scoop.

Freezing point depression of a solution is a colligative property associated with the number of dissolved molecules. The lower the molecular weight, the greater the ability of a molecule to depress the freezing point. Thus monosaccharides such as fructose or glucose produce a much softer ice cream than disaccharides such as sucrose. This limits the amount and type of sugar which one can successfully incorporate into the formulation.

Stabilising Ice Cream

The stabilisers are a group of compounds, usually polysaccharides, responsible for adding viscosity to the unfrozen portion of water and thus holding this water so that it cannot migrate within the product. Without the stabilisers, the ice cream would become coarse due to the migration of this free water and the growth of existing ice crystals. For a smooth consistency, ice crystals should be small. Large crystals lead to a coarse, grainy texture. Crystal size depends on how quickly the ice cream is frozen. Slow freezing promotes a larger number of nucleation sites and, consequently, a large number of smaller crystals. In the distribution channels of today's marketplace, the supermarkets, and so on, ice cream has many opportunities to warm up, partially melt some of the ice, and then refreeze as the temperature is once again lowered. This process is known as heat shock and as a result the ice cream becomes more icy tasting. Stabilisers help to prevent this.

Gelatine, a protein of animal origin, was used almost exclusively in the ice cream industry as a stabiliser but has gradually been replaced with polysaccharides of plant origin due to their increased effectiveness and reduced cost. The stabilisers in use today include: carboxymethyl cellulose, locust bean gum which is derived from the beans of exotic trees grown mostly in Africa, guar gum, from the guar bush, carrageenan, sodium alginate, etc. Often, two or more of these stabilisers are used in combination to lend synergistic properties to each other and improve their overall effectiveness.

The emulsifiers are a group of compounds in ice cream which aid in developing the appropriate fat structure and air distribution necessary for the smooth eating and good meltdown characteristics desired in ice cream. Earlier, egg yolks were used as emulsifiers. Today, two emulsifies predominate most of the ice cream formulations: (i) mono and di-glycerides, derived from the partial hydrolysis of fats or oils of animal or vegetable origin, and (ii) polysorbate 80, a product consisting of a glucose molecule bound to a fatty acid, oleic acid. Both of these compounds have hydrophobic regions, the fatty acids, and hydrophilic regions, either glycerol or glucose. Together, the stabilisers and emulsifiers make up less than one half per cent by weight of our ice cream. Ice crystals, the other major component of ice cream begin to form when the mixture is cooled after whipping.

Manufacture of ice cream

The steps involved are: (i) preparation of the mix, (ii) pasteurisation, (iii) homogenisation, (iv) ageing, (v) freezing, and (vi) hardening.

Preparation of the mix

The liquid ingredients are mixed and heated to about 43°C. Sugar and dry ingredients are added to the warm mix and dissolved. Gross particulates such as nuts or fruits are not added at this stage but added during the freezing step. The formulated mix should have proper viscosity, stability and handling characteristics.

Pasteurisation

The mix is pasteurised by batch or continuous heating process in equipment similar to those used in milk pasteurisation. HTST (79°–82°C for 25 seconds) or batch method (68°–71°C for about 30 minutes) may be used. Pasteurisation renders the mix free from harmful bacteria, brings into solution and aids in blending all the ingredients of the mix, improves flavour and keeping quality and also produces a more uniform product.

Homogenisation

The mix is homogenised at the same temperature as, it comes out of the pasteuriser. A two-stage homogeniser (2500 psi first stage and 600 psi at second stage) is used to breakdown the fat globules and clumps so that butter or cream formation and separation are prevented. Homogenisation also blends the ingredients thoroughly, improves the texture and palatability of the ice cream. It also reduces the ageing time, aids in obtaining the desired overrun and produces a more uniform product.

Ageing

The homogenised mix is cooled rapidly to about 4°C to prevent bacterial growth and held at this temperature for about 3 to 24 hours. Ageing provides time for the melted fat to solidify, the gelatin or other stabilisers to swell and combine with water. The milk proteins also swell with water and the viscosity of the mix is increased. These changes lead to quicken the whipping process to desired overrun in the freezer to give a smoother ice cream with desirable body and texture and also to slow down ice cream melting.

Freezing

The mix is now ready to be frozen. The cold mix at about 4°C is pumped to a batch or continuous freezer. The mix and air enter the freezing cylinders which are chilled by circulating refrigerant between double walls. The twin purposes of freezing operation are: (i) to freeze the mix to about –3°C, and (ii) to beat in and subdivide air cells. Freezing must be quick to prevent the growth of large sized ice crystals that would coarsen the texture and air cells must be small in size and evenly distributed to give a stable frozen foam. Scrapped surface freezer provided with a mixing element or dasher is used. The rotating dasher with its sharp scraper blades removes the layers of frozen ice cream off the inner freezer wall as it is formed. This prevents build-up of an insulating layer which would otherwise decrease the freezing efficiency of the freezer wall. The ice cream scrapings are mixed with the remaining mix in the freezer cylinder and thus serve as seed material for forming small ice crystals which speed-up the freezing process. The dasher's rods also beat air into the freezing mix.

The mix passing through the freezer cylinder is frozen and whipped to a temperature of about –3°C in about 30 seconds. At this temperature, all the water in the mix is not frozen and ice cream is semi-solid, in which condition it is easily pumped out of the cylinder as a continuous extrusion by the incoming unfrozen mix and the propelling action of the dasher. Fruit and flavouring nuts are added to soft ice cream coming out the freezer. The soft ice cream goes to a packaging machine where it may be packed in bulk containers or small packages for retail sale.

Hardening

The cartons are sent to the hardening chamber where the freezing process is completed. The temperature is maintained at –23° to –34°C and the remaining water freezes, making the ice cream firm within 24 hours. The ice cream is now ready for storage or delivery.

Physical structure of ice cream and possible defects

Changes in the physical structure are the causes of several common defects in the finished product. Ice cream is a foam containing air cells which constitute the overrun. The overrun gives the ice cream approximately twice the volume of the original mix. In the frozen ice cream the foam forms a film of the mix surrounding the air cells. The fat globules and frozen ice crystals are dispersed within the film or layer of the mix. As ice cream ages, the foam shrinks and the weakened film of mix collapses and thereby the ice cream loses volume. This can be excessive if the mix is low in solids content and constitutes a serious defect.

Fluctuating storage temperature permit repeated partial thawing and freezing and the ice cream becomes coarse and icy due to the formation of bigger sized ice crystals. Lactose, if present in excess, crystallises out and the ice cream becomes grain or sandy in texture.

Excessive and shrinkage occurs if the storage temperature is higher. Shrinkage due to mechanical compaction when ice cream is dipped from tubs to make cones results in dipping loss. Other textural defects include gummy, crumbly, curdy and watery characteristics due to poor mix formulations. Flavour defects include oxidised flavour and cooked flavour occur due to poor quality of the ingredients.

Ice cream may have the following composition: greater than 10 per cent milkfat and usually between 10 per cent and as high as 16 per cent fat in some premium ice creams: 9 to 12 per cent milk solids not fat: this component, also known as the serum solids, contains the proteins (caseins and whey proteins) and carbohydrates (lactose) found in milk: 12 to 16 per cent sweeteners: usually a combination of sucrose and glucose-based corn syrup sweeteners: 0.2 to 0.5 per cent stabilisers and emulsifiers: 55 to 64 per cent water which comes from the milk or other ingredients.

These compositions are percentage by weight. Since ice cream can contain as much as half air by volume, these numbers may be reduced by as much as half if cited by volume. In terms of dietary considerations, however, the percentages by weight are more relevant.

EMERGING PROCESSING AND PRESERVATION TECHNOLOGIES FOR MILK AND DAIRY PRODUCTS

Pasteurisation and, more recently, ultra-high-temperature (UHT) processing are the traditional methods used to eliminate pathogens with minimal detriment to the physical and chemical properties of milk. The main purpose of thermally processing raw milk is to make it safe for human consumption. The demand for better quality dairy products with longer shelf lives has prompted the industry to search for new means to enhance these two important properties. Several recent technologies have shown potential commercial applications for improving quality and extending the shelf life of milk and other dairy products. High-pressure processing (HPP) can inactivate vegetative bacteria in milk. Pulsed electric field (PEF) technology shows some potential in the pasteurisation of fluid milk. Irradiation has been an effective method for destroying pathogens but produces undesirable changes in sensory attributes and quality of dairy products. Modified atmosphere packaging (MAP) using CO_2 has an antimicrobial effect and inhibits the growth of some psychrotrophic bacteria in dairy products such as fluid milk, cheese, yogurt, ice cream mixes and sour cream. Membrane microfiltration has been applied successfully to reduce the microbial load of raw milk; the technique requires less thermal treatment and therefore improves milk quality. The antimicrobial effect of natural components of milk, such as lactoperoxidase, lactoferrin and xanthine oxidase, can also preserve dairy foods, thus increasing shelf life. The basic concepts of these technologies, their potential uses and limitations, and their possible effects on the quality and shelf life of dairy products are discussed in this section.

Processing Technologies

Heat treatment

Milk and dairy products are heat treated to inactivate pathogenic micro-organisms and some undesirable enzymes. This practice improves product safety and prolongs shelf life. The most common heat process is pasteurisation, which can be applied at different temperature and time conditions ranging from 63°C for 30 min to 100°C for 0.01 sec. Pasteurisation produces both irreversible and reversible changes in milk components and causes both desirable and undesirable effects. Heat treatment of milk increases the amount of colloidal phosphate, decreases Ca^{++}, hydrolyses phosphoric esters, isomerises lactose, decreases pH, increases titratable acidity, denatures serum proteins, inactivates enzymes, and forms free sulphhydryl groups that drop redox potential and degrades some vitamins. Changes of milk components by heat treatment largely depend on the combination of heating intensity and time duration.

High-temperature/short-time (HTST) pasteurisation is the most widely used treatment for preserving the quality and extending the shelf life of dairy products. HTST pasteurisation destroys all pathogenic micro-organisms but not bacterial spores. HTST processing also deteriorates the physical and chemical properties of the product. Plate heat exchanger systems are most commonly used for milk pasteurisation in modern industry.

During ultra-high-temperature (UHT) treatment, the product is held for a few seconds at a higher temperature (135° to 150°C) than with HTST pasteurisation. The two UHT methods are direct heating by steam injection or infusion and indirect heat transfer by heat exchange. The UHT process destroys all viable micro-organisms, including bacterial spores, and extends product shelf life. Additionally, UHT causes considerable changes in milk properties such as excessive heated flavour, phosphotase reduction, activation of spores or spore-forming bacteria, gelation, reactivation of lipase, increased viscosity and decreased nutritive value.

High-pressure processing

High-pressure processing (HPP) is a novel non-thermal food processing technology that uses extremely high pressure to kill vegetative micro-organisms. Inactivation of vegetative microbes through HPP may result from denaturation of deoxyribonucleic acid (DNA) replication and transcription, solidification of lipids, breakage of biomembranes or leakage of cell contents. Applications of HPP to food extend the shelf life without thermal denaturation; preserve nutritional value with retention of natural flavour, colour, texture and taste; and increase food safety.

High-pressure processing can operate within a wide range of conditions. High pressure machines can process volumes from 5 ml to 200 litres and operating pressures from 30,000 to 130,000 psi (200 to 900 MPa) for typically 30 seconds to a few minutes. The typical temperatures are 20° to 40°C, but in some cases the range can go from −20° to 80°C. Under HPP, food retains its original shape with minor cellular damage because pressure is applied uniformly in all directions. The effect of HPP on food characteristics depends on the applied pressure, temperature and duration.

Functional properties of food proteins such as hydration, gelation and emulsification characteristics are altered by disruption of protein-water interactions and protein-protein interactions. HPP breaks only hydrogen protein bonds, disrupts hydrophobic and electrostatic interactions, makes greater ionisation of molecules, and inactivates micro-organisms. Covalent bonds are not affected.

High-pressure processing has been used on dairy products. The process destroys micro-organisms in milk and reduces coagulation and ripening time in cheese. HPP technology increases viscosity and apparent elasticity of gel and thus decreases syneresis in yogurt. The effect of HPP on milk depends greatly on the properties and composition of the milk. UHT milk pressurised at 400 MPa and 50°C for 15 minutes resulted in a reduction of approximately 5 log (CFU/g) for *Escherichia coli* and 6 log for *Staphylococcus aureus* at 500 MPa. Besides destroying micro-organisms, HPP may alter the physical characteristics of milk. Pasteurised skim milk was HPP processed up to 700 MPa for 3 minutes at 20°C and kept constant for 22 minutes. The treatment increased the dynamic viscosity and surface hydrophobicity of milk. Milk turbidity and lightness decreased. The particle size started to decrease with increased pressure from 230 to 430 MPa and reached minimal size with pressure from 430 MPa and above. Because skim milk is a colloidal emulsion of casein particles, the functional properties of skim milk are largely dependent on the size of casein particles.

High-pressure processing technology was applied to investigate the accelerated ripening of gouda cheese at 14°C, 50 to 400 MPa, for 20 to 100 minutes and cheddar cheese at 25°C, 50 MPa, for 3 days. The results of those studies showed that HPP treatment using the conditions mentioned above did not accelerate ripening of the cheeses. However, Kolakowski reported that camembert cheese treated by HPP at 0 to 500 MPa obtained the highest degree of proteolysis at the pressure of 50 MPa for 4 hours. Kolakowski also mentioned that the number of micro-organisms in gouda and camembert cheeses decreased significantly by HPP at pressures above 400 MPa.

Another study concluded that increasing temperature accelerated cheese ripening as well as the risk of microbial spoilage. Accelerated cheese ripening was attributed to a combination of HPP and increased ripening temperature.

Processing of yogurt by HPP technology has also been investigated. The application of HPP at approximately 414 MPa at room temperature can extend shelf life or even produce shelf-stable yogurt. The continuous development of acidity after packaging, which can lead to syneresis, can be reduced by HPP. Tanaka and Hatanaka subjected yogurt to pressures of 200 to 300 MPa at 10 to 20°C for 10 minutes. The treatment did not modify the yogurt texture and did not reduce the numbers of viable lactic acid bacteria. Pressure above 300 MPa prevented overacidification; however, the numbers of viable lactic acid bacteria were reduced.

Pulsed electric field

Pulsed electric field (PEF) is a nonthermal processing technology that may have the potential to replace traditional thermal pasteurisation. The use of PEF technology in foods reduces pathogen levels while increasing shelf life; retaining original flavour, colour and nutritional properties; and improving protein functionalities. PEF processing involves the application of a short burst of high-voltage energy to a fluid as it flows between two inert electrodes. The complete PEF system consists of a fluid-handling section, high-voltage pulse generator and multiple-stage co-field PEF treatment chamber. The effect of PEF treatment on micro-organisms is known as electroporation. PEF causes swelling of the cell membrane, resulting in reversible or irreversible ruptures. The high-voltage pulsed electricity discharges that are induced into microbes in the food product develop pores that allow permeation of small molecules in cellular membranes, thus impairing cellular functions. Several factors influence PEF process efficiency. The effects of PEF treatment on inactivation of micro-organisms largely depend on process conditions such as electric field intensity, pulse width, treatment time and temperature, pulse wave shapes; microbial entities such as type, concentration and growth stage of micro-organisms; and treatment media, such as pH, antimicrobials, ionic compounds conductivity and medium ionic strength.

Studies about the effects of PEF on dairy products have been conducted on skim milk, whole milk and yogurt. Fluid milks containing *Escherichia coli*, *Salmonella dublin*, *Listeria innocua* and *Listeria monocytogenes* were processed at PEF conditions of 28.6 to 50 kV/cm, 1.5 to 100 µsec, 23 to 100 pulses and temperatures from 10° to 63°C. Although the PEF conditions were different, the studies reported 2.0 to 4.0 log (CFU/ml) reductions. A study investigated the application of PEF on raw milk by inoculating ultra-high-temperature (UHT) skim milk with *Pseudomonas fluorescens*, *Lactococcus lactis*, and *Bacillus cereus*. Smith reported that the PEF treatment caused 0.3 to 3.0 log reductions of *P. fluorescens*, *L. lactis* and *B. cereus* in UHT milk and total micro-organisms in raw milk. In all cases, PEF had a partial effect on the inactivation and destruction of micro-organisms in milk, and the survivability of the cells differed for various organisms. Other researchers reported 2.0 to 4.0 log reductions for *Escherichia coli* in skim milk, *Listeria innocua* in skim milk, *Listeria monocytogenes* (*scott A*) in pasteurised whole milk (3.5 per cent milk fat), and *Staphylococcus aureus* in simulated milk ultrafiltrate.

The log reduction of *Saccharomyces cerevisiae*, *Lactobacillus bulgaricus* and *Streptococcus thermophilus* in yogurt treated by PEF at 23 to 38 kV/cm, 100 µsec, 20 pulses and 63°C was investigated; the PEF treatment produced a 2.0 log reduction. These results suggest that the use of PEF has some limitations due to the difficulty of inactivating endospores and low conductivity in foods caused by solids. The microbial reduction achieved in the studies is not substantial enough to consider PEF treatments as a substitute for current pasteurisation methods of dairy products. However, the efficiency of PEF processing in microbial reduction in milk may be improved by employing longer treatment times and higher electric field strengths. Combination with other non-thermal techniques may be necessary for more efficient PEF treatment for the processing of fluid dairy products.

Irradiation

Food irradiation is the exposure of food to a source of ionising radiation energy. In general terms, radiation refers to exposure to or illumination by rays or waves of all types. Microwaves, infrared or ultraviolet light and X-rays are common sources of energy. Gamma (γ) radiation is the most common type of energy used in food irradiation. The application of irradiation to foods reduces the pathogenic potential of micro-organisms present because nucleic acids and macromolecules of food micro-organisms are very sensitive to ionisation. Irradiation disrupts the genetic material of living cell, destroys foodborne pathogens and reduces the number of spoilage micro-organisms. Ionisation in food caused by irradiation modifies the structure and composition of large and complicated molecules. Food irradiation also affects food components such as water, carbohydrate, lipid, protein, vitamins, minerals and other trace elements through reactive ions or free radicals, which combine with other ions to achieve a more stable state.

Irradiation of milk and dairy products has been investigated at a wide range of radiation energy intensities (0.07 to 2.5 kGy). Irradiation of milk started to be used during the 1930s in order to increase the vitamin D content in milk. The difference with today's irradiation methods was the use of ultraviolet (UV) light as the source of ionisation rather that γ-rays. Fluid milk and evaporated milk were irradiated with UV light. In most studies, dairy products have been exposed to high radiation doses suitable for sterilisation, causing the development of off flavours, aftertaste, and loss of vitamins A, B_1, and B_2. Irradiation treatment of milk and dairy products has created flavour problems due to sulphur compounds produced from milk protein fraction and oxidative rancidity from lipid fraction. The off-flavour production level in milk and cheese depended on their composition and the conditions of radiation and storage. Irradiation with a dose of 0.25 kGy at room temperature extended the shelf life of pasteurised milk stored at 4°C; however, the milk lost a certain amount of vitamin A, B_1, and B_2.

Irradiation of other dairy products includes cheese, frozen desserts, and caseinate films. Irradiation at an average dose of 2.5 kGy was an effective method for destroying pathogenic bacteria *Listeria monocytogenes* and *Salmonella* in camembert cheese without affecting enzyme activity and flavour. Gamma irradiation at a dose of 40 kGy at −78°C was sufficient to sterilise ice cream and frozen yogurt, but not for mozzarella or cheddar cheeses. The irradiation caused a decrease in overall acceptability of the product due to off flavour and after taste, but it had little effect on product colour or texture. Irradiation combined with modified atmosphere packaging or antioxidant was effective at preserving sensory properties of peppermint ice cream packed with helium and strawberry yogurt bars treated with ascorbyl palmitate. Water solubility and microbial degradation of caseinate films were reduced by gamma irradiation at 64 kGy dosage. The improved changes were associated with the higher number of cross-links on the film caused by irradiation.

Modified atmosphere packaging

Modified atmosphere packaging (MAP) is a technology used to extend the shelf life of fresh and processed food products. The MAP process consists of flushing the food packaging with antimicrobial gases just before sealing. Modified atmosphere packaging has been used successfully to extend the shelf life of solid dairy foods such as shredded cheese. In MAP, gas is added directly into liquids or semiliquid foods such as milk, yogurt, cottage cheese, sour cream and ice cream. The gas concentration used in MAP can vary from 40 to 1100 ppm, depending on the type of product and packaging characteristics.

Antibacterial agent carbon dioxide and inert nitrogen are the gases used in these technologies. Carbon dioxide is widely used to inhibit the growth of some psychrotrophic bacteria that deteriorate refrigerated food and to restrict the growth of typical aerobic Gram-negative spoilage bacteria. The gas enters microbial cells and lowers the pH, thus retarding the growth of microbes. The effectiveness of MAP in foods is improved with exclusion of the oxygen necessary for the growth of aerobic spoilage bacteria. Oxygen also causes oxidative rancidity and colour changes.

Several researchers have investigated MAP in cottage cheese. Flushing CO_2 gas into the headspace of plastic containers filled with cottage cheese inhibited the growth of yeasts, moulds and psychrotrophic bacteria for 112 days; however, flavour and texture were retained for only 45 days. The application of CO_2 gas above 750 ml/l in cottage cheese kept the quality and maintained the colour and flavour for 28 days at 4°C. MAP using 500 ml/l CO_2 gas in cottage cheese inhibited the growth of yeasts and fungi. *Pseudomonas* spp. and *Listeria monocytogenes* were inhibited in cottage cheese with 400 ml/l CO_2. CO_2 extended the shelf life of cottage cheese cream but caused a slight flavour alteration due to the CO_2 dissolved in the cream.

Modified atmosphere packaging has also been applied to other cheese products to maintain quality, inhibit micro-organism growth and extend shelf life. MAP with plain CO_2 was applied to whey cheeses stored at 4°C. Chemical composition was retained and lipolysis was inhibited completely. MAP with several ratio combinations was applied to cameros cheese to investigate its effect on shelf life and microbial quality. Gas ratios of 50:50 and 40:60 (CO_2:N_2) were the most effective in reducing proteolysis and lipolysis, which helped in retaining good sensory properties. These gases were also effective in inhibiting the growth of mesophiles, psychrotrophs, enterobacteriaceae and coli forms, thus extending shelf life.

Effective MAP technology is associated with proper storage temperature, proper amount of gas dissolved and high-barrier packaging. A disadvantage of MAP is that the gas applied dissipates quickly during modern processing.

Membrane filtration

Membrane filtration occurs when fluids and solvents are selectively transported and passed through a barrier by applying a driving force across the barrier. The membrane materials that act as the barrier can be organic polymers, metals, ceramics, layers of chemicals, liquids or gases. Membrane filtration has been used for the separation, concentration, demineralisation, fractionation or clarification of liquids. Membrane filtrations are classified by membrane types, pore sizes and process conditions into microfiltration (MF), nanofiltration (NF), ultrafiltration (UF) and reverse osmosis (RO). These membrane filtrations have been applied in the dairy industry for the removal of bacteria in milk, standardisation of milk, concentration of milk protein, fractionation of caseins, cheese-making and whey processing for many years. Membrane technologies have also been used in the dairy industry for new product development, improving product quality and enhancing process profitability. The effectiveness of a filtration system depends on the types and characteristics of membrane; therefore, the selection of membrane is important with respect to operating costs, energy requirements, reducing operating time, and increasing product quality.

Microfiltration is applied for the removal of bacteria from milk and cheese milk. It is also used in the preparation of casein-enriched cheese milk and to modify the α- and β-casein ratio of milk. MF of skim milk reduced bacteria by about 99.5 per cent, extended shelf life and retained the milk properties intact. Rodriguez Studied the effect of UF and MF technologies on the texture of semihard, low-fat cheese. The use of MF milk improved cheese texture and produced lower retention of whey protein as compared with UF membrane; however, the UF process produced better cheese yields than the MF process.

Nanofiltration membranes have high permeability of salts such as sodium chlorides and potassium chlorides and very low permeability for organic compounds such as lactose, protein and urea. These characteristics make NF suitable for dairy application. NF concentrates and demineralises whey at the same time, which traditionally was processed using evaporation or reverse osmosis followed by electrodialysis. With these properties, the use of NF reduces the cost of energy consumption and wastewater disposal considerably. Demineralisation of whey has been accomplished by NF.

Ultrafiltration and RO are widely used in cheese manufacturing and whey treatment. UF and RO have been used in whey concentration and the development of whey protein concentrates, and the UF process has been applied to making fresh cheeses and semihard cheeses. The use of UF processing in making low-fat cheddar cheese did not significantly improve flavour, body or texture characteristics. Aroma and flavour degradation were reported in cheeses made from UF concentrated milk. The advantages of UF milk in cheese-making are cheese yield increases of about 16 to 20 per cent, reduction of the quantity of coagulant used by 80 per cent, and decrease of biological oxygen demand (BOD) of the whey produced. RO concentrated 35,000 kg of whey fourfold, reducing the BOD of permeates.

Thus, the development and use of emerging technologies and new processing procedures have been shown to be promising. Most of them provide specific advantages to improve the shelf life and quality of dairy products; however, they also present some disadvantages and limitations. Several of these new technologies are still in experimental stages and may not fall under current food and drug administration (FDA) regulations associated with low-acid canned foods which relate only to processing procedures involving a thermal treatment to render the commercial sterility of the product. Although some of these nonthermal processes may have capabilities to produce shelf-stable products, public health concerns are significant. The FDA specifies that, 'any nonthermal process used to create a commercially sterile food product must result in a food product that has not been prepared, packed or held under unsanitary conditions whereby it may have become contaminated with filth or whereby it may have been rendered injurious to health. Consequently, the future applications and utilisation of nonthermal technologies and new processing procedures will depend greatly on more research results, economics and legal approval.

Chapter 7

Bakery and Cereal Products

INTRODUCTION

Cereals are the edible seeds of plants of the grass family. They can be grown in a large part of the world and provide the staple food for most of mankind. Cereals in their dry state are not subject to fermentation due to their low water content. Properly dried cereals contain less than 14 per cent water and this limits microbial growth and chemical changes during storage. However, on mixing grains or cereal flour with water or other water-based fluids, enzymatic changes occur that may be attributed to the enzymes inherent in the grain itself and/or to micro-organisms. These micro-organisms can either be those present as the natural contaminating flora of the cereal, or they can be added as a starter culture. This chapter will be mainly devoted to fermented bakery products made from wheat. However, on a global basis, many fermented cereal products are derived wholly or in part from other grains such as rice, maize, sorghum, millet, barley and rye. Different cereals differ not only in nutrient content, but also in the composition of the protein and carbohydrate polymers. The functional and sensory characteristics of products made from different cereals will therefore vary at the outset due to these factors. In addition to this, the opportunity to vary technological procedures and microbiological content and activity provides us with the vast range of fermented cereal products that are prepared and consumed in the world today.

CEREAL COMPOSITION

Carbohydrates are quantitatively the most important constituents of cereal grains, contributing 77–87 per cent of the total dry matter. In wheat, the carbohydrate in the endosperm is mainly starch, whereas the pericarp, testa and aleurone contain most of the crude and dietary fibre present in the grain. The pericarp, testa and aleurone also contain over half the total mineral matter. Whole meal flour is derived, by definition, from the whole grain and contains all its nutrients. When wheat is milled into flour, the yield of flour from the grain (extraction rate) reflects the extent to which the bran and the germ are removed and thereby determines not only the whiteness of the flour, but also its nutritive value and baking properties. Decreasing extraction rate results in a marked and nutritionally important, decrease in fibre, fat, vitamins and minerals. The protein content of different cereal grains varies between 7 and 20 per cent, governed not only by cereal genus, species or variety (i.e. genetically regulated), but also by plant growth conditions such as temperature, availability during plant growth of water and also of nitrogen and other minerals in the soil. There is an uneven distribution of different protein types in the different parts of the grain, so that although the protein concentration is not radically affected by milling, the proteins present in different milling fractions will vary.

147

Starch

The starch in cereals is contained in granules that vary in size, from 2–3 μm to about 30 μm according to grain species. Barley, rye and wheat have starch granules with a bimodal size distribution, with large lenticular and small spherical grains. Almost 100 per cent of the starch granule is composed of the polysaccharides amylose and amylopectin and the relative proportions of these polymers vary according not only to species of cereal, but also to variety within a species. However, both wheat and maize contain about 28 per cent amylose, but in wheat the ratio of amylose to amylopectin does not vary. The amylose molecule is essentially linear, with up to 5000 glucose molecules polymerised by α-1,4 linkages and only occasional α-1,6 linkages. Amylopectin is a much larger (up to 10^6 glucose units) and more highly branched molecule with approximately 4 per cent of α-1,6 linkages which cause branching in the α-1,4 glucosidic chain.

During milling of grains, some of the starch granules become damaged, particularly in hard wheat. The starch exposed in these broken granules is more susceptible to attack by amylases and also absorbs water much more readily. The degree of damage to the starch grains therefore dictates the functionality of the flour in various baking processes. When water is added to starch grains they absorb water and soluble starch leaks out of damaged granules. Heating of this mixture results in an increase in viscosity and a pasting of the starch, which on further heating leads to gelatinisation as the ordered crystalline structure is disrupted and water forms hydration layers around the separated molecules. The gelatinisation temperature of starch from different cereals varies from 55° to 78°C. partly due to the ratio of amylose to amylopectin. The gelatinisation of wheat starts at about 60°C. Despite the fact that there is not sufficient water to totally hydrate the starch in most bakery foods, the heat causes irreversible changes to the starch. On cooling a heated cereal product, some starch molecules reassociate, causing a firming of the product.

Nonstarch polysaccharides, the pentosan, which are principally arabinoxylans, comprise approximately 2–3 per cent of the weight of flour. They are derived from the grain cell walls and are polymers that may contain both pentoses and hexoses. They are able to absorb many times their own weight in water and contribute in baking by increasing the viscosity of the aqueous phase, but they may also compete with the gluten proteins for available water. Cereals also contain small amounts (1–3 per cent) of mono-, di- and oligosaccharides and these are important as an energy source for yeast at the start of dough fermentation.

Protein

Cereal proteins contribute to the nutritional value of the diet and therefore the composition and amount of protein present are inherently important. However, the protein content in cereals also has several important aspects in fermented bakery products. The amount and type of some of the proteins is important for the formation of an elastic dough and for its gas-retaining properties. Other proteins in cereals are enzymes with specific functions, not only for the developing germ, but also for various changes that take place from the processing of flour to bakery products.

Gluten proteins

The unique storage proteins of wheat are also the functional proteins in baking. The gliadins and glutenins, collectively called gluten proteins, make up about 80 per cent of the total protein in the grain and are mostly found in the endosperm. These proteins have very limited solubility in water or salt solutions, unlike albumins and globulins (Fig. 7.1). A good bread flour (known as 'strong' flour) must contain adequate amounts of gluten proteins to give the desired dough characteristics and extra gluten may be added to the bread formulation.

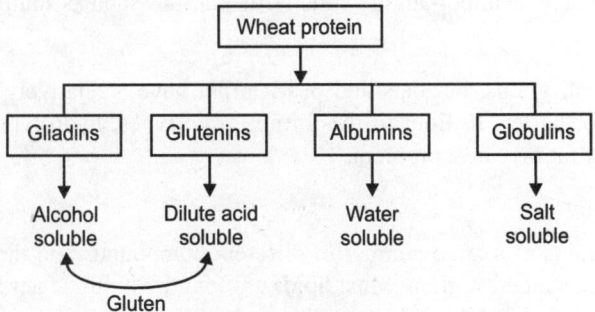

Fig. 7.1. Wheat proteins.

Enzyme proteins

The albumin and globulin proteins are concentrated in the bran, germ and aleurone.

Amylases

The primary function of starch-hydrolysing enzymes is to mobilise the storage polysaccharides to readily metabolised carbohydrates when the grain germinates.

α-amylase hydrolyses α-1,4 glycosidic bonds at random in the starch molecule chain but is unable to attack the α-1,6 linkages at the branching points on the amylopectin molecule. The activity of α-amylase causes a rapid reduction in size of the large starch molecule and the viscosity of a heated solution or slurry of starch is greatly decreased. It is most active on gelatinised starch, but granular starch is also slowly degraded.

β-amylase splits off two glucose units (maltose) at a time from the non-reducing end of the starch chain, thus providing a large amount of fermentable carbohydrate. β-amylase is also called a saccharifying enzyme since its action causes a marked increase in sweetness of the hydrated cereal. Neither the hydrolysis of amylopectin nor of amylose is completed by β-amylase, since the enzyme is not able to move past the branching points. The presence of both α- and β-amylases, however, leads to a much more comprehensive hydrolysis, since α-amylase produces several new reducing ends in each starch molecule. The level of α-amylase is very low in intact grain but increases markedly on germination, whereas β-amylase levels in intact and germinated grain are similar.

Flour containing too much α-amylase absorbs less water and therefore results in heavy bread. In addition, the dough is sticky and hard to handle and the texture of the loaf is usually faulty, having large open holes and a sticky crumb texture. However, some activity is required and bakers may add amylase either as an enzyme preparation or as wheat or barley malt in order to slightly increase loaf volume and improve crumb texture. The thermal stability of amylases from different sources dictates their activity during the baking process. Microbial amylases with greater thermal stability have been used in bread to decrease firming (retrogradation) upon storage since these enzymes are not fully denatured during baking.

Proteases

Proteinases and peptidases are found in cereals and their primary function is to make small amino nitrogen compounds available for the developing seed embryo during germination, when the levels of these enzymes also increase. However, whether these enzymes have a role in bread baking is not certain. Peptidases may furnish the yeast with soluble nitrogen during fermentation and a proteinase in wheat that is active at low pH may be important in acidic fermentations such as sourdough bread.

Lipases

Lipases are present in all grains, but oats and pearl millet have a relatively high activity of lipase compared with wheat or barley. In flour of the former grain types, hydrolytic rancidity of the grain lipids and added baking fat may be a problem.

Lipids

Lipids are present in grains as a large number of different compounds and they vary from species to species and also within each cereal grain. Most lipids are found within the germ. Wheat flour contains about 2.5 per cent lipids, of which about 1 per cent are polar lipids (tri- and diglycerides, free fatty acids and sterol esters) and 1.5 per cent are nonpolar lipids (phospholipids and galactosyl glycerides). During dough mixing, much of the lipid forms hydrophobic bonds to the gluten protein.

BREAD

Many different types of bread are produced in the world. Bread formulations and technologies differ both within and between countries due to both traditional and technological factors including: (i) which cereals are traditionally grown in a country and their suitability for bread baking, (ii) the status of bread in the traditional diet, (iii) changes in lifestyle and living standards, (iv) globalisation of eating habits, and (v) economic possibilities for investing in new types of bread-making equipment.

The basic production of most bread involves the addition of water to wheat flour, yeast and salt. Other cereal flours may be blended into the mixture and other optional ingredients include sugar, fat, malt flour, milk and milk products, emulsifiers and gluten (for further ingredients and their roles in bread (Table 7.1). The mixture is worked into an elastic dough that is then leavened by the yeast to a soft and spongy dough that retains its shape and porosity when baked. An exception to this is the production of bread containing 20–100 per cent rye flour, where the application of sourdough and low pH are required.

Table 7.1. Bread additives.

Dough Additive	Role
Cysteine, sodium sulphite and metabisulphite[a]	Reducing agent. Aids optimal dough development during mixing by disrupting disulphide (–S–S–) bonds. A 'dough relaxer'
Amylase	Releases soluble carbohydrate for yeast fermentation and Maillard browning reaction. Reduces starch retrogradation
Ascorbic acid	Oxidising agent. Strengthens gluten and increases bread volume by improving gas retention
Potassium iodate, calcium iodate; calcium peroxide; azodicarbonamide[a]	Fast-acting oxidants; oxidises flour lipids, carotene and converts sulphydryl (–SH) groups to disulphide (–S–S–) bonds
Potassium and calcium bromates[a]	Delayed-acting oxidants: Develops dough consistency, reduces proofing stage
Emulsifiers, strengtheners/conditioners and crumb softeners	Dispersion of fat in the dough. Increase dough extensibility. Interact with the gluten-starch complex and thereby retard staling

(Contd ...)

Dough Additive	Role
Soya flour	Increases nutritional value, bleaches flour pigments, increases in loaf volume increases crumb firmness and crust appearance, promotes a longer shelf life
Vital wheat gluten and its derivatives	Increases gluten content, used especially when mixing time or fermentation time is reduced. Water adsorbant. Improves dough and loaf properties
Hydrocolloids: Starch-based products from various plants	Regulates water distribution and water-holding capacity and thereby improves yield. Strengthens bread crumb structure and improves digestibility
Cellulose and cellulose-based derivatives	Source of dietary fibre
Salt	Enhances flavour (ca. 2% based on flour weight) and modifies mixing time for bread and rolls. Increases dough stability, firmness and gas retention properties. Raises starch gelatinisation temperature

[a] Not allowed in all countries.

Bread Formulation

The formulation of bread is determined by several factors. In a simple bread, the baking properties of the flour are of vital importance in determining the characteristics of the loaf using a given technology. In addition, the bread obtained from using poor bread flour or suboptimum technology may be improved by using certain additives (Table 7.1).

The major methods used to prepare bread are summarised in Fig. 7.2. In the straight dough method, all the ingredients are added together at the start of the process, which includes two fermentation steps and then two proofing steps. In the sponge and dough method, only part of the dry ingredients are added to the water and this soft dough undergoes a fermentation of about 5 hours before the remainder of the ingredients are added and the dough is kneaded to develop the structure. Although these processes are time consuming, their advantages are that they develop a good flavour in the bread and that the timing and technology of the processes are less critical. Mechanical dough development processes, such as the Chorleywood bread process developed in the United Kingdom in the 1960s, radically cut down the total bread-making time. The fermentation step is virtually eliminated and dough formation is achieved by intense mechanical mixing and by various additives that hasten the process. The resulting loaf has a high volume and a thin crust but lacks flavour and aroma. The trend is now away from this kind of process due to customer demand for more flavourful bread and reduced use of additives.

Development of Dough Structure

When wheat flour and water are mixed together in an approximately 3:1 ratio and kneaded, a viscoelastic dough is formed that can entrap the gas formed during the subsequent fermentation. The amount of water absorbed by the flour is dependent upon and therefore must be adjusted to, the integrity of the starch granules and the amount of protein present. A high proportion of damaged granules, as found in hard wheat flour, results in greater water absorption. The unique elastic property of the dough is due to the nature of the gluten proteins. Hydrated gliadin is sticky and extensible, whereas glutenin is cohesive and plastic. When hydrated during the mixing process, the gluten proteins unfold and bond to each other by forming a complex (gluten) as kneading proceeds, with an increasing number of cross-linkages between the protein molecules as they become aligned. Disulphide bonds (–S–S–) break and reform within and between the protein molecules during mixing.

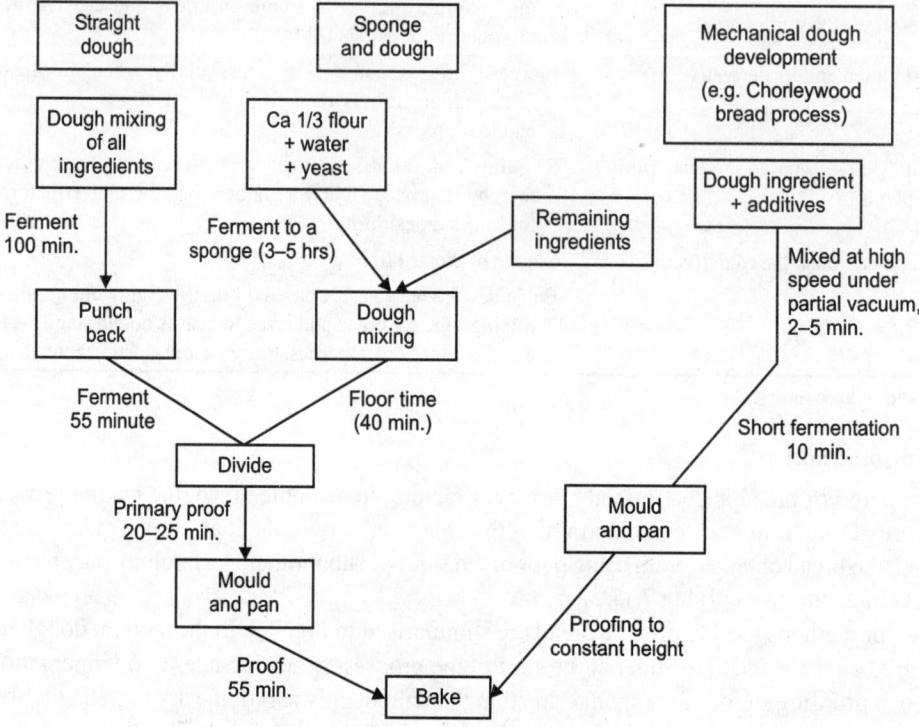

Fig. 7.2. Bread-processing methods.

Gluten does not form spontaneously when flour and water are mixed; energy must be provided, (i.e. in the actual mixing process) in order for the molecular bonds 10 break and reform as the gluten structure. At this point, the dough stiffens and becomes smooth and shiny. The gluten is now composed of protein sheets in which the starch granules are embedded. In addition, free polar lipids and glycolipids are incorporated in the complex by hydrophobic and hydrogen bonds. The properties of the dough are determined by the amount of protein present and by the relative proportions of the gluten proteins.

Another important part of the dough formation is the incorporation of air, in particular nitrogen. This forms insoluble bubbles in the dough that become weak points where carbon dioxide collects during the subsequent fermentation step. In the Chorleywood bread process, the dough is mixed under partial vacuum so that the incorporated bubbles expand and are then split into many small ones as mixing continues, thus giving a fine-pored loaf crumb after baking.

Dough Fermentation

During the fermentation step, several processes happen simultaneously and in order to produce a bread of the required quality characteristics, each of these processes must be optimised to that end.

Yeasts have been used to leaven bread for thousands of years, but only in comparatively recent times have pure cultures of the yeast *Saccharomyces* (*S.*) *cerevisiae* been added to the bread dough as a leavening agent. The commercial production of baker's yeast follows procedures similar to those used in the production of brewing, wine-making and distilling strains of this same species. Indeed, the baking industry was originally supplied with yeast waste from the brewing industry until about 1860. However, commercial production of yeast biomass specifically for the baking industry developed alongside an increasingly expanding manufacture of bread in commercial bakeries and the development of the technology that provided the great volumes required by the industry.

Commercial production of baker's yeast

Saccharomyces cerevisiae was originally produced commercially using grain mash as a growth substrate, but for economic reasons, it is now grown on sucrose-rich molasses, a by-product from the sugar cane or sugar beet refining industry. Nitrogen, phosphorous and essential mineral ions such as magnesium are added to promote growth. The production of the yeast biomass for the baking industry is multistage and takes about 10–13 hours at 30°C. *S. cerevisiae* shows the Crabtree effect, as its metabolism favours fermentative metabolism at high levels of energy-giving substrate, thus resulting in a low production of biomass. To avoid this, molasses is added incrementally towards the end of the production of yeast biomass and the mixture is vigorously aerated in order to promote respiration and avoid fermentative metabolism. At the end of the production, the yeast is allowed to 'ripen' by aeration in the absence of nutrients. This step synchronises the yeast cells into the stationary growth phase and also promotes an increase in the storage sugar trehalose in the cells, thus improving their viability and activity.

When the fermentation is complete, the amount of yeast is about 3.5–4 per cent w/v. The biomass is separated and concentrated by centrifugation and filtering. The yeast cream is then processed into pressed yeast or is dried.

Preparation of yeast

The most usual types of commercial yeast preparations are the following:
1. Cream yeast is a near liquid form of baker's yeast that must be kept at refrigerated temperatures. It may be added directly to the bakery product being made.
2. Compressed yeast is formed by filtering cream yeast under pressure to give approximately 30 per cent solids. It has a refrigerated shelf life of 3 weeks.
3. Active dry yeast (ADY) is produced by extruding compressed yeast through a perforated steel plate. The resulting thin strands are dried and then broken into short lengths to give a freeflowing granular product after further drying. Depending on the subsequent treatment and packaging. ADY may have a shelf life of over a year. However, ADY requires rehydration before application in dough and this can be a labourintensive operation in a large bakery. The product rehydrates best using steam or in water with added sugar at 40°C. Rehydration in pure water promotes leaching of cell contents and a reduction in the activity of the yeast.
4. High activity dry yeast (HADY) (instant active dry yeast, IADY) is a similar product, where improved drying techniques are used to give a product with smaller particle size that does not need to be rehydrated before use and can therefore be incorporated directly into bread dough without prior treatment.

Desirable properties of baker's yeast

Yeast plays a critically important role in leavened bread production and over the decades of commercial production, strains have been selected that give improved performance. Desirable characteristics include:
1. High CO_2 production during the dough fermentation due to high glycolytic rate.
2. The ability to quickly commence maltose utilisation when the glucose in the flour is depleted.

3. The ability to store high concentrations of trehalose, which gives tolerance to freezing and to high sugar and salt concentrations.
4. Tolerance to bread preservatives such as propionate.
5. Viability and retained activity during various storage conditions.

In the future, strains will probably be developed with even more useful properties. In particular, the flavour-forming properties will receive special attention.

Role of yeast in leavened bread

When yeast is incorporated into the dough, conditions allow a resumption of metabolic activity, although there is little actual multiplication of the yeast during shorter bread-making processes such as the straight dough and Chorleywood processes (Fig. 7.2). The yeast has been produced under aerobic (respiratory) conditions and is therefore adapted to this metabolism, but conditions very quickly become anaerobic in bread dough since the oxygen incorporated in the dough is soon depleted. The sugars are metabolised to pyruvate by glycolysis; pyruvate is then decarboxylated to acetaldehyde, thus producing carbon dioxide; and then ethanol is formed by reduction of acetaldehyde by $NADH_2$ (Fig. 7.3). For each molecule of glucose (or half molecule of maltose) that is metabolised, two molecules each of ethanol and carbon dioxide are produced. This fermentative metabolism is the prevalent pathway in *S. cerevisiae* in dough due both to the absence of oxygen and to the nonlimiting supply of fermentable sugar.

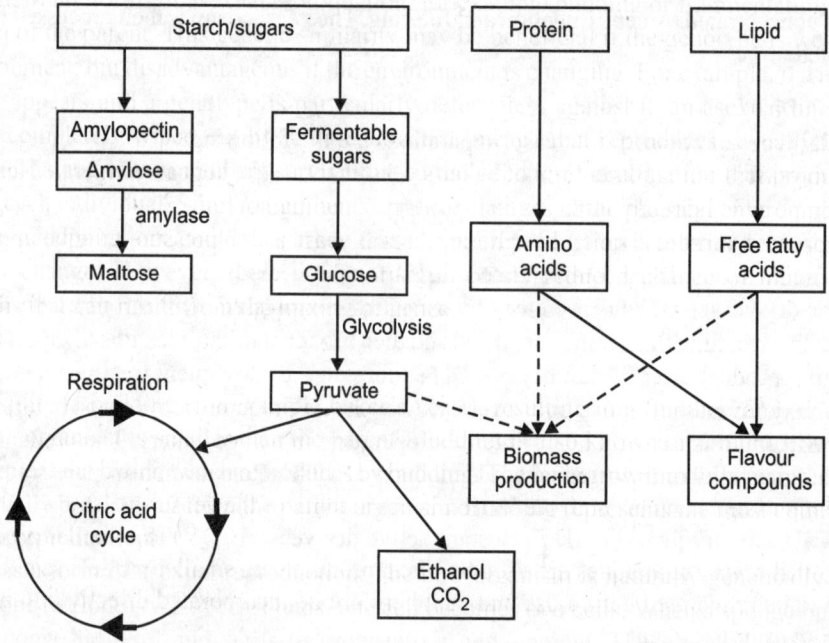

Fig. 7.3. Biochemical changes during fermentation of bread.

The amount of maltose available is a complex interaction between the amount of damaged starch, the level of amylases in the flour and the stage and length of the fermentation process. Maltose accumulates during the early stages of the fermentation because it is generated by amylase but is not metabolised by the yeast because the presence of glucose represses maltose utilisation.

When readily fermentable sugars (glucose and fructose) are exhausted, the yeast shows a lag in fermentation and then turns its metabolism to the maltose produced from the action of β-amylase on starch. If sucrose has been added in the bread formulation (e.g. 4 per cent), this is fermented in preference to maltose and the lag in the fermentation may not be observed. High amounts of added sucrose (e.g. 20 per cent) significantly retard fermentation due to the high osmotic stress on yeast.

The products of yeast metabolism in dough fermentation vary considerably with pH. In bread, the pH is usually below 6.0, but above this, end products in addition to ethanol and CO_2 are formed, such as succinate, acetic acid and glycerol and less ethanol and CO_2 are formed. *S. cerevisiae* is also able to degrade proteins and lipids and several flavour compounds are produced (Fig. 7.3).

It is generally not considered that the yeast fermentation is important for bread flavour and aroma development in traditional bread processes. However, the modern mechanical dough development processes, where the fermentation stage has been radically reduced, produce bread with a flavour that is inferior to that produced by the traditional straight dough process.

This indicates that the yeast fermentation does make a positive contribution to bread flavour. Zehentbauer and Grosch showed that yeast level and fermentation time and temperature affected aroma in the crust of baguettes and they identified the flavour compounds 2-acetyl-l-pyrroline (roasty), methyl propanal and 2- and 3-methylbutanal (malty) and 1-octene-3-ol and (E)-2-nonenal (fatty). An increase in fermentation time allows for a development of flavour, but this trend is not really noticeable until much longer fermentation times are used, as in sourdough breads. There is not a clear borderline between regular bread and sourdough bread.

The production of ethanol and CO_2 is essential for the development of the desired bread crumb structure and several factors affect both the development of the dough and its leavening (Fig. 7.4). During fermentation, some of the CO_2 is lost to the atmosphere, but most either collects in the small pockets of air incorporated during dough mixing or is dissolved in the dough's aqueous phase. The amount that can be dissolved in the aqueous phase is dependent on temperature and is greater at lower temperatures. As the aqueous phase is already saturated with CO_2, it cannot escape from the bubbles by diffusion into the dough, so the bread begins to increase in volume. As the gas collects, the rheological properties of the dough allow it to expand in order to equalise the pressure that builds up. Ethanol reacts with the gluten to slightly soften it, allowing for easier expansion of the dough. It is important that CO_2 develop immediately after dough preparation and proceed at an adequate intensity. In addition, the dough must have the physical properties necessary to withstand dough manipulation and allow for gas retention, so that the optimal structure has been obtained for the final proof and baking.

Bread-Baking Process

When the bread has undergone the final proofing and is put in the oven, the outer surface rapidly starts to form the crust. A temperature gradient develops due to transfer of heat from the pan to the loaf and if the loaf is to achieve optimal properties, then the heat of the oven and the state of the bread proof need to be synchronised. Apart from the outer crust, no part of the bread ever becomes dry; therefore, despite oven temperatures of well over 200°C, the temperature in most of the loaf will not exceed 100°C. The primary rise in temperature increases the activity of the yeast and its production of CO_2. At the same time, the solubility of CO_2 decreases, ethanol and water evaporate and the gases increase in volume. This results in a marked increase in the volume of the dough, called 'oven spring'.

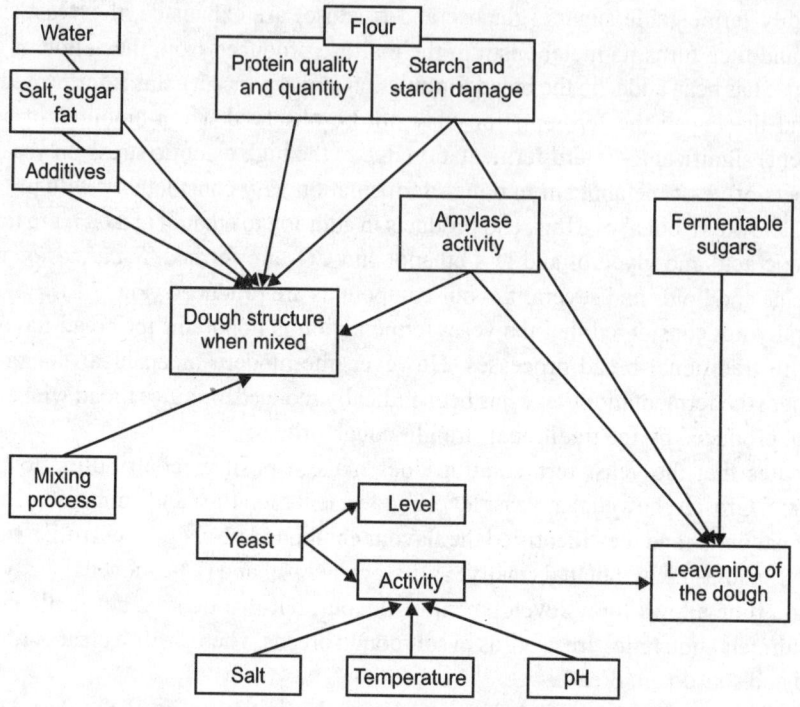

Fig. 7.4. Important factors for bread leavening.

As the temperature in the loaf continues to rise, several other changes take place. The yeast is increasingly inhibited and its enzymes are inactivated at about 65°C. The amylases in the dough are active until about 65–70°C is reached and a rapid increase in the amount of soluble carbohydrate takes place. Gelatinisation of starch occurs at 55–65°C and the water that this requires is taken from the gluten protein network, which then becomes more rigid, viscous and elastic until a temperature is reached at which the protein begins to coagulate. At this stage, the structure of the dough has changed to a more rigid structure due to denatured protein and gelatinised starch. These changes first occur near the crust and gradually move into the crumb as the heat is transferred inwards.

Towards the end of baking the temperature at the crust is much higher than 100°C. The crust becomes brown and aroma compounds, predominantly aldehydes and ketones, are formed, mainly from Maillard reactions. The formation of flavour compounds is two staged. First, compounds are formed from the fermentation itself and then during baking some of these compounds may react with each other or with the bread components to form other flavour compounds. Some other flavour compounds formed during the fermentation may be lost due to the high temperature, but those that remain gradually diffuse into the crumb after cooling. On further storage, the levels of flavour compounds decrease due to volatilisation. Over 200 different flavour and aroma compounds have been identified in bread.

Staling

The two main components of staling (firming of the bread crumb) are loss of moisture, mainly due to migration of moisture from the crumb to the crust (which becomes soft and leathery) and the retrogradation of starch. The major chemical change that occurs during staling is starch retrogradation, but a redistribution of water between the starch and the gluten also has been proposed. The gelatinisation of the starch that occurs during cooking or baking gradually reverses and the starch molecules form intermolecular bonds and crystallise, expelling water molecules and resulting in the firming of crumb texture. Starch retrogradation is a time and temperature dependent process and proceeds fastest at low temperatures, just above freezing point. Since the rearrangement of the starch molecules is facilitated by a high water activity, staling is retarded by the addition of ingredients that lower water activity (e.g. salt and sugar) or bind water (e.g. hydrocolloids and proteins). The staling rate can also be slowed by the incorporation of surfactants, shortening, or heat stable α-amylase. Freezing of baked goods also retards staling since the water activity is drastically lowered. Much of the firming of the loaf during cooling is due to retrogradation of the amylose whereas the slower reaction of staling is due, in addition, to retrogradation of amylopectin.

SOURDOUGH BREAD

When cereal flour does not contain gluten, it is not suitable for production of leavened bread in the manner described above. However, if rye flour, which is very low in gluten proteins, is mixed with water and incubated at 25–30°C for a day or two, there is a good possibility that first step of sourdough production will be started. This mixture will regularly develop fermentation with lactic acid bacteria (LAB) and yeasts. This forms the basis of sourdough production and this low-pH dough is able to leaven.

The use of cereal flour and water as a basis for spontaneous or directed fermentation products is common in many countries. In Africa, fermented porridge and gruel as well as their diluted thirst quenchers, are the main products of these natural fermentations, whereas Europeans and Americans and their descendants enjoy a variety of sourdough breads. In all these areas beers are also produced.

This great variety of fermented products has an historic prototype in the earliest reported leavened breads in Egypt about 1500 BC. Considering the simplicity of the process and the ease with which it succeeds, it has been suggested that peoples in several places must have shared this experience independently. It may be surmised that the experience with gruels and, porridge preceded the idea of making bread. Common bread fermented only with yeast appeared later in our history and it was a staple food in the Roman Empire. This also indicates that the Romans had wheat with sufficient gluten potential. It is possible to make leavened bread without gluten using sourdough and this bread has become a favourite among many peoples.

Advantages of Making Sourdough Bread

1. Sourdough bread does not have to contain high levels of gluten for successful leavening.
2. Low pH inhibits amylase and thereby, degradation of starch is avoided.
3. Sourdough improves the water-binding capacity of starch and the swelling and solubility of pentosans.
4. Sourdough bread has very good keeping quality and an excellent safety potential.
5. Less costly cereal flours can be used.
6. A different variety of flavour and taste attributes can be offered.
7. Sourdough bread can nutritionally compete with regular bread.
8. Phytic acid is degraded by phytase in flour and from lactic acid bacteria. This improves the availability of iron and other minerals.
9. Bread volume is increased, crumb quality is improved and staling is delayed.

Rye flour is very low in gluten proteins and instead, starch and pentosans make an important contribution to bread structure. The swelling and solubility of pentosans increase when LAB fermentation lowers pH. Gelatinisation of starch occurs at about 55°–58°C. Considering that the flour amylase has a temperature optimum around 50°–52°C, it is crucial that the amylase is actually inactivated in the pH range that is obtained during sourdough fermentation. When mixtures of wheat and rye flour are used for bread making, a sourdough process is necessary if the content of rye flour exceeds 20 per cent.

Rye and wheat flour contain phytic acid that binds minerals, particularly iron, that then become nutritionally unavailable. However, these cereals also contain phytases with pH optima around 5.0–5.5; thus phytate degradation is very good in fermented flour, where these phytate complexes are also more soluble. Lactic acid bacteria also appear to have some phytase activity.

As wheat flour is able to form gluten, some of the considerations about amylases and starch are not equally relevant when baking wheat bread. Nevertheless, wheat flour is often used in sourdough bread.

However, preferred qualities like improved keeping and safety potential as well as the increased variety of flavours appeal to many consumers. These desirable qualities are also praised because they represent an alternative natural preservation method.

Microbiology of Sourdough

An established, 'natural' sourdough is dominated by a few representatives of some bacteria and yeast species. This results from the selective ecological pressures exerted in the (rye) flour-water environment. Rye flour is an appropriate choice for this mixture because leavening of the dough is dependent on sourdough development. At the start of fermentation, a 50:50 (w/w) rye flour-water mixture at 25°–30°C will harbour approximately the following:

Mesophilic micro-organisms, aerobes	10^3–10^7 cfu/g
Lactic acid bacteria	<10 to 5×10^2 cfu/g
Yeast	10–10^3 cfu/g
Moulds	10^2 to 5×10^4 cfu/g

Among the mesophiles at the start, members of the Enterobacteriaceae dominate. Micro-organisms dominating in the sourdough after 1–2 days at 25°–30°C are as follows:

Lactic acid bacteria	10^9 cfu/g
Yeast	10^6 to 5×10^7 cfu/g

Some important properties of the rye flour-water environment determine that certain LAB and yeasts will compete most favourably. Lactobacilli have a superior ability to ferment maltose, they thrive despite limited iron due to the presence of phytic acid and they are able to grow at about pH 5.0 and lower.

Reports show that different LAB may be isolated from sourdoughs; however, *Lactobacillus sanfranciscencis* has been found most often. Table 7.2 presents some of the other *Lactobacillus* species that have been isolated from sourdough. The selection of yeasts may be even narrower, with *Candida milleri* often cited (Table 7.2). Several other species are isolated occasionally.

Table 7.2. Common representatives of lactic acid bacteria and yeasts isolated from mature sourdoughs.

	Heterofermentative	*Homofermentative*
Lactic acid bacteria	*Lactobacillus sanfranciscencis* (formerly *Lb. sanfrancisco*, *Lb. brevis* subsp. *lindneri*) *Lb. brevis*, *Lb. fructivorans*, *Lb. fermentum*, *Lb. pontis*, *Lb. sakei* (formerly *Lb. bavaricus*, *Lb. reuteri*)	*Lb. Plantarum* *Lb. delbrueckii*
Yeasts	*Candida milleri*, *C. krusei*, *Saccharomyces cerevisiae*, *S. exiguus Torulopsis holmii*, *T. candida*	

Starters

It is traditional bakers' practice to maintain a good sourdough over time by regular transfer, for example, every 8 hours. This is called 'rebuilding'. Such established cultures are referred to as Type I sourdoughs (Type I process) and a three-stage fermentation procedure is considered necessary to obtain an optimal sourdough. Each step is defined by specific dough yield, temperature and incubation time.

Dough yield is defined as:

$$\frac{(Flour + Water)\ by\ weight}{Flour\ by\ weight} = \times 100\ Dough\ yield$$

A high dough yield implies that a relatively large amount of water is used to make the dough; such a dough would conform with certain requirements in industrial production when there is a need to pump the dough. The lactobacilli and yeasts in Table 7.2 are all common in sourdoughs; however, the composition of starter cultures for Type I processes have been continuously stable maintained for many years and may be compared to certain mixed cultures in dairy technology. The LAB and yeasts in such cultures will be particularly well adjusted and adapted for the conditions in sourdoughs. In Germany, established natural sourdough starter cultures with a stable composition of *Lb. sanfranciscensis* and *Candida milleri* have been propagated for decades; they are marketed as 'Reinzuchtsauerteig'. When the sourdough process has been started through a one-stage or a three-stage procedure, a part of the optimised dough is withdrawn to start up the sourdough production for the next day. These sourdoughs are mentioned in different languages as Anstellgut (German), mother sponge (English), chef (French), masa madre (Spanish), madre (Italian).

Sourdoughs in Type II processes are used mainly for enhancing the flavour and taste of the regular bread. Addition of baker's yeast is required for efficient leavening. Type I sourdoughs are good alternatives as starters for the production of Type II sourdoughs. At the start of a production period, industrially large quantities of Type II sourdoughs may be stocked for portion-wise use over time. Sourdoughs for Type III processes are dried sourdough preparations.

Defined cultures have also been marketed: however, the suitability of Type I and Type II cultures appears to outcompete the alternatives offered. In addition to baker's yeast the conection of defined cultures comprise at least pure cultures of *Lb. brevis* (heterofermentative) and *Lb. delbruckii* and *Lb. Plantarum* (homofermentative). The homofermentative culture produce mainly lactic acid under anaerobic conditions, whereas the heterofermentative cultures will also produce acetic acid or ethanol and carbon dioxide. By controlling, if possible, the contributions from these different cultures, the relative amounts of acetic and lactic acids may be regulated. This important relationship

$$\frac{Lactic\ acid\ (mole)}{Acetic\ acid\ (mole)}$$

is called the fermentation quotient (FQ).

Relatively mild acidity will have an FQ about 4–9, whereas a more strongly flavoured rye bread, as produced in Germany, requires a much lower FQ, for example, 1.5–4.0.

Sourdough Processes

Several more or less traditional sourdough processes are practiced on a large scale in present-day bakery industry. One line comprises processes designed for baking with rye flour. They maybe the Type I processes mentioned above. The Berliner short-sour process, the Detmolder one-stage process and the

Lönner one-stage process are typical for central and northern Europe. In every case, the process is initiated by a starter culture, 2–20 per cent (often 9–10 per cent), in a rye flour-water (close to 50:50 w/w) mixture that is incubated for 3–24 hours at 20°–35°C, depending on the process. When the resulting sourdough is ready, bread making starts with an 'inoculation' of about 30 per cent sourdough together with rye flour, wheat flour, baker's yeast and salt. The final rye:wheat ratio is regularly 70:30 w/w. Dough yield is adjusted to satisfy handling (e.g. pumping) and microbial nutrition requirements.

Another line of sourdough processes comprises those for baking with wheat only. The San Francisco sourdough process is often mentioned in this connection. Italian wheat sourdough products, for example, Panettone, Colomba and Pandoro, are also very important. The starter for San Francisco sourdough is ideally rebuilt every 8 hours to maintain maximum activity. However, a mature sponge may be kept refrigerated for days with acceptable performance. For rebuilding the starter, sponge (40 per cent) is mixed with high-gluten wheat flour (40 per cent) and water (about 20 per cent) to ferment at bakery temperature. Final bread making requires a dough consisting of the ripe sourdough (9.2 per cent), regular wheat flour (45.7 per cent), water (44.2 per cent) and salt (0.9 per cent). Proofing for 7 hours follows, during which the pH decreases from about 5.3 to about 3.9. A sourdough starter culture for San Francisco French bread production commonly contains *Lb. sanfranciscensis* and *Candida holmii*.

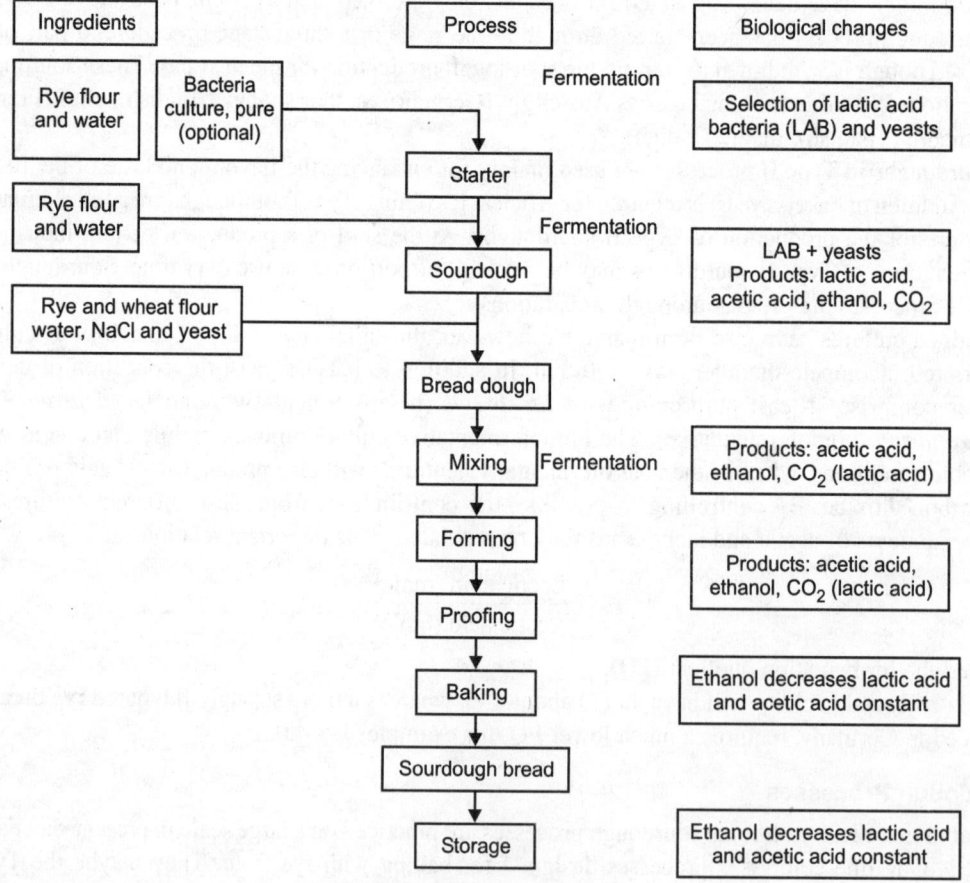

Fig. 7.5. The sourdough process.

Selection and Biochemistry of Micro-organisms in Sourdough

Sourdough breads based on rye or wheat flour or their mixtures enjoys a remarkable standing in many societies, either as established, traditional products or as 'innovative' developments for more natural products and a wider choice of flavours. Well-functioning and popular sourdough starters that have been maintained by simple rebuilding for decades and the re-establishment of the 'same' stable starter over and over again from a constant quality flour, are both expressions of stable ecological conditions. The simplicity of the procedures may be somewhat deceiving with respect to the actual complexity of these biological systems. In the following sections, metabolic events and biochemical aspects of sourdough fermentation will be discussed. Attention will be drawn to some of the more clear points about the metabolic events and other biochemical facts. The near future should bring us closer to a comprehensive understanding.

Carbohydrate metabolism

The development of a mixture (1:1) of rye flour or even wheat flour with water incubated some hours at 25°–30°C will almost inevitably lead to a microbiological population consisting of lactic acid bacteria (LAB) and yeasts. It may need rebuilding several times in order to stabilise it, but from then on the composition of the microflora may be constant for years, provided the composition of the flour and the conditions for growth are not changed much. Representative LAB and yeasts have been presented in Table 7.2. These micro-organisms have certain characteristics in common. First, the selected LAB are very efficient maltose fermenters, a prime reason why they competed so well in the first place. Several lactobacilli in sourdoughs, e.g. *Lb. sanfranciscensis*, *Lb. pontis*, *Lb. reuteri* and *Lb. fermentum*, harbor a key enzyme, maltose phosphorylase, which cleaves maltose (the phosphorolytic reaction) to glucose-1-phosphate and glucose. Glucose-1-phosphate is metabolised heterofermentatively via the phosphogluconate pathway, while glucose is excreted into the growth medium. Glucose repression has not been observed with these lactobacilli. Most of the yeast species identified in sourdoughs are, *per se*, maltose negative and will thus prefer to take up glucose when it is available. Other micro-organisms may experience glucose repression of the maltose enzymes, to the benefit of the sourdough lactobacilli. Among the yeasts, *S. cerevisiae*, which is maltose positive and transports maltose and hexoses very efficiently, cannot take up maltose due to glucose repression and will, as a consequence, be defeated from the sourdough flora. *S. cerevisiae* as baker's yeast is, however, used at the bread-making stage, but as an addition in the recipe. Additional yeast cells may also be necessary for fast and efficient CO_2 production, because the yeasts are relatively sensitive to acids, particularly to acetic acid, which is excreted by the heterofermentative lactobacilli that often dominate the LAB flora of the sourdough. *Candida milleri* (syn. *S. exiguus*, *Torulopsis holmii*) is common in sourdoughs for San Francisco French bread. This yeast tolerates the acetic acid from heterolactic fermentation and thrives on glucose and sucrose in preference to maltose; it thus appears to be a near ideal partner for *Lb. sanfranciscensis*.

Wheat and rye flour contain mainly maltose as a readily available carbohydrate, although rye flour has greater amylase activity and therefore has a greater potential for release of maltose. Early work in the United States on *Lb. sanfranciscensis* indicated that this organism would only ferment maltose. However, strains isolated in Europe appeared more diversified and some of them would ferment up to eight different sugars. Utilisation of maltose by *Lb. sanfranciscensis*, *Lb. pontis*, *Lb. reuteri* and *Lb. fermentum* through phosphorolytic cleavage with maltose phosphorylase is energetically very favourable and shows increased cell yield and excretion of glucose when maltose is available. In these conditions the cells have very low levels of hexokinase.

Cometabolism

Lactobacilli in sourdough production arc not only specialised for maltose fermentation they also exploit co-fermentations for optimised energy yield. *Lactobacillus sanfranciscensis, Lb. pontis* and *Lb. fermentum* all have mannitol dehydrogenase. Thus fructose may be used as an electron acceptor for the re-oxidation of NADH in maltose or glucose metabolism and then acetylphosphate may react on acetate kinase to yield ATP and acetate. The lactobacilli gain energetically and more acetic acid may contribute to the desirable taste and flavour of bread. In practical terms addition of fructose is used to increase acetate in the products, that is, lower FQ. Comparable regulation of acetate production may be achieved by providing citrate, malate or oxygen as electron acceptors, resulting in products like succinate, glycerol and acetate.

Proteolysis and amino compounds

In a sourdough, the flour contributes considerable amounts of amino acids and peptides; however, in order to satisfy nutritional requirements of growing LAB and provide sufficient amino compounds, precursors, for flavour development, some proteolytic action is necessary. The LAB have been suspected as the main contributors of proteinase and peptidase activities for release of amino acids in sourdoughs, although the flour enzymes may also have considerable input. In addition, lysis of microbial cells, particularly yeast cells, add to the pool of amino acids; a stimulant peptide containing aspartic acid, cysteine, glutamic acid, glycine and lysine that appears in the autolytic process of *C. milleri* has also been identified. *Lactobacillus sanfranciscensis* has been found to have a regime of intracellular peptidases, endopeptidase and proteinase, as well as a dipeptidase and proteinase in the cell envelope. Limited autolysis of lactobacillus populations in sourdoughs may add to the repertoire of enzymes that will release amino acids from flour proteins, including those from proline-rich gluten in wheat. Some of the enzymes have been purified for further characterisation and they express interesting activity levels at sourdough pH and temperatures.

The addition of exogenous microbial glucose oxidase, lipase, endoxylanase, α-amylase, or protease in the production of sourdough with 11 different LAB cultures showed positive effects on acidification rate and level for only three cultures, one *Leuconostoc citreum*, one *Lactococcus lactis* subsp, *lactis* and one *Lb. hilgardii*. *Lactobacillus hilgardii* with lipase, endoxylanase or α-amylase showed increased production of acetic acid. *Lactobacillus hilgardii* interacted with the different enzymes for higher stability and softening of doughs.

Recent work with *Lb. sanfranciscensis, Lb. brevis* and *Lb. alimentarius* in model sourdough fermentation showed, by using two-dimensional electrophoresis, that 37–72 polypeptides had been hydrolysed. The polypeptides varied over wide ranges of pls and molecular masses and they originated from albumin, globulin and gliadin, but not from glutenin. Free amino acid concentrations increased, in particular those of proline and glutamic and aspartic acid. Proteolysis by the lactobacilli had a positive effect on the softening of the dough. A toxic peptide for celiac patients, A-gliadin fragment 31–43, was degraded by enzymes from lactobacilli. The agglutination of human myelogenous leukemia-derived cells (K562) by toxic peptic-tryptic digest of gliadins was abolished by enzymes from lactobacilli.

Volatile compounds and carbon dioxide

Both yeasts and LAB contribute to CO_2 production in sourdough products, but the importance of the two varies. In bread production with only the (natural) sourdough microflora, the input from LAB may even be decisive for leavening because the counts and kinds of yeast may not be optimal for gas production. Relatively low temperature (e.g. 25°C) and low dough yield (e.g. 135) would select for

LAB activities and less yeast metabolism. More complete volatile profiles were obtained at higher temperatures (e.g. 30°C) and with a more fluid dough. Of course increasing the leavening time may give substantially richer volatile profiles. If baker's yeast, *S. cerevisiae*, is added to optimise and speed up the production process, the contribution from yeasts will dominate.

Bread made with chemical acidification without fermentation starter failed in sensory analysis. This indicates that fermentation with yeasts and LAB is important for good flavour, although high quality raw materials and proofing and baking are also decisive factors. Flavour compounds distinguishing the different metabolic contributions in sourdough are as follows:

1. Yeast fermentation (alcoholic): 2-methyl-1-propanol, 2,3-methyl-1-butanol.
2. LAB homofermentative: diacetyl, other carbonyls.
3. LAB heterofermentative: ethyl acetate, other alcohols and carbonyls.

Antimicrobial compounds from sourdough LAB

The primary antimicrobial compounds produced by sourdough LAB are lactic and acetic acid, diacetyl, hydrogen peroxide, carbon dioxide and ethanol and among these, the two organic acids continue to be the most important contributions for beneficial effects in fermentations.

Researchers in the field, of course, also consider and test possibilities that LAB may produce bacteriocins and other antimicrobials. Thus antifungal compounds from *Lb. plantarum* 21B have been identified, for example, phenyl lactic acid and 4-hydroxyphenyl lactic acid. Caproic acid from *Lb. sanfranciscensis* also has some antifungal activity.

A real broad-spectrum antimicrobial from *Lb. reuteri* is reuterin (β-hydroxypropionic aldehyde), which comes as a monomer and a cyclic dimer. Reutericyclin, which was isolated from *Lb. reuteri* LTH2584 after the screening of 65 lactobacilli, is a tetramic acid derivative. Reutericyclin inhibited Gram-positive bacteria (e.g. *Lactobacillus* spp., *Bacillus subtilis*, *B. cereus*, *Enterococcus faecalis*, *Staphylococcus aureas* and *Listeria innocua*) and it was bactericidal towards *B. subtilis*, *S. aureus* and *Lb. sanfranciscensis*. The ability to produce reutericyclin was stable in sourdough fermentations over a period of several years. Reutericyclin produced in sourdough was also active in the dough.

A few bacteriocins or bacteriocin-like compounds have also been identified, isolated and characterised. Bavaricin A from *Lb. sakei* MI401 was selected by screening 335 LAB strains, including 58 positive strains. Bavaricin A (and Bavaricin MN from *Lb. sakei* MN) have the N-terminal consensus motif of bacteriocin class IIA in common, comprise 41 and 42 amino acids, respectively and similar hydrophobic regions. Bavaricin A inhibits *Listeria* strains and some other Gram-positive bacteria but not *Bacillus* or *Staphylococcus*. Plantaricin ST31 is produced by *Lb. plantarum* ST. It contains 20 amino acids and the activity spectrum includes several Gram-positive bacteria but not *Listeria*. A bacteriocin-like compound, BLIS C57 from *Lb. sanfranciscensis* C57, was detected after screening 232 *Lactobacillus* isolates, including 52 strains expressing antimicrobial activity. BLIS C57 inhibits Gram-positive bacteria including *bacilli* and *Listeria* strains.

TRADITIONAL FERMENTED CEREAL PRODUCTS

Only two cereals, wheat and rye, contain gluten and are thereby suitable for the production of leavened bread, but many other food cereals are grown in the world. On a global basis, a great proportion of cereals are consumed as spontaneously fermented products, in particular in Africa, Asia and Latin America. Most fermented cereals are dominated by lactic acid bacteria (LAB) and the microflora associated with the grains, flour or any other ingredient, together with contamination from water, food-making equipment and the producers themselves, represent the initial fermentation flora. Malted flour is also an important source of micro-organisms. The changes that take place during the fermentation are due to both the metabolism of the micro-organisms present and the activity of enzymes in the cereal and these are in turn affected by the great variety of technologies that are used. The technology may be simple, involving little more than a mixing of flour with water and allowing it to ferment, or it may be extremely complex and involve many steps with obscure roles. Indigenous fermented foods are usually based upon raw materials that have a sustainable production in their country of origin and are therefore attracting increasing interest from researchers—both within pure and applied food science and also in anthropology. These ancient technologies often have deep roots in the culture of a country and there is increasing awareness of the importance of preserving these traditional foods. Many products are not yet described in the literature and knowledge of them is in danger of disappearing. It is, therefore, necessary to document the technologies used and to identify the fermenting organisms and the metabolic changes that are essential for the characteristics of the product. It is, however, often difficult to describe the sensory attributes of a product that is inherently variable.

In Africa, as much as 77 per cent of the total caloric consumption is provided by cereals of which rice, maize, sorghum and millet are most important. Cereals are also significant sources of protein. Most of the cereal foods consumed in Africa are traditional fermented products and are very important both as weaning foods and as staple foods and beverages for adults. In Asia, many products are based on rice and maize is most widely utilised in Latin America.

Indigenous fermented cereals can be classified according to raw material, type of fermentation, technology used, product usage, or geographical location. They can range from quite solid products such as baked flat breads to sour, sometimes mildly alcoholic, refreshing beverages.

Many factors have an influence on the characteristics of an indigenous product (Fig. 7.6). The choice of raw material may be primarily influenced by price and availability rather than by preference.

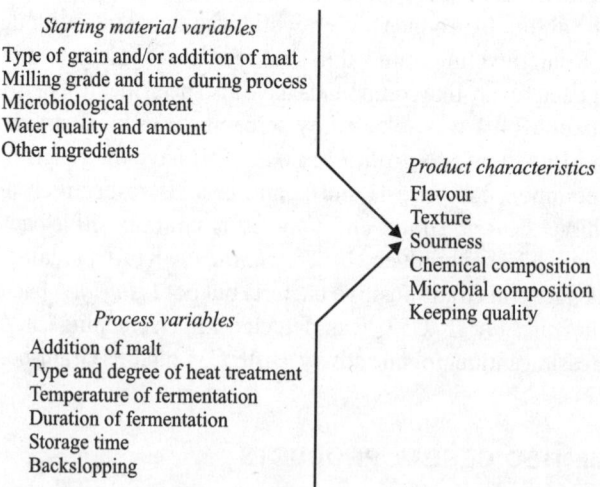

Starting material variables
Type of grain and/or addition of malt
Milling grade and time during process
Microbiological content
Water quality and amount
Other ingredients

Product characteristics
Flavour
Texture
Sourness
Chemical composition
Microbial composition
Keeping quality

Process variables
Addition of malt
Type and degree of heat treatment
Temperature of fermentation
Duration of fermentation
Storage time
Backslopping

Fig. 7.6. Important factors determining the characteristics of spontaneously fermented cereal products.

For instance Togwa, a Tanzanian fermented beverage, may be made from maize in the inland areas of Morogoro and Iringa, but from sorghum in the coastal areas of Dar es Salaam and Zanzibar. Similarly, the Ethiopian product borde may be made from several different grains according to availability—

sorghum, maize, millet, barley and also the Ethiopian cereal tef. The use of different grains obviously affects the sensory characteristics of a product and yet it may have the same name throughout the country. Some fermented cereal products also contain other ingredients. Idli is a leavened steamed cake made primarily from rice to which black gram dahl is added. This not only improves the nutritional quality, but in addition, the black gram imparts a viscosity, apparently specific for this legume, which may aid air entrapment during fermentation and thereby lighten the texture of the product. However, on a broader basis, the addition of legumes such as soyabean flour to fermented cereals has been suggested as an economically feasible way to generally improve the nutritional quality of cereal foods.

Some fermented cereal products are made using unmalted grain, with no extra addition of amylase, but they tend to either be very thick or of low nutritional density. Malted flour is added to many indigenous fermented cereals, a traditional technology that has far-reaching effects on several product characteristics. The addition of malt provides amylases (in particular α-amylase) that hydrolyse the starch, sweeten the product and also cause a considerable decrease in viscosity of the product after heat treatment. The malting process, the germination of grain following steeping in water, is associated with colossal microbiological proliferation and the organisms that develop during malting are a source of fermenting organisms. Many Asian products, for example koji, a Japanese fermented cereal or soyabean product, are first inoculated with a fungus, as a source of amylase, in order to liberate fermentable sugars from the cereal starch.

Many fermented cereals are multipurpose. A single product may be prepared in varying thicknesses and used as a fermented gruel for both adults and children, or it may be watered down and used as a fermented thirst-quenching beverage. As Wood remarked, the latter type of product makes a meaningful contribution to nutrition; the potential of their replacement by cola-type beverage would result in a serious negative impact on the nutrition of people in developing countries.

The use of fermented cereals as weaning foods in developing countries raises several important issues. Unfermented gruels deteriorate very rapidly in unhygienic conditions, especially if refrigeration is not available. They then represent a significant source of foodborne infections that annually claim the lives of millions of young children. Fermented malted cereal gruels have been shown on the whole to contain low numbers of pathogenic organisms since these are inhibited and killed by the low pH that rapidly develops in the product. Fermented cereals are therefore usually regarded as safer than their unfermented counterparts. A weaning food made from unmalted cereals may be a cause of malnutrition because its thick viscosity limits the nutritional intake of a small child. Addition of malted flour decreases the viscosity so that more food can be ingested. If the fermentation flora includes yeasts in addition to LAB, a measurable reduction of carbohydrate will occur due to the production of CO_2 and other volatile compounds. Analysis of fermented cereal products therefore shows that the protein:carbohydrate ratio is improved during the fermentation and this obviously has nutritional benefits.

Milling of cereals into flour is usually done prior to fermentation, but in some products, for example, borde (Ethiopia), wet milling is used. This technique can be used when mechanical grain mills are not available and if the product is required to be smooth and without bits of suspended bran. The starch is also liberated from the grain more thoroughly when slurried with water and sieved than if it has been previously dry milled.

A heat treatment step is found at some point in the production technology of most fermented cereal products and may involve boiling, steaming or roasting. The type of heating employed is likely to have an effect on the flavour of the product, certainly if the temperature attained is sufficient to promote Maillard reactions. The heat also gelatinises the starch, making it more susceptible to amylolytic enzymes, thus providing greater amounts of fermentable carbohydrates. However, at the same time, most of the natural contaminating (and potentially fermenting) flora and cereal enzymes are destroyed. Such products are also prone to contamination after the heat treatment step, and are thereby potentially unsafe should pathogenic organisms grow during the subsequent fermentation. The traditional solution to this is to use 'backslopping', the addition of some of a previous batch of the product and/or the addition of malted flour. Regular backslopping results in a selection of acid-tolerant organisms and functions as an empirical starter culture.

Fermentation usually takes place at ambient temperatures and this may cause seasonal variations in products due to selection of different micro-organisms at different temperatures. The duration of fermentation is largely a matter of personal choice, based on expected sensory attributes. Heat treatment after fermentation makes for a safer product, but it has the disadvantage of change of taste or loss of volatile flavour and aroma compounds.

Microflora of Spontaneously Fermented Cereals

Spontaneously acid-fermented cereal products may contain a variety of micro-organisms, but the flora in the final product is generally dominated by acid-tolerant LAB. Yeasts are also invariably present in large numbers when the fermentation is prolonged. A typical fermented cereal product contains approximately 10^9 and 10^7 cfu/g of product, of LAB and yeasts, respectively. However, since yeast cells are considerably larger than bacteria cells, their metabolic contribution to product characteristics is likely to be just as important as that of the LAB. The buffer capacity of cereal slurries is low and the pH therefore drops quickly as acid is produced. Pathogenic organisms are inhibited by a fast acid production, so the addition of starter cultures, either as a pure culture or by 'backslopping' promotes acid production and contributes to the safety of the fermented product.

The potential and the need for upgrading traditional fermentation technologies have initiated considerable research. In some recent studies of spontaneously fermented cereals, the LAB and yeasts have been isolated and identified as a first stage towards developing starter cultures for small-scale production of traditional fermented cereals. Muyanja recorded that bushera, a traditional Ugandan fermented sorghum beverage that contains high numbers of LAB, was usually consumed by children after one day of fermentation as 'sweet bushera'. After 2–4 days, the product became sour and alcoholic and was consumed by adults. However, the sweet bushera showed very high counts of coliforms and had a reputation for causing diarrhea. Clearly, the development of defined starter cultures would improve the safety of this and similar products.

Some recent examples of studies on the microbial flora of spontaneously fermented cereals are shown in Table 7.3. For each product, several different types of organisms have been isolated.

In other words, a specific product is not produced from fermentation by a specific organism or organisms. *Lb. plantarum* seems to be the most commonly isolated *Lactobacillus* species in fermented cereals. In addition, heterofermentative LAB such as leuconostocs, *Lb. brevis* and *Lb. fermentum* frequently occur. Yeasts are always present in spontaneously fermented products, but few studies have characterised the predominating species. However, Jespersen reported that *S. cerevisciae* is the predominant yeast in many African fermented foods and beverages.

All spontaneously fermented products contain, or have contained, many different types of micro-organisms. These have grown in the product and will have metabolised some of the cereal components, thereby making a contribution (positive or negative) with their metabolites to the overall sensory characteristics of that product. However, studies on spontaneously fermented products have focused on

LAB and yeasts since these organisms are often associated with other, better known, fermented products and have a history of safe use in food. Stanton proposed that the nature of the substrate (raw material) and the technology used to produce fermented foods are the predominating factors that determine the development of micro-organisms and, thereby, the properties of a product.

Table 7.3. Lactic acid bacteria and yeasts isolated from some traditional fermented cereal products.

Product (country of origin)	Cereal basis	Most prevalent Species of LAB	Species of yeast
Togwa (Tanzania)	Various	*Lb. brevis, Lb. cellobiosus, Lb. Plantarum*	*P. orientalis* *S. cerevisiae*
		W. confusa	*C. pelliculosa*
		P. pentosaceus	*C. tropicalis*
Bushera (Uganda)	Sorghum, millet	*Lb. brevis; E. faecium* *Ln. mesenteroides* subsp. *mesenteroides*	NR
Ogi (Nigeria)	Maize	*Lb. reuleri, Lb. leichmanii, Lb. plantarum. Lb. casei, Lb. fermentum, Lb. brevis, Lb. alimentarius, Lb. buchneri, Lb. jensenii*	*S. cereviseae* and *candida mycoderma*
Pozol (Mexico)	Maize	*Streptococcus* spp.	
		Lb. plantarum, Lb. fermentum	
		Lb. brevis	*C. mycoderma*
		Ln. mesenteroides	*S. cerevisiae, Rhodotorula* spp.
		Lc. lactis, Lc. raffinolactis	
Borde (Ethiopia)	Various	*Lb. brevis*	NR
		W. confusa	
		P. pentosaceus	
Idli (India)	Rice and blackgram beans	*Leuconostocs* spp. *Enterococcus faecalis*	*Saccharomyces* spp.

Note: *Lb. lactobacillus*; *Ln., Leuconostoc*; *L., Lactococcus*; *P., Pediococcus, E., Enterococcus*; *W., Weisella*; *S., Saccharomyces*; *l., lsa*; NR, Not recorded.

Desirable Properties of the Fermenting Microflora

The most important property of a starter culture for a fermented cereal is the ability to quickly produce copious amounts of lactic acid in order to achieve a rapid decline in pH and retard the growth of pathogens and other undesirable organisms. Some workers have sought amylolytic LAB strains, as this could remove the need for using the highly contaminated malted flour in a product. The starter should also be able to hydrolyse the cereal protein in order to obtain the amino acids sufficient for rapid growth and it should produce desirable and product-typical aroma and flavour compounds, but not off-flavours. Some products are characterised by a foaming consistency and heterofermentative organisms (LAB or yeasts) are required for this property. Bacteriocin-producing strains have also been sought in an attempt to increase the microbiological safety of the products. Starter cultures must also be commercially propagable and be able to survive preservation methods without loss of viability, activity or metabolic traits.

Microbiological and Biochemical Changes in Traditional Fermented Cereals

Few studies have been made on the biochemical changes that take place in traditional fermented cereals. Mugula analysed samples of naturally fermented togwa made from sorghum and maize, to which togwa was backslopped and malt was added. The development of groups of micro-organisms, organic acids, soluble carbohydrates and volatile components was studied during the 24 hours fermentation. Maltose and glucose increased during the first part of the fermentation due to the action of cereal amylases, but later were reduced as the growth of LAB and yeasts increased. The pH dropped from around 5.0 to 3.2 in 24 hours and this was mirrored by a rise in lactic acid to about 0.5 per cent. Ethanol and secondary alcohols and aldehydes increased during the secondary part of the fermentation. Malty flavours are typical for fermented cereal products and may be produced during grain malting. Secondary aldehydes and alcohols are responsible for these flavours and may also originate from microbial metabolism of the branched-chain amino acids leucine, isoleucine and valine. These compounds are produced by yeasts, some LAB and probably also by other micro-organisms in the product.

Many spontaneously fermented cereals also have a very short shelf life, since fermentation continues in the absence of refrigeration. Off-flavours, in particular vinegary notes, are a common problem. The very low pH in fermented cereal products may be sensorially compensated for by saccharification by β-amylase.

FERMENTED PROBIOTIC CEREAL FOOD

A probiotic food is a live bacterial food supplement, which when ingested, may improve the well-being of the host in a variety of ways by influencing the balance of the host's intestinal flora. Most probiotic bacteria have been isolated from the healthy human intestine and are members of the genus *Lactobacillus*, but some products may contain *Bifidobacterium* spp. or the yeast *Saccharomyces boulardii*. While the potential benefits of probiotic bacteria have been generally accepted for many decades, it is only in comparatively recent years that research has been able to scientifically document the beneficial medical effect due to some specific strains. There is now strong scientific evidence that specific strains of probiotic micro-organisms are able to:

1. Show a prophylactic action against and alleviate diarrhoea caused by bacterial and viral infections, radiation therapy or the use of antibiotics.
2. Suppress undesirable bacteria in the gut with beneficial results for patients with conditions such as irritable bowel syndrome and ulcerative colitis.
3. Influence the immune system, showing positive results four infant atopic eczema and other allergies.

Indeed, in addition to the list above, other effects have been proposed; the lowering of blood cholesterol; the prevention of acute respiratory infections, *Helicobacter pylori* infections and colonisation by potential pathogens in intensive care units in hospitals; relief of constipation and a protection against the development of various forms of cancer. However, so far, convincing proof for the efficacy of probiotics against these problems has not been obtained. The positive effects that have been documented have led to a great interest from food manufacturers and consumers alike. The main motivation for consuming probiotic products is said to be the developing consumer trend towards healthy living though natural foods and medicines and a trend away from the use of antibiotics and the incorporation of chemical additives in food. As the beneficial effects of probiotic foods become scientifically accepted, there will be increasing pressure from food manufacturers on the authorities to allow health claims to be used in product advertising. Probiotic fermented milks were the first probiotic products to be produced commercially and are available in many countries.

Some fermented probiotic cereal products are now being prepared and marketed (Table 7.4) and may have an appeal for those who do not consume dairy products.

Table 7.4. Fermented probiotic cereal foods.

Type of product (commercial name)	Cereal constituent	Probiotic constituent
Fermented fruit flavoured cereal drink (Pro Viva)	Oat + malted barley flour	*Lb. plantarum* 299v
Fermented cereal drink	Oat 'milk'	*Lb. reuteri*; *lb. acidophilus*; *B. bifidus*
Fruit flavoured cereal pudding (Yosa)	Oat flour	*Lb. acidophilus*; *B. bifidus*
Cereal-based weaning food	Maize + malted barley flour	*Lb. acidophilus* *Lb. rhamnosus* 'GG' *Lb. reuteri*

Note: *Lb = Lactobacillus*; *B = Bifidobacterium.*

Oats are a popular basis for probiotic cereal foods. This choice is due to the healthy image of oats with respect to soluble and insoluble fibre content and the potential to reduce blood cholesterol due to β-glucans. A prebiotic is a compound, usually an oligosaccharide, that reaches the colon undigested by the host's enzymes and selectively favours the growth of probiotic bacteria. Such compounds include, fructooligosaccharides lactulose, and inulin. It has been suggested that the best probiotic results may be obtained by using a combination of a prebiotic (such as oats) and a probiotic organism. In this way, the total physiological effect of the food could be increased.

In order for a probiotic product to have a physiological effect, it has been suggested that it should contain at least 10^6 cfu/g product and that daily intake should be at least 100 g. The final acidity in the product has been shown to be of critical importance for the survival of probiotic bacteria during storage. Many probiotic bacteria do not tolerate a pH below 4.0 and fermented cereals frequently reach this pH due to the poor buffering capacity of the substrate. In addition, the physiological state of the probiotic organisms at the time of storage also determines their survival. Organisms that show poor growth during a fermentation period are more likely to die out during cold storage. This necessitates careful formulation of the product as well as selection of the right probiotic culture.

The choice of a substrate for a probiotic food is partially governed by the tolerance of the food towards heat pasteurisation or even sterilisation before fermentation and cereal mixtures lend themselves well to this treatment. Probiotic products require fermentation at around 37°C for 8 to 18 hours, depending on substrate. The suitability of such conditions for the growth of pathogenic organisms necessitates strict adherence to hygiene both before and during fermentation. A fast lactic acid development in the product during fermentation is a critical step and the growth of probiotic organisms in cereal products is growth of probiotic organisms in cereal products is greatly stimulated by the addition of malted flour (either of the same grain or of barley malt) or milk, due to the increased availability of fermentable sugars, peptides and amino acids. For probiotic weaning foods, the use of malt has a further advantage since at a given viscosity, the product has a higher nutritional density.

Probiotic cereal foods are in their infancy and the future will probably see further development in this type of product. New strains with proven probiotic efficacy and good flavour-forming abilities will increase the range of probiotic products available.

CONTAMINATION, PRESERVATION AND SPOILAGE OF CEREALS AND CEREAL PRODUCTS

Contamination

The exteriors of harvested grains contain some of the natural flora that they had while growing, plus contamination from soil and other sources. Freshly harvested grains contain loads of a few thousand to millions of bacteria per gram and from none to several hundred thousand mould spores and, perhaps, spores of smuts and rusts. Bacteria are mostly in the families *Pseudomonadaceae*, *Micrococcaceae*, *Lactobacillaceae* and *Bacillaceae*. If the grains are stored under moist conditions, moulds may grow and produce numerous spores. Scouring and washing of the grains removes part of the micro-organisms, but most of the micro-organisms are removed with the outer portions of the grain during milling. The milling processes, especially bleaching, reduce numbers of organisms, but there then is a possibility of contamination during other procedures, such as blending and conditioning.

Bacteria in wheat flour include spores of *Bacillus*, coliform bacteria and a few representatives of the genera *Achromobacter*, *Flavobacterium*, *Sarcina*, *Micrococcus*, *Alcaligenes* and *Serratia*. Mould spores are chiefly those of aspergilli and penicillia, with also some of *Alternaria*, *Cladosporium* and other genera. Numbers of bacteria vary widely from a few hundred per gram to millions. Most samples of white wheat flour from the retail market contain a few hundred to a few thousand bacteria per gram and average about twenty to thirty bacillus spores per gram and fifty to one hundred mould spores. Patent flours usually give lower counts than straight or clear and numbers decrease with storage of the flour. Higher counts usually are obtained on prepared flours and still higher (8000 to 12,000 per gram on the average) on graham and whole-wheat flours which contain also the outer parts of the wheat kernel and are not bleached. Corn meal often contains from 5000 to 70,000 bacteria per gram and 1000 to 4,00,000 moulds. Malts, because of incubation in a moist condition, contain high numbers of bacteria, usually in the millions per gram.

The surface of a freshly baked loaf of bread is practically free of viable micro-organisms but is subject to contamination by mould spores from the air during cooling and before wrapping. During slicing contamination may take place from micro-organisms in the air, on the knives or on the wrapper. Cakes are similarly subject to contamination. Spores of bacteria able to cause ropiness in bread will survive the baking process.

Preservation

Most cereals and cereal products have such a low moisture content that little difficulty is encountered in the prevention of the growth of micro-organisms as long as the foods are kept dry. Such materials are stored in bulk or in containers so as to keep out vermin, especially insects and rodents, resist fire and avoid rapid changes in temperature and hence increase in moisture. A storage temperature of about 40° to 45°F (4.4° to 7.2°C) is recommended for the dry products. Many bakery products, e.g. breads, rolls, cakes, pastries, pies and canned mixes, contain enough moisture to be subject to spoilage unless special preservative methods are employed or turnover is rapid.

Asepsis

As in other food industries, the adequate cleansing and sanitisation of equipment is essential for reasons of both sanitation and preservation. Improperly sanitised equipment may be a source of rope bacteria and the acid-forming bacteria that cause sourness of doughs. Bread, cakes and other baked goods that may be subject to spoilage by moulds should be protected against contamination by mould spores. Protection of bread is especially important. The bread leaves the oven free of live mould spores should be cooled promptly in an atmosphere free of them, sliced with sporefree knives and wrapped without delay.

Use of heat

Bakery products may be sold unbaked, partially baked or fully baked. The complete baking process ordinarily destroys all bacterial cells, yeasts and mould spores, but not spores of the rope-forming or other bacteria; yet it has been reported that mould spores in proofer cloths in bakeries can build up enough heat resistance to survive baking. Unbaked or partially baked products usually are kept on the retailer's shelf for only a short period or are kept cool during longer storage. Some special breads, e.g. Boston brown bread or nut bread, have been successfully canned.

Use of low temperatures

Although ordinary room temperatures are used by most housewives for the storage of baked goods, keeping times could be lengthened and risk of food poisoning lessened if really warm temperatures, such as those of hot kitchens or summer weather, were avoided and the foods were stored in a cool place or even in the refrigerator. The freezing-storage of bakery goods is on the increase. Unbaked or partially baked products, waffles, cheese cake, ice-cream pie, fish, poultry and meat pies now often are frozen. Bread and rolls can be stored successfully for months in the frozen condition.

Use of chemical preservatives

Sodium and calcium propionates (0.1 to 0.32 per cent of the weight of the flour) are used routinely by many bakers, mostly in bread but sometimes in other products, to delay or prevent mould growth and ropiness. Sorbic acid has been recommended as a substitute for propionate. Acidification of the dough, usually with acetic acid, has been employed to combat rope.

Use of Irradiation

In bakeries, ultraviolet rays have been used to destroy or reduce numbers of mould spores in dough and proof rooms, on the knives of slicing machines, in the room where the bread is packaged and on the surface of bread, cakes and other bakery products. The application of radio-frequency radiations to loaves of bread to reduce the likelihood of mould spoilage has been reported and ionising radiations, gamma and cathode rays, have been applied experimentally for the preservation of baked goods.

Spoilage

Cereal grains and meals and flours made from them, should not be subject to microbial spoilage if they are prepared and stored properly because their moisture content is too low to support even the growth of moulds. If, however, these products are moistened above the minimum for microbial growth, that growth will follow. A little moistening will permit only mould growth, but more moisture will allow the growth of yeasts and bacteria.

Cereal grains and meals

Since cereal grains and meals ordinarily are not processed so as to greatly reduce their natural flora of micro-organisms, they are apt to contain moulds, yeasts and bacteria which are ready to grow if enough moisture is added. In addition to starch, which is unavailable to many organisms, these grains contain some sugar and available nitrogen compounds, minerals and accessory growth substances; and the amylases will release more sugar if the grains are moistened and proteinases will yield more available nitrogenous foods. A little added moisture will result in growth of moulds at the surface where air is available. A wet mash of the grains or mash of the meals will undergo an acid fermentation, chiefly by the lactic acid and coliform bacteria normally present on plant surfaces. This may be followed by an alcoholic fermentation by yeasts as soon as the acidity has increased enough to favour them. Finally moulds and perhaps film yeasts will grow on the top surface, although acetic acid bacteria, if present, may oxidise the alcohol to acetic acid and inhibit the moulds.

Flours

The dry cleaning and washing of grains and the milling and sifting of flour reduce the content of micro-organisms, but the important kinds still are represented in whole-grain flours, such as whole-wheat or buckwheat and the spoilage would be similar to that described for cereal grains and meals.

White wheat flour, however, usually is bleached by an oxidising, agent, such as an oxide of nitrogen, chlorine, nitrosyl chloride, or benzoyl peroxide and this process serves to reduce microbial numbers and kinds. A moisture content of flour of less than 13 per cent has been reported to prevent the growth of all micro-organisms. Other workers claim that 15 per cent permits good mould growth and over 17 per cent the growth of both moulds and bacteria. Therefore, slight moistening of white flour brings about spoilage by moulds. Because of the variations in microbial content of different lots of flour, the type of spoilage in a flour paste is difficult to predict. If acid-forming bacteria are present, an acid fermentation begins, followed by aloholic fermentation by yeasts if they are there and then acetic acid by *Acetobacter* species. This succession of changes would be more likely in freshly milled flour than in flour that had been stored for a long period with a consequent reduction in kinds and numbers of micro-organisms. In the absence of lactics and coliforms, micrococci have been found to acidify the paste and in their absence species of Bacillus may grow, especially aerobacilli which produce lactic acid, gas, alcohol, acetoin and small amounts of esters and other aromatic compounds. It is characteristic of most flour pastes to develop an odour of acetic acid and esters.

Bread

During fermentations taking place in the doughs for various kinds of bread, it was noted that some changes caused by micro-organisms are desirable and are even necessary in the making of certain kinds of bread. The acid fermentation by lactics and coliform bacteria that is normal in flour pastes or doughs may, however, be too extensive if too much time is permitted, with the result that the dough and bread made from it may be too 'sour'. Excessive growth of proteolytic bacteria during this period may destroy some of the gas-holding capacity so essential during the rising of the dough and produce what is called a 'sticky' dough. Sticky doughs, however, are usually the result of overmixing or gluten breakdown by reducing agents, e.g. glutathione. There also is the possibility of the production by micro-organisms of undesirable flavours other than the sourness.

The chief types of microbial spoilage of baked bread are mouldiness and ropiness, usually termed 'mould' and 'rope'.

Mould

Moulds are the most common and hence the most important cause of the spoilage of bread and, in fact, of most bakery products. The temperatures attained in the baking procedure usually are high enough to kill all mould spores in and on the loaf, so that moulds must reach the outer surface or penetrate after baking. They can come from the air during cooling or thereafter, from handling or from wrappers and usually initiate growth in the crease of the loaf and between the slices of sliced bread.

Chief moulds involved in the spoilage of bread are the so-called 'bread mould', *Rhizopus nigricans*, with its white cottony mycelium and black dots of sporangia; the green-spored *Penicillium expansum* or *P. stoloniferum*; *Aspergillus niger* with its greenish- or purplish-brown to black conidial heads and yellow pigment diffusing into the bread; and *Monilia* (*Neurospora*) *sitophila*, whose pink conidia give a pink or reddish colour to its growth. Species of *Mucor* or *Geotrichum* or any of a large number of species of other genera of moulds may develop. Mould spoilage is favoured by: (i) heavy contamination after baking, due, for example, to air heavily laden with mould spores, a long cooling time, considerable air circulation, or a contaminated slicing machine, (ii) slicing, in that more air is introduced into the loaf; (iii) wrapping, especially if the bread is warm when wrapped, and (iv) storage in a warm, humid place. There is little growth of commercial importance on bread crust in a relative humidity below 90 per cent. Bread with 6 per cent of milk solids retains moisture somewhat better than milk-free bread and hence there is less moisture between loaf and wrapper and hence less moulding, but there is not enough effect to be of much practical importance. Moulding often begins within a loaf of sliced bread, where more moisture is available than at the surface, especially in the crease.

Various methods are employed to prevent mouldiness of bread: (i) prevention of contamination of bread with mould spores in so far as is practicable. The air about the bread is kept low in spores by removal of possible breeding places for moulds, such as returned bread, or walls and equipment. Spore-laden flour dust from other parts of the bakery has been incriminated in causing increased mouldiness of bread. Filtration and washing of air to the room and irradiation of the room and more especially the air by means of ultraviolet rays cut down contamination, (ii) prompt and adequate cooling of the loaves before wrapping to reduce condensation of moisture beneath the wrapper, (iii) ultraviolet irradiation of the surface of the loaf and of slicing knives, (iv) destruction of moulds on the surface by electronic heating, (v) keeping the bread cool to slow down mould growth, or freezing and storage in the frozen condition to prevent growth entirely, and (vi) incorporation in the bread dough of some mycostatic chemical.

Most commonly employed now is sodium or calcium propionate at the rate of 0.1 to 0.3 per cent of the weight of the flour, a treatment that also is effective against rope. Sorbic acid, up to 0.3 per cent, has been suggested as a substitute for propionate but is not permitted by present standards. An older remedy was the addition of vinegar or acetate to the dough or treatment of the exterior of the loaf with vinegar.

Rope

Ropiness of bread is fairly common in home-baked bread, especially during hot weather, but it is comparatively rare in commercially baked bread because of preventive measures now employed. Ropiness is caused by a mucoid variant of *Bacillus subtilis* or *B. licheniformis*, formerly called *B. mesentericus*, *B. panis* and other species names. The spores of these species can withstand the temperature of the bread during baking, which does not exceed 100°C and can germinate and grow in the loaf if conditions are favourable. The ropy condition apparently is the result of capsulation of the bacillus, together with hydrolysis of the flour proteins (gluten) by proteinases of the organism and of starch by amylase to give sugars that encourage rope formation. The area of ropiness is yellow to brown in colour and is soft and sticky to the touch. In one stage the slimy material can be drawn out into long threads when the bread is broken and pulled apart. The unpleasant odour is difficult to characterise, although it has been described as that of decomposed or over ripe melons. First the odour is evident, then discolouration and finally softening of the crumb, with stickiness and stringiness.

The production of ropiness is favoured by the following factors: (i) heavy contamination of the dough with spores of the causative bacillus, chiefly from the ingredients. Of these, the flour is likely to be the heaviest source of spores of the rope organism and for that reason flours are tested for their content of spores of mesophilic bacteria. The yeast, dry milk, sugar, malt and malted products also have been reported to be sources of spores of rope bacteria, (ii) contamination of the dough from equipment or of the bread by slicing knives. Spores of *B. subtilis* may build up on equipment, if trouble has been encountered previously, (iii) slow cooling of the bread after baking. This favours rapid germination of spores and multiplication of vegetative cells in the bread, (iv) lack of acidity in the bread. *B. subtilis* is favoured by pH values near neutrality and is increasingly inhibited as the acidity is increased (pH drops) toward pH 5.0, and (v) storage of bread in a warm, humid atmosphere. This is more likely to happen in the home than elsewhere during the hot months of summer. Bread containing spores may develop the defect at temperatures above 90°F (32.2°C), when the spores would not cause spoilage if the bread were kept at lower temperatures for the usual period before use.

Methods for preventing ropiness of bread are readily inferred from the conditions favouring it: (i) use of ingredients of the dough that are low in numbers of spores of the rope bacterium. Some can be purchased with this low content specified, (ii) adequate cleansing and sanitising of equipment coming in contact with the dough to prevent contamination from this source. Slicing knives also should be kept free from the bacterial spores, (iii) prompt cooling of the loaves after baking, (iv) use of a dough formula that will result in a pH of 5.0 to 5.15 in the bread. This has been accomplished by the addition of acetic, tartaric, citric, or lactic acid, or acid phosphate, but acidification must be used with caution or the rising of the dough will be adversely affected, (v) addition of 0.1 to 0.3 per cent of sodium or calcium propionate (or sorbic acid) on the basis of the weight of the flour. This probably is the best preventive procedure and, as has been pointed out, also inhibits growth of moulds, and (vi) storage of the bread at a cool temperature. This, in itself, may be enough to prevent ropiness during the normal period of holding bread, if the original contamination of rope spores was not heavy. Freezing bread and storing it in the frozen condition will prevent ropiness entirely.

A number of methods have been suggested for testing flour or other ingredients for the presence of spores of rope bacteria. Most reliable is a bread-baking and incubation test. A plate count of spores of mesophilic *bacillus* species has been employed where a flour suspension is pasteurised at 80°C for 10 minute and plated quantitatively. A count of 20 or more spores per 100 gram of flour is considered objectionable. Another method employs quantitative dilutions of the flour in nutrient broth followed by incubation at 37°C for 48 hours. A grayish-white surface pellicle on the broth is indicative of the growth of a Bacillus species. Other, less successful methods have been recommended. Ropiness also can occur in doughnuts, brown bread and cakes.

Red bread

Red or 'bloody', bread is striking in appearance but rare in occurrence. The red colour results from the growth of pigmented bacteria, usually *Serratia marcescens*, an organism that often is brilliantly red on starchy foods. In ancient times the mysterious appearance of apparent drops of blood was considered miraculous. Necessary for the phenomenon is the accidental contamination of the bread with the red organisms and unusually moist conditions to favour their growth. Moulds, such as *Monilia sitophila*, previously mentioned, may impart a pink to red colour to bread. A red colour in the crumb of dark bread has been caused by *Oidium* (*Geotrichum*) *aurantiacum*.

Chalky bread

Chalky bread, also uncommon in occurrence, is so named because of white, chalklike spots. The defect has been blamed on the growth of yeastlike fungi, *Endomycopsis fibuliger* and *Trichosporon* variable.

Cakes and other bakery products

Moulds are the chief cause of the microbial spoilage of cakes and other bakery products. Methods of prevention are similar to those listed for bread. Ultraviolet irradiation of the surfaces of cakes before wrapping and packaging has been successful in reducing mould spoilage and propionates can be employed for most kinds of cake, but not for some of the fruit pies. Sorbic acid is effective in preventing mould growth on cakes. As has been indicated, ropiness can develop in cakes or doughnuts; the cause and methods of prevention are similar to those for bread.

Staling of bakery products

The deterioration of bread, cakes, pies and other bakery products called 'staling' is due mostly to physical changes during holding and not to micro-organisms. Freezing and storage in the frozen condition is an effective method of preventing the changes.

Macaroni and Tapioca

Swelling of moist macaroni has been reported to be caused by gas production by bacteria resembling *Aerobacter cloacae*. During the drying of macaroni on paper a mould of the genus *Monilia* has been found responsible for purple streaks at the contact points with the paper. The appearance of these defects is uncommon, however, despite the long, slow drying process and few reports of spoilage have been made.

Tapioca, prepared from the root starch of cassava, will spoil if moistened.

Chapter 8

Beer

INTRODUCTION

The word beer comes from the Latin word *Bibere* (to drink). It is a beverage whose history can be traced back to between 6000 and 8000 years and the process, being increasingly regulated and well controlled because of tremendous strides in the understanding of it, has remained unchanged for hundreds of years. The basic ingredients for most beers are malted barley, water, hops and yeast; indeed, the 500-year-old Bavarian purity law (the *Reinheitsgebot*) restricts brewers to these ingredients for beer to be brewed in Germany. Most other brewers worldwide have much greater flexibility in their production process opportunities, yet the largest companies are ever mindful of the importance of tradition.

Compared to most other alcoholic beverages, beer is relatively low in alcohol. The highest average strength of beer [alcohol by volume (ABV) indicates the millilitres of ethanol per 100 ml of beer] in any country worldwide is 5.1 per cent and the lowest is 3.9 per cent. By contrast, the ABV of wines is typically in the range 11–15 per cent.

OVERVIEW OF MALTING AND BREWING

Brewer's yeast *Saccharomyces* can grow on sugar anaerobically by fermenting it to ethanol (Fig. 8.1):

$$C_6H_{12}O_6 \rightarrow 2C_2H_5OH + 2CO_2$$

while malt and yeast contribute substantially to the character of beers, the quality of beer is at least as much a function of the water and, especially, of the hops used in its production.

Barley starch supplies most of the sugars from which the alcohol is derived in the majority of the world's beers. Historically, this is because, unlike other cereals, barley retains its husk on threshing and this husk traditionally forms the filter bed through which the liquid extract of sugars is separated in the brewery. Even so, some beers are made largely from wheat while others are from sorghum.

The starch in barley is enclosed in a cell wall and proteins and these wrappings are stripped away in the malting process (essentially a limited germination of the barley grains), leaving the starch largely preserved. Removal of the wall framework softens the grain and makes it more readily milled. Not only that, unpleasant grainy and astringent characters are removed during malting.

In the brewery, the malted grain must first be milled to produce relatively fine particles, which are for the most part starch. The particles are then intimately mixed with hot water in a process called mashing. The water must possess the right mix of salts. For example, fine ales are produced from waters with high levels of calcium while famous pilsners are from waters with low levels of calcium.

Typically mashes have a thickness of three parts water to one part malt and contain a stand at around 65°C, at which temperature the granules of starch are converted by gelatinisation from an indigestible granular state into a 'melted' form that is much more susceptible to enzymatic digestion. The enzymes that break down the starch are called the amylases. They are developed during the malting process, but only start to act once the gelatinisation of the starch has occurred in the mash tun. Some brewers will have added starch from other sources, such as maize (corn) or rice, to supplement that from malt. These other sources are called adjuncts. After perhaps an hour of mashing, the liquid portion of the mash, known as wort, is recovered, either by straining through the residual spent grains or by filtering through plates. The wort is run to the kettle (sometimes known as the copper, even though they are nowadays fabricated from stainless steel) where it is boiled, usually for around 1 hour. Boiling serves various functions, including sterilisation of wort, precipitation of proteins (which would otherwise come out of solution in the finished beer and cause cloudiness), and the driving away of unpleasant grainy characters originating in the barley. Many brewers also add some adjunct sugars at this stage, at which most brewers introduce at least a proportion of their hops.

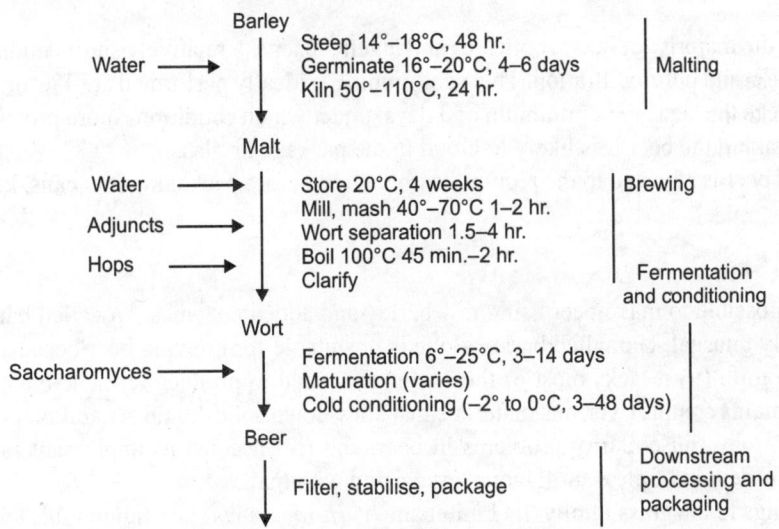

Fig. 8.1. Overview of malting and brewing.

The hops have two principal components: resins and essential oils. The resins (so-called α-acids) are changed ('isomerised') during boiling to yield iso-α-acids, which provide the bitterness to beer. This process is rather inefficient. Nowadays, hops are often extracted with liquefied carbon dioxide and the extract is either added to the kettle or extensively isomerised outside the brewery for addition to the finished beer (thereby avoiding losses due to the tendency of the bitter substances to stick on to yeast). The oils are responsible for the 'hoppy nose' on beer. They are very volatile and if the hops are all added at the start of the boil, then all of the aroma will be blown up the chimney (stack). In traditional lager brewing, a proportion of the hops is held back and only added towards the end of boiling, which allows the oils to remain in the wort. For obvious reasons, this process is called late hopping. In traditional ale production, a handful of hops is added to the cask at the end of the process, enabling a complex mixture of oils to give a distinctive character to such products. This is called dry hopping. Liquid carbon dioxide can be used to extract oils as well as resins and these extracts can also be added late in the process to make modifications to beer flavour.

After the removal of the precipitate produced during boiling ('hot break', 'trub'), the hopped wort is cooled and pitched with yeast. There are many strains of brewing yeast and brewers carefully look after their own strains because of their importance in determining brand identity. Fundamentally brewing yeast can be divided into ale and lager strains, the former type collecting at the surface of the fermenting wort and the latter settling at the bottom of a fermentation (although this differentiation is becoming blurred with modern fermenters). Both types need a little oxygen to trigger off their metabolism, but otherwise the alcoholic fermentation is anaerobic. Ale fermentations are usually complete within a few days at temperatures as high as 20°C, whereas lager fermentations at temperatures as low as 6°C can take several weeks. Fermentation is complete when the desired alcohol content has been reached and when an unpleasant butterscotch flavour, which develops during all fermentations, has been mopped up by yeast. The yeast is harvested for use in the next fermentation.

In traditional ale brewing, the beer is now mixed with hops, some priming sugars and with isinglass finings from the swim bladders of certain fish, which settle out the solids in the cask.

In traditional lager brewing, the 'green beer' is matured by several weeks of cold storage, prior to filtering.

Nowadays, the majority of beers, both ales and lagers, receive a relatively short conditioning period after fermentation and before filtration. This conditioning is ideally performed at −1°C or lower (but not so low as to freeze the beer) for a minimum of 3 days, under which conditions more proteins drop out of the solution, making the beer less likely to cloud in the package or glass.

The filtered beer is adjusted to the required carbonation before packaging into cans, kegs or glass or plastic bottles.

Barley

Although it is possible to make beer using raw barley and added enzymes (so-called barley brewing), this is extremely unusual. Unmalted barley alone is unsuitable for brewing beer because: (i) it is hard and difficult to mill, (ii) it lacks most of the enzymes needed to produce fermentable components in wort, (iii) it contains complex viscous materials that slow down solid-liquid separation processes in the brewery, which may cause clarity problems in beer, and (iv) it contains unpleasant raw and grainy characters and is devoid of pleasant flavours associated with malt.

Barley belongs to the grass family. Its Latin name is *Hordeum vulgare*, though this term tends to be retained for six-row barley (discussed later), with *Hordeum distichon* being used for two-row barley. The part of the plant of interest to the brewer is the grain on the ear. Sometimes this is referred to as the seed, but individual grains are generally called kernels or corns. A schematic diagram of a single barley corn is shown in Fig. 8.2.

Four components of the kernel are particularly significant:
1. The embryo, which is the baby plant.
2. The starchy endosperm, which is the food reserve for the embryo.
3. The aleurone layer, which generates the enzymes that degrade the starchy endosperm.
4. The husk (hull), which is the protective layer around the corn. Barley is unusual amongst cereals in retaining a husk after threshing and this tissue is traditionally important for its role as a filter medium in the brewhouse when the wort is separated from spent grains.

The first stage in malting is to expose the grain to water, which enters an undamaged grain solely through the micropyle and progressively hydrates the embryo and the endosperm. This switches on the metabolism of the embryo, which sends hormonal signals to the aleurone layer, triggers that switch on the synthesis of enzymes responsible for digesting the components of the starchy endosperm. The digestion products migrate to the embryo and sustain its growth.

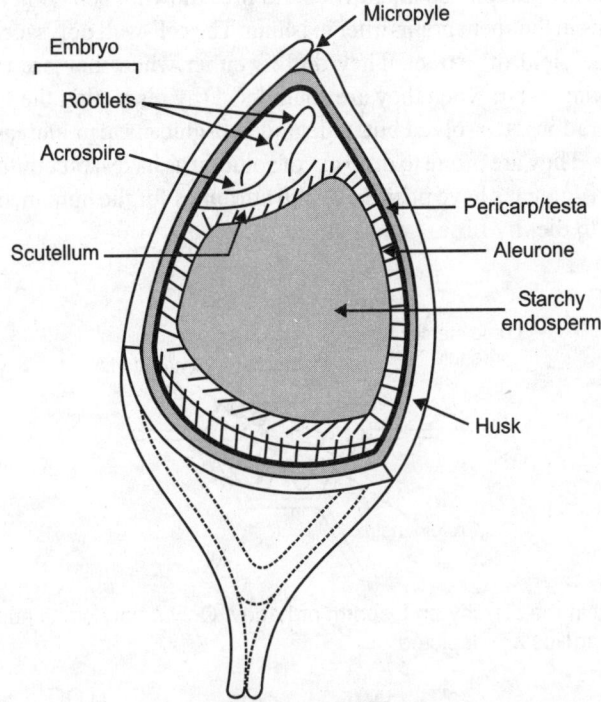

Fig. 8.2. A barley corn.

The aim is controlled germination, to soften the grain, remove troublesome materials and expose starch without promoting excessive growth of the embryo that would be wasteful (malting loss). The three stages of commercial malting are:

1. Steeping, which brings the moisture content of the grain to a level sufficient to allow metabolism to be triggered in the grain.
2. Germination, during which the contents of the starchy endosperm are substantially degraded ('modification') resulting in a softening of the grain.
3. Kilning, in which the moisture is reduced to a level low enough to arrest modification.

The embryo and aleurone are both living tissues, but the starchy endosperm is dead. It is a mass of cells, each of which comprises a relatively thin cell wall (approximately 2 μm) inside which are packed many starch granules amidst a matrix of protein (Fig. 8.3). This starch and protein (and also the cell-wall materials) are the food reserves for the embryo. However, the brewer's interest in them is as the source of fermentable sugars and assimilable amino acids that the yeast will use during alcoholic fermentation. The wall around each cell of the starchy endosperm comprises 75 per cent β-glucan, 20 per cent pentosan, 5 per cent per cent protein and some acids, notably acetic acid and the phenolic acid, ferulic acid. The β-glucan comprises long linear chains of glucose units joined through β-linkages. Approximately 70 per cent of these linkages are between C-1 and C-4 of adjacent glucosyl units (so-called β 1-4 links, just as in cellulose) and the remainder are between C-1 and C-3 of adjacent glucoses (β 1-3 links, which are not found in cellulose) (Fig. 8.4). These 1-3 links disrupt the structure of the β-glucan molecule and make it less ordered, more soluble and digestible than cellulose. Much less is known about the pentosan (arabinoxylan, Fig. 8.5) component of the wall, and it is generally believed that it is less easily solubilised and difficult to breakdown when compared with the β-glucan, and that it largely remains in the spent grains after mashing. The cell-wall polysaccharides are problematic because they restrict the yield of extract. They do this either when they are insoluble (by wrapping around the starch components) or when they are solubilised (by restricting the flow of wort from spent grains during wort separation). Dissolved but undegraded β-glucans also increase the viscosity of beer and slow down filtration. They are prone to drop out of solution as hazes, precipitates or gels. Conversely it has been claimed that β-glucans have positive health attributes for the human, by lowering cholesterol levels and contributing to dietary fibre.

Fig. 8.3. A single cell within the starchy endosperm or barley. Only a very small number of the multitude of small and large starch granules are depicted.

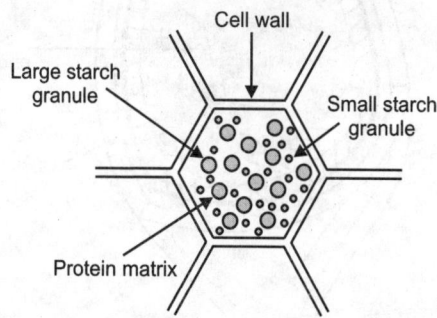

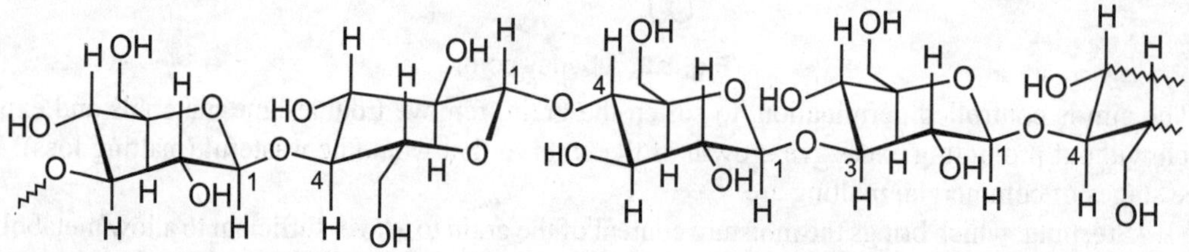

Fig. 8.4. Mixed linkage β-glucan in the starchy endosperm cell wall of barley. The 1-3 linkages occur every third or fourth glucosyl, although there are 'cellulosic' regions wherein there are longer sequences of 1-4 linked glucosyls ~indicates that the chain continues in either direction molecular weights of these glucans can be many millions.

The enzymic breakdown of β-glucan during the germination of barley and later in mashing is in two stages: solubilisation and hydrolysis. Several enzymes (collectively the activity is referred to by the trivial name 'solubilase') may be involved in releasing β-glucan from the cell wall, including esterases that hydrolyse ester bonds believed to cement polysaccharides, perhaps to the protein-rich middle lamella. The most recent evidence, however, is that the pentosan component encloses much of the glucan (Fig. 8.6), and accordingly pentosanases are efficient solubilases. This is despite the observations that pentosans are less digestible than glucans. β-glucans are hydrolysed by endo-β-glucanases (*endo* enzymes hydrolyse bonds inside a polymeric molecule, releasing smaller units, which are subsequently broken down by *exo* enzymes that chop off one unit at a time, commencing at one end of the molecule). These enzymes convert viscous β-glucan molecules to non-viscous oligosaccharides comprising three or four glucose units. Less well-understood enzymes are responsible for converting these oligosaccharides to glucose. There is little if any β-glucanase in raw barley, it being developed during the germination phase of malting in response to gibberellins. Endo-β-glucanase is extremely sensitive to heat, meaning that it is essential that malt is kilned very carefully to conserve this enzyme if it is necessary that it should complete the task of glucan degradation in the brewhouse. This is especially important if the brewer is using β-glucan-rich adjuncts such as unmalted barley, flaked barley and roasted barley. It is also the reason why brewers often employ a low temperature start to their mashing processes. Alternatively, some brewers add exogenous heat-stable β-glucanases of microbial origin.

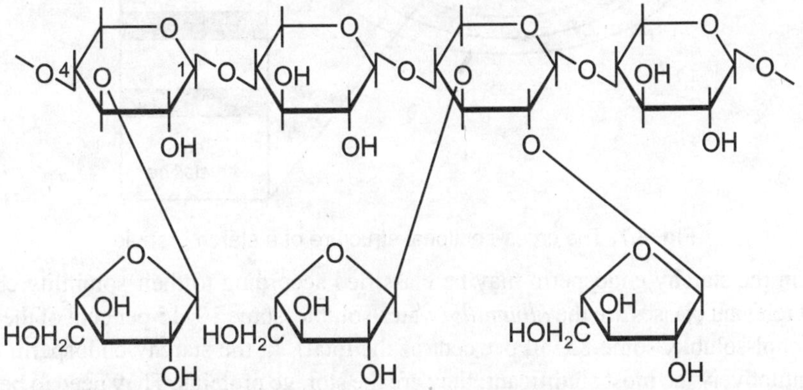

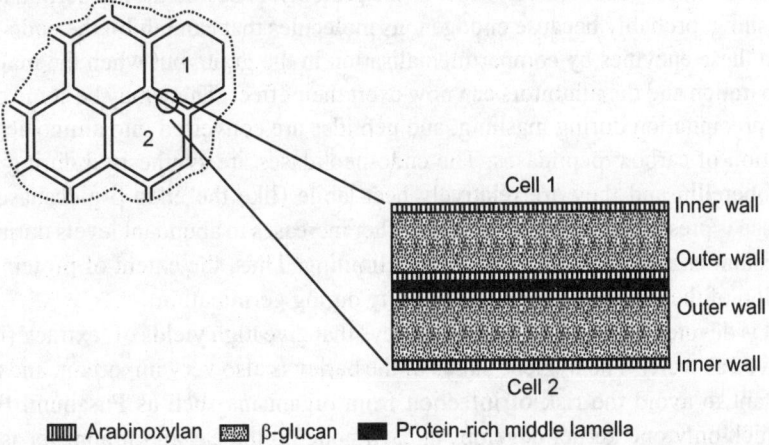

Fig. 8.5. Pentosans in the walls of barley comprise a linear backbone of β 1 → 4 linked xylosyl residues with arabinose attached through either α1 → 2 or α1 → 3 bonding. Although not depicted here, the arabinose residues are variously esterified with either ferulic acid or acetic acid.

Cell 1
Inner wall
Outer wall
Outer wall
Inner wall
Cell 2

▦ Arabinoxylan ▨ β-glucan ▮ Protein-rich middle lamella

Fig. 8.6. Current understanding of the structure or the cell walls or barley endosperm. Walls surrounding adjacent cells are cemented by a protein-rich middle lamella. To this is attached arabinoxylan, within which is the β-glucan.

The starch in the cells of the starchy endosperm is in two forms: large granules (approximately 25 μm) and small granules (5 μm). The structure of granules is quite complex, having crystalline and amorphous regions (Fig. 8.7).

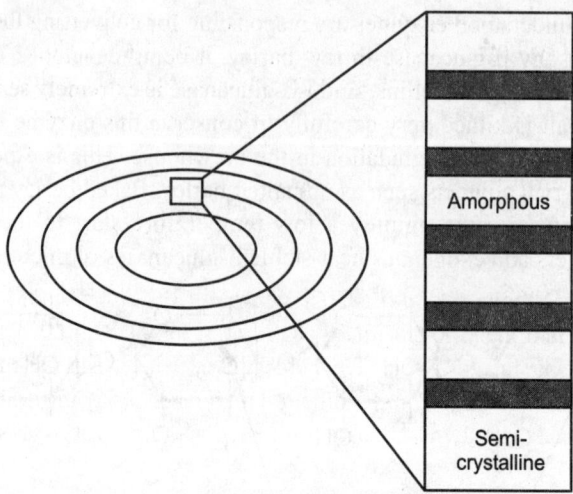

Fig. 8.7. The cross-sectional structure of a starch granule.

The proteins in the starchy endosperm may be classified according to their solubility characteristics. The two most relevant classes are the *albumins* (water-soluble, some 10–15 per cent of the total) and the *hordeins* (alcohol-soluble, some 85–90 per cent of the total). In the starchy endosperm of barley, the latter are quantitatively the most significant: they are the storage proteins. They need to be substantially degraded in order that the starch can be accessed and amino acids (which will be used by the yeast) generated. Their partial degradation products can also contribute to haze formation via cross-linking with polyphenols. Excessive proteolysis should not occur, however, as some partially degraded protein is required to afford stable foam to beer. Most of the proteolysis occurs during germination rather than subsequent mashing, probably because endogenous molecules that can inhibit the endo-proteinases are kept apart from these enzymes by compartmentalisation in the grain, but when the malt is milled, this disrupts the separation and the inhibitors can now exert their effect. There may be some ongoing protein extraction and precipitation during mashing, and peptides are converted into amino acids at this stage through the action of carboxypeptidases. The endo-peptidases are synthesised during germination in response to gibberellin and they are relatively heat-labile (like the endo-β-glucanases). Substantial carboxypeptidase is present in raw barley and it further increases to abundant levels during germination. It is a heat-resistant enzyme and is unlikely to be limiting. Thus, the extent of protein degradation is largely a function of the extent of proteinase activity during germination.

Much effort is devoted to breeding malting barleys that give high yields of 'extract' (i.e. fermentable material dissolved as wort). The hygiene status of the barley is also very important, and pesticide usage may be important to avoid the risk of infection from organisms such as Fusanum. Barleys may be two-row, in which only one kernel develops at each node on the ear and it appears as if there is one kernel on either side of the axis of the ear, or six-row in which there are three corns per node. Obviously there is less room for the individual kernels in the latter case and they tend to be somewhat twisted and smaller and therefore less desirable. Farmers are restricted in how much nitrogenous fertiliser they can use because the grain will accumulate protein at the expense of starch in the endosperm, and it is the starch (*ergo* fermentable sugar) that is especially desirable. Maltsters pay a 'malting premium' for the right variety, grown to have the desired level of protein. There must be some protein present, as this is the fraction of the grain which includes the enzymes and which is the origin of amino acids (for yeast metabolism) and foam polypeptide. The amount of protein needed in malt will depend on whether the brewer intends to use some adjunct material as a substitute for malt. For example, corn syrup is a rich source of sugar but not of amino acids, which will need to come from the malt.

Dead grain will not germinate, so batches of barley must pass viability tests. Most barley in the Northern Hemisphere is sown between January and April and is referred to as Spring Barley. The earlier the sowing, the better the yield and lower the protein levels because starch accumulates throughout the growing season. In locales with mild winters, some varieties (Winter Barleys) are sown in September and October. Best yields of grain are in locales where there is a cool, damp growing season allowing steady growth, and then fine, dry weather at harvest to ripen and dry the grain. Grain grown through very hot, dry summers is thin, poorly filled and has high nitrogen. Malting barley is grown in many countries such as Canada, Germany, Russian Fed, France, Spain, Turkey, USA, UK, Ukraine and Australia.

Grain arrives at the maltings by road or rail and, as the transport waits, the barley will be weighed and a sample tested for viability, nitrogen content and moisture. Expert evaluation will also provide a view on how clean the sample is in terms of weed content and whether the grain 'smells sweet'. Once accepted, the barley will be cleaned and screened to remove small grain and dust, before passing into a silo, perhaps via a drying operation in areas with damp climates. Grain should be dry to counter infection and outgrowth.

It is essential that the barley store is protected from the elements, yet it must also be ventilated, because barley, like other cereals, is susceptible to various infections, for example, Fusarium, storage fungi such as *Penicillium* and *Aspergillus*, Mildew and pests, for example, aphids and weevils.

Steeping is probably the most critical stage in malting. If homogeneous malt is to be obtained (which will go on to 'behave' predictably in the brewery), then the aim must be to hydrate the kernels in a batch of barley evenly. Steeping regimes are determined on a barley-by-barley basis by small-scale trials but most varieties need to be taken to 42–46 per cent. Apart from water, barley needs oxygen in order to support respiration in the embryo and aleurone. Oxygen access is inhibited if grain is submerged for excessive periods in water, a phenomenon which directly led to the use of interrupted steeping operations. Rather than submerge barley in water and leave it, grain is steeped for a period of time, before removing the water for a so-called 'air-rest' period. Then a further steep is performed and so on. Air rests serve the additional purpose of removing carbon dioxide and ethanol, either of which will suppress respiration. A typical steeping regime may involve an initial steep to 32–38 per cent moisture (lower for more water-sensitive barleys). The start of germination is prompted by an air rest of 10–20 hours, followed by a second steep to raise the water content to 40–42 per cent. Emergence of the root tip 'chitting' is encouraged by a second air rest of 10–15 hours before the final steep to the target moisture. The entire steeping operation may take 48–52 hours.

Gibberellic acid (GA, itself produced in a commercial fermentation reaction from the fungus *Gibberella*) is added in some parts of the world to supplement the native gibberellins of the grain. Although some users of malt prohibit its use, GA can successfully accelerate the malting process. It is sprayed on to grain at levels between 0.1 and 0.5 ppm as it passes from the last steep to the germination vessel. The hormones migrate to the aleurone to regulate enzyme synthesis, for the most part to promote the synthesis of enzymes that breakdown successively β-glucan, protein and starch. The gibberellin first reaches the aleurone nearest to the embryo and therefore, enzyme release is initially into the proximal endosperm. Breakdown of the endosperm (modification), therefore, passes in a band from proximal to distal regions of the grain.

Traditionally, steeped barley was spread out to a depth of up to 10 cm on the floors of long, low buildings and germinated for periods up to 10 days. Men would use rakes either to thin out the grain ('the piece') or pile it up depending on whether the batch needed its temperature lowered or raised: the aim was to maintain it at 13°–16°C. Very few such floor maltings survive because of their labour intensity, and a diversity of pneumatic (mechanical) germination equipment is now used. Newer germination vessels are circular, made of steel or concrete, with capacities of as much as 500 tonnes and with turning machinery that is microprocessor-controlled. A modern malting plant is arranged in a tower format, with vessels vertically stacked, steeping tanks uppermost.

Germination in a pneumatic plant is generally at 16°–20°C. Once the whole endosperm is readily squeezed out and if the shoot initials (the acrospire) are about three-quarters the length of the grain (the acrospire grows the length of the kernel between the testa and the aleurone and emerges from the husk at the distal end of the corn), then the 'green malt' is ready for kilning.

Through the controlled drying (kilning) of green malt, the maltster is able to:
1. Arrest modification and render malt stable for storage.
2. Ensure survival of enzymes for mashing.
3. Introduce desirable flavour and colour characteristics and eliminate undesirable flavours.

Drying should commence at a relatively low temperature to ensure survival of the most heat-sensitive enzymes (enzymes are more resistant to heat when the moisture content is low). This is followed by a progressive increase of temperature to effect the flavour and colour changes (Maillard reaction) and complete drying within the limited turnaround time available (typically under 24 hours). There is a great variety of kiln designs, but most modern ones feature deep beds of malt. They have a source of heat for warming incoming air, a fan to drive or pull the air through the bed, together with the necessary loading and stripping systems. The grain is supported on a wedge-wire floor that permits air to pass through the bed, which is likely to be up to 1.2 metres deep. Newer kilns also use 'indirect firing', in that the products of fuel combustion do not pass through the grain bed, but are sent to exhaust, the air being warmed through a heater battery containing water as the conducting medium. Indirect firing arose because of concerns with the role of oxides of nitrogen present in kiln gases that might have promoted the formation of nitrosamines in malt. Nitrosamine levels are now seldom a problem in malt.

Lower temperatures will give malts of lighter colour and will tend to be employed in the production of malts destined for lager-style beers. Higher temperatures, apart from giving darker malts, also lead to a wholly different flavour spectrum. Lager malts give beers that are relatively rich in sulphur compounds, including DMS. Ale malts have more roast, nutty characters. For both lager and ale malts, kilning is sufficient to eliminate the unpleasant raw, grassy and beany characters associated with green malt.

When kilning is complete, the heat is switched off and the grain is allowed to cool before it is stripped from the kiln in a stream of air at ambient temperatures. On its way to steel or concrete hopper bottomed storage silos, the malt is 'dressed' to remove dried rootlets, which go to animal feed.

Some malts are produced not for their enzyme content but rather for use by the brewer in relatively small quantities as a source of extra colour and distinct types of flavour. These roast malts may also be useful sources of natural antioxidant materials. There is much interest in these products for the opportunities they present for brewing new styles of beer.

Mashing: The Production of Sweet Wort

Sweet wort is the sugary liquid that is extracted from malt (and other solid adjuncts used at this stage) through the processes of milling, mashing and wort separation. Larger breweries will have raw materials delivered in bulk (rail or road) with increasingly sophisticated unloading and transfer facilities as the size increases. Smaller breweries will have malt, etc. delivered by sack.

The conscientious brewer will check the delivery and the vehicle it came in for cleanliness and will representatively sample the bulk. The resultant sample will be inspected visually and smelled before unloading is permitted. Most breweries will spotcheck malt deliveries for key analytical parameters to enable them to monitor the quality of a supplier's material against the agreed contractual specification. Grist materials are stored in silos sized according to brewhouse throughput.

Milling

Before malt or other grains can be extracted, they must be milled. Fundamentally the more extensive the milling, the greater the potential there is to extract materials from the grain. However, in most systems for separating wort from spent grains after mashing, the husk is important as a filter medium. The more intact the husk, the better the filtration. Therefore, milling must be a compromise between thoroughly grinding the endosperm while leaving the husk as intact as possible.

There are fundamentally two types of milling: dry milling and wet milling. In the former, mills may be either roll, disk or hammer. If wort separation is by a lauter tun (discussed later), then a roll mill is used. If a mash filter is installed, then a hammer (or disk) mill may be employed because the husk is much less important for wort separation by a mash filter. Wet milling, which was adopted from the corn starch process, was introduced into some brewing operations as an opportunity to minimise damage to the husk on milling. By making the husk 'soggy', it is rendered less likely to shatter than would a dry husk.

Mashing

Mashing is the process of mixing milled grist with heated water in order to digest the key components of the malt and generate wort containing all the necessary ingredients for the desired fermentation and aspects of beer quality. Most importantly it is the primary stage for the breakdown of starch.

The starch in the granules is very highly ordered, which tends to make the granules difficult to digest. When granules are heated (in the case of barley starch beyond 55°–65°C), the molecular order in the granules is disrupted in a process called gelatinisation. Now that the interactions (even to the point of crystallinity) within the starch have been broken down, the starch molecules become susceptible to enzymic digestion. It is for the purpose of gelatinisation and subsequent enzymic digestion that the mashing process in brewing involves heating. Although 80–90 per cent of the granules in barley are small, they only account for 10–15 per cent of the total weight of starch. The small granules are substantially degraded during the malting process, whereas degradation of the large granules is restricted to a degree of surface pitting. (This is important, as it is not in the interests of the brewer (or maltster) to have excessive loss of starch, which is needed as the source of sugar for fermentation.) The starch in barley (as in other plants) is in two molecular forms: amylose, which has very long linear chains of glucose units, and amylopectin, which comprises shorter chains of glucose units that are linked through side chains.

Several enzymes are required for the complete conversion of starch to glucose. α-Amylase, which is an endo enzyme, hydrolyses the $\alpha1$–4 bonds within amylose and amylopectin. β-Amylase, an *exo* enzyme, also hydrolyses $\alpha1$–4 bonds, but it approaches the substrate (either intact starch or the lower molecular weight 'dextrins' produced by α-amylase) from the non-reducing end, chopping off units of two glucoses (i.e. molecules of maltose). Limit dextrinase is the third key activity, attacking the $\alpha1$–6 side chains in amylopectin.

α-Amylase develops during the germination phase of malting. It is extremely heat resistant, and also present in very high activity; therefore, it is capable of extensive attack, not only on the starch from malt but also on that from adjuncts added in quantities of 50 per cent or more. β-Amylase is already present in the starchy endosperm of raw barley, in an inactive form through its association with protein Z. It is released during germination by the action of a protease (and perhaps a reducing agent). β-Amylase is considerably more heat-labile than α-amylase, and will be largely destroyed after 30–45 minutes of mashing at 65°C. Limit dextrinase is similarly heat sensitive.

Furthermore, it is developed much later than the other two enzymes, and germination must be prolonged if high levels of this enzyme are to be developed. It is present in several forms (free and bound): the bound form is both synthesised and released during germination. Like the proteinases, there are endogenous inhibitors of limit dextrinase in grain, and this is probably the main factor which determines that some 20 per cent of the starch in most brews is left in the wort as non-fermentable dextrins. Although it is possible to contrive operations that will allow greater conversion of starch to fermentable sugar, in practice, many brewers seeking a fully fermentable wort add a heat-resistant glucoamylase (e.g. from *Aspergillus*) to the mash (or fermenter). This enzyme has an *exo* action like β-amylase, but it chops off individual glucose units.

There are several types of mashing which can broadly be classified as infusion mashing, decoction mashing and temperature-programmed mashing. Whichever type of mashing is employed, the vessels these days are almost exclusively fabricated from stainless steel (once they were copper). What stainless steel loses in heat transfer properties is made up for in its toughness and ability to be cleaned thoroughly by caustic and acidic detergents. Irrespective of the mashing system, most mashing systems (apart from wet milling operations) incorporate a device for mixing the milled grist with water (which some brewers call 'liquor'). This device, the 'pre-masher', can be of various designs, the classic one being the Steel's masher, which was developed for the traditional infusion mash tun (Fig. 8.8).

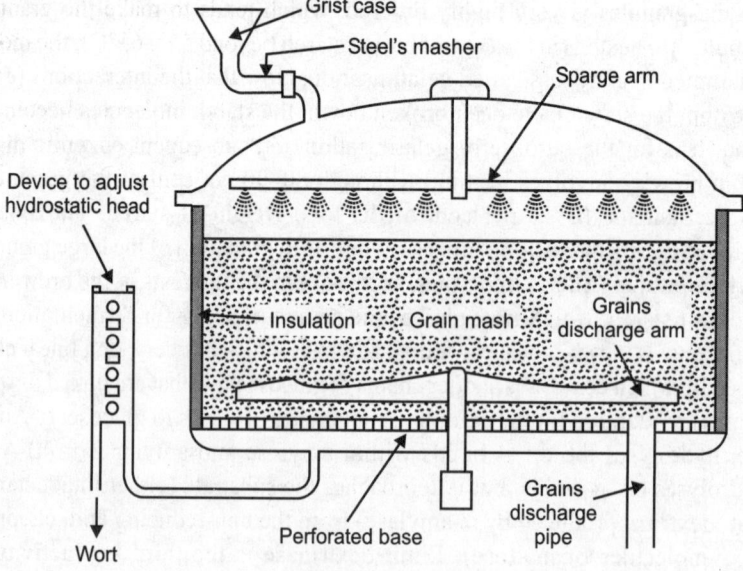

Fig. 8.8. A mash tun.

Infusion mashing is relatively uncommon, but still championed by traditional brewers of ales. It was designed in England to deal with well-modified ale malts that did not require a low temperature start to mashing in order to deal with residual cell-wall material (β-glucans). Grist is mixed with water (a typical ratio would be three parts solid to one part water) in a Steel's masher en route to the preheated mash tun, with a single holding temperature, typically 65°C, being employed. This temperature facilitates gelatinisation of starch and subsequent amylolytic action. At the completion of this 'conversion', wort is separated from the spent grains in the same vessel, which incorporates a false bottom and facility to regulate the hydrostatic pressure across the grains bed. The grist is sparged to enable leaching of as much extract as possible from the bed. Decoction mashing was designed on the mainland continent of Europe to deal with lager malts which were less well-modified than ale malts. Essentially it provides the facility to start mashing at a relatively low temperature, thereby allowing hydrolysis of the β-glucans present in the malt, followed by raising the temperature to a level sufficient to allow gelatinisation of starch and its subsequent enzymic hydrolysis. The manner by which the temperature increase was achieved was by transferring a portion of the initial mash to a separate vessel where it was taken to boiling and then returned to the main mash, leading to an increase in temperature. This is a rather simplified version of the process, which traditionally involved several steps of progressive temperature increase. Temperature-programmed mashing: Although there are some adherents to the decoction-mashing protocol, most brewers nowadays employ the related but simpler temperature-programmed mashing. Again, the mashing is commenced at a relatively low temperature, but subsequent increases in temperature are effected in a single vessel (Fig. 8.9) by employing steam-heated jackets around the vessel to raise the temperature of the contents, which are thoroughly mixed to ensure even heat transfer. Mashing may commence at 45°–50°C, followed by a temperature rise of 1°C.min^{-1} until the conversion temperature (63°–68°C) is reached. The mash will be held for perhaps 50 minutes to 1 hour, before raising the temperature again to the sparging temperature (76°–78°C). High temperatures are employed at the end of the process to arrest enzymic activity, to facilitate solubilisation of materials and to reduce viscosity, thereby allowing more rapid liquid-solid separation.

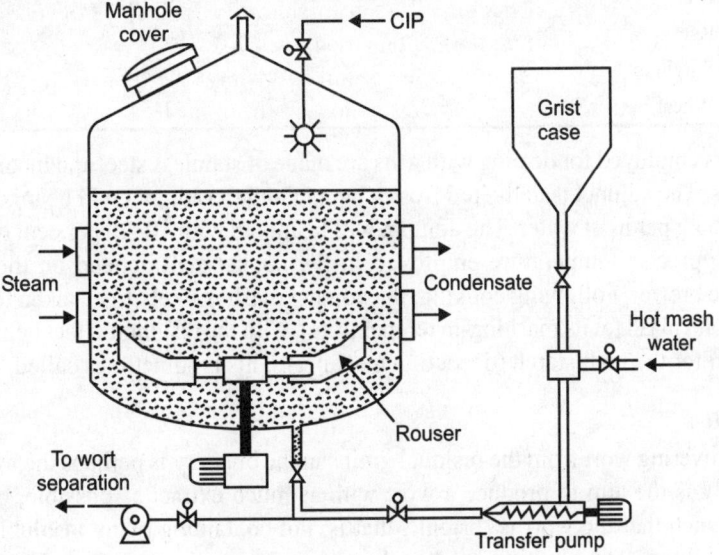

Fig. 8.9. A mash converter.

Adjuncts

The decision whether to use an adjunct or not is made on the basis of cost (does it represent a cost advantageous source of extract, compared to malted barley?) and quality (does the adjunct provide a quality benefit, in respect of flavour, foam or colour?). Liquid adjuncts (sugars/syrups) are added in the wort boiling stage (discussed later). A series of solid adjuncts may be added at the mashing stage because they depend on the enzymes from malt to digest their component macromolecules. Solid adjuncts may be based on other cereals as well as barley: wheat, corn (maize), rice, oats, rye and sorghum. In turn, these adjuncts can be in different forms: raw cereal (barley, wheat); raw grits (corn, rice, sorghum); flaked (corn, rice, barley, oats); micronised or torrefied (corn, barley, wheat); flour/starch (corn, wheat, sorghum) and malted (apart from barley this includes wheat, oats, rye and sorghum).

A key aspect of solid adjuncts is the gelatinisation temperature of the starch (Table 8.1). A higher gelatinisation temperature for corn, rice and sorghum means that these cereals need treatment at higher temperatures than do barley, oats, rye or wheat. If the cereal is in the form of grits (produced by the dry milling of cereal in order to remove outer layers and the oil-rich germ), then it needs to be 'cooked' in the brewhouse. Alternatively, the cereal can be preprocessed by intense heat treatment in a micronisation or flaking operation. In the former process, the whole grain is passed by conveyor under an intense heat source (260°C), resulting in a 'popping' of the kernels (puffed breakfast cereals). In flaking, grits are gelatinised by steam and then rolled between steam-heated rollers. Flakes are not required to be milled in the brewhouse, but micronised cereals are.

Table 8.1. Gelatinisation temperatures of starches from different cereals.

Source	Gelatinisation temperature (°C)
Barley	61–62
Corn	70–80
Oats	55–60
Rice	70–80
Rye	60–65
Sorghum	70–80
Wheat	52–54

Cereal cookers employed for dealing with grits are made of stainless steel and incorporate an agitator and steam jackets. The adjunct is delivered from a hopper and the adjunct will be mixed with water at a rate of perhaps 15 kg per hl of water. The adjunct will be mixed with 10–20 per cent of malt as a source of enzymes. The precise temperature employed in the cooker will depend on the adjunct and the preferences of the brewer. Following cooking, the adjunct mash is likely to be taken to boiling and then mixed with the main mash (at its mashing-in temperature), with the resultant effect being the temperature rise to conversion for the malt starch (decoction mashing). This is sometimes called 'double mashing'.

Wort separation

Traditionally, recovering wort from the residual grains in the brewery is perhaps the most skilled part of brewing. Not only is the aim to produce a wort with as much extract as possible, but many brewers prefer to do this such that the wort is 'bright', that is, not containing many insoluble particles which may present difficulties later. All this needs to take place within a time window, for the mashing vessel must be emptied in readiness for the next brew.

Irrespective of the system employed for mash separation (traditional infusion mash tun, lauter tun, or mash filter), the science dictating rate of liquid recovery is the same and is defined by Darcy's equation:

$$\text{Rate of liquid flow} = \frac{\text{Pressure} \times \text{bed permeability} \times \text{filteration area}}{\text{Bed depth} \times \text{wort viscosity}}$$

And so the wort will be recovered more quickly if the device used to separate the wort has a large surface area, is shallow and if a high pressure can be employed to force the liquid through. The liquid should be of as low viscosity as possible, as less viscous liquids flow more readily. Also the bed of solids should be as permeable as possible. Perhaps the best analogy here is to sand and clay. Sand comprises relatively large particles around which a liquid will flow readily. To pass through the much smaller particles of clay, though, water has to take a much more circuitous route and it is held up. The particle sizes in a bed of grains depend on certain factors, such as the fineness of the original milling and the extent to which the husk survived milling (discussed earlier). Furthermore, a layer (teig or oberteig) collects on the surface of a mash, this being a complex of certain macromolecules, including oxidatively cross-linked proteins, lipids and cell-wall polysaccharides, and this layer has a very fine size distribution analogous to clay. (The oxidative cross-linking of the proteins is exactly akin to that involved in bread dough.) However, particle size also depends on the temperature, and it is known that at the higher temperatures used for wort separation (e.g. 78°C), there is an agglomeration of very fine particles into larger ones past which wort will flow more quickly.

Lauter tun

Generally this is a straight-sided round vessel with a slotted or wedged wire base and run-off pipes through which the wort is recovered (Fig. 8.10). Within the vessel there are arms that can be rotated about a central axis. These arms carry vertical knives that are used as appropriate to slice through the grains bed and facilitate run-off of the wort. Water can be sparged onto the grain to ensure collection of all the desired soluble material. The spent grains are shipped off site to be used as cattle food.

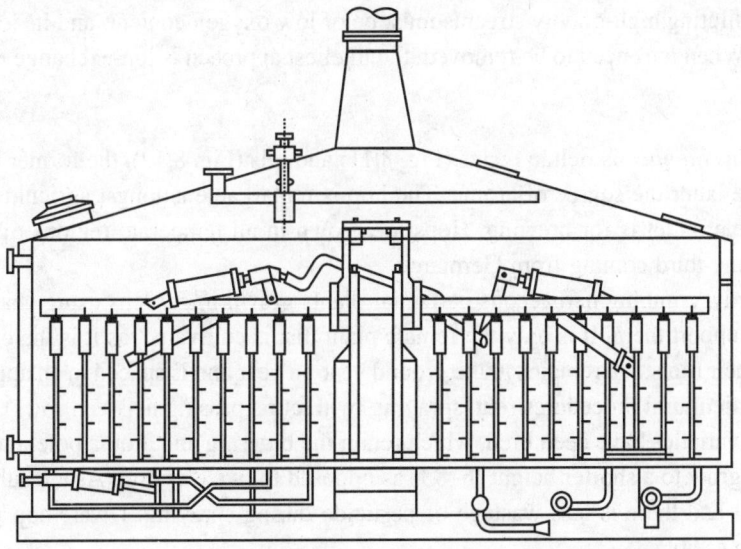

Fig. 8.10. A lauter tun.

Mash filters

Increasingly, modern breweries use mash filters. These operate by using plates of polypropylene to filter the liquid wort from the residual grains. Accordingly, the grains serve no purpose as a filter medium and their particle sizes are irrelevant. The high pressures that can be used in the squeezing of the plates together overcome the reduced permeability due to smaller particle sizes (the sand versus clay analogy used earlier). Furthermore, the grains bed depth is particularly shallow (2–3 inches), being nothing more than the distance between the adjacent plates.

Water

Since water represents at least 90 per cent of the composition of most beers, it will clearly have a major direct impact on the product, particularly in terms of flavour and clarity. The nature of the water, however, exerts its influence much earlier in the process, through the impact of the salts it contains on enzymic and chemical processes, through the determination of pH, etc.

Water in breweries comes either from wells owned by the brewer or from municipal supplies; especially in the latter instance, the water will be subjected to clean-up procedures, such as charcoal filtration, to eliminate undesirable taints and colours. The water in some places is very hard, while in some places it is soft.

The water composition can be adjusted, either by adding or by removing ions. Thus, calcium levels may be increased in order to promote the precipitation of oxalic acid as oxalate, to lower the pH by reaction with phosphate ions ($3Ca^{2+} + 2HPO_4^{2-} \rightarrow Ca_3(PO_4)_2 + 2H^+$) and to promote amylase action. (The optimum pH for mashing is between 5.2 and 5.4.) The alkalinity of water used for sparging (alkalinity is largely determined by the content of carbonate and bicarbonate) may be reduced to less than 50 ppm in order to limit the extraction of tannins. Ions such as iron and copper must be as low as possible to preclude oxidation. Furthermore, water may need to be of different standards for different purposes. The microbiological status of water used for slurrying yeast or for use downstream generally is important. Water used for diluting high-gravity streams must be of low oxygen content, and its ionic composition will be critical. When ions need to be removed, the likeliest approach is ion-exchange resin technology.

Hops

The hop, *Humulus lupulus*, is rich in resins (Fig. 8.11) and oils (Fig. 8.12), the former being the source of bitterness, the latter the source of aroma. The hop is remarkable amongst agricultural crops in that essentially its sole outlet is for brewing. Hops are grown in all temperate regions of the world, with approximately one-third coming from Germany.

Hops are hardy, climbing herbaceous perennial plants grown in gardens using characteristic string frameworks to support them. It is only the female plant that is cultivated, as it is the one that develops the hop cone. Their rootstock remains in the ground year on year and is spaced in an appropriate fashion for effective horticultural procedures (e.g. spraying by tractors passing between rows). In recent years, so-called dwarf varieties have been bred, which retain the bittering and aroma potential of 'traditional' hops but which grow to a shorter height (6–8 ft as opposed to twice as big). As a result, they are much easier to harvest and there is less wastage of pesticide during spraying. Dwarf hop gardens are also much cheaper to establish.

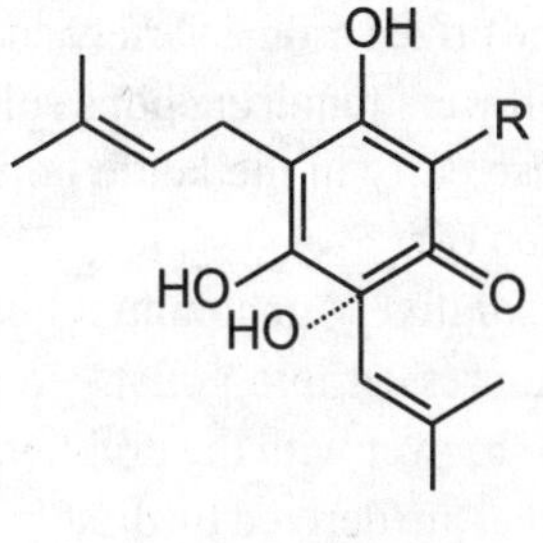

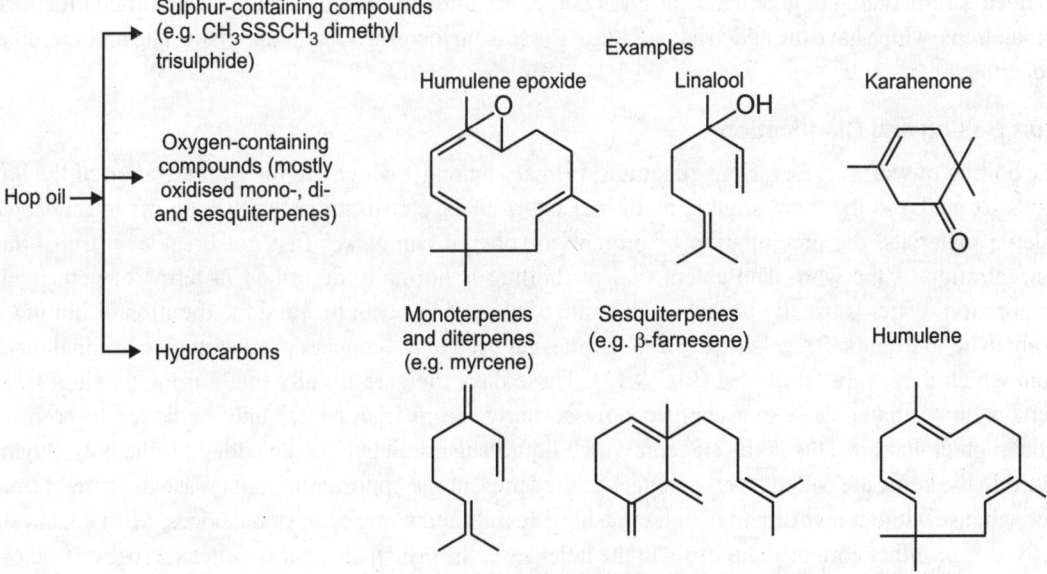

Name	Side chain (R)
Humulone	—CO·CH$_2$·CH(CH$_3$)$_2$ isovaleryl
Cohumulone	—CO·CH(CH$_3$)$_2$ isobutyryl
Adhumulone	—CO·CH(CH$_3$)·CH$_2$·CH$_3$ 2-methylbutyryl

Fig. 8.11. Hop resins.

Fig. 8.12. Hop oils.

Hops are susceptible to a wide range of diseases and pests. The most serious problems come from *Verticillium* wilt, downy mildew, mould and the damson-hop aphid. Varieties differ in their susceptibility to infestation and have been progressively selected on this basis. Nonetheless, it is frequently necessary to apply pesticides, which are always stringently evaluated for their influence on hop quality, for any effect they may have on the brewing process and, of course, for their safety.

Hops are generally classified into two categories: aroma hops and bittering hops. All hops are capable of providing both bitterness and aroma. Some hops, however, such as the Czech variety Saaz, have a relatively high ratio of oil to resin and the character of the oil component is particularly prized. Such varieties command higher prices and are known as aroma varieties. They are seldom used as the sole source of bitterness and aroma in a beer: a cheaper, higher α-acid hop (a bittering variety) is used to provide the bulk of the bitterness, with the prized aroma variety added late in the boil for the contribution of its own unique blend of oils. Those brewers requiring hops solely as a source of bitterness may well opt for a cheaper variety, ensuring its use early in the kettle boil so that the provision of bitterness is maximised and unwanted aroma is driven off.

The use of whole cone hops is comparatively uncommon nowadays. Many brewers use hops that have been hammer-milled and then compressed into pellets. In this form they are more stable, more efficiently utilised and do not present the brewer with the problem of separating out the vegetative parts of the hop plant. Some use hop extracts that are derived by dissolving the resins in liquid carbon dioxide, followed by a chemical isomerisation if the bitterness is to be added to the finished beer rather than in the boiling stage. Recent years have been marked by an enormous increase in the use of such pre-isomerised extracts after they have been modified by reduction. One of the side chains on the iso-α-acids is susceptible to cleavage by light; it then reacts with traces of sulphidic materials in beer to produce 2-methyl-3-butene-1-thiol (MBT), a substance that imparts an intensely unpleasant skunky character to beer. If the side chain is reduced, it no longer produces MBT. For this reason, beers that are destined for packaging in green or clear glass bottles are often produced using these modified bitterness preparations, which have the added advantage of possessing increased foam-stabilising and antimicrobial properties.

Wort Boiling and Clarification

The boiling of wort serves various functions, primary amongst which are the isomerisation of the hop resins (α-acids) to the more soluble and bitter iso-α-acids, sterilisation, the driving off of unwanted volatile materials, the precipitation of protein/polyphenol complexes (as 'hot break' or 'trub') and concentration of the wort. The extent of wort boiling is normally described in terms of percentage evaporation. Water is usually boiled off at a rate of about 4 per cent hr^{-1} and the duration of boiling is likely to be 1–2 hours. Brew kettles are sometimes referred to as 'coppers', reflecting the original metal from which they were fabricated (Fig. 8.13). These days they are usually made from stainless steel. Certain fining materials (e.g. a charged polysaccharide from Irish Moss) may be added to promote protein precipitation. This is the stage at which liquid sugar adjunct can be added (Table 8.2). Sugars added in the kettle are called 'wort extenders': they present the opportunity to increase the extract from a brewhouse without investment in extra mashing vessels and wort separation devices. Most sugars are derived from either corn or sugar cane. In the latter case, the principal sugar is either sucrose or fructose plus glucose if the product has been 'inverted'. There are many different corn sugar products, differing in their degree of hydrolysis and therefore fermentability. Through the controlled use of acid but increasingly of starch-degrading enzymes, the supplier can produce preparations with a full range of fermentabilities depending on the needs of the brewer: from 100 per cent glucose through to high dextrin.

After boiling, wort is transferred to a clarification device. The system employed for removing insoluble material after boiling depends on the way in which the hopping was carried out. If whole hop cones are used, clarification is through a hop jack (hop back), which is analogous to a lauter tun, but in this case the bed of residual hops constitutes the filter medium. If hop pellets or extracts are used, then the device of choice is the whirlpool, a cylindrical vessel, into which hot wort is transferred tangentially through an opening 0.5–1 metre above the base (Fig. 8.14). The wort is set into a rotational flux, which forces trub to a pile in the middle of the vessel.

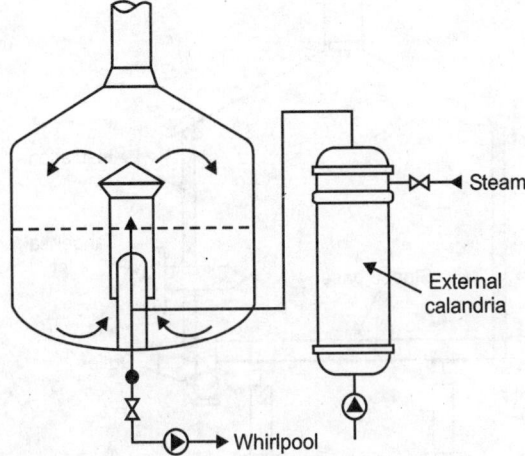

Fig. 8.13. Kettle: Wort in this design is siphoned through the external heating device (calandria), thus ensuring an efficient and highly turbulent boil.

Table 8.2. Brewing sugars.

Type	Carbohydrate distribution (%)
Cane	Sucrose predominantly
Invert	Glucose (50), fructose (50)
Dextrose	Glucose (100)
High conversion (acid + enzyme)	Glucose (88), maltose (4), maltotriose (2), dextrin (6)
Glucose chips	Glucose (84), maltose (1), maltotriose (2), dextrin (13)
Maize syrup	Glucose (45), maltose (38), maltotriose (3), dextrin (14)
Very-high maltose	Glucose (5), maltose (70), maltotriose (10), dextrin (15)
High conversion (acid)	Glucose (31), maltose (18), maltotriose (13), dextrin (38)
High maltose	Glucose (10), maltose (60), dextrin (30)
Low conversion	Glucose (12), maltose (10), maltotriose (10), dextrin (68)
Maltodextrin	Maltose (1.5), maltotriose (1.5), dextrin (95)
Malt extract	Comparable to brewer's wort—also contains nitrogenous components

The products dextrose through maltodextrin are customarily derived by the selective hydrolysis of corn (maize)-derived starch by acid and enzymes to varying extents.

Wort Cooling

Almost all cooling systems these days are of the stainless steel plate heat exchanger type, sometimes called 'paraflows' (Fig. 8.15). Heat is transferred from the wort to a coolant, either water or glycol depending on how low the temperature needs to be taken. At this stage, it is likely that more material will precipitate from solution ('cold break'). Brewers are divided on whether they feel this to be good or bad for fermentation and beer quality. The presence of this break certainly accelerates fermentation and, therefore, it will directly influence yeast metabolism. As in so much of brewing, the aim should be consistency: either consistently 'bright worts' or ones containing a relatively consistent level of trub.

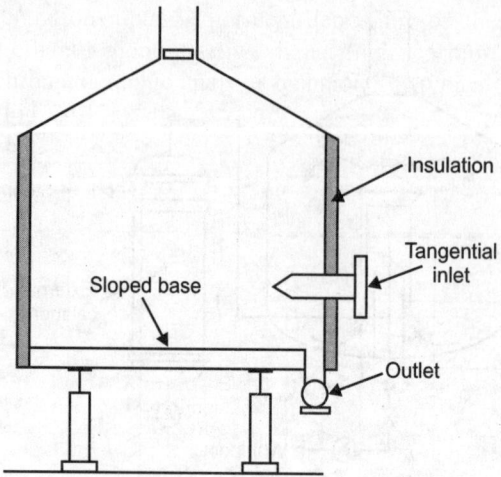

Fig. 8.14. A 'whirlpool' (hot wort residence vessel).

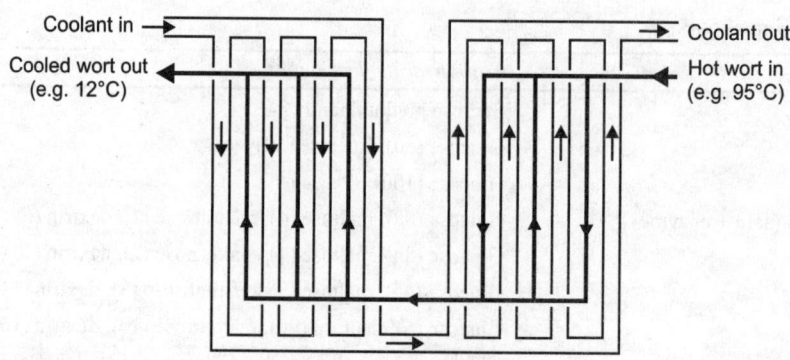

Fig. 8.15. Heat exchanger.

Yeast

Brewing yeast is *Saccharomyces cerevisiae* (ale yeast) or *Saccharomyces pastorianus* (lager yeast). There are many separate strains of brewing yeast, each of which is distinguishable phenotypically [e.g. in the extent to which it will ferment different sugars, or in the amount of oxygen it needs to prompt its growth, or in the amounts of its metabolic products (i.e. flavour spectrum of the resultant beer), or its behaviour in suspension (top versus bottom fermenting, flocculent or non-flocculent)] and genotypically, in terms of its DNA fingerprint.

The fundamental differentiation between ale and lager strains is based on the ability or otherwise to ferment the sugar melibiose (Fig. 8.16): ale strains cannot whereas lager strains can because they produce the enzyme (α-galactosidase) necessary to convert melibiose into glucose and galactose. Ale yeasts also move to the top of open fermentation vessels and are called top-fermenting yeasts. Lager yeasts drop to the bottom of fermenters and are termed bottom-fermenting yeasts. Nowadays it is frequently difficult to make this differentiation, when beers are widely fermented in similar types of vessel (deep cylindro-conical tanks) which tend to equalise the way in which yeast behave in suspension.

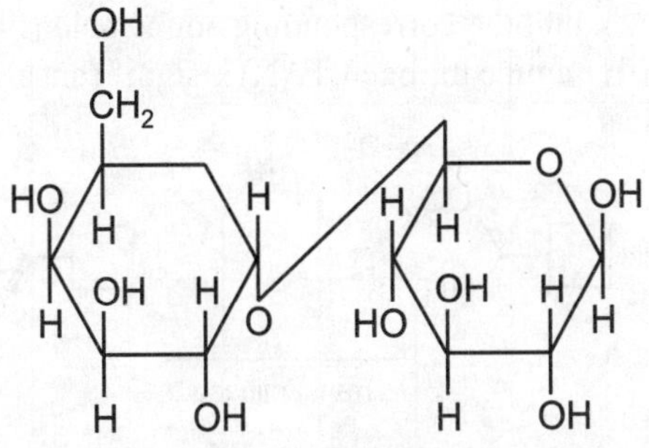

Fig. 8.16. Melibiose.

When presented with wort, yeast encounters a selection of carbohydrates which, for a typical all-malt wort, will approximate to maltose (45 per cent), maltotriose (15 per cent), glucose (10 per cent), sucrose (5 per cent), fructose (2 per cent) and dextrin (23 per cent). The dextins (maltotetraose and larger) are unfermentable. The other sugars will ordinarily be utilised in the sequence sucrose, glucose, fructose, maltose, and lastly maltotriose, though there may be some overlap (Fig. 8.17). Sucrose is hydrolysed by an enzyme (invertase) released by the yeast outside the cell, and then the glucose and fructose enter the cell to be metabolised. Maltose and maltotriose also enter, through the agency of specific permeases. Inside the cell they are broken down into glucose by an α-glucosidase. Glucose represses the maltose and maltotriose permeases.

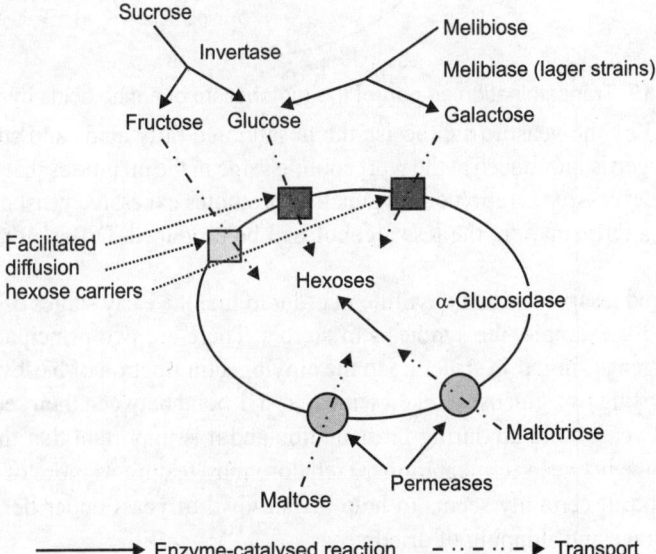

Fig. 8.17. The uptake of sugars by brewing yeast.

The principal route of sugar utilisation in the cell is the EMP pathway of glycolysis. Brewing yeast derives most of the nitrogen it needs for synthesis of proteins and nucleic acids from the amino acids in the wort. A series of permeases is responsible for the sequential uptake of the amino acids. It is understood that the amino acids are transaminated to keto acids and held within the yeast until they are required, when they are transaminated back into the corresponding amino acid (Figs 8.18 and 8.19). The amino acid spectrum and level in wort (free amino nitrogen, FAN) is significant as it influences yeast metabolism leading to flavour-active products.

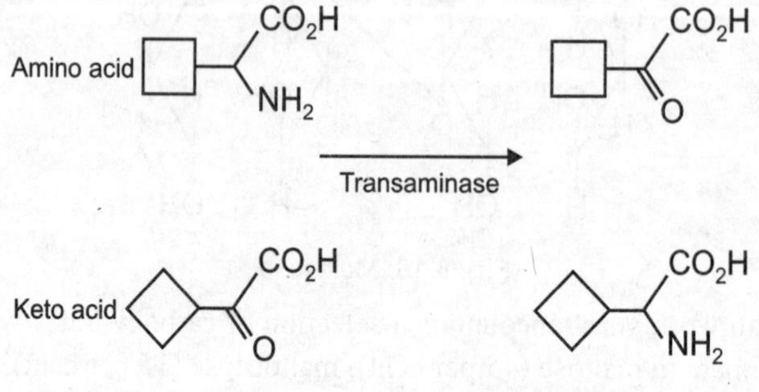

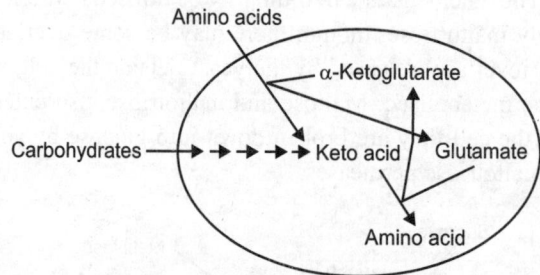

Fig. 8.18. The principle of transamination.

Fig. 8.19. Transamination as part of the metabolism of amino acids by yeast.

Oxygen is needed by the yeast to synthesise the unsaturated fatty acids and sterols it needs for its membranes. This oxygen is introduced at the wort cooling stage in the quantities that the yeast requires — but no more, because excessive aeration or oxygenation promotes excessive yeast growth, and the more yeast is produced in a fermentation, the less alcohol will be produced. Different yeasts need different amounts of oxygen.

Yeast uses its stored reserves of carbohydrate in order to fuel the early stages of metabolism when it is pitched into wort, for example, the synthesis of sterols. There are two principal reserves: glycogen and trehalose. Glycogen is similar in structure to the amylopectin fraction of barley starch. Trehalose is a disaccharide comprising two glucoses linked with an α-1,1 bond between their reducing carbons. The glycogen reserves of yeast build up during fermentation and it is important that they are conserved in the yeast during storage between fermentations. Trehalose may feature as more of a protection against the stress of starvation. It certainly seems to help the survival of yeast under dehydration conditions employed for the storage and shipping of dried yeast.

Pure yeast culture was pioneered by Hansen at Carlsberg in 1883. By a process of dilution, he was able to isolate individual strains and open up the possibility of selecting and growing separate strains for specific purposes. Nowadays brewers maintain their own pure yeast strains. While it is still a fact that some brewers simply use the yeast grown in one fermentation to 'pitch' the following fermentation, and that they have done this for many tens of years, it is much more usual for yeast to be repropagated from a pure culture every 4–6 generations. (When brewers talk of 'generations', they mean successive fermentations; strictly speaking, yeast advances a generation every time it buds, and therefore there are several generations during any individual fermentation.)

Large quantities of yeast are needed to pitch commercial-scale fermentations. They need to be generated by successive scale-up growth from the master culture (Fig. 8.20). Higher yields are possible if fed-batch culture is used. This is the type of procedure used in the production of baker's yeast. It takes advantage of the Crabtree effect, in which high concentrations of sugar drive the yeast to use it fermentatively rather than by respiration. When yeast grows by respiration, it captures much more energy from the sugar and therefore produces much more cell material. In fed-batch culture, the amount of sugar made available to the yeast at any stage is low. Together with the high levels of oxygen in a well-aerated system, the yeast respires and grows substantially. The sugar is 'dribbled in' and the end result is a far higher yield of biomass, perhaps four-fold more than is produced when the sugar is provided in a single batch at the start of fermentation.

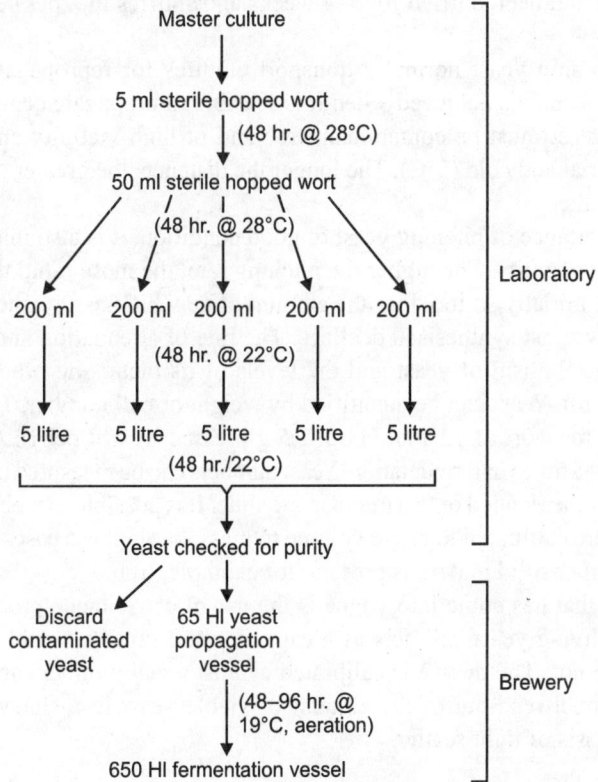

Fig. 8.20. Yeast propagation.

The majority of brewing yeasts are resistant to acid (pH 2.0–2.2) and so the addition of phosphoric acid to attain this pH is very effective in killing bacteria with which yeast may become progressively contaminated from fermentation to fermentation. Many brewers use such an acid washing of yeast between fermentations.

There are two key indices of yeast health: viability and vitality. Both should be high if a successful fermentation is to be achieved. Viability is a measure of whether a yeast culture is alive or dead. While microscopic inspection of a yeast sample is useful as a gross indicator of that culture (e.g. presence of substantial infection), quantitative evaluation of viability needs a staining test. The most common is the use of methylene blue: viable yeast decolourises it, dead cells do not. Although a yeast cell may be living, it does not necessarily mean that it is healthy. Vitality is a measure of how healthy a yeast cell is. Many techniques have been advanced as an index of vitality, but none has been accepted as definitive.

Preferably yeast is stored in a readily sanitised room that can be cleaned efficiently and which is supplied with a filtered air supply and possesses a pressure higher than the surroundings in order to impose an outwards vector of contaminants. Ideally it should be at or around 0°C. Even if storage is not in such a room, the tanks must be rigorously cleaned, chilled to 0–4°C and have the facility for gently rousing (mixing) to avoid hot spots. Yeast is stored in slurries ('barms') of 5–15 per cent, solids under 6 inches of beer, water or potassium phosphate solution. An alternative procedure is to press the yeast and store it at 4°C in a cake form (20–30 per cent dry solids). Pressed yeast may be held for about 10 days, water slurried and beer slurried for 3–4 weeks and slurries in 2 per cent phosphate, pH 5 for 5 weeks.

Brewers seeking to ship yeast normally transport cultures for repropagation at the destination. However, greater consistency is achieved when it is feasible to propagate centrally and ship yeast for direct pitching. Such yeast must be contaminant-free and of high viability and vitality, washed free from fermentable material and cold (0°C). The longer the distance, the greater the recommendation for low moisture pressed cake.

Apart from the importance of pitching yeast of good condition, it is also important that the amount pitched is in the correct quantity. The higher the pitching rate, the more rapid the fermentation. As the pitching rate increases, initially so too does the amount of new biomass synthesised, until at a certain rate, the amount of new yeast synthesised declines. The rate of attenuation and the amount of growth directly impacts the metabolism of yeast and the levels of its metabolic products (i.e. beer flavour) hence the need for control. Yeast can be quantified by weight or cell number. Typically some 10^7 cells per ml will be pitched for wort of 12°Plato (1.5–2.5 g pressed weight per l). At such a pitching rate, lager yeast will divide 4–5 times in fermentation. Yeast numbers can be measured using a haemocytometer, which is a counting chamber loaded onto a microscope slide. It is possible to weigh yeast or to centrifuge it down in pots which are calibrated to relate volume to mass, but in these cases it must be remembered that there are usually other solid materials present, for example, trub.

Another procedure that has come into vogue is the use of capacitance probes that can be inserted in-line. An intact and living yeast cell acts as a capacitor and gives a signal whereas dead ones (or insoluble materials) do not. The device is calibrated against a cell number (or weight) technique and therefore allows the direct read-out of the amount of viable yeast in a slurry. Other in-line devices quantify yeast on the basis of light scatter.

Brewery Fermentations

Primary fermentation is the fermentation stage proper in which yeast, through controlled growth, is allowed to ferment wort to generate alcohol and the desired spectrum of flavours. Increasingly brewery fermentations are conducted in cylindro-conical vessels (Fig. 8.21). The fermentation is regulated by control of several parameters, notably the starting strength of the wort (°Plato, which approximates to percentage sugar by weight, or Brix), the amount of viable yeast ('pitching rate'), the quantity of oxygen introduced and the temperature. Fermentation is monitored by measuring the decrease in specific gravity (alcohol has a much lower specific gravity than sugar).

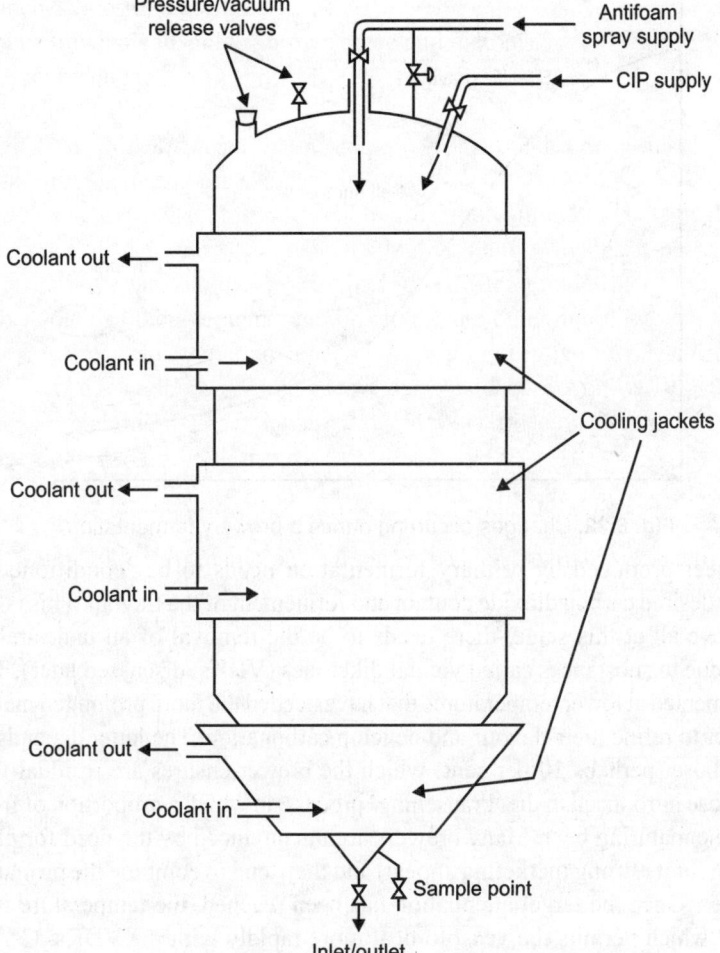

Fig. 8.21. A cylindro-control fermentation vessel.

Ales are generally fermented at a higher temperature (15°–20°C) than lagers (6°–13°C) and therefore attenuation (the achievement of the finished specific gravity) is achieved more rapidly. Thus, an ale fermenting at 20°C may achieve attenuation gravity in 2 days, whereas a lager fermented at 8.5°C may take 10 days. The temperature has a substantial effect on the metabolism of yeast, and the levels of a flavour substance like iso-butanol will be 16.5 and 7 mg l^{-1}, respectively, for the ale and the lager. Some brewers add zinc (e.g. 0.2 ppm) to promote yeast action—it is a cofactor for the enzyme alcohol dehydrogenase. During fermentation, the pH falls because yeast secretes organic acids and protons. A diagram depicting the time course of fermentation can be found in Fig. 8.22.

Surplus yeast will be removed at the end of fermentation, either by a process such as 'skimming' for a traditional square fermenter employing top fermenting yeast, or from the base of a cone in a cylindro-conical vessel. This is not only to preserve the viability and vitality of the yeast, but also to circumvent the autolysis and secretory tendencies of yeast that will be to the detriment of flavour and foam. There will still be sufficient yeast in the beer to effect the secondary fermentation.

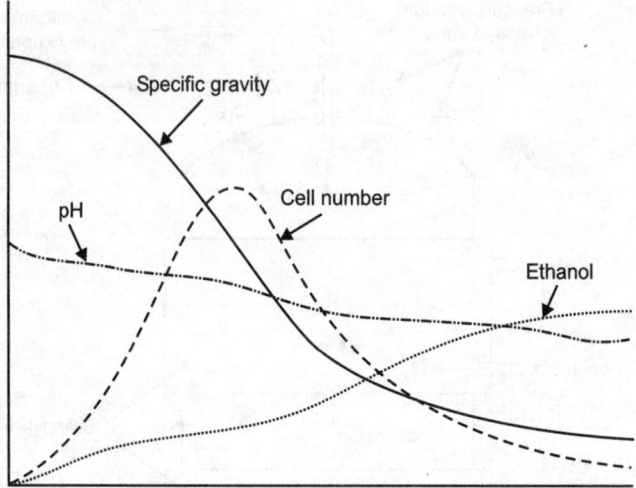

Fig. 8.22. Changes occurring during a brewery fermentation.

The 'green' beer produced by primary fermentation needs to be 'conditioned', in respect of establishment of a desired carbon dioxide content and refinement of the flavour. This is called secondary fermentation. Above all at this stage, there needs to be the removal of an undesirable butter-scotch flavour character due to substances called vicinal diketones (VDKs; discussed later). Traditionally it is the lager beers fermented at lower temperatures that have needed the more prolonged maturation (storage: 'lagering') in order to refine their flavour and develop carbonation. The latter depends on the presence of sugars, either those (perhaps 10 per cent) which the brewer ensures are residual from the primary fermentation or those introduced in the 'krausening' process, in which a proportion of freshly fermenting wort is added to the maturing beer. Many brewers are unconvinced by the need for prolonged storage periods (other than for its strong marketing appeal) and they tend to combine the primary and secondary fermentation stages. Once the target attenuation has been reached, the temperature is allowed to rise (perhaps by 4°C), which permits the yeast to deal more rapidly with the VDKs. Carbonation will be achieved downstream by the direct introduction of gas.

Once the secondary fermentation stage is complete (and the length of this varies considerably between brewers), then the temperature is dropped, ideally to −1° or −2°C to enable precipitation and sedimentation of materials which would otherwise cause a haze in the beer. The sedimentation of yeast is also promoted in this 'cold conditioning' stage, perhaps with the aid of isinglass finings (Fig. 8.23). These are solutions of collagen derived from the swim bladders of certain species of fish from the South China Seas. Collagen has a net positive charge at the pH of beer, whereas yeast and other particulates have a net negative charge. Opposite charges attracting, the isinglass forms a complex with these particles and the resultant large agglomerates sediment readily because of an increase in particle size. Sometimes, the isinglass finings are used alongside 'auxiliary finings' based on silicate, the combination being more effective than isinglass alone. Some brewers centrifuge to aid clarification.

For the most part, fermenters these days are fabricated from stainless steel and will be lagged and feature jackets that allow coolant to be circulated (the heat generated during fermentation is sufficient to effect any necessary warming—so the temperature is regulated by balancing metabolic heat with cooling afforded by the coolant in the jacket, which may be water, glycol or ammonia depending on how much refrigeration is demanded). Modern vessels tend to be enclosed, for microbiological reasons. However, across the world there remain a great many open tanks. Cylindro-conical vessels can have a capacity of up to 13000 hl and are readily cleaned using CIP operations.

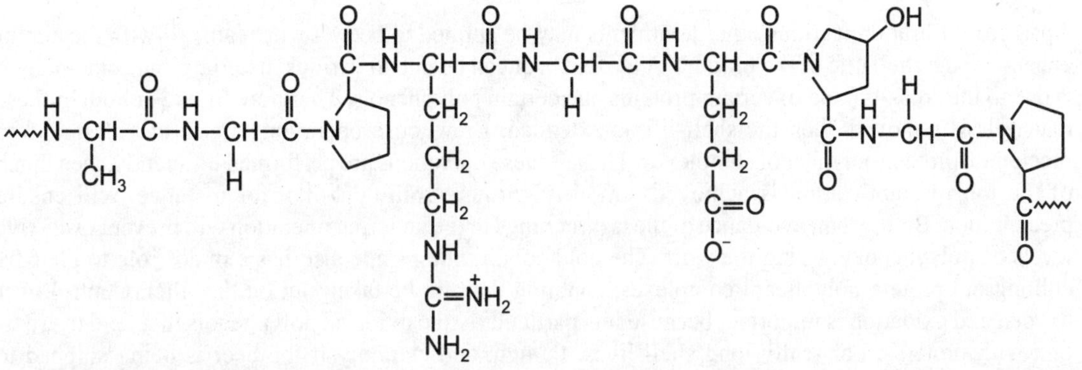

Fig. 8.23. A typical repeating structure in the collagen polypeptide chain that, when dissolved in partially degraded forms, represents isinglass. The amino and imino acid residues in this particular sequence are ~alanyl-prolyl-arginyl-glycyl-glutamyl-hydroxyprolyl-prolyl~.

Only one company, in New Zealand, practises continuous fermentation. Many brewers nowadays maximise the output by fermenting wort at a higher gravity than necessary to give the target alcohol concentration, before diluting the beer downstream with deaerated water to 'sales gravity' (i.e. the required strength of the beer in package). This is called 'high-gravity brewing'. There are limits to the strength of wort that can be fermented. This is because yeast becomes stressed at high sugar concentrations and when the alcohol level increases beyond a certain point. Brewing is unusual amongst alcohol production industries in that it reuses yeast for ensuing fermentations. Excluded from this are those beers in which very high alcohol levels are developed (e.g. the barley wines). The yeast is stressed in these conditions and will not be reusable. This is the reason why wine fermentations, for instance, involve 'one trip' yeast. This is also the reason why, in the production of sweeter fortified wines, alcohol is added at the start of fermentation in order to hinder the removal of sugars.

Filtration

After a period of typically 3 days minimum in 'cold conditioning', the beer is generally filtered. Diverse types of filter are available, perhaps the most common being the plate-and-frame filter which consists of a series of plates in sequence, over each of which a cloth is hung. The beer is mixed with a filter-aid porous particles which both trap particles and prevent the system from clogging. Two major kinds of filter aid are in regular use: kieselguhr and perlite. The former comprises fossils or skeletons of primitive organisms called diatoms. These can be mined and classified to provide grades that differ in their permeability characteristics. Particles of kieselguhr contain pores into which other particles (such as those found in beer) can pass, depending on their size. Perlites are derived from volcanic glasses crushed to form microscopic flat particles. They are better to handle than kieselguhr, but are not as efficient as filter aids. Filtration starts when a pre-coat of filter aid is applied to the filter by cycling a slurry of filter aid through the plates. This pre-coat is generally of quite a coarse grade, whereas the filter-aid (the body feed) which is dosed into the beer during the filtration proper tends to be a finer grade. It is selected according to the particles within the beer that need to be removed. If a beer contains a lot of yeast, but relatively few small particles, then a relatively coarse grade is best. If the converse applies, then a fine grade with smaller pores will be used.

Stabilisation of beer

Apart from filtration, various other treatments may be applied to beer downstream, all with the aim of enhancing the shelf-life of the product. A haze in beer can be due to various materials, but principally it is due to the cross-linking of certain proteins and certain polyphenols. Therefore, if one or both of these materials is removed, then the shelf-life is extended. Brewhouse operations are in part designed to precipitate protein-polyphenol complexes. Thus, if these operations are performed efficiently, then much of the job of stabilisation is achieved. Good, vigorous, 'rolling' boils, for instance, will ensure precipitation. Before that, avoidance of the last runnings in the lautering operation will prevent excessive levels of polyphenol entering the wort. The cold conditioning stage also has a major role to play, by chilling out protein-polyphenol complexes, enabling them to be taken out on the filter. Control over oxygen and oxidation is important because it is particularly the oxidised polyphenols that tend to cross-link with proteins. For really long shelf-lives, though, and certainly if the beer is being shipped to extremes of climate, additional stabilisation treatments will be necessary. Polyphenols can be removed with PVPP. Protein can be precipitated by adding tannic acid, hydrolysed using papain (the same enzyme from paw paw that is used as meat tenderiser) or, and most commonly, adsorbed on silica hydrogels and silica xerogels.

Gas Control

Final adjustment will now be made to the level of gases in the beer. As we have seen, it is important that the oxygen level in the bright beer is as low as possible. Unfortunately, whenever beer is moved around and processed in a brewery, there is always the risk of oxygen pick-up. For example, oxygen can enter through leaky pumps. A check on oxygen content will be made once the bright beer tank (filtered beer is bright beer) is filled and, if the level is above specification (which most brewers will set at 0.1–0.3 ppm), oxygen will have to be removed. This is achieved by purging the tank with an inert gas, usually nitrogen, from a sinter in the base of the vessel. The level of carbon dioxide in a beer may either need to be increased or decreased. The majority of beers contain between two and three volumes of CO_2, whereas most brewery fermentations generate 'naturally' no more than 1.2–1.7 volumes of the gas. The simplest and most usual procedure by which CO_2 is introduced is by injection as a flow of bubbles as beer is transferred from the filter to the bright beer tank. If the CO_2 content needs to be dropped, this is a more formidable challenge. It may be necessary for beers that are supposed to have a relatively low carbonation and, as for oxygen, this can be achieved by purging. However, concerns about 'bit' production have stimulated the development of gentle membrane-based systems for gas control. Beer is flowed past membranes, made from polypropylene or polytetrafluoroethylene, that are water-hating and therefore do not 'wet-out'. Gases, but not liquids, will pass freely across such membranes, the rate of flux being proportional to the concentration of each individual gas and dependent also on the rate at which the beer flows past the membrane.

Packaging

The packaging operation is the most expensive stage in the brewery, in terms of raw materials and labour. Beer will be brought into specification in the Bright Beer Tank (sometimes called the Fine Ale Tank or the package release tank). The carbonation level may be higher (e.g. by 0.2 volume) than that specified for the beer in package, to allow for losses during filling.

Although beer is relatively resistant to spoilage, it is by no means entirely incapable of supporting the growth of micro-organisms. For this reason, most beers are treated to eliminate any residual brewing yeast or infecting wild yeasts and bacteria before or during packaging. This can be achieved in one of two ways: pasteurisation or sterile filtration. Pasteurisation can take one of two forms in the brewery: flash pasteurisation for beer pre-package and tunnel pasteurisation for beer in can or bottle. The principle in either case, of course, is that heat kills micro-organisms. One PU is defined as exposure for 1 minute at 60°C. The higher the temperature, the more rapidly the micro-organisms are destroyed. A 7°C rise in temperature leads to a ten-fold increase in the rate of cell death. The pasteurisation time required to kill organisms at different temperatures can be read off from a plot. Typically, a brewer might use 5–20 PU but higher 'doses' may be used for some beers, for example, low alcohol beers which are more susceptible to infection. In flash pasteurisation, the beer flows through a heat exchanger (essentially like a wort cooler acting in reverse), which raises the temperature typically to 72°C. Residence times of between 30 and 60 seconds at this temperature are sufficient to kill off virtually all microbes. Ideally there will not be many of these to remove: good brewers will ensure low loadings of micro-organisms by attention to hygiene throughout the process and ensuring that the prior filtration operation is efficient. Tunnel pasteurisers comprise large heated chambers through which cans or glass bottles are conveyed over a period of minutes, as opposed to the seconds employed in a flash pasteuriser. Accordingly, temperatures in a tunnel pasteuriser are lower, typically 60°C for a residence time of 10–20 min. An increasingly popular mechanism for removing micro-organisms is to filter them out by passing the beer through a fine mesh filter. The rationale for selecting this procedure rather than pasteurisation is as much for marketing reasons as for any technical advantage it presents: many brands of beer these days are being sold on a claim of not being heat-treated, and therefore, free from any 'cooking'. In fact, provided the oxygen level is very low, modest heating of beer does not have a major impact on the flavour of many beers, although those products with relatively subtle, lighter flavour will obviously display 'cooked' notes more readily than will beers that have a more complex flavour character. The sterile filter must be located downstream from the filter that is used to separate solids from the beer. Sterile filters may be of several types, a common variant incorporating a membrane formed from polypropylene or polytetrafluoroethylene and with pores of between 0.45 and 0.8 μm.

Filling bottles and cans

Bottles entering the brewery's packaging hall are first washed and, if they are returnable bottles (i.e. they have been used previously to hold beer), they will need a much more robust cleaning and sterilisation, inside and out, involving soaking and jetting with hot caustic detergent and thorough rinsing with water. The beer coming from the bright beer tanks is transferred to a bowl at the heart of the filling machine. Bottle fillers are machines based on a rotary carousel principle. They have a series of filling heads: the more the heads, the greater the capacity of the filler. The bottles enter on a conveyor and, sequentially, each is raised into position beneath the next vacant filler head, each of which comprises a filler tube. An air-tight seal is made and, in modern fillers, a specific air evacuation stage starts the filling sequence. The bottle is counter-pressured with carbon dioxide, before the beer is allowed to flow into the bottle by gravity from the bowl. The machine will have been adjusted so that the correct volume of beer is introduced into the vessel. Once filled, the 'top' pressure on the bottle is relieved, and the bottle is released from its filling head. It passes rapidly to the machine that will crimp on the crown cork but, en route, the bottle will have been either tapped or its contents 'jetted' with a minuscule amount of sterile water in order to fob the contents and drive off any air from the space in the bottle between the surface of the beer and the neck (the 'headspace'). Next stop is the tunnel pasteuriser if the beer is to be pasteurised after filling, but if sterile filtration is used, the filler and capper are likely to be enclosed in a sterile room. The bottles now head off for labelling, secondary packaging and warehousing.

Putting beer into cans has much in common with bottling. It is the container, of course, that is very different—and definitely one trip. Cans may be of aluminium or stainless steel, which will have an internal lacquer to protect the beer from the metal surface and *vice versa*. Cans arrive in the canning hall on vast trays, all pre-printed and instantly recognisable. They are inverted, washed and sprayed, prior to filling in a manner very similar to the bottles.

Once filled, the lid is fitted to the can basically by folding the two pieces of metal together to make a secure seam past which neither beer nor gas can pass.

Filling kegs

Kegs are manufactured from either aluminium or stainless steel. They are containers generally of 100 litres or less, containing a central spear. Kegs, of course, are multi-trip devices. On return to the brewery from an 'outlet' they are washed externally before transfer to the multi-head machine in which successive heads are responsible for their washing, sterilising and filling. Generally they will be inverted as this takes place. The cleaning involves high-pressure spraying of the entire internal surface of the vessel with water at approximately 70°C. After about 10 seconds, the keg passes to the steaming stage, the temperature reaching 105°C over a period of perhaps half a minute. Then the keg goes to the filling head, where a brief purge with carbon dioxide precedes the introduction of beer, which may take a couple of minutes. The discharged keg is weighed to ensure that it contains the correct quantity of beer and is labelled and palleted before warehousing.

Quality of Beer

Flavour

The flavour of beer can be split into three separate components: taste, smell (aroma) and texture (mouthfeel).

There are only four proper tastes: sweet, sour, salt and bitter. They are detected on the tongue. A related sense is the tingle associated with high levels of carbonation in a drink: this is due to the triggering of the trigeminal nerve by carbon dioxide. This nerve responds to mild irritants, such as carbonation and capsaicin (a substance largely responsible for the 'pain delivery' of spices and peppers).

Carbon dioxide is also relevant insofar as its level influences the extent to which volatile molecules will be delivered via the foam and into the headspace above the beer in a glass.

The sweetness of a beer is due, of course, to its level of sugars, either those that have survived fermentation or those introduced as primings.

The principal contributors to sourness in beer are the organic acids that are produced by yeast during fermentation. These lower the pH: it is the H^+ ion imparted by acidic solutions that causes the sour character to be perceived on the palate. Most beers have a pH between 3.9 and 4.6.

Saltiness in beer is afforded by sodium and potassium, while of the anions present in beer, chloride and sulphate are of particular importance. Chloride is said to contribute a mellowing and fullness to a palate, while sulphate is felt to elevate the dryness of beer.

Perhaps the most important taste in beer is bitterness, primarily imparted by the iso-α-acids derived from the hop resins.

Many people believe that they can taste other notes on a beer. In fact they are detecting them with the nose, the confusion arising because there is a continuum between the back of the throat and the nasal passages. The smell (or aroma) of a beer is a complex distillation of the contribution of a great many individual molecules. No beer is so simple as to have its 'nose' determined by one or even a very few substances. The perceived character is a balance between positive and negative flavour notes, each of which may be a consequence of one or a combination of many compounds of different chemical classes. The 'flavour threshold' is the lowest concentration of a substance which is detectable in beer.

The substances that contribute to the aroma of beer are diverse. They are derived from malt and hops and by yeast activity (leaving aside for the moment the contribution of contaminating microbes). In turn there are interactions between these sources, insofar as yeast converts one flavour constituent from malt or hops into a different one, for example.

Various alcohols influence the flavour of beer (Table 8.3), by far the most important of which is ethanol, which is present in most beers at levels at least 350-fold higher than any other alcohol. Ethanol contributes directly to the flavour of beer, registering a warming character. It also influences the flavour contribution of other volatile substances in beer. Because it is quantitatively third only to water and carbon dioxide as the main component of beer, it is not surprising that it moderates the flavour impact of other substances. It does this by affecting the vapour pressure of other molecules (i.e. their relative tendency to remain in beer or to migrate to the headspace of the beer). The higher alcohols in beer are important as the immediate precursors of the esters, which are proportionately more flavour active (see Table 8.4). And so it is important to be able to regulate the levels of the higher alcohols produced by yeast if ester levels are also to be controlled.

Table 8.3. Some alcohols in beer.

Alcohol	Flavour threshold (mg l^{-1})	Perceived character
Ethanol	14,000	Alcoholic
Propan-1-ol	800	Alcoholic
Butan-2-ol	16	Alcoholic
Iso-amyl alcohol	50	Alcohol, banana, vinous
Tyrosol	200	Bitter
Phenylethanol	40–100	Roses, perfume

Table 8.4. Some esters in beer.

Ester	Flavour threshold (mg l^{-1})	Perceived character
Ethyl acetate	33	Solventy, fruity, sweet
Iso-amyl acetate	1.0	Banana
Ethyl octanoate	0.9	Apples, sweet, fruity
Phenylethyl acetate	3.8	Roses, honey, apple

The higher alcohols are produced during fermentation by two routes: catabolic and anabolic. In the catabolic route, yeast amino acids taken-up from the wort by yeast are transaminated to α-keto-acids, which are decarboxylated and reduced to alcohols:

$$RCH(NH_2)COOH + R^1COCOOH \rightarrow RCOCOOH + R^1CH(NH_2)COOH \qquad ... (8.1)$$

$$RCOCOOH \rightarrow RCHO + CO_2 \qquad ... (8.2)$$

$$RCHO + NADH + H^+ \rightarrow RCH_2OH + NAD^+ \qquad \qquad ... (8.3)$$

The anabolic route starts with pyruvate (the end point of the EMP pathway proper), the higher alcohols being 'side shoots' from the synthesis of the amino acids valine and leucine (Fig. 8.24). The penultimate stage in the production of all amino acids is the formation of the relevant keto acid which is transaminated to the amino acid. Should there be conditions where the keto acids accumulate, they are then decarboxylated and reduced to the equivalent alcohol. Essentially, therefore, the only difference between the pathways is the origin of the keto acid: either the transamination product of an amino acid assimilated by the yeast from its growth medium or synthesised *de novo* from pyruvate.

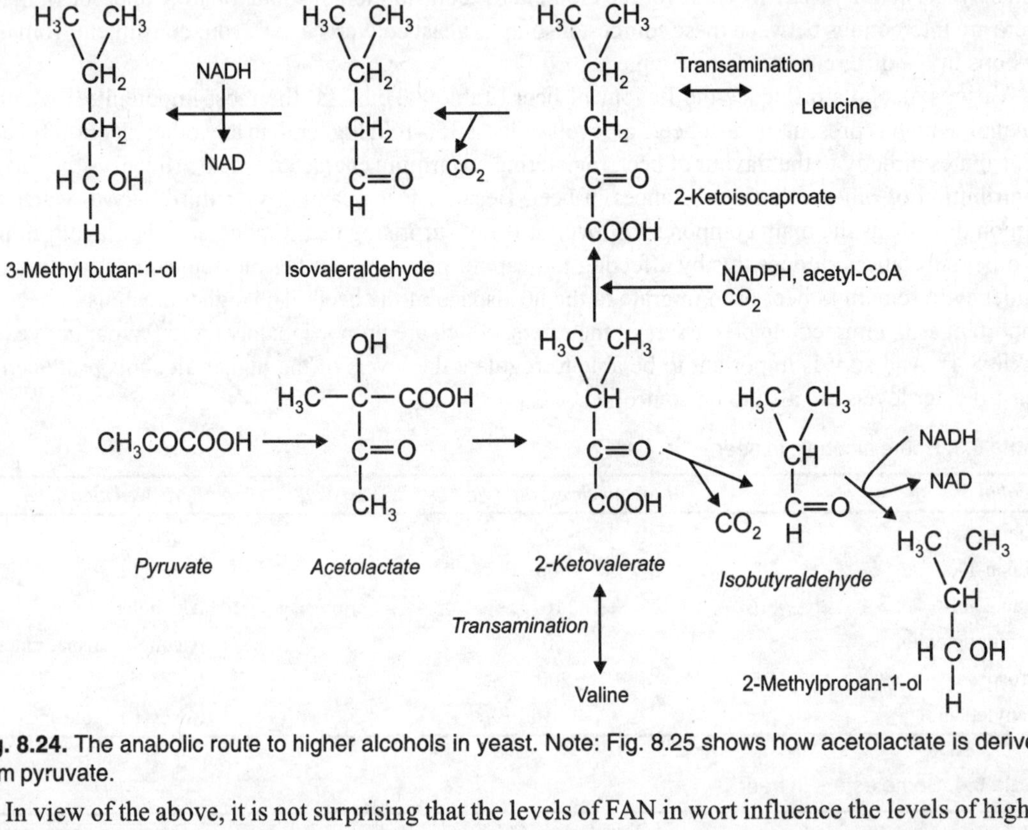

Fig. 8.24. The anabolic route to higher alcohols in yeast. Note: Fig. 8.25 shows how acetolactate is derived from pyruvate.

In view of the above, it is not surprising that the levels of FAN in wort influence the levels of higher alcohols formed. Higher alcohol production is increased at both excessively high and insufficiently low levels of assimilable nitrogen available to the yeast from wort. If levels of assimilable N are low, then yeast growth is limited and there is a high incidence of the anabolic pathway. If levels of N are high, then the amino acids feedback to inhibit further synthesis of them and therefore the anabolic pathway becomes less important. However, there is a greater tendency for the catabolic pathway to 'kick in'.

Even more important than FAN levels, though, is the yeast strain, with ale strains producing more of these compounds than lager strains. Fermentations at higher temperatures increase higher alcohol production. Conditions favouring increased yeast growth (e.g. excessive aeration or oxygenation) promote higher alcohol formation, but this can be countered by application of a top pressure on the fermenter. The reasons why increased pressure has this effect are unclear, but it has been suggested that it may for some reason be due to an accumulation of carbon dioxide. Whatever the reason, it is pertinent to mention that beer produced in different sizes and shapes of vessel, displaying different hydrostatic pressures, do produce higher alcohols (and thereof esters) to different extents. This can be a problem for product matching between breweries (e.g. in franchise brewing operations).

Various esters may make a contribution to the flavour of beer (Table 8.4). The esters are produced from their equivalent alcohols (ROH), through catalysis by the enzyme alcohol acetyl transferase (AAT), with acetyl-coenzyme A being the donor of the acetate group:

$$ROH + CH_3COSCoA \rightarrow CH_3COOR + CoASH$$

Clearly the amount of ester produced will depend *inter alia* on the levels of acetyl-CoA, of alcohol and of AAT. Esters are formed under conditions when the acetyl-CoA is not required as the prime building block for the synthesis of key cell components. In particular, acetyl-CoA is the starting point for the synthesis of lipids, which the cell requires for its membranes. Thus, factors promoting yeast production (e.g. high levels of aeration/oxygenation) lower ester production, and *vice versa*.

However, perhaps the most significant factor influencing the extent of ester production is yeast strain, some strains being more predisposed to generating esters than others. This may relate to the amount of AAT that they contain. The factors that dictate the level of this enzyme present in a given yeast strain are not fully elucidated, but it does seem to be present in raised quantities when the yeast encounters high-gravity wort, and this may explain the disproportionate extent of ester synthesis under these conditions.

Whereas the esters and higher alcohols can make positive contributions to the flavour of beer, few beers (with the possible exception of some ales) are helped by the presence of VDKs, diacetyl and (less importantly) pentanedione (Table 8.5). Elimination of VDKs from beer depends on the fermentation process being well-run. These substances are offshoots of the pathways by which yeast produces the amino acids valine and isoleucine (and therefore there is a relationship to the anabolic pathway of higher alcohol production).

Table 8.5. VDKs in beer.

VDK	Flavour threshold mg l^{-1})	Perceived character
Diacetyl	0.1	Butterscotch
Pentanedione	0.9	Honey

The pathway for diacetyl production is shown in Fig. 8.25 because it is more significant (with respect to diacetyl being present at higher levels and with a lower flavour threshold). The precursor molecules leak out of the yeast and break down spontaneously to form VDKs. Happily, the yeast can mop up the VDK, provided it remains in contact with the beer and is in good condition.

Reductases in the yeast reduce diacetyl successively to acetoin and 2,3-butanediol, both of which have much higher flavour thresholds than diacetyl.

Many brewers allow a temperature rise at the end of fermentation to facilitate more rapid removal of VDKs. Others introduce a small amount of freshly fermenting wort later on as an inoculum of healthy yeast (a process known as *Krausening*). Persistent high diacetyl levels in a brewery's production may be indicative of an infection by *Pediococcus* or *Lactobacillus* bacteria. If the ratio of diacetyl to pentanedione is disproportionately high, then this indicates that there is an infection problem.

In many ways the most complex flavour characters in beer are due to the sulphur-containing compounds. There are many of these in beer (Table 8.6) and they make various contributions. Thus, many ales have a deliberate hydrogen sulphide character, not too much, but just enough to give a nice 'eggy' nose. Lagers tend to have a more complex sulphury character. Some lagers are relatively devoid of any sulphury nose. Others, though, have a distinct DMS character, while some have characters ranging from cabbagy to burnt rubber. This range of characteristics renders substantial complexity to the control of sulphury flavours.

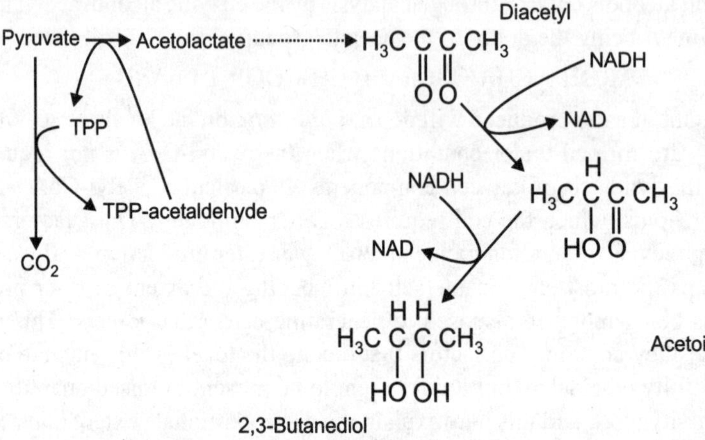

Fig. 8.25. The production and elimination of diacetyl by yeast.

Table 8.6. Some sulphur-containing substances in beer.

S-containing compound	Flavour threshold (mg l^{-1})	Perceived character
Hydrogen sulphide	0.005	Rotten eggs
Sulphur dioxide	25	Burnt matches
Methanethiol	0.002	Drains
Ethanethiol	0.002	Putrefaction
Propanethiol	0.0015	Onion
Dimethyl sulphide	0.03	Sweetcorn
Dimethyl disulphide	0.0075	Rotting vegetables
Dimethyl trisulphide	0.0001	Rotting vegetables, onion
Methyl thioacetate	0.05	Cooked cabbage
Diethyl sulphide	0.0012	Cooke vegetable garlic
Methional	0.25	Cooked potato
3-Methyl-2-butene-1-thiol	0.000004–0.001	Lightstruck, skunky
2-Furfurylmercaptan	–	Rubber

All of the DMS in a lager ultimately originates from a precursor, S-methylmethionine (SMM), produced during the germination of barley (Fig. 8.26). SMM is heat sensitive and is broken down rapidly whenever the temperature gets above about 80°C in the process. Thus, SMM levels are lower in the more intensely kilned ale malts and, as a result, DMS is a character more associated with lagers. SMM leaches into wort during mashing and is further degraded during boiling and in the whirlpool. If the boil is vigorous, most of the SMM is converted to DMS and this is driven off. In the whirlpool, though, conditions are gentler and any SMM surviving the boil will be broken down to DMS but the latter tends to stay in the wort. Brewers seeking to retain some DMS in their beer will specify a finite level of SMM in their malt and will manipulate the boil and whirlpool stages in order to deliver a certain level of DMS into the pitching wort. During fermentation, much DMS will be lost with the gases, so the level of DMS required in the wort will be somewhat higher than that specified for the beer. There is another complication, insofar as some of the SMM is converted into a third substance, DMSO, during kilning. This is not heat-labile but is water-soluble. It gets into wort at quite high levels and some yeast strains are quite adept at converting it to DMS.

COOH
|
H$_2$NCH
|
CH$_2$
|
H$_3$C-$\overset{+}{S}$-CH$_2$
|
CH$_3$

S-methylmethionine

Synthesised in barley
embryo during germination

Heat* →

Homoserine

+

H$_3$C-S-CH$_3$

Dimethyl sulphide

2 / 1 →

O
↑
H$_3$C-S-CH$_3$

Dimethyl sulphoxide

*e.g. malt kilning, wort boiling

1. At curing temperature in kilning
2. By yeast/bacterial metabolism

Fig. 8.26. The origin of DMS in beer.

Hydrogen sulphide (H$_2$S) can also be produced by more than one pathway in yeast. It may be formed by the breakdown of amino acids such as cysteine or peptides like glutathione, or by the reduction of inorganic sources such as sulphate and sulphite (Fig. 8.27). Once again, yeast strain has a major effect on the levels of H$_2$S that are produced during fermentation. For all strains, more H$_2$S will be present in green beer if the yeast is in poor condition, because a vigorous fermentation is needed to purge H$_2$S. Any other factor that hinders fermentation (e.g. a lack of zinc or vitamins) will also lead to an exaggeration of H$_2$S levels in beer. Furthermore, H$_2$S is a product of yeast autolysis, which will be more prevalent in unhealthy yeast.

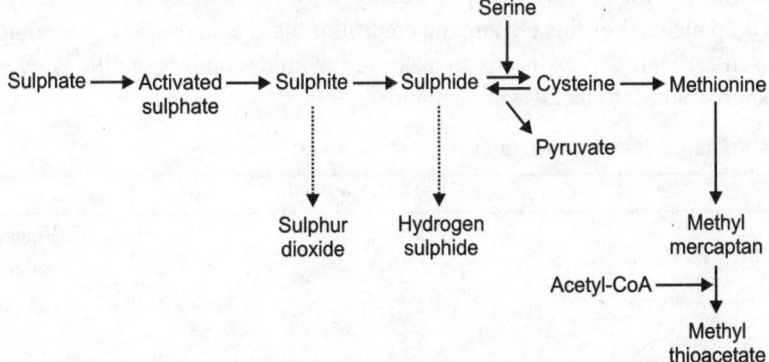

Fig. 8.27. The origins of other sulphur-containing volatiles in beer.

When the bitter iso-α-acids are exposed to light, they break down, react with sulphur sources in the beer and form a substance called 3-methyl-2-butene-1-thiol (MBT), which has an intense skunky character and is detectable at extremely low concentrations. There are two ways of protecting beer from this: do not expose beer to light or else bitter using chemically modified bitter extracts, the reduced iso-α-acids.

The addition of hops during beer production not only contributes much of the resulting bitterness, but also imparts a unique so-called 'hoppy' aroma. This attribute comes from the complex volatile oil fraction of hops. Most of the component substances do not survive the brewing process intact and are chemically transformed into as yet poorly defined compounds. Certainly, there does not appear to be one compound solely responsible for hop aroma in beer, although several groups (e.g. sesquiterpene epoxides, cyclic ethers and furanones) have been strongly implicated.

The point at which hops are added during beer production determines the resulting flavour that they impart. The practice of adding aroma hops close to the end of boiling (late hopping) still results in the substantial evaporation of volatile material, but of the little that remains, much is transformed into other species (e.g. the hop oil component humulene can be converted to the more flavour-active humulene epoxide). Further changes then occur during fermentation, such as the transesterification of methyl esters to their ethyl counterparts. The resultant late hop flavour is rather floral in character and is generally an attribute more associated with lager beers.

In a generally distinct practice, hops may be added to the beer right at the end of production. This process of dry hopping gives certain ales their characteristic aroma. The hop oil components contributed to beer by this process are very different to those from late hopping, with mono- and sesquiterpenes surviving generally unchanged in the beer.

Malty character in beer is due in part at least to isovaleraldehyde, which is formed by a reaction between one of the amino acids (leucine) and reductones in the malt. The toffee and caramel flavours in crystal malts and the roasted, coffee-like notes found in darker malts are due to various complex components generated from amino acids and sugars that cross-react during kilning—the Maillard reaction.

Acetaldehyde, which is the immediate precursor of ethanol in yeast, has a flavour threshold of between 5 and 50 mg l^{-1} and imparts a 'green apples' flavour to beer. High levels should not survive into beer in successful fermentations, because yeast will efficiently convert the acetaldehyde into ethanol. If levels are persistently high, then this is an indication of premature yeast separation, poor yeast quality or a Zymomonas infection.

The short-chain fatty acids (Table 8.7) are made by yeast as intermediates in the synthesis of the lipid membrane components. For this reason, the control of these acids is exactly analogous to that of the esters (discussed earlier): if yeast needs to make fewer lipids (under conditions where it needs to grow less), then short-chain fatty acids will accumulate.

Table 8.7. Some short-chain fatty acids in beer.

Fatty acid	Flavour threshold (mg l^{-1})	Perceived character
Acetic	175	Vinegar
Propionic	150	Acidic, milky
Butyric	2.2	Cheesy
3-Methyl butyric	1.5	Sweaty
Hexanoic	8	Vegetable oil
Octanoic	15	Goaty
Phenyl acetic	2.5	Honey

Some beers (e.g. some wheat beers) feature a phenolic or clove-like character. This is due to molecules such as 4-vinylguaiacol (4-VG), which is produced by certain *Saccharomyces* species, including *Saccharomyces diastaticus*. Its unwanted presence in a beer is an indication of a wild yeast infection. 4-VG is produced by the decarboxylation of ferulic acid by an enzyme that is present in *S. diastaticus* and other wild yeasts, but not in brewing strains other than a few specific strains of *S. cerevisiae*, namely the ones prized in Bavaria for their use in wheat beer manufacture. A further undesirable note is a metallic character which, if present in beer, is most likely to be due to the presence of high levels (>0.3 ppm) of iron. One known cause is the leaching of the metal from filter aid.

The flavour of beer changes with time. There is a decrease in bitterness (due to the progressive loss of the iso-α-acids), an increase in perceived sweetness and toffee character and a development of a cardboard note. It is the cardboard note that most brewers worry about in connection with the shelf-life of their products. Cardboard is due to a range of carbonyl compounds, which may originate in various precursors, including unsaturated fatty acids, higher alcohols, amino acids and the bitter substances. Most importantly, their formation is a result of oxidation, hence the importance of minimising oxygen levels in beer and, perhaps, further upstream.

Any drinker who has ordered a beer containing nitrogen gas will appreciate that one can talk of the mouthfeel and texture of beer. N_2 not only imparts a tight, creamy head to a beer, but it also gives rise to a creamy texture. More specifically, the partial replacement of carbon dioxide with nitrogen gas suppresses several beer flavour attributes, such as astringency, bitterness, hop aroma as well as the reduction in the carbon dioxide 'tingle'. Other components of beer, such as the a stringent polyphenols, may also play a part. Physical properties, such as viscosity, are influenced by residual carbohydrate in the beer and might also contribute to the overall mouthfeel of a product. It is thought that turbulent flow of liquids between the tongue and the roof of the mouth results in increased perceived viscosity and therefore enhanced mouthfeel.

Foam

A point of difference between beer and other alcoholic beverages is its possession of stable foam. This is due to the presence of hydrophobic (amphipathic) polypeptides, derived from cereal, that cross-link with the bitter iso-α-acids in the bubble walls to counter the forces of surface tension that tend to lead to foam collapse.

Gushing

Foaming can be taken to excess, in which case the problem which manifests itself in small pack is 'gushing', that is, the spontaneous generation of foam on opening a package of beer. This is due to the presence of nucleation sites in beer that cause the dramatic discharging of carbon dioxide from solution. These nucleation sites may be particles of materials like oxalate or filter aid, but most commonly gushing is caused by intensely hydrophobic peptides that are produced from Fusarium that can infect barley unless precautions are taken.

Spoilage of Beer

Compared with most other foods and beverages beer is relatively resistant to infection. There are several reasons for this, namely the presence of ethanol, a low pH, the relative shortage of nutrients (sugars, amino acids), the anaerobic conditions and the presence of antimicrobial agents, notably the iso-α-acids.

The most problematic gram-positive bacteria are lactic acid bacteria belonging to the genera *Lactobacillus* and *Pediococcus*. At least ten species of lactobacillus spoil beer. They tolerate the acidic conditions. Some species (e.g. *Lactobacillus brevis* and *Lactobacillus plantarum*) grow quickly during fermentation, conditioning and storage, while others (e.g. *Lactobacillus lindner*) grow relatively slowly. Spoilage with lactobacilli is especially problematic during the conditioning of beer and after packaging, resulting in a silky turbidity and off-flavours. Pediococci are homofermentative. Six species have been identified, the most important being *Pediococcus damnosus*. Such infection generates lactic acid and diacetyl. The production of polysaccharide capsules can cause ropiness in beer.

Many gram-positive bacteria are killed by iso-α-acids. These agents probably disrupt nutrient transport across the membrane of the bacteria, but only when they are present in their protonated forms (i.e. at low pH). This is one of the reasons why a beer at pH 4 will be more resistant to infection than one at pH 4.5. Some Gram positives are resistant to iso-α-acids and most gram negatives are.

Important gram-negative bacteria include the acetic acid bacteria (*Acetobacter*, *Gluconobacter*); Enterobacteriaceae (*Escherichia*, *Aerobacter*, *Klebsiella*, *Citrobacter*, *Obesumbacterium*); *Zymomonas*, *Pectinatus* and *Megasphaera*. Acetic acid bacteria produce a vinegary flavour in beer and a ropy slime. It is most often found in draft beer, where there is a relatively aerobic environment close to the beer, for example, in partly emptied containers. Enterobacteriaceae are aerobic and cannot grow in the presence of ethanol. They are a threat in wort and early in fermentation and they produce cabbagy/vegetable/eggy aromas. *Zymomonas* is a problem with primed beers (it uses invert sugar or glucose, but cannot use maltose). Although it has a metabolism reminiscent of *Saccharomyces* (it's actually used to produce alcoholic beverages in some countries), it does tend to produce large amounts of acetaldehyde. Major beer styles and their origin are given in Table 8.8.

Table 8.8. Major beer styles.

Style	Origin	Notes
Ales and stouts		
Bitter (pale) ale	England	Dry hop, bitter, estery, malty, low carbonation (on draught), copper colour
India pale ale	England	Similar, but substantially more bitter
Alt (n.b. Alt means 'old')	Germany	Estery, bitter, copper colour
Mild (brown) ale	England	Darker than pale ale, malty, slightly sweeter, lower in alcohol
Porter	England	Dark brown/black, less 'roast' character than stout, malty
Stout	Ireland	Black, roast, coffee-like, bitter
Sweet stout	England	Caramel-like, brown, full-bodied
Imperial stout	England	Brown/black, malty, alcoholic
Barley wine	England	Tawny/brown, malty, alcoholic, warming
Kölsch	Germany	Straw/golden colour, caramel-like, medium bitterness, low hop aroma
Weizenbier (wheat beer)	Germany	Hefeweissens retain yeast (i.e. turbid). Kristalweissens are filtered. Very fruity, clove-like, high carbonation
Lambic	Belgium	Estery, sour, 'wet horse-blanket', turbid. Lambic may be mixed with cherry (krick), peach (peche), raspberry (framboise), etc. Old lambic blended with freshly fermenting lambic = gueuze

(Contd ...)

Style	Origin	Notes
Saison	Belgium	Golden, fruity, phenolic, mildly hoppy
Lagers		
Pilsener	Czech	Golden/amber, malty, late hop aroma
Bock	Germany	Golden/brown, malty, moderately bitter
Helles	Germany	Straw/golden, low bitterness, malty, sulphury
Märzen (meaning 'March' for when traditionally brewed)	Germany	Diverse colours, sweet malt flavour, crisp bitterness
Vienna	Astro-Hungaria	Red-brown, malty, toasty, crisply bitter
Dunkel	Germany	Brown, malty, roast-chocolate
Schwarzbier	Germany	Brown/black, roast malt, bitter
Rauchbier	Germany	Smokey
Malt liquor	USA	Pale colour, alcoholic, slightly sweet, low bitterness

ENZYMES IN BREWING

Enzymes are proteins with a special structure capable of accelerating the breakdown of different substrates. They act as catalysts to increase the speed of a chemical reaction without themselves undergoing any permanent chemical change. They are not used up in the reaction or appear as reaction products.

Enzymes bind temporarily to the substrate, thereby lowering the amount of activation energy, enabling the reaction to occur faster and at lower temperatures. Like most chemical reactions, the rate of an enzyme-catalysed reaction increases as the temperature is raised. A 10°C rise in temperature will increase the activity of most enzymes by 50 to 100 per cent. Variations in reaction temperature as small as 1°–2°C may introduce changes of 10–20 per cent in the results.

In the case of enzymatic reactions, this is complicated by the fact that high temperatures adversely affect many enzymes. The reaction rate increases with temperature to a maximum level, then abruptly falls off with further increase of temperature. Many enzymes start to become denatured at temperatures above 40°C. Over a period of time, enzymes will be deactivated, at even moderate temperatures. Storage of enzymes at 5°C or below is generally the most suitable.

Enzymes are equally affected by changes in pH. The optimum pH value will vary greatly from one enzyme to another. Most of the brewing enzymes have an optimum pH in the range 4.5 to 6.0, which is the operating range of most brewing processes. Concentration of enzyme used, with reference to the substrate concentration, plays an important role. With an excess concentration of substrate, such as starch in a brewers' wort, there is a linear effect of increasing the enzyme concentration upon the reaction rate. Hence, if all other factors are kept constant, malts with higher enzymatic power will break down starch faster. It has been shown that if the amount of the enzyme is kept constant and the substrate concentration is gradually increased, the reaction velocity will increase until it reaches a maximum. After this point, increases in substrate concentration will not increase the velocity.

In addition to temperature and pH, there are other factors, such as ionic strength, which can affect the enzymatic reaction. Each of these physical and chemical parameters must be considered and optimised, in order for an enzymatic reaction to be accurate and reproducible.

Biochemical Changes During Brewing

Enzymes are essential in catalysing the biochemical changes, which occur in the brewing process. There are two principal processes of interest to the brewer:

1. The breakdown of carbohydrate, principally starch, in malted barley, to sugars.
2. The fermentation of sugars and other nutrients by yeast, under anaerobic conditions, to release energy and produce ethanol, as a metabolic by-product.

These biological reactions are catalysed by enzymes from the barley and yeast respectively. Barley is able to produce all the enzymes needed to degrade starch, β-glucan, pentosans, lipids and proteins, which are the major compounds of concern to the brewer.

During malting, the barley corn is allowed to germinate and produce enzymes for breaking down the cell walls in the corn and release energy stored as starch in the endosperm. The starch is present as concentric granules surrounded by a protein matrix, and has to be broken down during mashing before the enzyme amylases can gain access.

Three principal enzymic reactions occur in malt during the mashing process. The principal reaction is the hydrolysis of starch to sugars by α and β-amylase. Before enzyme hydrolysis can occur, it is necessary to exceed the starch gelatinisation temperature of malt. Therefore, it is necessary to select the optimum conditions for the saccharifying enzymes to operate. This is achieved by stabilising the enzymes by:

1. Optimising pH at mashing (usually between pH5 and 6).
2. Adding calcium ions to stabilise the enzyme.
3. Using thick mash (high concentration substrate to insulate the enzymes against denaturing).
4. Optimising temperature to favour the activity of both the α and β-amylase.

The amylase enzymes break the α-1,4 links in amylose and amylopectin to give a mixture of glucose, maltose, maltotriose and higher sugars called dextrins, which are unfermentable, to give a wort (malt derived sugar solution), which is fermentable up to 70 per cent.

α-amylase produces random hydrolyses of starch to dextrins; while β-amylase attacks the starch and dextrins from the reducing end, stripping off pairs of sugar molecules (maltose).

By varying the mashing temperature, it is possible to preferentially favour one enzyme reaction over the other and hence influence the fermentability of the wort, with the lower temperatures giving higher fermentable worts.

Apart from starch, barley contains a number of non-starch polysaccharides, principal being β-glucan (~75 per cent of the cell wall). The molecule has a distinctive linear structure containing 70 per cent β-1,4 linkages and 30 per cent β-1,3 linkages. Mostly it is water soluble, but a proportion is bound covalently to cell wall proteins. If there is insufficient degradation of the cell walls, then enzymic access to the protein and starch will be restricted, and the extract from the malt is reduced.

Although much of the necessary β-glucanase activity occurs during malting, there is inevitably some survival of cell wall material (even in the most fully modified malt). This will be exacerbated if adjuncts such as barley and wheat are also used. Consequently, it is necessary to ensure the continued activity of β-glucanase during mashing. If the large viscous β-glucan molecules are not broken down during malting or mashing, other process problems can also occur. These include:

1. Reduced extract recovery.
2. High wort viscosity.
3. Poor run off performance.
4. Beer filtration problems.
5. Beer haze problems.

Most brewers are very careful in selecting malt with low β-glucan levels, and it is common practice in many breweries to add exogenous β-glucanase to decrease wort and beer viscosity and to improve filterability. Advantage of addition of β-glucanase can be shown by an increasing in filter flow rate and decrease in wort viscosity.

Hydrolysis of proteins and polypeptides

While about 95 per cent of the starch from malt is solubilised by the end of mashing, only about 35–40 per cent of the malt protein (total nitrogen) is solubilised. This is referred to as the TSN (total soluble nitrogen) in an unboiled wort. The principal enzymes involved in the breakdown of malt proteins are:

1. Endoproteases, which break the large protein molecules into polypeptide chains.
2. Exopeptidases, which attack polypeptides, stripping off small polypeptides to produce amino acids.

Endopeptidases have a low optimum temperature and hence with high temperature mashing most of the protein breakdown will have taken place during the malting process. They randomly attack the protein. Exopeptidases are able to withstand higher temperatures and release the amino acids from the polypeptide chains.

There are two principal groups of exopeptidase enzymes:

1. Carboxypeptidase which attacks the proteins from the carbonyl end. This enzyme is not present in raw barley, but is rapidly produced during steeping and is active at normal mash pH. Optimum conditions for its use are: pH 3.9–5.5; temperature: 45°–50°C; and inactivation temperature: 70°C.
2. Aminopeptidase, which attacks the proteins from the amino end, is much less active at mash pH and does not play a significant role in protein breakdown during mashing. Optimum conditions for its use are: pH: 4.8–5.2; temperature: 50°C; inactivation temperature: >70°C.

Most of the proteolysis occurs during malting. It is impossible to completely compensate for a nitrogen deficiency in malt by introducing a prolonged mash stand at <50°C without adding exogenous enzymes. Nitrogenous materials account for 5–6 per cent of wort solids, which is equivalent to around 30–40 per cent of the total nitrogen in malt. Good yeast growth and rapid fermentation requires 160 mg/l of free amino nitrogen (at 12°P wort) depending on the yeast strain.

Carboxypeptidases can release amino acids in mashing, provided the endopeptidase has broken down the protein substrate during the malting process. The optimum temperature to produce free amino nitrogen production is 50°C. Proteins in the mash dissolve at these low temperatures and then precipitate at 65°C, which can inhibit lautering. Excessive proteolysis in malting and mashing will reduce foam stability and the pH of a normal mash is not optimal for proteolysis.

Proteins Found in Wort

Much of the surplus protein is left behind in the spent grains, but when oxidised can form a protein 'scum', which causes run off problems. Some of the soluble proteins play an essential role as enzymes, catalysing the reactions described above.

Polypeptides

These are long-chain sequences of relatively high molecular weight amino acids. There are two important groups in brewing: Hydrophobic polypeptides, which make up beer foam; and acidic polypeptides, which can combine with polyphenols to produce hot and cold break, and if not removed, these contribute to colloidal instability in beer. This group of compounds is also probably important in contributing to the texture and mouth-feel of the beer.

Peptides

These are short chain sequences of amino acids, usually 2 to 10 units long, and probably have a minor effect on body and mouth-feel.

Amino acids

These make up 10–15 per cent of the TSN and are an essential source of nutrient for yeast growth. The usual concentration of soluble free amino nitrogen (FAN) in wort is required to be above 160-mg/l; lower levels can lead to a defective fermentation.

In addition to their role in yeast growth, amino acids are also involved in a number of metabolic pathways, producing significant flavour active compounds, which contribute to the final flavour of the beer. The activity of proteolytic enzymes is effected by temperature of mashing, which, in turn, will effect the total nitrogen, amino nitrogen, head retention and shelf life stability.

Fermentation

Yeasts are able to respire anaerobically, but under anaerobic conditions they can only partially break down sugar molecules to ethanol to release energy in the form of ATP (adenosine triphosphate).

The role of yeast in the fermentation is that of a living catalyst, effecting the reaction without becoming part of the finished product. During the course of the fermentation, the yeast cells grow and replicate up to five times. Although the yeast gains its energy from the sugar, which it converts to alcohol it can only utilise simple sugars. The sugars are taken up in a specific order, with the monosaccharides, glucose and fructose used first, together with sucrose.

Although the latter is a disaccharide, it behaves like a monosaccharide, since it is broken down to glucose and fructose outside the cell, through the action of the yeast enzyme invertase. Once the wort glucose level falls, the yeast starts to use the disaccharide, maltose, which is usually the most abundant sugar in brewers, wort. Maltose has to be transported into the cell, where it is broken down to glucose. Lastly most yeast strains can utilise the trisaccharide, maltotriose, but only slowly.

Brewing strains of yeast cannot generally ferment the longer chained or branched sugars (called dextrins), which persist in to the finished beer as unfermentable extract to give the beer body and mouth-feel. As well as sugars, yeast requires nitrogen, which in wort comes from the malt, in the form of soluble amino nitrogen.

A healthy fermentation yeast requires more than 160 mg/l of soluble nitrogen. If there is insufficient soluble nitrogen, for example when high cereal or sugar adjunct are used, then additional nitrogen may be required in the form of simple ammonium salts. Table 8.9 shows the action of enzymes.

Table 8.9. Action of enzymes.

Type of enzyme	Action	Principal sugars produced
Heat stable alpha amylase	Endo 1,4 alpha bonds	Reduces viscosity, maltodextrins
Alpha amylase and alpha glucoamylase	α-1,4 bonds and α-1,4 and 1,6 bonds	Maltose syrup
Alpha amylase and pullulanase	α-1,4 bonds and α-1,6 bonds	Very high maltose syrup

Syrup manufacture

A number of brewers use brewing syrups, which are manufactured from hydrolysed starch solution. Since the starch is not malted, microbial exogenous enzymes have to be used and by selecting different enzyme combinations the syrup producer can control the composition and fermentability of the syrup.

Brewing

As already discussed, beer is produced by mixing crushed barley malt and hot water in a large copper mash. Besides malt, adjuncts such as maize, sorghum, rice and barley or pure starch itself, are added to the mash. The mash is filtered in a lautertun. The resulting liquid, sweet wort, is run off to the copper where it is boiled with hops.

The hopped wort is cooled and transferred to the fermentation vessels where yeast is added. After the fermentation, the so-called green beer, is matured before the final filtration and bottling. This is a much-simplified account of making beer.

The traditional source of enzymes used for the conversion of cereals into beer is barley malt, one of the key ingredients in brewing. If too little enzyme activity is present in the mash, there will be several undesirable consequences, such as:

1. Too low yield of extract.
2. Longer time for wort separation.
3. Slower rate of fermentation.
4. Lower alcohol content.
5. Inferior flavour.
6. Lower stability.

Enzymes are used to supplement malt's own enzymes in order to prevent these problems.

Rossari biotech has developed a compounded formulation—Fermross BR—combining benefits of various enzymes to ensure:

1. Optimal and efficient liquefaction of adjuncts.
2. Accelerate rate of fermentation.
3. Shorten the beer maturation time.
4. Allow cheaper raw materials for beer manufacture.

Brewing with Adjuncts

Malt is the traditional source of α-amylase for the liquefaction of adjuncts. Nevertheless, it needs to be supplemented with heat stable α-amylase to ensure:

1. More predictable and simpler liquefaction of adjuncts, shorter process time and increased productivity.
2. The malt enzymes are preserved for subsequent saccharification process, resulting in a better wort and beer quality.
3. Eliminating the malt from the adjunct cooker, rendering more freedom in balancing volumes and temperatures in the mashing programme, while using high adjunct ratio.

Brewing with Barley

Traditionally, the use of barley has been limited to 10–20 per cent of the grist when using high-quality malts. Low-quality malts need to be supplemented with extra enzyme activity, to maintain adequate brewing performance.

Brewers may add Fermross BR blend of thermo stable α-amylase, β-glucanase and protease at the mashing-in stage or later, separately as required.

Wort separation and beer filtration are two common bottlenecks in brewing. Poor lautering reduces production capacity and lowers extract yields. A thorough breakdown of β-glucans and pentosans during mashing is essential for fast wort separation. Non-degraded β-glucans and pentosans carried over into the fermenter reduce the beer filtration capacity. Fermross BR improves wort separation thereby increasing rate of filtration.

Enzymes in Improving Fermentation

Improvements in fermentability for various substrates can be achieved by adding Fermross BR which contains α-amylase, at the start of fermentation, together with a glucoamylase at mashing-in. Fungal α-amylases produce maltose and dextrins, whereas glucoamylase produces glucose from both linear and branched dextrins. The alcohol content is an important parameter that brewers must control. The amount of alcohol in a beer is controlled by the level of fermentable sugar in the extract; which in turn, is controlled by the amount of amylases in the mash, and the saccharifying enzymes used during fermentation.

Yeast needs proteins in order to multiply. If the level of available amino nitrogen is less, the fermentation is poor, leading to inferior beer quality. Fermross BR contains a neutral protease, when added at mashing-in, raise the level of free amino nitrogen. This is beneficial when working with poor malts or with high adjunct ratios.

Diacetyl Control

Beer is said to be mature for racking when the diacetyl level drops below 0.07 ppm. Diacetyl gives beer an off-flavour like buttermilk. During 'maturing' diacetyl content drops to a level where it can't be tasted.

Diacetyl is formed by oxidative decarboxylation of α-acetolactate during primary fermentation, which is removed again by the yeast, during beer maturation by conversion to acetoin; which is almost tasteless.

By adding Fermross BR, which contains an enzyme α-acetolactate decarboxylase at the beginning of the primary fermentation, it is possible to convert α-acetolactate directly into acetoin. Most of the α-acetolactate is degraded before it has a chance to oxidise and thus less diacetyl is formed. Thus, use of Fermross BR shortens or completely eliminates the maturation period. The brewery enjoys greater fermentation and maturation capacity without investing in new equipment.

Chapter 9

Wine and Cider

INTRODUCTION

The Merriam-Webster's dictionary defines wine as the usually fermented juice of a plant product (as a fruit) used as a beverage. While in rural communities in countries such as Great Britain wines have from time immemorial been produced from all manner of plant materials (and not only fruits). The discussion in the present chapter to the products of commercial entities furnishing wines is based on the grape (Fig. 9.1).

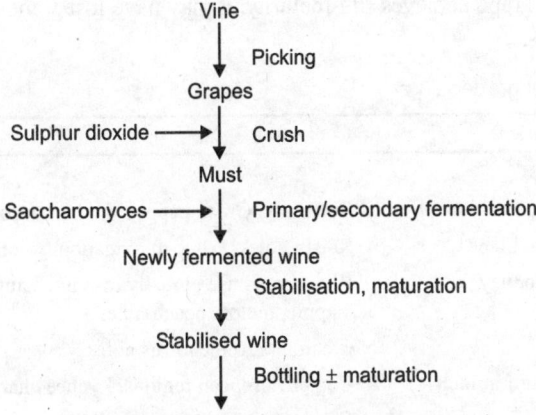

Fig. 9.1. An overview of wine making.

The importance of sound viticulture as a precursor to wines of excellence is unequivocally accepted as a truth in wine making companies worldwide. More so than for beer is the belief held that it is not possible to make an excellent product unless there is similar excellence in the source of fermentable carbohydrate. Most wineries tend to grow their own grapes or buy them from nearby vineyards.

The ideal climate for growing wine grapes is where there is no summer rain, it is hot or at least warm during the day, there are cool nights and little risk of frost damage. The great grape-growing and wine regions are Italy, France, Spain, United States, Argentina, Germany, South Africa, Australia, Chile, Romania. A benchmark figure for the yield of wine from one metric ton of grapes would be around 140–160 gal. As red grapes are fermented on the skins and therefore are less demanding in the pressing stage, the yield is some 20 per cent higher than for whites.

Wine grapes belong to the genus *Vitis*. Within the genus, the main species are *vinifera* (by far the most important), *lubruscana* and *rotundifolia*. Commercial vines tend to be *Vitis vinifera* grafter onto rootstocks of the other *Vitis* species. Of course within the species is a diversity of varieties (cultivars)—for example, *V. vinifera* var. Cabernet Sauvignon.

It takes approximately 4–5 years from the first planting to yield the first truly good crop of grapes. The scion (top) of the vine and the rootstock to which it is grafted must be selected on the basis of compatibility, one with the other and the combination with the local soil and climate. Other key issues that come to bear in viticulture are the availability of sunlight, depth of the soil, its nutrient and moisture content and how readily it drains.

Some regions are especially susceptible to diseases such as Pierce's disease and phylloxera (an insect that attacks rootstock and which is prevalent, for instance, in the Eastern United States but now also in California).

Vines should go dormant in order to survive cold winters. Cool autumn conditions with light or medium frosts allow the vine to store enough carbohydrate for good growth in the ensuing spring. There may be 500–600 or more vines per acre. New vines are trained up individual stakes in the first growing season, Only one shoot is trained in each instance with the others being pinched off. Pruning of vines takes place in winter months after the vines have proceeded to dormancy and the canes have hardened and turned brown. It is important to match grape variety to the location and to the style of wine. A variety may develop certain characteristics earlier depending on how warm the growing region is. Accordingly, when that grape achieves full maturity, it may have lost some of that character. Table 9.1 summarises varietal issues.

Table 9.1. Some varieties of grape.

Type	Example	Comments
White cultivars		
Messiles	Sauvignon blanc	Bordeaux. Green pepper and herbaceous notes
Muscats	Muscat blanc	Raisin notes. Prone to oxidation, so often made into dessert wines
Noiriens	Chardonnay	Widespread use globally; use in champagne production. Wines have apple, melon, peach notes
Parellada		Catalonia. Apple/citrus notes
Rhenans	Gewurztraminer	Cooler European regions. Lychee characters
Riesling		German origin. Rose and pine notes
Viura		Rioja. Butterscotch and banana
Red cultivars		
Carmenets	Cabernet Sauvignon Merlot	Bordeaux. Tannic. Blackcurrant aroma lighter in character
Nebbiolo		Italy Acid, tannic. Truffle, tar and violet notes
Noiriens	Pinot Noir	Beet, cherry, peppermint notes when optimal
Sangiovese		Chianti. Cherries, violets, liquorice
Serines	Syrah	France (n.b. Shiraz in Spain). Tannic, peppery aromas
Tempranillo		Spain, especially Rioja. Also grown in Argentina. Jam, citrus, incense notes
Zinfandel		California. Also used for light blush wines

There is some understanding (though far from complete) of the chemistry involved in varietal differences. For instance, methyl anthranilate is found in Lambrusca, 2-methoxy-3-isobutylpyrazine in Cabernet Sauvignon, damascenone in Chardonnay (Fig. 9.2). For muscats there are terpenes such as linaloöl and geraniol and there are terpenols in White Riesling. Some of these are found in the form of complexes with sugars known as glycosides (Fig. 9.3). Yeast produces enzymes called glycosidases that sever the link between the flavour-active molecule and the sugar over time, illustrating the time dependence of flavour development in this type of wine.

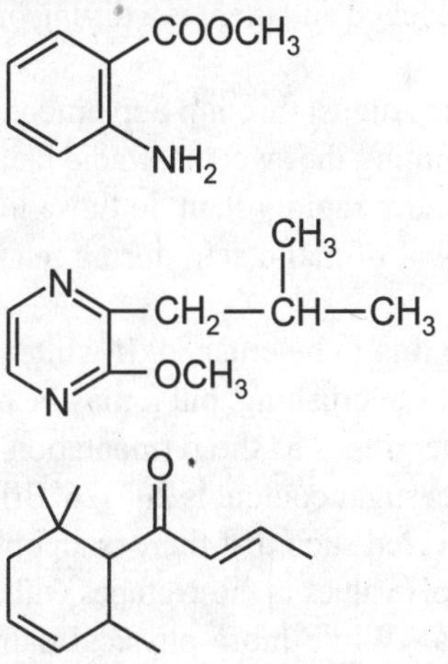

Methyl anthranilate

2-Methoxy-3-isobutylpyrazine

Damascenone

Fig. 9.2. Some compounds responsible for varietal differences in wines.

Sugar–aglycone —Glycosidase→ Sugar + aglycone

(Sugar–aglycone: Glycoside)

Examples of aglycones: terpenes and terpenols

For example, geraniol

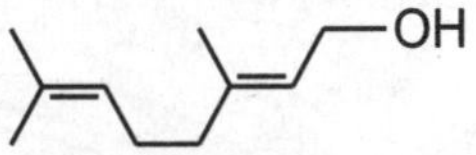

Fig. 9.3. Glycosides and glycosidases.

Unless a soil is extremely acidic or alkaline or suffers from deficient drainage, the soil type *per se* is unlikely to be a major issue with regard to grape quality. Any deficiencies in nitrogen level will need to be corrected by adding N, avoiding excess so as not to promote wasteful growth of non-grape tissue or increase the risk of spoilage and development of ethyl carbamate.

The local climate also influences the susceptibility of the vines to infestation. If there are rains in summer months or if the vineyard is afforded excessive irrigation, there is an increased risk of powdery or downy mildew. Excess water uptake by grapes can also cause berries to swell and burst, which in turn enables rot and mould growth. Over-watering leads to excessive cane growth and delays the maturation of the fruit. In regions where infestation and infection are a particular problem, it is likely that some form of chemical treatment will be necessary. *Botyritis cinerea* is common where summer rains are prevalent. Winemakers refer to it as grey mould when regarded in an unfavourable light but as 'noble rot' when deemed desirable. The contamination leads to oxidation of sugars and depletion of nitrogen, as well as reduction of certain desirable flavours. However, the character of certain wines depends on this infection, for example, the Sauternes from France.

Of particular alarm in some grape-growing regions is Pierce's disease. This is caused by the bacterium *Xylella fastidiosa* and is spread by an insect known as the glassy-winged sharpshooter. It is prevalent in North and Central America, and is of annual concern in some Californian vineyards. It appears to be restricted to regions with mild winters. The sharpshooter feeds on xylem sap and transmits bacteria to the healthy plant. The water-conducting system is blocked and there is a drying or 'scorching' of leaves, followed by the wilting of grape clusters.

Harvesting of grapes is usually in the period from August through September and October. The time of harvesting has a significant role to play in determining the sweetness/acid balance of grapes. Grapes grown in warm climates tend to lose their acidity more rapidly than do those in cooler environs. This loss of acidity is primarily due to respiratory removal of malic acid during maturation. The other key acid, tartaric, is less likely to change in level.

Ripe fruit should be picked immediately before it is to be crushed. If white grapes are picked on a hot day, they should be chilled to less than 20°C prior to crushing, but it may be preferable to pick them by night. However, this is not the same for red wine grapes as the fermentation temperature is higher. Fruit destined for white table wine is picked when its sugar content is 23°–26°Brix. Grapes for red table wine have a longer hang time. These values are selected such that there is an optimal balance between alcohol yield, flavour and resistance to spoilage. The pH values in these grapes will be 3.2–3.4 and 3.3–3.5, respectively. Harvesting is increasingly mechanical. While more physical damage occurs, it can be performed under cooler night-time conditions which is desirable, especially for white cultivars. Sulphur dioxide may be added during mechanical harvesting.

Payment is made on the basis of the measured Brix content of the fruit, measured by a hydrometer or, more usually, by a refractometer. A commercial specification will also state the maximum weight of non-grape material that can be tolerated (perhaps 1–2 per cent) and that the berries should be free from mould and rot. For many winemakers, it has been decided that growing their own grapes is prudent. However, the buying in of some material from other suppliers does allow financial flexibility. The structure of the grape is illustrated in Fig. 9.4.

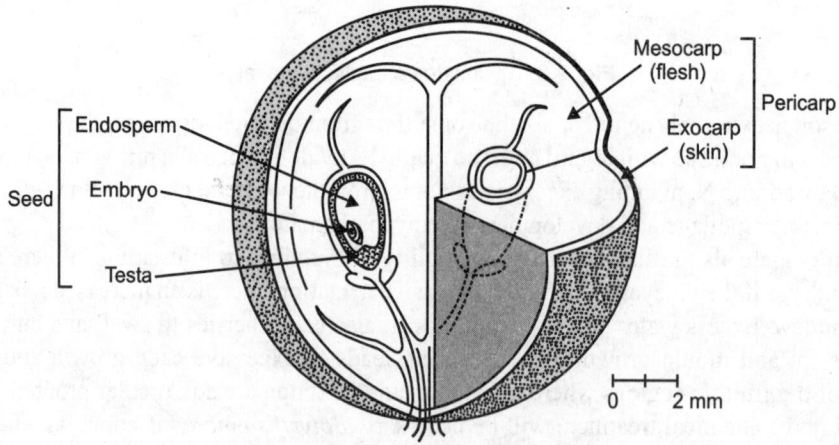

Fig. 9.4. The structure of the grape.

The main features are the skin and the flesh. The skin comprises an outer 1-cell deep epidermis and an inner 4–20-cell deep hypodermis, which is the origin of the colour and most of the flavour compounds in the grape. Sugar and acid are concentrated in the flesh. The sugar content may reach as high as 28 per cent. Tartaric and malic acids account for 70 per cent of the total acids in the grape.

GRAPE PROCESSING

Nowadays the vessels used for extracting grapes and fermenting wine are fabricated from stainless steel and are jacketed to allow temperature regulation. These tanks are subject to in place cleaning, usually a caustic regime incorporating sequestering agents, followed by the use of sanitisers.

Grapes are moved by screw conveyors from the receiving 'bin' to the stemmer-crusher. They pass from there either to a drainer, a holding tank or (in the case of red grapes) directly to the fermenter.

Stemming and Crushing

Stems are not usually left in contact with crushed grapes so as to avoid off-flavours. This is not uniformly the case. Pinot noir, then, is sometimes fermented in the presence of stems in order to garner its distinct peppery character. Stemmer-crushers frequently employ a system of rapidly spinning blades, but may have a roller-type design. In either case, there is an initial crushing into a perforated drum arrangement that separates grape from stem.

The aim is even breakage of grapes. If grapes are soft or shrivelled, they are tougher to break open. Excessive force will lead to too much skin and cell breakage, and in turn in the release of unwanted enzymes and buffering materials that maintain too high a pH. There will also be problems later on in the clarification stage. It is also important to avoid damaging seeds in order that tannins are not excessively released.

It is not necessary to separate the juice from skins immediately for red wine, but is so for white or blush wines. The colour is located in the skin as polyphenolic molecules called anthocyanins. Blush wines are lighter than rose wines. For the latter, overnight contact between juice and skin with a modest fermentation (perhaps a fall in Brix of 1–5) allows the appropriate extraction of anthocyanins. After rose or blush juice has been separated from the skins, it should be protected from oxidation by the addition of sulphur dioxide (SO_2). SO_2 addition to the crusher depends on several factors, notably whether mould or rot is present and also what the surface area to volume ratio is in the tank (i.e. the likelihood of air ingress). If the grapes are not infected and the area to volume is low, then SO_2 may perhaps be avoided. However, in this instance, the juice should be settled at a low temperature ($<12°C$). The rapid separation of skin and juice for white wines also minimises the pick-up of astringent tannins. The process may also impact other flavour compounds, for example, the flavours that impact Muscat. For certain grapes/wines, therefore, there is a balance to be maintained in terms of oxygen availability, SO_2 use, contact time and temperature.

Although seldom used for wines of quality, 'thermovinification' may be used to enhance colour recovery in some wines. The technique involves rapid heating and cooling of crushed grapes. The heat kills the cells, allowing pigments to be released, which may result in undesirable flavours.

Botrytis produces an enzyme called laccase that oxidises red pigments, developing a brown colouration. In these circumstances, heating before vinification may be used to destroy the enzyme. Another enzyme that oxidises polyphenols –PPO– is located in the grape *per se*, but it is inhibited by SO_2.

During fermentation, the pH should be maintained below 3.8. Wines then tend to ferment more evenly, there is a reduced likelihood of malolactic fermentation and the wine develops better sensory properties. Furthermore, at higher pH, SO_2 is less inhibitory to wild yeast. Maintaining this low pH is especially important for white wines. Prolonged contact with the grape skin causes lower total acidity through precipitation of potassium acid tartrate. The pH may be lowered to 3.25–3.35 by the addition of tartaric acid.

Drainers and Presses

Drainers are basically screen-based systems. Presses differ according to the severity of their operations. Membrane or bag presses are very gentle and leave little sediment. By contrast, bladder presses are often used on account of their rapidity, but the juice tends to contain higher solids levels.

The extent to which Maillard reactions can occur during processing is controlled by attention to temperature, pH and the type of sugar. These reactions occur for the most part at around 15 per cent moisture.

Oxidative reactions may occur, with the major substrates being caffeoyl tartaric acid (caftaric acid; Fig. 9.5), p-coumaroyl tartaric acid and feruloyl tartaric acid. These are the precursors in PPO-catalysed browning reactions for those wines that have minimum skin contact. To accelerate juice settling so as to obtain a clearer product, pectic enzyme is frequently added at the crushing stage to minimise the level of pectin, which originates in the wall material of the grape (Fig. 9.6). The enzyme also allows easier pressing and affords higher yields.

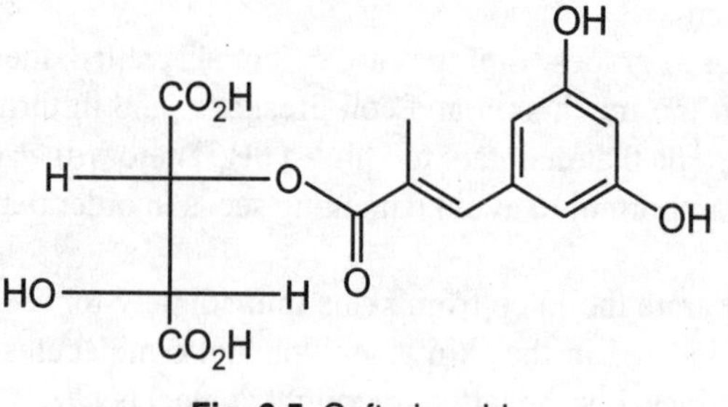

Fig. 9.5. Caftaric acid.

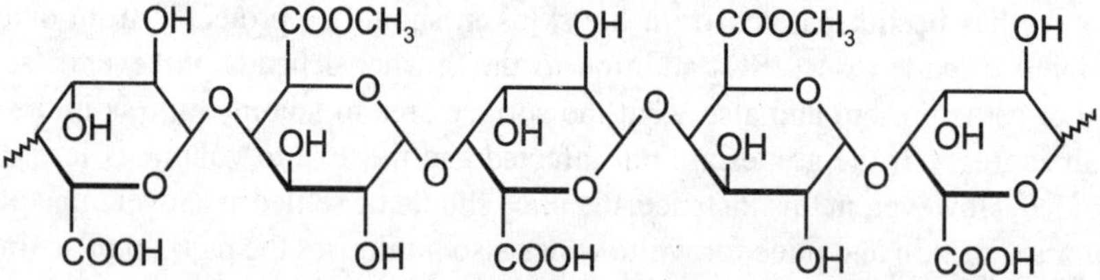

Fig. 9.6. The repeating unit of pectin: lengthy sequences of anhydrogalacturonic acid partly esterified with methanol.

FERMENTATION

Juice

Once the juice has separated from the skins, it is held overnight in a closed container. Thereafter it is racked off (or centrifuged), prior to the addition of yeast. Winemakers generally aim to leave some solids as a surface for the yeast to populate (or perhaps as a nucleation site to allow CO_2 release, as is the case for the residual cold break in brewery fermentations). Failing this, they may add diatomaceous earth or bentonite.

In locations where the grapes do not ripen well owing to a short growing season, it may be necessary to add sugar (sucrose), but only up to a maximum of 23.5°Brix. Such a practice is illegal in some locales, for example, California.

The typical composition of the grapes from which the juice is derived is given in Table 9.2.

Table 9.2. Composition of grapes (percentage of the fresh weight).

Component	Range
Water	70–85
Glucose	8–13
Fructose	7–12
Pentoses	0.01–0.05
Pectins	0.01–0.1
Tartaric acid	0.2–1.0
Malic acid	0.1–0.8
Citric acid	0.01–0.05
Acetic acid	0.0–0.02
Anthocyanins	0.0–0.05
Tannins	0.01–0.1
Amino acids	0.01–0.08
Ammonia	0.001–0.012
Minerals	0.3–0.5

Diverse sugars, notably glucose and fructose, are present in essentially equal quantities in mature grapes. Sucrose is hydrolysed at the low pH values involved and this is further promoted by invertase. Total reducing sugars will usually amount to <250 g l^{-1}.

The organic acids are predominately tartaric acid in grapes grown in warmer climates and malic acid in grapes from colder climates (Fig. 9.7).

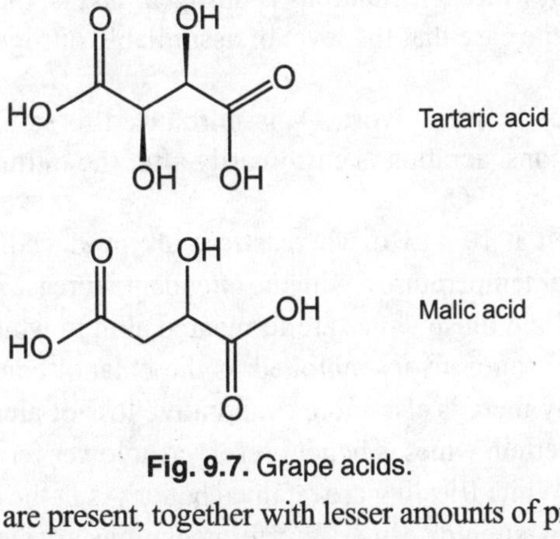

Fig. 9.7. Grape acids.

Amino acids and ammonia are present, together with lesser amounts of proteins (<20 to >100 mg l^{-1} in the juice). The latter presents a risk to the colloidal stability of wine. Although vitamins are present in only small amounts, they are generally sufficient for yeast. A diversity of phenolic compounds is present, and these can be classified as catechins, flavonols and flavanones (Fig. 9.8). The main inorganic cation in juice is potassium, from <400 to >2000 mg l^{-1}.

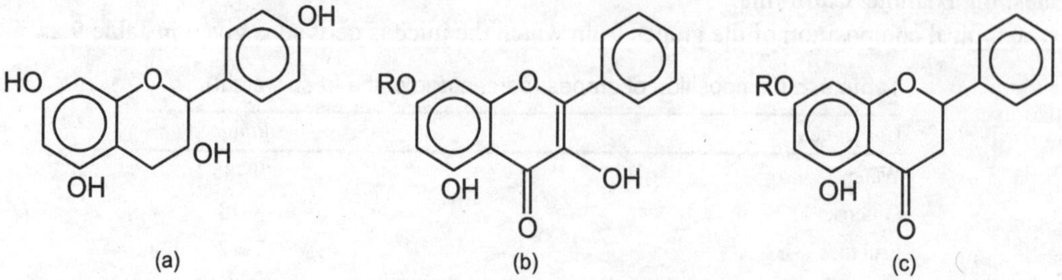

Fig. 9.8. Some polyphenolic species. (a) catechin, (b) flavonol and (c) flavanone.

Yeast

The relevant species are *Saccharomyces cerevisiae* and *Saccharomyces bayanus* (Table 9.3).

Table 9.3. Yeasts for fermenting wine.

Saccharomyces cerevisiae
Saccharomyces bayanus
Zygosaccharomyces bailii
Schizosaccharomyces pombe
Torulaspora delbrueckii (flor yeast)

Contrary to commercial-scale brewing, dried yeast is extensively employed in wine making, where the precise nuances of yeast strain seem to be deemed less important than is the case for beer.

Pesticides employed on the grapes can inhibit yeast. Clarification of the must eliminates most of them, but bentonite or carbon treatment may also be employed. However, ironically, the most common inhibitor of fermentation is SO_2.

The chief limiting factor in wine fermentations is nitrogen, that is, the amino acid level in the must. Accordingly, it is frequently the case that the level of assimilable nitrogen is increased by the addition of diammonium phosphate.

As for the fermentation of brewer's wort, O_2 is introduced to satisfy the demands of the yeast. However, for wine fermentations, aeration is customarily after the introduction of yeast so as to avoid the scavenging of the oxygen by PPO.

White wines are fermented at 10°–15°C whereas reds are produced at 20°–30°C. Fermentation is inherently more rapid at higher temperatures, with the attendant increase in production of flavour active volatiles such as esters. Rose and blush wines are fermented akin to white wines.

Fermentation tends to be progressively inhibited as the ethanol concentration rises, especially at higher temperatures. Naturally there is also more evaporative loss of alcohol at higher temperatures.

The varietal character of certain wines is better preserved at lower fermentation temperatures. Thus, for example, the terpenols in White Riesling are retained better. As in the case of beer, high levels of the undesirables such as hydrogen sulphide can arise if fermentations are sluggish.

In all cases, fermentation should be complete within 20–30 days. The progress of fermentation is monitored by measuring the decline in Brix value.

Wine is usually racked off the yeast once fermentation is complete. However, some wine makers leave the wine in contact with the yeast for several months, perhaps with intermittent rousing, in order that materials should be released from yeast, beneficially impacting flavour.

Colour and flavour extraction from red grapes is maximised by mixing either by pumping or by stirring. Usually pumping over (of half of the total vessel contents) is performed twice per day. Extraction is also greater at higher temperatures and increased ethanol concentrations.

A technique traditional for Beaujolais wines is *Maceration carbonique*, which leads to wines with distinct estery, 'pear drop' characteristics. Whole grape clusters are exposed to an atmosphere of CO_2. The sugar converts to ethanol (about 2.5 per cent ABV), with the accompanying production of several phenolic compounds. The initial phase of fermentation in the whole grapes is conducted at 30°–32°C. The weight of the berries, together with the action of the developed ethanol and carbon dioxide, break down the grape cells and colour is extracted. After 8–11 days, the grapes are pressed and the juice obtained is combined with that which is free running. The whole is fermented to dryness at 18°–20°C. Then SO_2 is added and the wine is clarified.

FILTRATION AND STABILISATION

Clarification

White wines are either centrifuged or treated with bentonite, which will also adsorb protein. Bentonite is a clay that contains high levels of aluminium and silica. Sometimes it is substituted by silica gels of the type extensively used in brewing.

Casein may be added to remove phenols, which can also be achieved by PVPP. Isinglass is also sometimes used as a fining agent. Red wines are primarily fined in order to reduce their astringency. Fining agents include gelatine egg white and isinglass.

Filtration

Contrary to most beers, this is relatively uncommon and only performed on an as-needs basis, either to recover wine from lees (i.e. the residual solid material) after cold stabilisation treatments or immediately before bottling. Microbial threats may be eliminated by membrane filtration.

Stabilisation

One of the biggest threats to wine is oxidative browning. The ingress of oxygen after fermentation should be minimised. Sometimes 'pinking' of white wines in bottle is prevented by adding ascorbic acid. But the chief antioxidant is SO_2, by reacting with the active peroxides in wine

$$H_2O_2 + SO_2 \rightarrow H_2O + SO_3$$

Metal ions, such as iron, which potentiate the conversion of oxygen into activated forms such as peroxide are removed by casein or citrate.

The sulphur dioxide must be in a free, unbound form at concentrations between 15 and 25 mg l^{-1}.

Any hydrogen sulphide present in wine may be eliminated by the addition of low levels of copper

$$CuSO_4 + H_2S \rightarrow CuS \downarrow + H_2SO_4$$

Certain inorganic precipitates can be thrown in wine, with tartrate being a key problem. This is avoided by cold treatment of the wine. Protein hazes are avoided by the use of chilling and bentonite.

Maintaining wine in an anaerobic state and with 20–30 mg l^{-1} SO$_2$ is generally sufficient to prevent spoilage by most bacteria and yeast. Furthermore, when fermented to dryness, most white wines are relatively resistant to spoilage.

USE OF OTHER MICRO-ORGANISMS IN WINE PRODUCTION

Red wines usually undergo a malolactic fermentation, effected by the lactic acid bacteria Pediococcus (homofermentative), Leuconostoc (heterofermentative), Oenococcus (heterofermentative) and Lactobacillus (either). In this process, malic acid is degraded to lactic acid with an attendant decrease in total acidity and a net increase in pH. The bacteria concerned prefer a relatively high pH and tend to be inhibited by SO$_2$. They also do not perform well at too low a temperature. For an effective malolactic fermentation, the wine should have a pH of 3.25–3.5 a total SO$_2$ level below 30 ppm and zero free SO$_2$. The malolactic fermentation formerly depended on the microflora native to the process, but in most instances nowadays the specific bacterial strains required are seeded into the vessel.

Grapes from warm climates tend to contain less malic acid and therefore benefit less from such a fermentation than do grapes from relatively cold areas. A further type of natural fermentation effected in the production of some wines is the application of certain yeasts (formerly believed to be *Torulaspora delbrueckii* but likelier to be *S. cerevisiae*) growing as a film on the surface in the production of 'flor' sherry. The main impact is the production of acetaldehyde.

CHAMPAGNE/SPARKLING WINE

The best such wines are produced from the juice of Pinot noir or Chardonnay grapes. There must be rigorous avoidance of colour development, hence the extensive use of SO$_2$, bentonite and PVPP.

Fermentation in bottle is effected by a culture of *S. bayanus* that is flocculent and able to perform at high alcohol concentrations. The parent wine, invert sugar and yeast are delivered into pressure-resistant bottles sporting a lip for the application of a crown cork. A 2.5-cm headspace will be left in the bottle before it is laid on its side and held at 12°C. The wine will ferment to dryness over a period of several weeks but may be left for more than a year for the achievement of best quality.

There follows the process of 'riddling' in which the yeast is worked into the neck of the bottle. The yeast is loosened by hitting the bottom of the bottle with a rubber mallet or by using a shaking device. Then the bottle is put neck down into a rack at an angle of 45°. The bottle is rotated a quarter turn daily until the yeast sediment has all arrived at the cap. Then the inverted bottle is chilled to 0°C and carried through a brine bath cold enough to yield a frozen plug of wine about 3.5 cm long. The cap is removed and as the ice plug is forced out, it scrapes the yeast with it. The bottle is immediately turned upright again, refilled with wine containing sugar and some SO$_2$, corked and labelled.

In an alternative approach, very cold riddled wine is completely removed from bottles, pooled and cold stabilised under pressure. It is filtered and returned to bottles for corking and labelling as 'sparking wine'. Certain wines are carbonated simply by bubbling with carbon dioxide prior to packaging.

AGEING

Contrary to most beers, wines tend to benefit from ageing, which is performed either in tank, barrel or bottle. The extent of ageing is likely to be less for white wines than for reds. During the ageing of wines, there is careful monitoring of colour, aroma, taste and the level of SO$_2$.

The flavour of white wine is very largely determined by the esters produced during fermentation. Some chardonnays are aged in oak barrels, from which some characteristics are derived (Table 9.4).

Diverse oaks may be used in ageing, with relevant compounds increasing in level being guaiacol, eugenol and furfuryl alcohol (Fig. 9.9). Burgundy and Loire whites are left on the lees for up to 2 years.

Table 9.4. Examples of compounds developing in alcoholic beverages aged in oak.

Cyclotene

Dihydromaltol

Ellagic acid

4-Ethylguaiacol

Ethyl maltol

4-Ethylphenol

Eugenol

Furaneol

Furfural

Gallic acid

Hydroxymethyl furfural

β-Ionone

Maltol

5-Methylfurfural

β-Methyl-γ-octalactone

Norisoprenoids

Syringaldehyde

Vanillin

Note: Flavour changes occurring during ageing are not solely due to extraction of substances from the wood. Other significant events include oxidation, evaporation and chemical reactions leading to the production of new compounds.

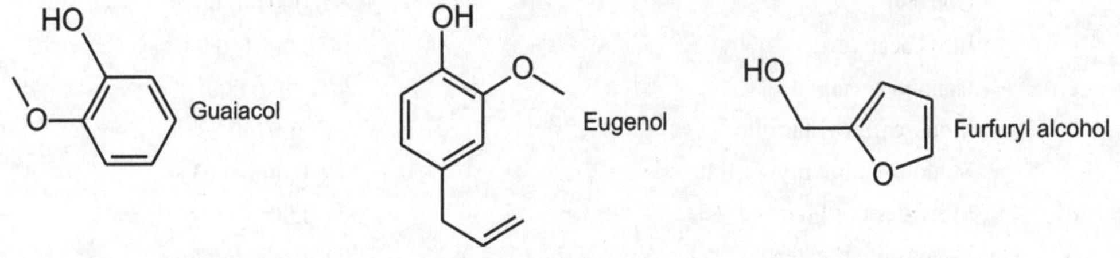

Fig. 9.9. Wood-derived flavour compounds.

Red wines, having undergone their malolactic fermentation are then aged. Bordeaux wines are held 2 years in barrel. By comparison, zinfandel ageing should not be excessively prolonged in order to retain the raspberry character.

PACKAGING

Residual oxygen in wine is removed by sparging with nitrogen gas. Careful control of oxygen levels is effected during the bottling operation *per se*. Some winemakers add sorbic acid as an antimicrobial preservative for sweet table wines. If such an additive is to be avoided, then more attention must be paid to cold filling and sterility.

Table 9.5 presents an approximate summary of the main chemical components of wine.

Table 9.5. The major components of table wine.

Component	Range (g l^{-1})
Ethanol	80–110
Methanol	0–0.3
Propanol	0.007–0.07
Isobutyl alcohol	0.007–0.17
Active amyl alcohol	0.019–0.1
Isoamyl alcohol	0.08–0.35
1-Hexanol	0.001–0.012
2-Phenylethanol	0.005–0.07
2,3-Butanediols	0.015–1.6
Sorbitol	0.005–0.39
Mannitol	0.08–1.4
Erythritol	0.03–0.27
Arabitol	0.013–0.33
Glycerol	1.1–23
Malic acid	0–6.0
Tartaric acid	0.5–4.0
Succinic acid	0.5–1.3
Citric acid	0–0.3
Acetaldehyde	0.003–0.49
Acetoin	0.0007–0.138
Diacetyl	0.0001–0.0075
Ethyl acetate	0.0001–0.23
Isoamyl acetate	0–0.009
Mono-caffeoyl tartrate	0.07–0.23
Mono-p-coumaroyl tartrate	0.008–0.03
Mono-feruloyl tartrate	0.001–0.016
Various other esters	Various, but low
Total amino acids	0.37–4.2
Protein	2–2.5
Tannins	0.05–2.5
Histamine	0–0.49
Tyramine	0–0.012
Potassium	0.09–2
Sodium	0.003–0.3
Nitrate	0.0–0.05

TAINTS AND GUSHING

Cork taints on wine can come from several sources. Trichloroanisole affords a musty or mouldy character, geosmin an earthy note and 2-methylisoborneol a chlorophenolic aroma (Fig. 9.10). They are due to chlorine treatment of corks with subsequent methylation by bacteria and moulds. It is advisable to keep corks at very low moisture content (5–7 per cent) in order to minimise this problem. Of course metal or plastic-lined caps do not present this risk—but are widely unfavoured in view of their lesser aesthetic appeal. Taints may also arise from wooden vessels employed in the winery.

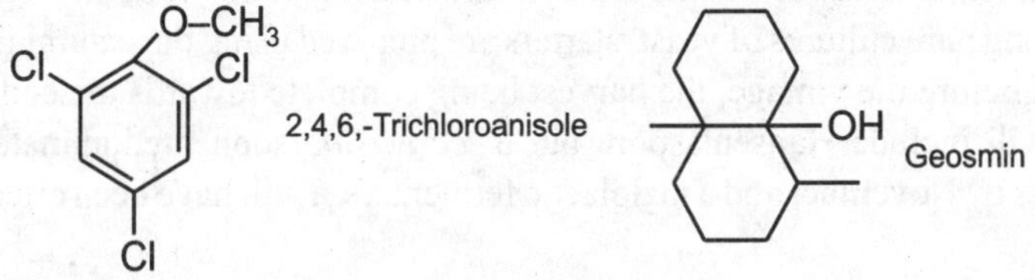

Fig. 9.10. Wine taints.

Gushing in wine may arise due to microscopic mould growth. As for beer, the shelf life of wine is greatly enhanced by cool temperature of storage.

FORTIFIED WINES

Fortified wines are those in which fermented, partially fermented or unfermented grape must is enriched with wine-derived spirit. According to the European Union (EU) regulations, such liquor wines are those with an acquired alcohol content of 15–22 per cent by volume and a total alcohol content of at least 17.5 per cent by volume. The chief fortified wines are sherry (originating in Spain, notably Jerez de la Frontera, which is in the southern province of Cadiz), port (from Portugal and made from grapes produced in or around the upper valley of the River Douro in the north of the country) and madeira (from the Portuguese archipelago of Madeira).

The wine fortification technology originated in such regions because the local soil and climate were not well suited to the production of wines of inherent excellence. The process also allowed protection against microbial infection during the storage and shipment of products.

Sherry is only made from white grapes, but port and madeira may be produced from either red or white grapes. In no instance is a single product made from a mixture of the two grape types. Wines upon which sherry is based tend to be dry and the fortification occurs post-fermentation. If the sweetness needs to be increased, it is through the addition of grape-derived products downstream. Such additions usually comprise wines that have been fortified at the start of fermentation: by adding alcohol at the start of fermentation, yeast action is arrested and accordingly there is retention of sugar.

Port is usually fortified approximately halfway through the primary fermentation, and so tends to be sweeter than sherry through the preservation of unfermented sugars.

Madeira may be fortified through either route depending on the sweetness targeted in the product.

The wines used to make sherry derive much of their character from ageing in oat 'butts'. Sometimes, however, there is the development of *flor*, a film of yeast on the surface. This yeast may comprise the primary fermenting yeast but may also include other adventitious yeasts from diverse genera.

In contrast, characteristics derived from the grape are substantially more important for wines going into port, especially red port. Much of the character of madeiras develops in the estufagem process, which is a heating of the product at, say, 50°C for 3 months.

Sherry, port and madeira are each blended to the target quality during maturation. Sherry and madeira are fortified using an essentially neutral spirit containing at least 96 per cent ABV and which is continuously distilled from the wine or from related products (the lees or the pomace). Fortification of port is with wine spirit (76–78 per cent ABV). This spirit does contain substances such as alcohols, esters and carbonyl-containing compounds that contribute directly to the flavour of port.

Sherry

Nowadays fermentation is likely to be in open cylindrical tanks (500–1000 hl) regulated to ca. 25°C. Rather than employing pure cultures of yeast, starters are prepared using the natural flora on a proportion of grapes harvested before the vintage, the harvest being complete towards the end of September. The initial population will include Hanseniaspora but *S. cerevisiae* soon predominates. Fermentation is completed to dryness by November and a malolactic fermentation will have been effected by endogenous lactic acid bacteria.

Post-fermentation, the young wines are racked from the lees and fortified with spirit (>95 per cent ABV) produced by the distillation of wine and its by-products (lees, pomace). The spirit is first mixed with an equal volume of wine and settled for some 3 days before using to fortify the main wine.

This procedure leads to less generation of turbidity than does addition of undiluted spirit. The young unaged wines are classified into either *finos* or *olorosos* depending on their characteristics. Finos are dry, light and pale gold in colour and have an alcohol content of 15.5–16.5 per cent. They are matured under flor yeast, which tends to develop when the grapes are exposed to cool westerlies when grown on soils rich in calcium carbonate. Olorosos, which are matured in the absence of flor yeast, are dry, rich dark mahogany wines with full noses and alcoholic contents of 21 per cent. The higher levels of poly phenolics in these wines suppress flor development.

Newly fermented wines are left to mature unblended for approximately 1 year. They then pass to a blending process (the 'solera' system), in which the aim is to introduce product consistency. It comprises a progressive topping up of older butts of wine with younger wines.

A sherry must be aged for a minimum of 3 years before sale. During ageing, flor prevents air from accessing the sherry, and so microbial spoilage and oxidative browning is prevented. If there is no flor, as in olorosos, then oxidative browning can occur. Amontillado sherries are produced with an initial flor maturation followed by ageing in the absence of flor, so oxidation and esterification reactions are prevalent in that style of sherry. The flor process leads to a decrease in volatile acidity and glycerol, as well as an increase in the level of acetaldehyde, the latter meaning that fino sherries have a distinct apple note. Other flavour compounds associated with sherries include 4,5-dimethyl-3-hydroxy-2-(5$_H$)-furanone, which affords a nutty character to sherry matured under flor and trans-3-methyl-4-hydroxyoctanoic acid lactone, which emerges from the oak and offers the woody note found in many sherries.

Fino sherries are not usually sweetened, are matured for 3–8 years and have alcohol contents of 15.5–17 per cent ABV. Olorosos and Amontillados are generally sweetened and reach 17–17.5 per cent ABV. Sherries may be fined, traditionally with egg white although increasingly with isinglass or gelatine. They may be centrifuged before filtering and may also be stabilised by treatment with bentonite.

Finally they are cooled through a heat exchanger and ultra-cooler to reach a temperature between −8° and −9°C, holding there for 10–14 days to chill out colloidally unstable material. Finely ground potassium bitartrate may be added to promote the nucleation of this material. Finally, the sherry is membrane-filtered to eliminate microbes and some solids, prior to bottling.

Port

Much of the port produced these days is fermented in closed tanks at ca. 16°C with facility for turning the contents. Must is run-off after 2-3 days of fermentation at which point most of the sugars have been converted into alcohol. Fermentation is inhibited by the addition of grape brandy with wine becoming port officially at 19–20 per cent ABV.

Red wines destined for ruby will have been aged for 3–5 years in wood. Those going to tawny will have been aged in wood for more than 30 years. Vintage ports are from wines of a single harvest that are judged to be of outstanding quality. They will be aged in wood for 2–3 years and then the ageing completed in bottle for at least 10 years.

A major contributor to the ageing changes in ruby and tawny is the polymerisation of anthocyanins. This is not only partly through oxidative cross-linking, but also through that induced by acetaldehyde. Other significant aldehydes include the furfurals and lignin degradation products from wood, such as vanillin, syringaldehyde, cinnamaldehyde and coniferaldehyde (Fig. 9.11). Phenols such as guaiacol, eugenol and 4-vinylphenol are also extracted from wood during maturation. Other changes include increases in the level of glycerol and decreases in the levels of citric acid and tartaric acid, the latter by the deposition of potassium hydrogen tartrate. In the acidic, high ethanol wines, esters are produced by the reaction of ethanol with acetic, lactic, malic, succinic and tartaric acids.

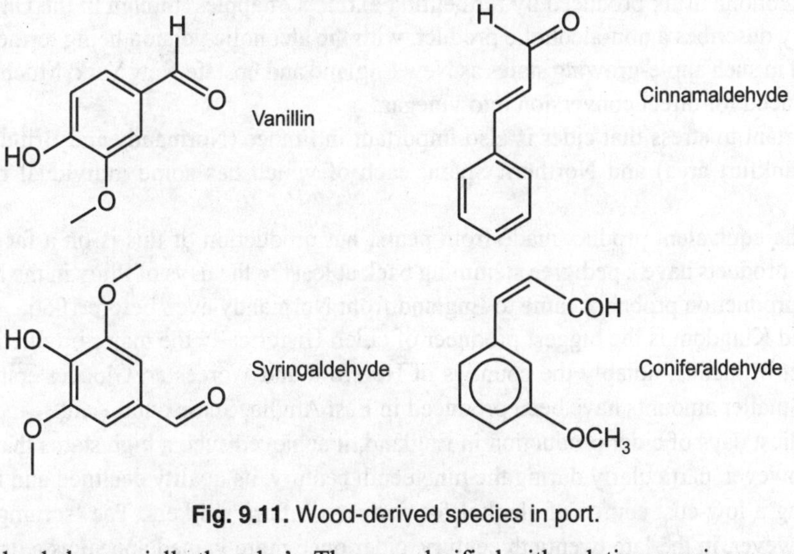

Fig. 9.11. Wood-derived species in port.

Ports are blended, especially the ruby's. They are clarified with gelatine, casein or egg white. White ports will be treated with bentonite, and centrifugation is sometimes employed. Rubies and younger tawnies are cold stabilised by holding at −8°C for 1 week. Alternatively, the chilled wine is passed continuously through a crystallising tank containing a concentrated suspension of crystals of potassium bitartrate. Then the wine is filtered with diatomaceous earth followed by sheet, cartridge or membrane filtration.

Madeira

Fermentation may be in various types of vessel, ranging from wooden casks to stainless steel fermenters, but generally there is no temperature control, so 35°C may be reached or perhaps exceeded. Starter cultures are not employed. Fortification to 17–18 per cent ABV is either immediate, to prevent malolactic fermentation and the action of endogenous acetic acid bacteria, or delayed 2–3 months, in which case volatile acidity is likely to have increased.

The heating stage is effected after increasing the sweetness by approximately 2°–9°Brix using either a fortified grape juice, concentrated grape must or hydrolysed corn syrup. Heating is by circulating hot water around the product, either using a stainless steel coil in the tank or through a jacket. Heating is typically in concrete at 40°–50°C for at least 3 months. A brown hue is produced, together with caramelisation aromas and a soft palate arising from the impact on phenolics. The estufagem process must be conducted during the first 3 years.

Madeiras are mostly aged in wood. Vintage madeiras must come from a single variety in a single year and must be aged for more than 20 years in wood and at least 2 years in bottle. Blending of madeira is a simplified version of the port system.

Many madeiras are charcoal-treated to remove the more extreme characteristics developed during the heating stage. They are fined with casein, treated with bentonite and held at –8°C for 1 week before filtration using diatomaceous earth and ensuing sheet or sheet-plus cartridge filtration.

CIDER

Cider is an alcoholic drink produced by fermenting extracts of apples, though in the United States the term generally describes a non-alcoholic product, with the alcoholic version being termed 'hard cider' and produced in such apple-growing states as New England and upstate New York. Much of the latter is actually produced for direct conversion into vinegar.

It is important to stress that cider is also important in France (Normandy and Brittany), Germany (the Trier/Frankfurt area) and Northern Spain, each of which has some individual manufacturing approaches.

Perry is the equivalent product made from pears, but production of this is on a far smaller scale. Both of these products have a pedigree stemming back at least to the days of Pliny in the Mediterranean basin. Cider production probably came to England from Normandy even before 1066.

The United Kingdom is the biggest producer of cider. Historically the major production areas have been the West Midlands, notably the counties of Hereford and Worcester, Gloucestershire, Somerset and Devon. Smaller amounts have been produced in East Anglia, Sussex and Kent.

In the earliest days of cider production in England, it achieved such a high status that it was a peer for wines. However, particularly during the nineteenth century, its quality declined and it assumed the status of being a low-cost source of alcohol for peripatetic farm workers. The 'scrumpy' image was assumed. However, in the late twentieth century, cider once more gained appeal as a drink of quality, including for young people.

The biggest selling style of cider is as a clear carbonated, light flavoured beverage in bottle or can with an alcohol content of between 1.2 per cent, and 85 per cent ABV. Increasingly there is a trend towards chaptalisation—that is, the addition of sugars or syrups prior to fermentation to supplement the carbohydrate derived from apple. For the most part, modern ciders may comprise only 30–50 per cent apple juice.

New product development has been rife in the cider industry in recent years. Thus, *inter alia* there have been higher alcohol variants, 'white' ciders stripped of their colour, so-called ice versions and ciders flavoured with diverse other components.

When served on draught, cider is essentially a competitor for beer, primarily the lager-style products. However, there are styles of draught cider that are much more akin to cask conditioned ales. Nonetheless, there is probably a closer match between cider making and wine making than there is with brewing.

In France, ciders tend to be of lower alcohol content and distinctly sharp in flavour. Those from the Asturias region of Spain are somewhat vinegary and foamy, while those from Germany tend to have relatively high alcohol content.

Apples

The starting material for cider production is raw apples. A classification for these is offered in Table 9.6.

Table 9.6. Types of cider apples.

Type of apple	Tannin content (%)	Acid content (%)
Bittersharp	>0.2	>0.45
Bittersweet	>0.2	<0.45
Sharp	<0.2	>0.45
Sweet	<0.2	<0.45

It is not necessarily the case that cider must be made from true cider apples. For example, cider has been made successfully from Bramley apples. Frequently the substrate derived directly from the apple is supplemented with apple juice concentrate (AJC).

There are several advantages to using true cider varieties. They tend to have high sugar contents, of up to 15 per cent. They display a range of acidities, from 0.1 to 1 per cent. Their fibrous structure makes it easier to effect pressing and with higher yields of juice. It is possible to store them over a period of several weeks without losing texture, during which period their starch converts into sugar. Finally, they have a high tannin content (perhaps ten-fold higher than in dessert apples), this being important for body and mouthfeel. The polyphenols also inhibit breakdown of pectin, rendering the pulp from bittersweet apples less slimy and therefore easier to process.

The polyphenolics in apples comprise a range of oligomeric procyanidins based on the flavanoid (−)-epicatechin (Fig. 9.12). Also present are the phenolic acids chlorogenic and *p*-coumaroyl quinic acid, as well as the glycosides, phloretin glucoside and xyloglucoside (Fig. 9.13).

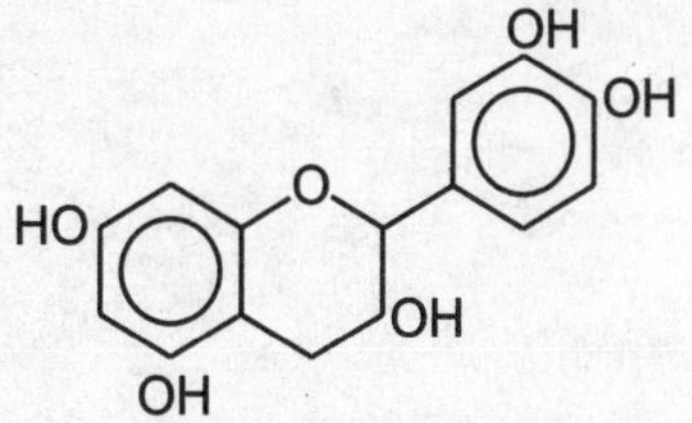

Fig. 9.12. Epicatechin.

The cider orchards are different for cider apples. The aesthetic appeal of the appearance and size of the fruit is relatively unimportant when compared with apples that are intended to be sold as eating fruit. Of more significance is the ease with which they can be harvested. The apples are for the most part grown on bush trees with more than 30 per acre. Cropping is biennial.

Most of the larger cider making companies possess their own orchards. They also enter into contracts with outside growers for a proportion of their raw material. Cider is usually produced from more than a single cultivar in order to achieve the preferred balance of acidity, sweetness and astringency/bitterness (Table 9.7). The gross composition of cider varieties is actually not very dissimilar to that of other apples and leads to a pressed juice with an overall composition given in Table 9.8.

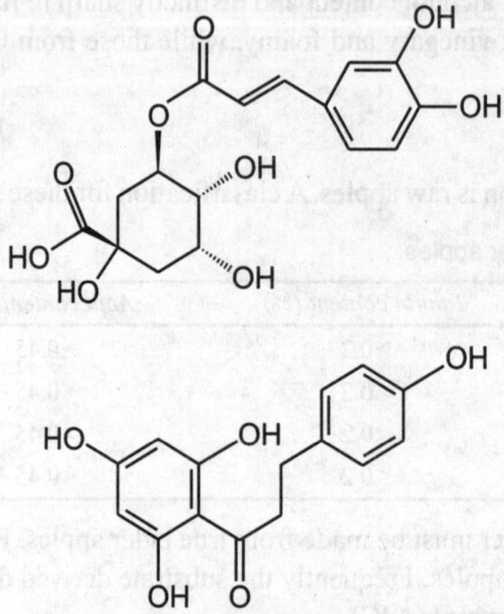

Chlorogenic acid

Phloretin

Fig. 9.13. Phenolic species derived from apples.

Table 9.7. Cider apple cultivars.

Bittersharp	Sharp
Brown Snout	Brown's apple
Bulmer's Foxwhelp	Frederick
Chisel Jersey	Reinette Obry
Kingston Black	
Bittersweet	Sweet
Ashton Brown	Northwood
Chisel Jersey	Sweet Alford
Dabinett	Sweet Copping
Ellis Bitter	
Harry Master's Jersey	
Major	
Medaille d'Or	
Michelin	
Taylor's	
Tremlett's Bitter	
Vilberie	
Yarlington Mill	

Table 9.8. Major components of cider apple juice.

Component	Range
Fructose	70–110 g/l
Glucose	15–30 g/l
Sucrose	20–45 g/l
Pectin	1–10 g/l
Amino acids	0.5–2 g/l
Potassium	1.2 g/l
pH	3.3–3.8
Phenolics and polyphenolics	1–2.5 g/l

The most likely limiting factor will be the assimilable nitrogen content, depending on the nutrient status of the trees in the orchard. By contrast, the total polyphenol content of apples tends to be inversely related to this nutrient status.

AJC is now extensively used in cider making. Typically it has a concentration of 70°Brix, the high osmotic pressure meaning that it can be stored for long periods and therefore purchased at economically favourable times. Sometimes, however, AJC made from true bittersweets is in short supply and it may be produced in-house. Alternatively, the apple juice may be supplemented with cane or beet sugar or hydrolysed corn syrup.

Milling and Pressing

Apples are used when fully ripe and are customarily stored for several weeks so as to convert all of the starch into fermentable sugar. The apples are sorted and washed with the aim of eliminating debris and any rotten fruit.

Formerly the apples were crushed by stone or wooden rollers with an ensuing pressing in rack and cloth. The pulp was layered in woven synthetic clothes that alternated with wooden racks, the arrangement being referred to as a 'cheese'. Straw was used to separate the layers. The cheese was then stripped down and the pomace mixed with water 10 per cent by weight before repressing. The residual pomace was used as animal feed or for pectin production.

In modern cider making facilities, a high-speed grater mill feeds a hydraulic piston press. Within the press are compressible chambers, with many flexible ducts that are enclosed in nylon socks. When the piston is compressed, it forces juice through the ducts. There may be a second extraction by water. When the piston is withdrawn, the dry pomace falls away readily. Yields are much higher (75 per cent+) and there are much lower levels of suspended solids in the apple juice. The juice is afforded a coarse screening before it is run to tanks fabricated from fibreglass, stainless steel, polyethylene or wood.

Fermentation

Some blending of juices may occur prior to fermentation and additions made. In particular, there may be a blending with sugars or AJC, to arrive at a specific gravity of 1.08–1.1. The FAN level may be raised to 100 mg l^{-1} by the addition of ammonium sulphate or ammonium phosphate. Thiamine may be added, perhaps at 0.2 ppm, but this must be separate from the addition of sulphite as the latter will destroy it. Other B vitamins that are required are pantothenate (2.5 ppm), pyridoxine (1 ppm) and biotin

(7.5 ppb). Such materials are especially likely to be limiting if the cidermaker is using significant quantities of AJC or sugars.

Another potential problem with AJC is the generation of O and N containing heterocyclics within it (by Maillard reactions), which are inhibitors of yeast. They can be removed by the treatment of AJC with activated charcoal. If the apple juice and its additions are too 'bright', then it will be necessary to add some solids (e.g. bentonite) to act as nucleation sites, the escaping CO_2 relieving inhibition of the yeast and also serving to maintain agitation in the fermenter. We have already encountered this for the fermentations of beer and wine. Pectolytic enzymes are sometimes added to initial fruit pulp or to the juice immediately prior to fermentation.

SO_2 is traditionally added to prevent the growth of contaminating micro-organisms (Table 9.9). It is less critical from that aspect with the advent of dried wine yeast, but it is still important from a flavour perspective and is not without significance for antimicrobial protection. The effectiveness of SO_2 increases as the pH decreases because it is the undissociated form of bisulphite which has the antimicrobial properties. The pH is lowered to less than 3.8 by the addition of malic acid prior to the addition of sulphite.

Table 9.9. The quantity of sulphur dioxide that should be added to cider apple juice.

pH	SO_2 to be added (mg l^{-1})
3.0–3.3	75
3.3–3.5	100
3.5–3.8	150
>3.8	150 (after blending or acid addition to achieve a pH <3.8)

Healthy fruit generally will only contain low levels of sulphite-binding agents and should have sufficient SO_2 to offer effective resistance to spoilage before addition of yeast. If, however, the fruit is in less good condition, then it may contain materials such as 5-ketofructose or diketogluconic acid as a result of bacterial activity. This type of substance binds SO_2 and therefore reduces the endogenous protectant level. Furthermore, if ascorbic acid is oxidised to 1-xylosone, this also binds SO_2. Finally, if AJC is depectinised, this will yield galacturonic acid that will also diminish SO_2.

In traditional cider making, the yeast was delivered adventitiously with the fruit or the equipment (Saccharomyces does not naturally inhabit cider apples—but it is to be found on presses). SO_2 suppresses the growth of most microbes other than Saccharomyces. Traditionally a succession of micro flora in juice that had not been sulphited was involved in metabolising apple juice to cider. Saccharomyces was significant relatively late in the process. The introduction of SO_2, however, rendered Saccharomyces as being vastly more important in the process. Since the 1960s, though, the vast majority of cider fermentations have been seeded. Juice should be held at <10°C prior to the addition of that yeast in order to prevent native flora from kicking off fermentation. Many of the cultures now added were originally isolated from the cider factories themselves, but some cidermakers use wine yeasts with well-defined characteristics, including the spectrum of flavour compounds that they produce and their flocculation behaviour. Since the 1980s, there has been widespread use of active dried wine yeast, which simply needs mixing with warm water, freeing the cidermaker from the need for in-house propagation. Some will employ an aerobic yeast incubation period so as to ensure that the yeast membranes are in good condition in order that the yeast will be capable of effecting very high levels of alcohol production.

Frequently the inoculum is a mixture of *Saccharomyces pastorianus* and *Saccharomyces bayanus*. The former is felt to give a lively start to the fermentation, whereas the latter performs better later in the process, and ferments to dryness.

Where temperature control is effected (this is not universal), this is likely to be within the range 15°–25°C. If the fermentation displays sluggishness, then a portion of the goods may be warmed to 25°C by pumping through a heat exchanger. Most fermentations will be complete in 2 weeks.

Ciders are subjected to a malolactic fermentation as in the case of some wines. This is effected by heterofermentative *Leuconostoc oenos*, together with other lactobacilli. This is favoured if there is no sulphiting in fermentation and storage and also by autolysis of yeast when the cider is allowed to stand unracked on its lees. As sulphiting is so widespread these days, the malolactic fermentation is probably less significant than it once was. Furthermore, there is a lessening tendency to leave cider on the lees. In the malolactic fermentation, there is a conversion of malic to lactic acid and the release of carbon dioxide. The resultant cider will tend to have a more rounded, complex flavour that is less acidic. The process is inhibited if the pH is too low. A range of sulphite-binding compounds are produced during fermentation, but the most potent binder of SO_2 is acetaldehyde (Fig. 9.14). Essentially, until all of this is bound to SO_2, no free SO_2 can remain to bind other components. Indeed, SO_2 bound to carbonyls such as acetaldehyde has little antimicrobial action, which is why cidermakers try to minimise the level of carbonyls. The addition of thiamine reduces the production of pyruvate and of α-ketobutyrate. Pantothenate can reduce the production of acetaldehyde.

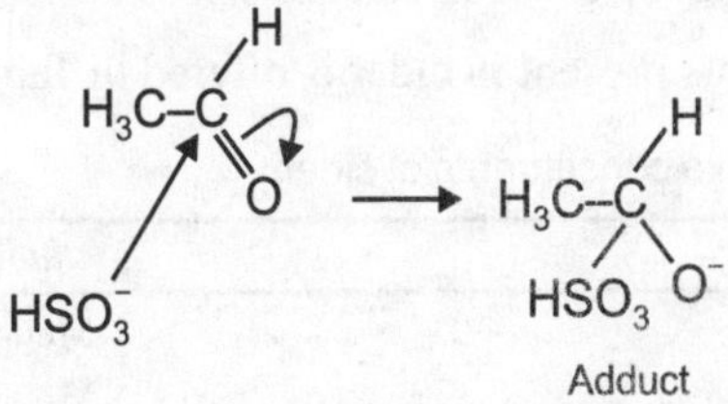

Fig. 9.14. Adduct formation.

Cider Colour and Flavour

The colour of cider arises through the oxidation of polyphenols in the juice. It can be regulated by the addition of sulphite. If the latter is added immediately after pressing, then nearly all colour development is suppressed due to binding of sulphite to the quinoidal forms of the polyphenolics. If SO_2 is added later, there is less reduction of colour because the quinones have become more intimately cross-linked. The colour decreases during fermentation because of the reducing nature of yeast.

Maillard browning reactions can occur during the storage of AJC, and these coloured products cannot be dealt with by yeast. The colour of finished cider is standardised by the addition of caramel or other permitted colourants. The colour is removed from speciality products like white ciders by the action of adsorbents such as activated carbon.

The traditional high bitterness and astringency of ciders originate with the procyanidins. Procyanidins with a degree of polymerisation (DP) 2–4 are bitter and are referred to as 'hard tannins'. Those with a DP of 5–7 are astringent ('soft tannins'). The relative delivery of bitterness and astringency depends both on the apple cultivar and on how the apples are processed. Oxidised polyphenols adsorb (become tanned) onto the apple pulp and this suppresses both astringency and bitterness. If oxidation occurs in the absence of the pulp, then there is a relative transition from bitterness to astringency as the units polymerise. Alcohol tends to enhance bitterness but suppresses astringency.

As in the case of beer and wine, the yeast produces a range of volatile components (e.g. esters), and key variables are yeast strain, fermentation temperature, and the clarity and nutrient composition of the fermentation feedstock. Higher quality apple cultivars tend to give juice containing lower levels of assimilable nitrogen, and the attendant slower fermentation rates may be associated with enhanced flavour delivery. For instance, levels of 2-phenylethanol may be increased. Cloudy juices will ferment to give increased levels of fusel oils.

There are several nonvolatile glycosidic complexes in apples that are hydrolysed by endogenous glycosidases when the fruit is disrupted. The malolactic fermentation results in the production of diacetyl which can afford a desirable buttery note to some ciders.

Spicy and phenolic notes arise from ethylphenol and ethyl catechol that come from phenolic acid precursors (Fig. 9.15). These are major contributors to the bittersweet flavours of well-made traditional ciders. However, at high levels, they give characters reminiscent of barnyards, possibly due to the slow growth of Brettanomyces in storage.

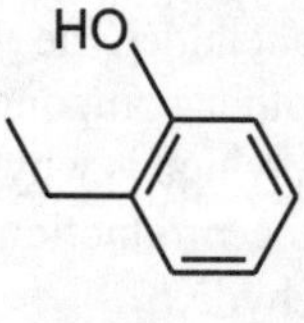

HO

2-Ethyl phenol

Fig. 9.15. A source of spiciness in cider.

A listing of volatile components present in cider is offered in Table 9.10.

Table 9.10. Volatile constituents of cider.

Iso-amyl alcohol	*Methionol*
Benzaldehyde	2-Methyl-butan-1-ol
Iso-butanol	3-Methyl-butan-1-ol
n-Butanol	2-Methylpropanol
Decanal	Nonanoic acid
δ-Decalactone	Nonanol
Decan-2-one	Octanoic acid
Diethyl succinate	Octanol
Ethyl acetate	Iso-pentanol
Ethyl benzoate	2-Phenylethanol
Ethyl decanoate	2-Phenylethyl acetate
Ethyl dodecanoate	*n*-Propanol
Ethyl guaiacol	sec-Pentanol
Ethyl hexanoate	Undecanal
Ethyl-2-hydroxy-4-methyl pentanoate	
Ethyl lactate	
Ethyl-2-methylbutyrate	
Ethyl octanoate	
n-Hexanol	
Hexanoic acid	
Hexyl acetate	

Post-fermentation Processes

Racking consists of removing the newly fermented cider from its lees. In modern cidermaking, this may occur relatively soon and in the absence of maturation, prior to blending and packaging. More traditional processing has the cider left on the lees for several weeks, with racking into tanks for months of storage with minimum contact with air. The malolactic fermentation may be encouraged, in which case sulphiting is avoided at this point.

Initial clarification of cider is by natural settling, by fining (bentonite, gelatine, chitosan, isinglass), or by centrifugation. Alternatively, a combination of these may be used.

The ciders will be filtered before packaging and may be blended, aided by expert tasting. If fermentation was to a higher-than-target alcohol content, then the cider will be thinned by the addition of water, and sugar or malic acid may be added, as well as of course carbon dioxide.

Final filtration is by powder, sheet and/or membrane filtration. There is increasing use of cross-flow microfiltration (Fig. 9.16). Most ciders are pasteurised and carbonated en route to final pack.

Typically 50 ppm SO_2 will be added to give a free SO_2 level of 30 ppm, but the precise figures will depend on the level of endogenous binding compounds present in the cider. If the cider is destined for cans, then SO_2 levels must be lower because as little as 25 ppm can cause damage to the lacquer layer and to the production of hydrogen sulphide.

Ascorbic acid may be added, but these days there is less use for sorbic acid as it is only fully effective in the presence of SO_2 and, further, it is only active against yeast and not bacteria.

Problems with cider

Cider sickness, caused by infection through *Zymomonas anaerobia* is now very uncommon, as it is countered by the lower pHs (<3.5) and reduced tendency to have residual sugar in the product. Symptoms include an aroma of banana skins and a white turbidity due to the acetaldehyde produced reacting with polyphenols to form insoluble complexes.

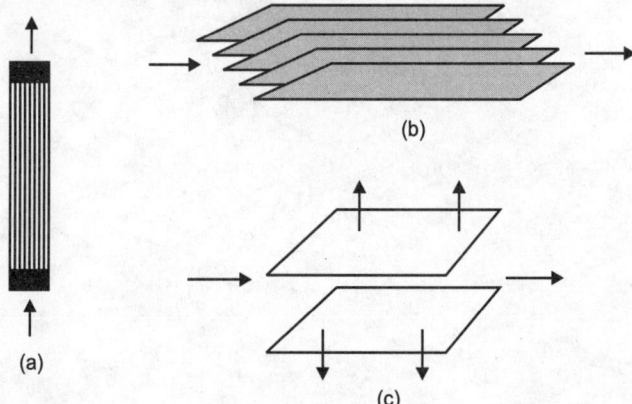

Fig. 9.16. Cross-flow microfiltration. The cider flows through multiple bundles of porous membranes. Particles, including micro-organisms, are held back by the membranes, with the clarified liquid emerging at right angle to the direction of flow, the continuous nature of which ensures that particles do not adhere to the pores and plug them.

Mousiness in cider is due to isomers of 2-acetyl or ethyl tetrahydropyridine (Fig. 9.17) produced by lactic acid bacteria or Brettanomyces under aerobic conditions. Detection of the flavour depends on reaction of the compounds with saliva, with the acidity of the saliva releasing the compounds from the base forms where they are not detected. Thus, simple smelling of cider will not tell whether there is a problem or not.

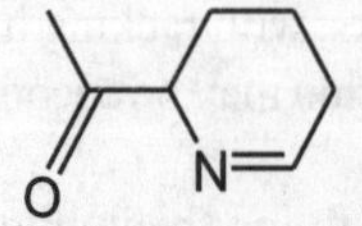

2-Acetyltetrahydropyridine

Fig. 9.17. A source of mousiness in cider.

Ropiness in cider is due to the production by lactic acid bacteria of a polymeric glucan that increases the viscosity of the cider, which appears to be oily when poured due to the movement of the slimy glucan.

Lactic acid bacteria may also break down glycerol. They produce 3-hydroxypropanal which spontaneously dehydrates to generate acrolein that has a bitter taste and a pungent aroma (Fig. 9.18).

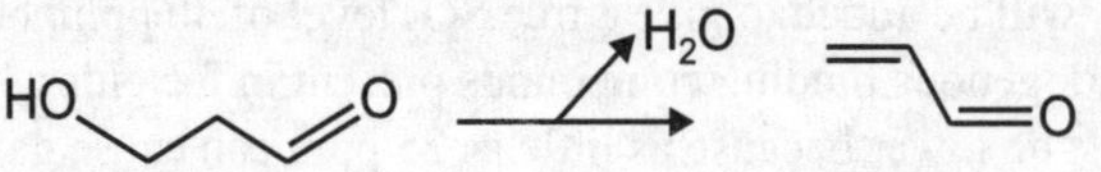

H_2O

3-Hydroxypropanal   Acrolein

Fig. 9.18. A source of pungent bitterness in cider.

Chill hazes in cider are due to complex formation between polyphenols and polysaccharides, and to a lesser extent, with the very low levels of proteins. This is promoted by iron and copper, the levels of which should be minimised.

Chapter 10

Distilled Alcoholic Beverages

INTRODUCTION

The principal distilled beverages are those derived from either grain (whiskies), grapes, (cognac, armagnac, brandy) or molasses (rum).

A distilled beverage, liquor, or spirit is a drinkable liquid containing ethanol that is produced by means of distilling fermented grain, fruit or vegetables. This excludes undistilled fermented beverages such as beer and wine.

Beer and wine were historically limited to a maximum alcohol content of about 15 per cent ABV. Most yeasts cannot reproduce when the concentration of alcohol is higher than 15 per cent; consequently, fermentation ceases at that point, preventing the production of more alcohol.

The term spirit refers to a distilled beverage that contains no added sugar and has at least 20 per cent ABV. Popular spirits include brandy, fruit brandy (aka eau-de-vie), gin, rum, tequila, vodka and whisky.

Distilled beverages that are bottled with added sugar and added flavourings, such as Grand Marnier, Frangelico and American schnapps, are liqueurs. In common usage, the distinction between spirits and liqueurs is widely unknown or ignored; consequently all alcoholic beverages other than beer and wine are generally referred to simply as spirits.

Fortified wines are created by adding a distilled beverage (usually brandy) to a wine.

WHISKY

Whisky (spelled this way for Scotch, but as whiskey for Irish and other forms of the product) is a distilled beverage made from cereals and normally matured in oak. It is subject to a great deal of legislation and custom.

Europian Union (EU) regulations state that it can be made from any cereal aided by starch-degrading enzymes with distillation to less than 94.8 per cent ABV, with ensuing maturation in wooden casks of less than 700 l in volume for a period in excess of 3 years for sale at a strength in excess of 40 per cent ABV. UK legislation dictates that Scotch whisky must be produced in Scotland, the enzymes must be entirely derived from malt and the only permitted addition is caramel. The United States, Japan and Canada have their own legislative peculiarities that will not be discussed here.

The major cereals used for the manufacture of whisky are barley, wheat, rye and corn (maize). Malted barley is employed as a source of flavour and enzymes, which are not only responsible for converting the barley starch but also that of adjuncts to fermentable sugars. The main analytical criteria for whisky malts are their diastatic power, α-amylase and extract, especially when they are being used alongside adjunct. The malts may be 'peated', that is, flavoured with the smoke from peat burnt on the kiln. Such malts are classified on their content of phenols.

Rye (*Secale montanum*) is quite widely used in Eastern Europe and former USSR, and is sometimes malted. Wheat (*Triticum vulgare*) has largely replaced corn in Scotch grain whiskies as the cost of importing grain from the United States became prohibitive and it is also used in some American whiskies. However, in the United States, corn (*Zea mays*) is especially widely used.

Malt is essentially mashed as in the case for beers, with clear wort being important to prevent burning on the stills. Wort from unmalted grain, however, is not separated from the spent grains because modern continuous distillation processes do not demand it. Fermentation and distillation are effected with all of the grain materials still present.

For malt whisky, mashes of water: grist ratio of 4:1 will be mixed in at 64.5°C, the malt having been broken in a roller mill. Although modern malt distilleries are changing over to the use of lauter tun technology, traditional distillery mash tuns feature rotating paddles to mix the mash and these will be employed for approximately 20 minutes before allowing the mash to stand for 1 hour. The worts will then be collected before addition of a second water (70°C; 2 m^3 per ton) and collection of those worts, followed by waters at 80°C (4 m^3 per ton) and 90°C (2 m^3 per ton). The first and second worts are cooled by a paraflow heat exchanger to approximately 19°C and diverted to a fermenter or wash back. The third and fourth worts are pooled as part of the mashing water for the next mash. Unlike for the brewing of beer, there is no boiling of worts.

The initial processing in the production of grain whiskies is significantly different from that of malt whiskies. Indeed it is not unheard of for distilleries to work with unmilled grain, in which case prolonged cooking is a necessity. For the most part, however, the first stage in production is the hammer milling of the cereal. The desire is fine particles that are readily extracted by water. The cereal is mashed with 2.5 parts water (or recycled weak worts or 'backset', which is a portion of the stillage from the distillation process that has had its solids removed. The latter is felt to deliver yeast nutrients). The mash, typically at 40°–45°C, is agitated to ensure that there is no sticking together of grist ('balling'). Some malted barley is likely to be included as a source of enzymes. The slurry is now pumped to a cooker (pressure vessel) wherein the mash is mixed and injected with steam, to achieve gelatinisation of the cereal. The temperature will be raised to 130°–150°C and held there for a relatively short period of time. Mixing is essential to avoid charring and excessive browning (Maillard) reactions. The contents of the cooker are now discharged to a flash cooling vessel, the sudden fall in pressure being referred to as 'blow-down'. The impact of this is to release any residual bound starch from the grain matrix. The temperature falls rapidly to around 70°C. The slurry is mixed with a separate slurry of malt (10–15 per cent of the total grist bill) that may be at 40°C, but alternatively may be at the conversion temperature for starch (65°–70°C). The malt enzymes then catalyse not only the hydrolysis of the malt starch but also that from the cooked grain. Food grade enzymes will also be added—and to some extent there may still be the use of green (unkilned) malt as a source of enzymes. Mashing will typically be for up to 30 minutes. Although the wort was formerly separated from the grains, this tends not to be done now in grain distilleries, and the whole mash contents are transferred to the fermenter. There is no boiling, so enzymes can continue to work. Furthermore, it also means that the fermenter contents can be more concentrated than would be the case otherwise. The downside to this is the risk of fouling of stills.

Fermentation of whisky was formerly performed widely with the surplus yeast generated in brewery fermentations. However, specific strains particularly suited to whisky production have been developed and these are supplied by yeast manufacturers in bulk for commercial use. Hybrids emerged not only from the ale strain *Saccharomyces cerevisiae* but also from the 'wild yeast' *Saccharomyces diastaticus*, which produces a spectrum of enzymes fully capable of hydrolysing starch to fermentable sugar. Thus, the distilling strains enable high alcohol yield. The strains may also be selected on the basis of their ability to produce esters. Yeast is supplied either as compressed moist yeast, as 'cream yeast' or, increasingly, as dried yeast. Quality considerations of the yeast (viability, etc.) are just as for brewing.

Fermentation on a small scale may be in closed wooden barrels, but on a larger scale, it will be in stainless steel vessels known as washbacks. Unlike in breweries, there is little temperature control during fermentation, other than to target the initial temperature, which may typically be in the range 19°–22°C. The temperature may go as high as 34°C during fermentation, hence the need for ale-based strains rather than lager-based ones. Typically the fermentation is complete within 40–48 hours. Some advocate holding a few hours prior to distillation in order to ensure that the endogenous lactic acid bacteria have an opportunity to enhance flavour.

Distillation

The stills used in the production of whisky are of two types: batch and continuous. Batch (or pot) stills employ double or triple distillation and generate a highly flavoured spirit. Continuous stills provide lighter flavoured spirits that are mostly employed in blending.

Pot stills are traditionally of copper, which may reduce the sulphuriness of the whisky (Fig. 10.1). The still comprises three major parts: the pot, which holds the liquid to be distilled; a swan neck and lyne arm; and a condenser. The precise design of the swan neck/lyne has a considerable impact on the reflux pattern obtained and hence on the flavour.

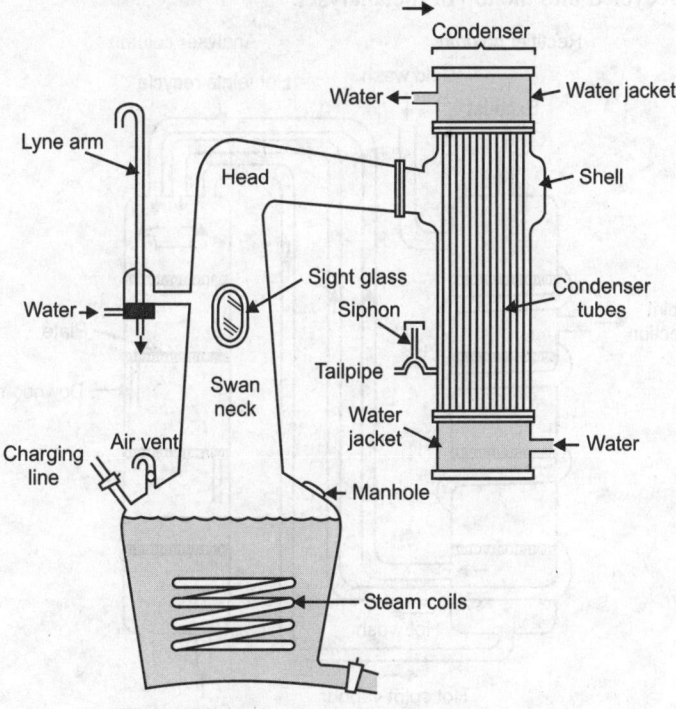

Fig. 10.1. A pot still.

The pot is heated either directly or indirectly. In the former case, an agitator may be present to prevent charring. Pots can be of diverse shapes, but in traditional Scotch whisky production, there are two stills: the wash still and the spirit still. All of the fermenter contents (the 'wash' will typically be 8 per cent ABV) are transferred to the wash still and boiled for between 5 and 6 hours to render a distillate known as 'low wines' which has an alcohol strength of 20–25 per cent ABV. This is subsequently transferred to a smaller spirit still. The spirit coming over from this can be divided into three components: the foreshots, the middle cut and the feints. The charge to the spirit still is a mix of foreshots and feints and low wines to a net alcohol concentration of less than 30 per cent ABV. The foreshots emerge first from the still, the feints last. They contain the undesirable highly volatile and least volatile components, respectively. They are recycled for re-distillation. The foreshots represent perhaps the first 30 minutes of the distillation and are collected in the feints receiver until the opening distillate strength of 85 per cent has fallen to 75 per cent. At this point, the spirit is judged to be potable and is collected in the spirits receiver. Collection proceeds for up to 3 hours, with the alcohol dropping to 60–72 per cent ABV. Thereafter the flow is diverted once more to the feints receiver and collection may continue until the alcohol reaches as little as 1 per cent ABV. Continuous distillation takes place in column stills, the most famous of which being that designed by Aeneas Coffey (Fig. 10.2). It comprises two adjacent columns. The wash is preheated by passing it through the tube in the second column (rectifier). Thence it is fed into the first column (analyser) near the top and steam is passed in at the base of the column. As the wash falls, volatiles are stripped from it and these emerge from the top of the column, passing to the rectifier column. Alcohol separates from water at the base. The spirit is removed towards the top of the rectifier. The final cut is taken off from the base of the column. Foreshots (from the top) and feints (from the base) are recycled into the top of the analyser.

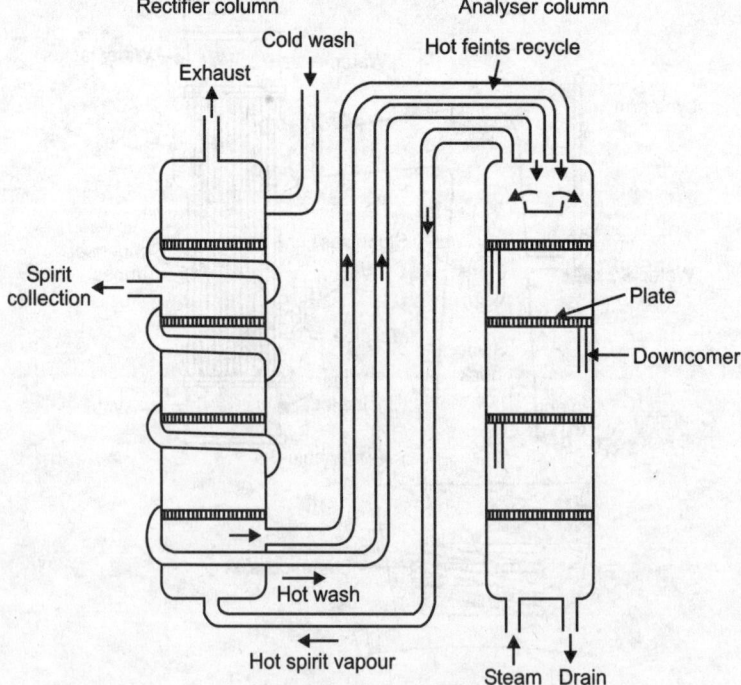

Fig. 10.2. A Coffey still.

Inside the column is a series of plates with holes that permit the upwards flow of vapour. The plates are linked by downcomers that alternate on opposite sides of the plates such that the descending liquid is obliged to flow across each plate. After distillation, new distillates are diluted (e.g. to 58–70 per cent ABV) before filling in oak casks.

The residue from the distillation process is called 'pot ale'. In grain distilleries, it is mixed with spent grains and yeast, whereas in malt distilleries, it is blended with grains and thence despatched for animal feed.

Whiskies are matured in oak casks. Whereas American bourbon and rye whiskies are put into new oak casks, Scotch, Irish and Canadian whiskies are filled into casks that have previously been employed for Bourbon or for sherry. For the most part they comprise 50 litre butts. Whisky casks are either of American white oak (which are used for Fino and Amontillado Sherries) or Spanish oak (used for Oloroso Sherry). The bourbon casks used for Scotch whiskies must be filled at least once with bourbon and the whiskies must have been in the cask for at least 4 years. Ageing of whisky in most countries must be for at least 3 years. There is a significant loss of alcohol by evaporation in this time, referred to as the 'angel's share'. In the maturation there is the development of mellowness and a decrease of harshness. Flavours associated with mature whisky are vanilla, floral, woody, spicy and smooth. The undesirable flavours that dissipate are sour, oily, sulphury and grassy. Various components are extracted from the wood, including those developed by wood charring. The major flavour components of whisky are listed in Table 10.1.

Table 10.1. Flavour constituents of whisky.

Main congeners	Ethyl octadecanoate
Acetaldehyde	Ethyl octanoate
Ethyl acetate	4-Ethyl guaiacol
Isobutanol	2-Ethylphenol
Methanol	4-Ethylphenol
2-Methyl butanol	Ethyl undecanoate
3-Methyl butanol	Eugenol
n-Propanol	Furfural
	Furfuryl formate
Other congeners	Gallic acid
Acetyl furan	Guaiacol
Benzaldehyde	Hexadecanol
Butanol	Hexanol
Coniferaldehyde	5-Hydroxymethyl furfural
m-, o-, p-Cresol	Isoamyl acetate
Decanoic acid	Isoamyl alcohol
Decanol	Isoamyl decanoate
Diethoxypropane	Isoamyl octanoate
Diethyl succinate	cis-Oak lactone
Dimethyl disulphide	trans-Oak lactone

(Contd ...)

Dimethyl sulphide	Octanol
Dimethyl trisulplude	Phenol
Dodecanoic acid	Phenylethanol
Dodecanol	Phenylethyl acetate
Ellagic acid	Phenylethyl butanoate
3-Ethoxypropanal	Scopoletin
Ethyl butanoate	Synapaldehyde
Ethyl decanoate	Syringealdehyde
Ethyl dodecanoate	Syringic acid
Ethyl hexadecanoate	Tetradecanoic acid
Ethyl hexadecenoate	Triethoxypropane
Ethyl hexanoate	Vanillic acid
Ethyl lactate	Vanillin
Ethyl nonanoate	3,5-Xylenol

Usually the lighter bodied spirits generated on a continuous still are blended with a range of heavier bodied spirits coming either from batch stills or by distillation to lower ethanol concentrations in column stills. In the decantation process, the various whiskies are decanted into troughs by which they flow to a blending vat wherein they are mixed by mechanical agitator and compressed air. Then 'de-proofing water' is added to take the product to its final strength.

In Scotland, the final products may be a blend of whiskies from more than ten grain distilleries and up to a hundred malt distilleries. There is an astonishing interaction and cooperation between separate companies to enable this. The blending is deliberately complex so that the unavailability of one or two whiskies in any single blending will not be noticeable. In other countries where there are far fewer distilleries, batch-to-batch variation must be achieved by varying conditions within the distilleries themselves—for example, the grist or the fermentation and distillation conditions.

Most whisky is filtered. Insoluble fractions, notably lignins and long chain esters of fatty acids, are removed by cooling to as low as –10°C and filtration, typically in plate and frame devices with diatomaceous earth as filter aid.

Whiskey Variants

Bourbon (United States) is made principally from corn (maize) plus added rye and barley and is aged in charred barrels. A close relative is Tennessee whiskey (United States), which is produced using a sour mash process. Canadian whisky (Canada) is a light product from rye and malted rye, with some corn and malted barley. Corn whiskey (United States) is from maize and is aged in barrels that have not been charred. Rye whiskey (United States) is from rye mixed with corn and barley and is aged in newly charred oak barrels.

COGNAC

The grape vines employed for the base wine for cognac production are nearly all from Charente and the adjacent regions of Deux-Sèvres and Dordogne. Furthermore, the grape varieties must be either Ugni blanc, Colmbard or Folle Blanc, with the exception that up to 10 per cent can be wines from Jurancon blanc, Semillon, Montils, Blanc ramè or Select.

Ugni blanc is by far the major variety, affording wine high in acidity and relatively low in alcohol which renders it most suitable for distillation. But suffice to say here that the microflora employed for fermentation is endogenous, with one report suggesting that more than 650 yeasts are involved. The belief is that active dry yeast (ADY) leads to the production of inferior products. Sulphur dioxide is not employed. Fermentation is relatively fast, the wines being maintained on the lees and subjected to malolactic fermentation. The sooner the distillation after fermentation, the better the quality of the product as there is less development of ethyl butyrate and acrolein (from the decomposition of glycerol).

The distillation employed in the production of cognac is known as the Charente process. The still must have a capacity of less than 30 hl, which means that the maximum practical working volume is no more than 25 hl. The vessel must be heated by an open fire.

Two successive distillations yield a spirit of <72 per cent ABV. In the first stage, 27–30 per cent ABV is achieved. In the further distillation of this, three major fractions are generated: the heads, the heart (spirit cut) and the seconds. The heads, comprising 1–2 per cent of the total, contain the most volatile components and are considered detrimental. The most 'noble' components are in the heart and herein is the cognac spirit to be matured. The seconds are recycled.

The nature of the wood employed for ageing of cognac has great significance. The fineness of the grain impacts the extent to which phenolics and other tannins are extracted, as does the shape and size of the barrel made from that wood and the extent to which the wood is charred in the shaping process. The wood is generally dried in the open air for over 3 years. New spirit is introduced to this new wood for a period of 8–12 months before transferring to older barrels, thereby avoiding the pick up and development of excessive astringent and bitter characteristics. Oxygen enters through the stave and is used by enzymes contributed by moulds in reactions that have a role in the ageing process. There is also volatile loss through the stave. The changes in key wood-derived volatiles that result from different periods of ageing are given in Table 10.2.

Table 10.2. Changes in volatiles in cognac during different periods of ageing in wood.

	Concentration (mgl^{-1})		
Component	0.7 years	5 years	13 years
Coniferaldehyde	3.7	5.9	6.7
Gallic acid	4.6	9.0	15.3
Sinapaldehyde	9.5	17.8	17.0
Syringaldehyde	2.3	8.9	17.6
Syringic acid	0.6	2.6	7.0
Vanillic acid	0.3	1.4	2.8
Vanillin	0.9	4.4	8.8

Several batches will be blended during ageing. New distillates at 70 per cent ABV are lowered in successive stages to the 40 per cent ABV level at which the product is bottled.

Armagnac and Wine Spirits

Armagnac is in South West France. The three main vinestocks used for armagnac are as for cognac, with Ugni blanc again being preferred on account of a reduced risk of rot as it comes to maturity rapidly. The wines must be distilled in the Appellation area, with the maximum content of distilled alcohol allowed being 72 per cent ABV. Again, the use of sulphur dioxide is forbidden. Two types of still are used: the continuous Armagnac still and two-stage pot stills. Continuous armagnac stills are fabricated from copper and are operated as described by Bertrand. Operational variables are the rate of wine flow and the heating regimen. Heating is always by open fire, although nowadays it will probably be fuelled by propane gas rather than by wood. Just as for whisky, the three components emerging from a still are heads, body and tailings.

The two-stage pot still is comparable with that used for cognac. Wine spirits are usually aged in oak casks. Coarse-grained wood is preferred because more oxygen can then enter to polymerise tannins. Oxygen ingress is also important for the oxidation of some of the alcohol to acetic acid, which in turn reacts with alcohol to generate flavoursome esters during ageing. A comparison of the key analytical parameters for armagnac, cognac and brandy is given in Table 10.3.

Table 10.3. An analytical comparison of wine spirits.

Parameter	Cognac	Armagnac	Brandy
Alcohol (% ABV)	40.04	41.4	45.46
Total acidity (as acetic acid)	103.6	153.9	31.46
Volatile acidity (as acetic acid)	59.3	106.5	19.06
Aldehydes	19.3	23.3	25.33
Esters	72.9	109.6	54.8
Higher alcohols	444.4	441.4	258.4
Total volatile substances	632	682.1	357.5

Apart from alcohol, units are g hr l^{-1}.

Expert blending is performed and the alcohol concentration lowered to a minimum of 40 per cent by the addition of distilled water. Caramel may be added to enhance colour. The product is held at −5°C for 1 week prior to filtration through cellulose.

Brandy is obtained from wine spirits blended or not with wine distillates distilled to less than 94.8 per cent ABV, such distillates not exceeding 50 proof maximum in the final product. The product is aged in oak for more than 1 year, unless the casks hold less than 1000 litres in which case ageing must be for a minimum of 6 months. According to Bertrand, the making of brandy is an opportunity to salvage defective wines or deal with production surpluses, although top quality brandies may be made from wine specifically produced for the purpose. Brandies must be >37.5 per cent ABV.

RUM

Rum primarily originated in the Caribbean, although the first references to liqueurs obtained from sugar cane are from India. Sugar cane was introduced to the Caribbean by Christopher Columbus in 1493.

The chief producing countries are Barbados and Santo Domingo. Nowadays the coastal planes of Guyana (Demerara) are rich in estates producing sugar cane (*Saccharum officinarum*).

At harvest time the fields of sugar cane are set alight in order to sanitise the soil, the stems are scorched in this process and the canes subsequently wither and are harvested by machete, a strategy thought to yield a superior product when compared with rum made from cane harvested by machine.

The canes are topped to remove the leafy parts and the cane then ferried to mills. There is considerable contamination with *Leuconostoc mesenteroides*, which produces a gum that causes problems during extraction. It is important to avoid delays between cutting and mining, and the maximum time elapse should be less than 24 hours.

During processing, the canes are cut and crushed and the juice limed, clarified and evaporated. Various fractions are generated, but the key product for rum is molasses. Four to five ions of molasses are typically obtained per 100 tons cane.

The nature of the molasses depends on cane variety, soil type, climate, cultivation and harvesting conditions. They are delivered hot to the distillery either by pipe or by tanker and are stored at 45°C. The molasses are pumped at 85°–88°Brix and are mixed with water in line. Lighter flavour rums may incorporate cane juice (12–16 per cent w/v sucrose).

Formerly adventitious yeasts were used to effect fermentation, but nowadays pure cultures of *S. cerevisiae*, *S. bayanus* and *Schizosaccharomyces pombe* are used. They are propagated from slopes by successively scaled up incubations using sucrose as the carbon source.

Prior to fermentation, the molasses are diluted to 45°Brix and their temperature elevated to 70°C in order to destroy contaminating organisms. The pH is lowered by the addition of sulphuric acid and the whole clarified by putting into a conical-bottomed settling tank, from which the sludge can be decanted from the cone. Ammonium sulphate is added as a source of nitrogen.

Fermentation is conducted at 30°–33°C in cylindroconical vessels that may be closed or open. The final sugar content will be 16°–20°Brix and this is reached in 24 hours with an alcohol yield of 5–7 per cent ABV. Some high-gravity fermentations nowadays furnish 10–13 per cent ABV.

Distillation is conducted in pot stills that were traditionally of copper or wood but now more likely to be fabricated from stainless steel. As for whisky, there are also column stills of stainless steel or copper (Coffey stills).

Pot stills afford heavier rums that need prolonged maturation, whereas the column stills are employed for lighter rums, or to generate the neutral spirits that can be used for the production of gin and vodka. Distillates are collected at 80–94 per cent ABV for rums and >96 per cent for neutral spirits.

Pot distillation of rum is exactly analogous to the techniques used in the production of whisky. The pot is charged with wash at approximately 5.5 per cent ABV and the retort charged with low wines at 51–52 per cent ABV from the previous distillation. The fractions obtained are heads, spirits and feints. The heads are rich in esters and are collected for the initial 5 minutes in the low wines receiver. The ensuing spirits are collected for 1.5–2 hours at 85 per cent ABV. When the emerging strength drops to 43 per cent ABV, the flow is again diverted to the low wines receiver in order to collect the feints. Distillation is completed when the distillate approaches some 1 per cent ABV.

Column distillation allows ten times more output than does pot distillation and is performed exactly analogously to the whisky process.

Rum is aged in Bourbon oak casks. It is racked at 83–85 per cent ABV. As the main production locale is tropical, ageing is quite rapid and may be complete within 6 months. There may first have been a blending of light rums produced in column stills with heavier rums out of pots. Furthermore, there may be transfers between casks for successive maturation periods. Finally rum is chilled to –10°C and filtered to remove fatty acid esters prior to dilution to final strength and packaging.

Chapter 11

Flavoured Spirits

INTRODUCTION

Vodka ('little water') is essentially pure alcohol in water, though flavoured variants are available. Gin comprises distilled alcohol flavoured with a range of botanicals. In the same stable come Genever (like gin, flavoured with juniper), Aquavit (caraway and/or dill), Anis (aniseed, star anise, fennel) and Ouzo (aniseed, mastic).

VODKA

Vodka comprises pure unaged spirit distilled from alcoholic matrices of various origins and usually filtered through charcoal. It is defined in the EU as a:

'Spirit drink produced by either rectifying ethyl alcohol of agricultural origin or filtering it through activated charcoal.

Vodka is a distilled beverage. It is a clear liquid consisting mostly of water and ethanol purified by distillation—often multiple distillation—from a fermented substance, such as grain (usually rye or wheat), potatoes or sugar beet molasses. An insignificant amount of other substances such as flavouring or unintended impurities is also commonly added.

Vodka usually has an alcohol content of 35 to 50 per cent by volume. The classic Russian, Lithuanian and Polish vodka is 40 per cent (80 proof). This can be attributed to the Russian standards for vodka production introduced in 1894 by Alexander III. According to the Vodka Museum in Moscow, Russian chemist Dmitri Mendeleev (more famous for his work in developing the periodic table) found the perfect percentage to be 38. However, since spirits in his time were taxed on their strength, the percentage was rounded up to 40 to simplify the tax computation. At strengths less than this, vodka drunk neat (without ice and not mixed with other liquids) can taste 'watery', while strengths above 40 per cent may give the taste of vodka more 'burn'. Some governments set a minimum alcohol content for a spirit to be called 'vodka'. For example, the European Union sets a minimum of 37.5 per cent alcohol by volume.

Although vodka is traditionally drunk neat in the Eastern European and Nordic countries of the 'vodka belt', its popularity elsewhere owes much to its usefulness in cocktails and other mixed drinks, such as the bloody mary, the screwdriver, the white russian, the vodka tonic and vodka martini.

Materials added in the production of vodka include sugar at up to 2 g l^{-1} and citric acid at up to 150 mg l^{-1}. Some vodkas have glycerol or propylene glycol added to enhance the mouthfeel. Amongst the flavoured vodkas are ones infused with pepper, a Polish product in which buffalo grass is steeped in the spirit and a Russian variant in which the vodka is treated with apple and pear tree leaves, brandy and port. The neutral alcohol base is frequently produced quite separately from the vodka *per se*, perhaps by a different company. It is chiefly produced from cereals (e.g. corn, wheat) but other sources of fermentable carbohydrate include beet and molasses in Western countries, cane sugar in South America and Africa, and potatoes in Poland and Russia.

The fermentation is, of course, effected by *Saccharomyces cerevisiae*, notably distillers' strains. The alcohol is purified and concentrated by continuous stills with 2–5 columns. The first of these is a 'wash column' that separates alcohol from the wash. The second major column is the 'rectifier' in which alcohol is concentrated. There may be a 'purifier' between the wash column and the final rectifier.

The wash column distillate is introduced halfway up the extractive distillation column and water (approximately 20 times more than wash) is fed in at the top. This procedure impacts the volatilisation of components of the wash and encourages the removal of volatiles. Ethanol mostly leaves with water at the base of the column, prior to concentration in the final rectification column.

Treatment with activated carbon is either by using a dispersion of purified charcoal in a tank prior to its removal by filtration or by passing the spirit through columns that contain charcoal in granular form.

Production

Vodka may be distilled from any starch/sugar-rich plant matter; most vodka today is produced from grains such as sorghum, corn, rye or wheat. Among grain vodkas, rye and wheat vodkas are generally considered superior. Some vodka is made from potatoes, molasses, soyabeans, grapes, sugar beets and sometimes even by-products of oil refining or wood pulp processing. In some Central European countries like Poland some vodka is produced by just fermenting a solution of crystal sugar and yeast. In the European Union there are talks about the standardisation of vodka, and the vodka belt countries insist that only spirits produced from grains, potato and sugar beet molasses be allowed to be branded as 'vodka', following the traditional methods of production.

Distilling and filtering

A common property of vodkas produced in the United States and Europe is the extensive use of filtration prior to any additional processing, such as the addition of flavourants. Filtering is sometimes done in the still during distillation, as well as afterwards, where the distilled vodka is filtered through charcoal and other media. This is because under U.S. and European law vodka must not have any distinctive aroma, character, colour or flavour. However, this is not the case in the traditional vodka producing nations, so many distillers from these countries prefer to use very accurate distillation but minimal filtering, thus preserving the unique flavours and characteristics of their products.

The 'stillmaster' is the person in charge of distilling the vodka and directing its filtration. When done correctly, much of the 'fore-shots' and 'heads' and the 'tails' separated in distillation process are discarded. These portions of the distillate contain flavour compounds such as ethyl acetate and ethyl lactate (heads) as well as the fusel oils (tails) that alter the clean taste of vodka. Through numerous rounds of distillation, or the use of a fractioning still, the taste of the vodka is improved and its clarity is enhanced. In some distilled liquors such as rum and baijiu, some of the heads and tails are not removed in order to give the liquor its unique flavour and mouth-feel. Repeated distillation of vodka will make its ethanol level much higher than legally allowed. Depending on the distillation method and the technique of the stillmaster, the final filtered and distilled vodka may have as much as 95–96 per cent ethanol. As such, most vodka is diluted with water prior to bottling. This level of distillation is what truly separates a rye-based vodka (for example) from a rye whisky; while the whisky is generally only distilled down to its final alcohol content, vodka is distilled until it is almost totally pure alcohol and then cut with water to give it its final alcohol content and unique flavour, depending on the source of the water.

Flavouring

Apart from the alcoholic content, vodkas may be classified into two main groups: clear vodkas and flavoured vodkas. From the latter ones, one can separate bitter tinctures, such as Russian Yubileynaya (anniversary vodka) and Pertsovka (pepper vodka).

While most vodkas are unflavoured, many flavoured vodkas have been produced in traditional vodka-drinking areas, often as home-made recipes to improve vodka's taste or for medicinal purposes. Flavourings include red pepper, ginger, fruit flavours, vanilla, chocolate (without sweetener), and cinnamon. In Russia and Ukraine, vodka flavoured with honey and pepper is also very popular. Ukrainians produce a commercial vodka that includes St John's Wort. Poles and Belarusians add the leaves of the local bison grass to produce Zubrówka (Polish) and Zubrovka (Belarusian) vodka, with slightly sweet flavour and light amber colour. In Poland, a famous vodka containing honey is called Krupnik.

This tradition of flavouring is also prevalent in the Nordic countries, where vodka seasoned with herbs, fruits and spices is the appropriate strong drink for midsummer seasonal festivities. In Sweden, there are forty-odd common varieties of herb-flavoured vodka (kryddat brännvin).

In Poland there is a separate category, nalewka, for vodka-based spirits with fruit, root, flower or herb extracts, which are often home-made or produced by small commercial distilleries. Its alcohol content is between 15 to 75 per cent. The Finnish vodka 'Finlandia' was the first vodka company to mass produce flavoured Vodka.

The Poles make a very pure (95 per cent, 190 proof) rectified spirit (Polish language: spirytus rektyfikowany). Technically a form of vodka, it is sold in liquor stores, not pharmacies. Similarly, the German market often carries German, Hungarian, Polish, and Ukrainian-made varieties of vodka of 90 to 95 per cent alcohol content. A Bulgarian vodka, Balkan 176°, is 88 per cent alcohol.

Other processing

Due to the low freezing point of alcohol, vodka can be stored in ice or a freezer without any crystallisation of water. In countries where alcohol levels are generally low (the USA for example, due to alcohol taxes varying with alcohol content), individuals sometimes increase the alcohol percentage by a form of freeze distillation.

If the alcohol level is low enough and the freezer cold enough (significantly below the freezing point of water), solid crystals will form which are mostly water (actually a dilute solution of alcohol). If these 'ice' crystals are removed, the remaining vodka will be enriched in alcohol.

Vodka and the EU

The recent success of grape-based vodka in the United States has prompted traditional vodka producers in the vodka belt countries of Poland, Finland, Lithuania and Sweden to campaign for EU legislation that will categorise only spirits made from grain or potatoes as 'vodka' rather than spirits made from any ethyl alcohol—provided, for example, by apples and grapes. This proposition has provoked heavy criticism from south European countries, which often distil used mash from wine-making into spirits; although higher quality mash is usually distilled into some variety of pomace brandy, lower-quality mash is better turned into a neutral-flavoured spirits instead. Any vodka then not made from either grain or potatoes would have to display the products used in its production. This regulation was adopted by the European Parliament on June 19, 2007.

Vodka consumed in sufficient amounts can be lethal—as can any alcoholic beverage—and can cause dehydration, digestive irritation, and other symptoms associated with a hangover. These are inherent properties of ethanol, even if to a lesser degree than the methanol, fusel oils, and other alcohols which are absent in pure vodka.

In some countries black-market vodka or 'bathtub' vodka is widespread because it can be produced easily and avoid taxation. However, severe poisoning, blindness, or death can occur as a result of dangerous industrial ethanol substitutes being added by black-market producers. In March 2007, BBC News UK made a documentary to find the cause of severe jaundice among imbibers of the 'bathtub' vodka. The cause was found to be an industrial disinfectant (Extrasept) added to the vodka by the illegal distillers because of its high alcohol content and low price of acquisition. Death toll estimates list at least 120 dead and more than 1,001 poisoned. The death toll is expected to rise due to the chronic nature of the cirrhosis that was causing the jaundice.

GIN

The word gin is a corruption of *genievre*. Gin is a spirit flavoured with juniper berries. Distilled gin is made by redistilling white grain spirit which has been flavoured with juniper berries. Compound gin is made by flavouring neutral grain spirit with juniper berries without redistilling and can be considered a flavoured vodka.

The most common style of gin, typically used for mixed drinks, is London dry gin. London dry gin is made by taking a neutral grain spirit (usually produced in a column still) and redistilling after the botanicals are added. In addition to juniper, it is usually made with amounts of citrus botanicals like lemon and bitter orange peel. Other botanicals that may be used include anise, angelica root and seed, orris root, licorice root, cinnamon, coriander and cassia bark. Plymouth Gin has a different recipe, and is made without the bitter botanicals of London dry gin. It has lemon and orange, angelica, anise, cardamom, coriander and Juniper. Bitter lemon and orange are not used.

Distilled gin evolved from the Dutch spirits jonge and oude Jenever or Genever (young and old Dutch gin), Plymouth gin, and Old Tom gin. Sloe gin is a common ready-sweetened form of gin that is traditionally made by infusing sloes (the fruit of the blackthorn) in gin. Similar infusions are possible with other fruits, such as damsons.

A well-made gin will be relatively dry compared to other spirits. Gin is often mixed in cocktails with sweeter ingredients like tonic water or vermouth to balance this dryness.

In the ED, a drink can be called gin if it is produced by addition to ethanol (of agricultural origin) natural (or nature-identical) flavourants such that the taste is predominantly one of juniper. 'Compounded gin' is made by adding essences to ethanol and this cannot be called gin.

The alcohol for gin may come from grain, molasses, potato, grape or whey-based fermentations.

The prime traditional flavourants are the juniper berry (*Juniperus communis*), coriander seed (*Coriandrum sativum*) and Angelica (*Archangelicum officinalis*), together with the peel of orange and lemon. Other materials may also be used in the formulation of gins and these include cassia bark, cubeb beris, liquorice, orris, almonds and grains of paradise.

Water quality is critical for the production of gin and, as for beer, this explains the traditional locales where the drink was first made and became popular. These days, as for beer, water purification and salt adjustment protocols mean that the production region is of no significance.

Gin is produced in copper pot stills similar to those used in the production of whisky. Nowadays they tend to be steam-heated rather than direct fired. The still is charged with water prior to adding alcohol to the desired concentration which is typically 60 per cent ABV. The botanics are added either loose or suspended in a bag. The still is closed and heated.

The 'heads' emerge first, followed by the main fraction, of some 80 per cent ABV, which is collected as gin. The 'tails' comprise the later fractions in which alcohol concentration is falling. They are collected with maximum heating and are combined with the heads as 'feints' to be purified in a separate distillation or alternatively sent to the alcohol supplier.

Sloe gin is produced by steeping berries of the sloe (*Prunus spinosa*) in gin. The mix is sweetened with sugar, filtered and bottled. Nowadays flavourants may be employed in place of the berries *per se*.

Pimms is based on a secret recipe and is compounded from gin and liqueurs.

Cocktails with gin

Perhaps the best-known gin cocktail is the Martini, traditionally made with gin and dry vermouth. Other gin-based drinks include: (i) allen—gin with lemon juice and Maraschino liqueur, (ii) gimlet—gin and lime juice, (iii) gin and juice—gin and orange juice, (iv) gin and tonic, (v) gin fizz, (vi) gin rickey—gin, lime juice and carbonated water, (vii) gin bucket, (viii) the last word, (ix) London mule, the gin version of a Moscow mule, (x) maiden's prayer, (xi) negroni, (xii) old etonian, (xiii) orange blossom—plymouth gin and orange juice, (xiv) pimm's cup, (xv) pink gin, (xvi) ramos gin fizz, (xvii) salty dog, (xviii) satan's whiskers, (xix) Singapore sling, (xx) Tom collins, and (xxi) white lady.

Gin is often combined with a number of other mixers.

Brands of Gin

Notable brands

1. Aviation: full and weighty mouth feel, Pacific Northwest inspired flavours of earth and spice, uniquely cool finish.
2. Beefeater: First produced in 1820.
3. BOLS Damrak Amsterdam: Dutch jenever.
4. Bombay Sapphire: distilled with ten botanicals.
5. Boodles British gin.
6. Booth's: first produced in 1790 by Sir Felix Booth.
7. Bulldog gin: infused with Poppy and Dragon Eye.
8. Citadelle: 19 exotic botanicals, made in Cognac, France.
9. Cork dry gin: First distilled at the watercourse distillery in Cork city in 1793, now Ireland's best selling gin.
10. Damrak: Sweet candied citrus aromas with a spicy licorice and a juniper edge.
11. Gilbey's gin.
12. Ginebra San Miguel: produced in the Philippines.
13. Gordon's: 'by appointment to Her Majesty Queen Elizabeth II of Great Britain.
12. Greenall's.
13. G'vine: based on an Ugni Blanc base spirit and infused with green grape flowers.
14. Hendrick's gin: An unusual gin made in Scotland, infused with cucumber and rose petals.
15. Old Tom gin.

16. Plymouth: first distilled in 1793.
17. Seagram's gin.
18. South gin: from New Zealand using New Zealand-native manuka berries and kawa kawa leaves.
19. Steinhäger.
20. Tanqueray.
21. Uganda Waragi: triple distilled Ugandan Waragi gin.
22. Whitley Neill gin: Small batch Super-premium gin distilled with Baobab fruit and Cape Gooseberries.

List of cocktails

A cocktail is a mixed drink typically made with a distilled beverage (such as gin, vodka, whiskey, tequila, or rum) that is mixed with other ingredients. If beer is one of the ingredients, the drink is called a beer cocktail.

Cocktails usually contain one or more types of liqueur, juice, fruit, sauce, honey, milk or cream, spices or other flavourings. Cocktails may vary in their ingredients from bartender to bartender, and from region to region. Two creations may have the same name but taste very different because of differences in how the drinks are prepared.

Varieties of cocktails: (i) cocktails with absinthe, (ii) cocktails with beer, (iii) cocktails with brandy or cognac, (iv) cocktails with cachaça, (v) cocktails with gin, (vi) cocktails with rum, (vii) cocktails with sake, (viii) cocktails with tequila, (ix) cocktails with vodka, (x) cocktails with whiskey/whisky or bourbon, (xi) cocktails with wine, sparkling wine, or port, (xii) cocktails with a liqueur as the primary ingredient, (xiii) cocktails with less common spirits, (xiv) bitters (as a primary ingredient), (xv) schnapps, (xvi) other, and (xvii) historical classes of cocktails.

LIQUEUR

A liqueur is an alcoholic beverage that has been flavoured with fruit, herbs, nuts, spices, flowers or cream and bottled with added sugar. Liqueurs are typically quite sweet; they are usually not aged for long but may have resting periods during their production to allow flavours to marry.

In some parts of the world people use the words cordial and liqueur interchangeably. Though in these places the two expressions both describe liqueurs made by redistilling spirits with aromatic flavourings and are usually highly sweetened, there are some differences. While liqueurs are usually flavoured with herbs, cordials are generally prepared with fruit pulp or juices.

Liqueurs date back centuries and are historical descendants of herbal medicines, often those prepared by monks, as Chartreuse or Bénédictine. Liqueurs were made in Italy as early as the 13th century and their consumption was later required at all treaty signings during the middle ages.

Nowadays, liqueurs are made worldwide and are served in many ways: by themselves, poured over ice, with coffee, mixed with cream or other mixers to create cocktails, etc. They are often served with or after a dessert. Liqueurs are also used in cooking.

Some liqueurs are prepared by infusing certain woods, fruits or flowers, in either water or alcohol, and adding sugar or other items. Others are distilled from aromatic or flavouring agents. The distinction between liqueur and spirits (sometimes liquors) is not simple, especially since many spirits are available in a flavoured form today. Flavoured spirits, however, are not prepared by infusion. Alcohol content is not a distinctive feature. At 15–30 per cent, most liqueurs have a lower alcohol content than spirits, but some liqueurs have an alcohol content as high as 55 per cent. Dessert wine, on the other hand, may taste like a liqueur, but contains no additional flavouring. Anise liqueurs have the interesting property of turning from transparent to cloudy when added to water: the oil of anise remains in solution in the presence of a high concentration of alcohol, but crystallises out when the alcohol concentration is reduced. Layered drinks made by floating different-coloured liqueurs in separate layers are attractive. Each liqueur is poured slowly into a glass over the back of a spoon or down a glass rod, so that the liquids of different densities remain unmixed, creating a striped effect. The word liqueur comes from the Latin liquifacere ('to liquefy'). A representative list of liqueur is given in Table 11.1.

Table 11.1. Some liqueurs and speciality alcoholic products.

Product	Notes	Country of origin
Absinthe	Brandy flavoured with sweet almonds and apricots	France
Advocaat	Brandy-base. Egg yolks, sugar and vanilla	Holland
Amaretto	Apricot kernel and bitter almond flavour	Italy
Anis	Anise/star anise/fennel flavour	Diverse
Arrack	Distillation of alcohol from grapes, sugar cane, rice or dates. Word means 'sweat'	Arabic
Bailey's	Irish whiskey and chocolate	Ireland
Benedictine	Brandy flavoured with 27 plants (including cardamom, cinnamon, cloves, juniper, nutmeg, tea, myrrh) and sugar. Coloured using saffron and caramel	France
Campari	Red product made by blending 68 herbs with quinine, Chinese rhubarb, cinchona bark and orange peels	Italy
Cassis	Macerated blackcurrants in neutral spirits and brandy	France
Chartreuse	Blend of 130 herbs and honey in brandy	–
Cherry brandy	Distilled juice of cherries, fermented in presence of crushed cherry stones, perhaps blended with Armagnac	Mainland Europe
Cointreau	Blend of distillates from bitter and sweet orange peel, plus sugar	France
Drambuie	Scotch whisky suffused with herbs, spices and heather honey	Scotland
Grande Marnier	Cognac blended with distillates of bitter orange and sugar	France
Malibu	Light rum/coconut	Barbados
Ouzo	Aniseed and fennel and mastic distilled in copper stills <1000 L	Greece
Pernod	Spirit base suffused with star anise, fennel, camomile, coriander, veronica and other herbs	France
Sambuca	Anis, star anise, elderflower, invert sugar	Italy
Southern comfort	Grain-based spirit containing peach and orange and sugar	United States
Tia Maria	Cane spirit/rum base with coffee and spices and sugar	Jamaica

SAKE

Sake or saké is a Japanese alcoholic beverage made from rice.

This beverage is called sake in English, but in Japanese, sake or o-sake refers to alcoholic drinks in general. The Japanese term for this specific beverage is Nihonshu, meaning 'Japanese sake'. Sake is also referred to in English as rice wine. However, unlike true wine, in which alcohol is produced by fermenting the sugar naturally present in fruit, sake is made through a brewing process more like that of beer. To make beer or sake, the sugar needed to produce alcohol must first be converted from starch. But the brewing process for sake differs from beer brewing as well, notably in that for beer, the conversion of starch to sugar and sugar to alcohol occurs in two discrete steps, but with sake they occur simultaneously. Additionally, alcohol content also differs between sake, wine and beer. Wine generally contains 9–16 per cent alcohol and most beer is 3–8 per cent, whereas undiluted sake is 18–20 per cent alcohol, although this is often lowered to around 15 per cent by diluting the sake with water prior to bottling.

Brewing

Sake is produced by the multiple parallel fermentation of rice. The rice is polished to remove the protein and oils from the exterior of the rice grains, leaving behind starch. A more thorough milling leads to fewer congeners and generally a more desirable product.

Newly polished rice is allowed to 'rest' until it absorbs enough moisture from the air not to crack when immersed in water. After this resting period, the rice is washed clean of the rice powder produced during milling and is steeped in water. The length of the soak depends on the degree to which the rice was polished, from several hours or even overnight for an ordinary milling to just minutes for highly polished rice.

After soaking, the rice is boiled in a large pot or it is steamed on a conveyor belt. The degree of cooking must be carefully controlled; overcooked rice will ferment too quickly for flavours to develop well and undercooked rice will only ferment on the outside. The steamed rice is then cooled and divided for different uses (Fig. 11.1).

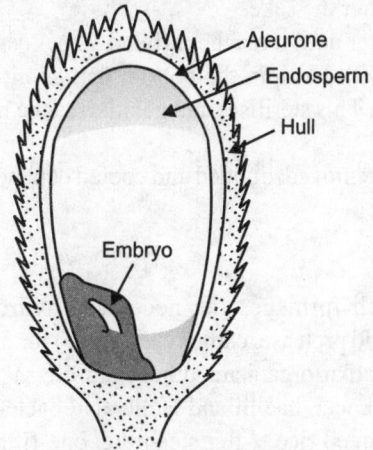

Fig. 11.1. A grain of rice.

Some of the steamed rice is taken to a culture room and inoculated with koji mould, (*Aspergillus oryzae*). The mould-laden rice is itself known as koji and is cultivated until the growth of the fungus reaches the desired level. This takes about two days.

When the koji is ready, the next step is to create the starter mash, known as shubo, or colloquially, moto. Koji rice, water and yeast are mixed together, and in the modern method, lactic acid is added to inhibit unwanted bacteria (in slower traditional methods, lactic acid occurs naturally). Next, freshly steamed rice is added and the yeast is cultivated over 10 to 15 days (in the modern method).

When the starter mash is ready, steamed rice, water, and more koji are added once a day for three days, doubling the volume of the mash each time. Staggering things this way allows the yeast to keep up with the increased volume. The mixture is now known as the main mash or moromi.

The main mash then ferments. This takes two to six weeks. With high-grade sake, fermentation is deliberately slowed by lowering the temperature to 10°C (50°F) or less.

Unlike malt for beer, rice for sake does not have the necessary amylase to convert starch to sugar and so must undergo a process of multiple fermentation, in which starch is converted to sugar by the koji, and sugar is converted to alcohol by yeast. With sake these two processes happen at the same time, not as separate steps, so sake is said to be made by multiple parallel fermentation.

After fermentation, sake is pressed to separate the liquid from the solids. With some sake, a small amount of distilled alcohol, called brewer's alcohol, is added before pressing in order to extract flavours and aromas that would otherwise stay in the solids. With cheap sake, a large amount of brewer's alcohol might be added to increase the volume of sake produced. Next, the remaining lees (a fine sediment) are removed, and the sake is carbon filtered and pasteurised. The sake is allowed to rest and mature and then it is usually diluted with water to lower the alcohol content from around 20 to 15 per cent or so, before finally being bottled.

Polishing, steeping and steaming

White rice with a slightly larger grain size than that generally used for food is reduced in weight by 25–30 per cent (or more than 50 per cent for some premium sakes) by the removal of outer layers. The latter jeopardise clarity and flavour and also impact the manner by which the mould grows. The more the polishing undertaken, the cleaner the sake.

The grain is then steeped in water until it reaches around 30 per cent moisture and is then transferred to a large wooden tub (koshiki) with holes in the bottom that admit steam. The mix is placed over a metal tub containing boiling water. This sterilises and gelatinises the rice, rendering it susceptible to the action of koji.

After 50–60 minutes the rice is removed, divided and cooled depending on which stage in the brewing process it is going to be used in.

Making koji

Koji comprises *A. oryzae*, which furnishes the necessary hydrolytic enzymes (α-glucosidase, glucoamylase, transglucosidase, acid protease, carboxypeptidase) for digesting the starch and the protein. The nature of the process is such that organisms other than the sake yeast will also develop. These include film-forming yeast, micrococci, bacilli and lactic acid bacteria. The rice employed for koji is more refined than the bulk of steamed rice. After steaming, one-fifth of the rice is removed from the koshiki and cooled to about 30°C. It is transferred to a double-walled solar-like room that retains heat. Dried spores of *A. oryzae* are scattered over the surface and kneaded in. Several hours later, the mix is transferred to shallow Japanese cedar wood trays (45 cm × 30 cm × 5.1 cm) that are put on shelves and covered with a cloth. As the koji mould grows, the temperature rises, so the mix is stirred twice every 4 hours. After 40–45 hours, the boxes are removed and advantage is taken of the low temperatures outside to stop the growth of koji. After cooling, the koji mix is light, dry and flaky and has a distinct aroma of horse chestnuts.

Making moto

The koji rice for making moto starter is basically treated in the same manner; however, the process is prolonged in order that even higher levels of enzymes are produced. Moto is the seed mash and represents less than 10 per cent of the total rice.

The longest standing method of moto production is mizu moto (bodai moto). Three kilograms of steamed rice already adventitiously infected with yeast from the air is sealed in a cloth bag and buried within uncooked polished rice (87 kg) to which is added 130 litres of water. After 4–5 days, the water becomes distinctly cloudy and bubbly and is sour. It is removed by filtration and the polished rice is steamed. A second mash is then produced with this yeasty water, all of the steamed rice and a further 40 kg of koji rice. The moto is ready for use after 5 days.

The disadvantage of this procedure is the emergence of high levels of lactic acid bacteria, causing the ensuing sake to be sour.

Since the 1920s the kimoto method has become the main approach to making moto. The mix comprises 75 kg steamed rice, 30 kg koji rice and 108 litre of water. This is divided in the early evening into 16 shallow wooden tubs, each of 70 cm diameter. Toji stir the mixture every 3–4 hours through the night (cooling by ambient chill air) and grind the moto the next day using long bamboo poles to which wooden panels are attached. The rice is rubbed against the bottom of the wooden tubs until the grains are reduced to approximately a third of their size and the mash comprises a thick paste. This procedure accelerates the activity of the koji.

The paste is transferred to a single large wooden vat and left for 2–3 days at 8°C. Then buckets of hot water are dropped into the mash, thereby raising the temperature and stimulating airborne yeasts into fermentation. The mix is maintained at 25°C and 20–25 days later, it is used as a starter for the main mash.

It is understood that in the early stages of the process, lactic acid bacteria prevent the growth of other, less desirable organisms. Later on the alcohol developed by yeast kills the lactic acid bacteria and any unwanted wild yeast.

Two other methods have evolved for making moto. The Yamahi process has the same principles as above, but there is an initial mixing of pure koji rice with water so as to accelerate saccharification before the addition of steamed rice. This has become the most popular method. The Sokujo process again has the same basic principle as for raw moto, but here the koji rice is mixed with water and lactic acid added to 5 per cent. At the same time, a pure culture of sake yeast is added to seed the fermentation. Steamed rice is mixed in before cooling and leaving for 2–3 days. Dakitaru is used to raise the temperature to 20°C. After 10–15 days, the mash is ready to use as a starter for the main mash.

Moromi

After the koji and moto are prepared, they are mixed over 4 days. This is traditionally in large wooden vats (7–20 kl). Increasingly large amounts of rice, koji rice and water are added to the moto on the first, third and fourth days. The addition rates (relative to moto) are 1:1 on the first day, 2:1 on the third day and 4:1 on the fourth day. Through the first and second days, the temperature is allowed to rise to 15°C and the whole is left uncovered. The endogenous acidity prevents the growth of spoilage bacteria. On the third day, the temperature is lowered to 9°–10°C and this further suppresses infection. After the fourth day addition, the ensuing 15–18 days represent a challenge for temperature control, unless the facilities are sufficiently modern to incorporate cooling.

Traditional brewers still operate in the winter months, with the use of slatted windows for cooling. In modern facilities, brewing can proceed around the year.

After 15–18 days, the mixture is filtered through weighted long narrow cotton sacks over a wooden 'sake boat' (sakafune). The sake trickles through a spigot at the base of the boat. The residual lees are sold for the pickling of vegetables and for use in cooking.

New sake is held for 10 days at a low temperature, during which time glucose and acid levels are enzymically lowered. Then it is pasteurised at 60°C and transferred to sealed vats, traditionally fabricated from Japanese cedar, where it will be held for 6–12 months. This allows a mellowing of the product which starts as being yellow, harsh and smelling of koji. During ageing, characters are developed in the sake from the wood.

After ageing there will be a blending ('marrying') followed by dilution with water to a final strength of 15–17 per cent ABV and bottling.

Modern sake making

In modern facilities, the vessels are likely to be fabricated from stainless steel. Rectified alcohol is likely to be employed as a proportion of the sake alcohol, and glucose, lactic acid and monosodium glutamate may also play a role in 'tripling the sake'. These are added to the final mash as a fourth addition. There is extensive use nowadays of the premier sake yeast strains, with cross-breeding to combine the best properties in a single strain.

In the latest moto processes at high temperature (koon toka mota), the moto mash is raised to 55°C for 5–8 hours. Lactic acid is added and the mix is cooled to 20°C prior to the addition of yeast. The entire process takes 5–7 days. It may be computer-controlled. Activated charcoal may be employed in place of sake boats.

A simplified overview of sake production is offered in Fig. 11.2.

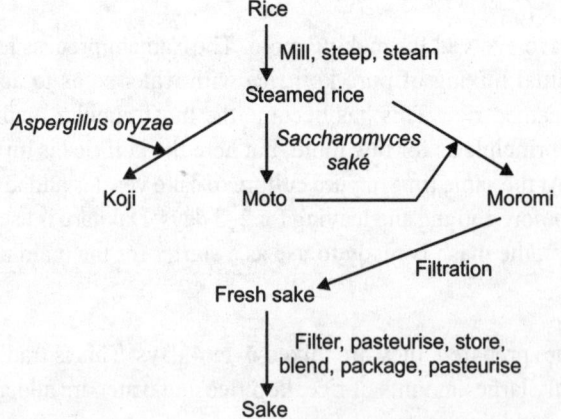

Fig. 11.2. Overview of sake production.

Flavour of sake

Apart from ethanol, significant contributors to the flavour of sake (derived via yeast metabolism) are other alcohols, esters and acids, including lactic acid from the moto stage (Table 11.2).

Table 11.2. Contributors to the flavour of sake.

Compound	Typical level (mg l⁻¹)
Propan-1-ol	120
Isoamyl alcohol	70–250
2-Phenylethanol	75
Isobutanol	65
Ethyl acetate	50–120
Ethyl caproate	10
Isoamyl acetate	10
Succinic acid	500–700
Malic acid	200–400
Citric acid	100–500
Acetic acid	50–200
Lactic acid	300–500

Serving temperature

Sakes are customarily served at 20°C when compared for taste. The sake is held in pitchers called tokkuri for pouring into cups known as sakazuki.

The precise manner by which sake is served depends very much on the season, any food that it is accompanying and on the type of sake. Many experts would be of the opinion that warming sake distorts the taste and should be avoided. However, another opinion is that dry sake is better warm (not hot). Nurukan means lukewarm (20°–40°C); kan is when sake is 40°–45°C (this is standard when sake is asked for warm); atsukan is when the sake is at 55°–60°C.

Varieties

Various types of sake offered for sale at a Japanese grocery in the United States. There are two basic types of sake: futsu-shu and tokutei meisho-shu. Futsu-shu, 'ordinary sake', is the equivalent of table wine and accounts for the majority of sake produced. Tokutei meisho-shu, 'special designation sake', refers to premium sakes distinguished by the degree to which the rice is polished and the added percentage of brewer's alcohol or the absence of such additives.

The three types of special designation sake are briefly discussed:

1. Honjozo-shu, in which a slight amount of brewer's alcohol is added to the sake before pressing, in order to extract extra flavours and aromas from the mash. This term was created in the late 1960s to distinguish it, a premium sake, from cheaply made liquors to which large amounts of distilled alcohol were added simply to increase volume. Sake with this designation must be made with no more than 116 litres of pure alcohol added for every 1,000 kilograms of rice.

2. Junmai-shu, 'pure rice sake', made from only rice, water and koji, with no brewer's alcohol or other additives. Before 2004, the Japanese government mandated that junmai-shu must be made from rice polished down to 70 per cent or less of its original weight, but that restriction has been removed.

3. Ginjo-shu, made from rice polished to 60 per cent or less of its original weight. Sake made from rice polished to 50 per cent or lower is called daiginjo-shu.

The term junmai can be added to ginjo or daiginjo, resulting in junmai ginjo and junmai daiginjo. However, as distilled alcohol is added in small amounts to ginjo and daiginjo to heighten the aroma, not to increase volume, a junmai daiginjo is not necessarily a better product than a daiginjo made with brewer's alcohol.

In addition to 'ordinary' sake and the special designations, there are many more types of sake.

Three ways to make the starter mash are given below:

1. Kimoto is the traditionally orthodox method for preparing the starter mash, which includes the laborious process of grinding it into a paste. This method was the standard for 300 years, but it is rarely used today.
2. Yamahai is a simplified version of the kimoto method, introduced in the early 1900s. Yamahai skips the step of making a paste out of the starter mash. That step of the kimoto method is known as yama-oroshi, and the full name for yamahai is 'yama-oroshi haishi', meaning 'discontinuation of yama-oroshi'. While the yamahai method was originally developed to speed production time, it is slower than the modern method and is now used only in speciality brews for the earthy flavours it produces.
3. Sokujo, 'quick fermentation', is the modern method of preparing the starter mash. Lactic acid, produced naturally in the two slower traditional methods, is added to the starter to inhibit unwanted bacteria. Sokujo sake tends to have a lighter flavour than kimoto or yamahai.

Different handling after fermentation:

1. Nigori or unfiltered sake.
2. Namazake is sake that has not been pasteurised. It requires refrigerated storage and has a shorter shelf-life than pasteurised sake.
3. Genshu is undiluted sake. Most sake is diluted with water after brewing, to lower the alcohol content from 18-20 per cent down to 14–16 per cent, but genshu is not.
4. Muroka means unfiltered. Note that this refers to sake that hasn't been carbon filtered, but which has been pressed and separated from the lees, and thus is clear, not cloudy. Carbon filtration can remove desirable flavours and odours as well as bad ones, thus muroka sake has stronger flavours than filtered varieties.
5. Nigorizake is cloudy sake. The sake is passed through a loose mesh to separate it from the mash. It isn't filtered thereafter and there is much rice sediment in the bottle. Before serving, the bottle is shaken to mix the sediment and turn the sake white or cloudy.
6. Seishu, 'clear/clean sake', is the Japanese legal definition of sake and refers to sake in which the solids have been strained out, leaving clear liquid. Thus nigorizake and doburoku are not seishu and therefore aren't actually sake under Japanese law. However, nigorizake can get seishu status by being strained clear and having lees put back in afterward.
7. Koshu is 'aged sake'. Most sake does not age well, but this specially made type can age for decades, turning yellow and acquiring a honeyed flavour.
8. Taruzake is sake aged in wooden barrels or bottled in wooden casks. The wood used is Cryptomeria, which is also inaccurately known as Japanese cedar. Sake casks are often broken open ceremonially for the opening of buildings, businesses, parties, etc. Because the wood imparts a strong flavour, premium sake is rarely used for this type.
9. Shiboritate, 'freshly pressed', refers to sake that has been shipped without the traditional six-month ageing/maturation period. The result is usually a more acidic, 'greener' sake.

10. Fukurozuri is a method of separating sake from the lees without external pressure, by hanging the mash in bags and allowing the liquid to drip out under its own weight. Sake produced this way is sometimes called shizukazake, meaning 'drip sake'.

11. Tobingakoi is when sake is pressed into 18-litre bottles ('tobin') and the brewer selects the best sake of the batch for shipping.

Others

1. Doburoku is the classic home-brew style of sake (although home brewing is illegal in Japan). It is created by simply adding koji mould or sake lees to steamed rice and water and letting the mixture ferment. The resulting sake is somewhat like a chunkier version of nigorizake.

2. Kuroshu is sake made from unpolished rice (i.e. brown rice), more like Chinese rice wine.

3. Teiseihaku-shu is sake with a deliberately high rice polishing ratio. It is generally held that the lower the rice polishing ratio (the per cent weight after polishing), the better the potential of the sake. However, beginning around 2005, teiseihaku-shu has been produced as a speciality sake made with high rice polishing ratios, usually around 80 per cent, to produce sake with the characteristic flavour of rice itself.

Some other terms commonly used in connection with sake:

1. Nihonshu-do, also called the Sake Meter Value, or SMV SMV $= (|1/\text{specific gravity}|-1) \times 1443$.

2. Specific gravity is measured on a scale weighing the same volume of water at 4°C and sake at 15°C. The sweeter the sake is, the lower the number gets. When the SMV was first used, 0 was designated the point between sweet sake and dry sake. Now +3 is considered neutral.

3. Seimai-buai is the rice polishing ratio, the percentage of weight remaining after polishing. Generally, the lower the number, the better the sake's potential. A lower percentage usually results in a fruitier sake, whereas a higher percentage will taste more like rice.

4. Kasu are pressed sake lees, the solids left after pressing and filtering. These are used for making tsukemono pickles, livestock feed and shochu, and as an ingredient in dishes like kasu soup.

Serving sake

Sake can be served in a wide variety of cups; here is a sakazuki (a flat, saucer-like cup), an ochoko (a small, cylindrical cup), and a masu (a wooden, box-like cup).

In Japan sake is served chilled, at room temperature, or heated, depending on the preference of the drinker, the quality of the sake, and the season. Typically, hot sake is a winter drink, and high-grade sake is not drunk hot, because the flavours and aromas will be lost. This masking of flavour is the reason that low-quality sake is often served hot. Sake is usually drunk from small cups called choko and poured into the choko from ceramic flasks called tokkuri. Saucer-like cups called sakazuki are also used, most commonly at weddings and other ceremonial occasions. Recently, footed glasses made specifically for premium sake have also come into use.

Another traditional cup is the masu, a box usually made of hinoki or sugi, which was originally used for measuring rice. In some Japanese restaurants, as a show of generosity, the server may put a glass inside the masu or put the masu on a saucer and pour until sake overflows and fills both containers.

Aside from being served straight, sake can be used as a mixer for cocktails, such as tamagozake, saketinis, nogasake or the sake bomb.

Storage

In general, it is best to keep sake refrigerated in a cool or dark room, as prolonged exposure to heat or direct light will lead to spoilage. Sake stored at room temperature is best consumed within a few months after purchase.

After opening the bottle of sake, it is best consumed within 2 or 3 hours. It is possible to store in the refrigerator, but it is recommended to finish the sake within 2 days. This is because once premium sake is opened, it begins to oxidise which affects the taste. If the sake is kept in the refrigerator for more than 3 days, it will lose its 'best' flavour. However, this does not mean it should be disposed of if not consumed. Generally, sake can keep very well and still taste just fine after weeks in the fridge. How long a sake will remain drinkable depends on the actual product itself, and whether it is sealed with a wine vacuum top.

Ceremonial use

A cask of sake before the kagami biraki. Sake is often consumed as part of Shinto purification rituals (compare with the use of grape wine in the Christian Eucharist). During World War II, kamikaze pilots drank sake prior to carrying out their missions.

In a ceremony called kagami biraki, wooden casks of sake are opened with mallets during Shinto festivals, weddings, store openings, sports and election victories, and other celebrations. This sake, called iwai-zake ('celebration sake'), is served freely to all to spread good fortune.

On the New Year many Japanese people drink a special sake called toso. Toso is a sort of iwai-zake made by soaking tososan, a Chinese powdered medicine, overnight in sake. Even children sip a portion. In some regions, the first sipping of toso is taken in order of age from younger to older.

Chapter 12

Meat and Meat Products

INTRODUCTION

Meat is animal flesh that is used as food. Most often, this means the skeletal muscle and associated fat, but it may also describe other edible tissues such as organs, livers, skin, brains, bone marrow, kidneys or lungs. The word meat is also used by the meat packing and butchering industry in a more restrictive sense — the flesh of mammalian species (pigs, cattle, etc.) raised and prepared for human consumption, to the exclusion of fish, poultry and eggs.

Originally meat was a term used to describe any solid food, but has now come to be applied, almost solely to animal flesh. As such, it has played a significant role in the human diet since the days of hunting and gathering, and animals (sheep) were first domesticated at the beginning of the Neolithic revolution around 9000 BC. Though abjured by some on moral or religious grounds, meat eating remains widely popular today. In the main, this is due to its desirable texture and flavour characteristics, although meat protein does also have a high biological value.

Meat consumption is often something of a status symbol and is generally far greater in wealthy societies. This is because large-scale meat production is a relatively inefficient means of obtaining protein. It requires agriculture to produce a surplus of plant proteins which can be fed to animals: with modern production techniques, it takes two kilos of grain to obtain 1 kilo of chicken, four for 1 kilo of pork and eight for 1 kilo of beef.

Though numerous species are used as a source of meat around the world, ranging from flying foxes to frogs and from kangaroos to crocodiles, the meat animals of principal importance in economic terms are cattle, pigs, sheep, goats and poultry.

STRUCTURE AND COMPOSITION

Edible animal flesh comprises principally the muscular tissues but also includes organs such as the heart, liver and kidneys. Most microbiological studies on meat have been conducted with muscular tissues and it is on these that the information presented here is based. Though in many respects the microbiology will be broadly similar for other tissues, it should be remembered that differences may arise from particular aspects of their composition and microflora.

Structurally muscle is made up of muscle fibres; long, thin, multi-nucleate cells bound together in bundles by connective tissue. Each muscle fibre is surrounded by a cell membrane, the sarcolemma, within which are contained the myofibrils, complexes of the two major muscle proteins, myosin and actin, surrounded by the sarcoplasm. The approximate chemical composition of typical adult mammalian muscle after *rigor mortis* is presented in Table 12.1. Its high water activity and abundant nutrients make meat an excellent medium to support microbial growth. Though many of the micro-organisms that grow on meat are proteolytic, they grow initially at the expense of the most readily utilised substrates—the water soluble pool of carbohydrates and nonprotein nitrogen. Extensive proteolysis only occurs in the later stages of decomposition when the meat is usually already well spoiled from a sensory point of view.

Table 12.1. Chemical composition of typical adult mammalian muscle after *rigor mortis*.

		% weight
Water	–	75.0
Protein	–	19.0
Myofibrillar	11.5	–
Sarcoplasmic	5.5	–
Connective	2.0	–
Lipid	–	2.5
Carbohydrate	–	1.2
Lactic acid	0.9	–
Glycogen	0.1	–
Glucose and glycolytic intermediates	0.2	–
Soluble non-protein nitrogen		1.95
Creatine	0.55	
Inosine mono phosphate	0.30	–
NAD/NADP Nucleotides	0.30	–
Nucleotides	0.10	–
Amino acids	0.35	–
Carnosine, anserine	0.35	–
Inorganic	–	0.85
Total soluble phosphorus	0.20	–
Potassium	0.35	–
Sodium	0.05	–
Magnesium	0.02	–
Other metals	0.23	–
Vitamins		

The carbohydrate content of muscle has a particularly important bearing on its microbiology. Glycogen is a polymer of glucose held in the liver and muscles as an energy store for the body. During life, oxygen is supplied to muscle cells in the animal by the circulatory system and glycogen can be broken down to provide energy by the glycolytic and respiratory pathways to yield carbon dioxide and water.

After death the supply of oxygen to the muscles is cut off, the redox potential falls and respiration ceases, but the glycolytic breakdown of glycogen continues leading to an accumulation of lactic acid and a decrease in muscle pH. Provided sufficient glycogen is present, this process will continue until the glycolytic enzymes are inactivated by the low pH developed. In a typical mammalian muscle the pH will drop from an initial value of around 7 to 5.4–5.5 with the accumulation of about 1 per cent lactic acid. Where there is a limited supply of glycogen in the muscle, acidification will continue only until the glycogen runs out and the muscle will have a higher ultimate pH. This can happen if the muscle has been exercised before slaughter but can also result from stress or exposure to cold. When the ultimate pH is above 6.2, it gives rise to dark cutting meat, a condition also known as dry, firm, dark (DFD) condition. Because the pH is relatively high, the meat proteins are above their isoelectric point and will retain much of the moisture present. The fibres will be tightly packed together giving the meat a dry, firm texture and impeding oxygen transfer. This, coupled with the higher residual activity of cytochrome enzymes, will mean that the meat has the dark colour of myoglobin rather than the bright red oxymyoglobin colour. The higher pH will also mean that microbial growth is faster so spoilage will occur sooner. Another meat defect associated with post-mortem changes in muscle carbohydrates is known as pale, soft, exudative (PSE) condition. This occurs mainly in pigs and has no microbiological implications but does give rise to lower processing yields, increased cooking losses and reduced juiciness. The PSE condition results when normal non-exercised muscle is stimulated just before slaughter leading to a rapid post-mortem fall in pH while the muscle is still relatively warm. This denatures sarcoplasmic proteins, moisture is expelled from the tissues which assume a pale colour due to the open muscle texture and the oxidation of myoglobin to metmyoglobin.

MICROBIOLOGY OF PRIMARY PROCESSING

The tissues of a healthy animal are protected against infection by a combination of physical barriers and the activity of the immune system. Consequently, internal organs and muscles from a freshly slaughtered carcass should be relatively free from micro-organisms. Microbial numbers detected in aseptically sampled tissues are usually less than 10 cfu kg^{-1}, although there is evidence that numbers can increase under conditions of stress and they will of course be higher if the animal is suffering from an infection. Since some animal diseases can be transmitted to humans, meat for human consumption should be produced only from healthy animals. Visual inspection before and after slaughter to identify and exclude unfit meat is the general rule, although it will only detect conditions which give some macroscopic pathological sign.

The most heavily colonised areas of the animal that may contaminate meat are the skin (fleece) and gastrointestinal tract. Numbers and types of organisms carried at these sites will reflect both the animal's indigenous microflora and its environment. The animal hide, for example, will carry a mixed microbial population of micrococci, staphylococci, pseudomonads, yeasts and moulds as well as organisms derived from sources such as soil or faeces. Organisms of faecal origin are more likely to be encountered on hides from intensively reared cattle or from those transported or held in crowded conditions.

With reasonable standards of hygienic operations, contamination of meat carcasses from processing equipment, knives and process workers is less important than contamination from the animals themselves. The greatest opportunity for this occurs during dressing, the stages during which the head, feet, hides, excess fat, viscera and offal generated from the bones and muscular tissues.

Skinning can spread contamination from the hide to the freshly exposed surface of the carcass through direct contact and via the skinning knife or handling. Washing the animal prior to slaughter can reduce microbial numbers on the hide but control is most effectively exercised by skilful and hygienic removal of the hide. The viscera contain large numbers of micro-organisms, including potential pathogens, and great care must be taken to ensure the carcass is not contaminated with visceral contents either as a result of puncture or leakage from the anus or oesophagus during removal.

After dressing, carcasses are washed to remove visible contamination. This will have only a minor effect on the surface microflora, although bactericidal washing treatments such as hot water (80°C), chlorinated water (50 mg l^{-1}) or dilute lactic acid (1–2 per cent) have been shown to reduce the surface microflora by amounts varying between about 1 and 3.5 log cycles.

After dressing the carcass is cooled to chill temperatures during which cold shock may cause some reduction in numbers. At chill temperatures, microbial growth among the survivors is restricted to those psychrotrophs present and these can be further inhibited by the partial surface drying that takes place. Surface numbers of bacteria at the end of dressing will typically be of the order of 10^2–10^4 cfu cm^{-2}. Counts are generally higher in sheep carcasses than beef and higher still in pigs which are processed differently, the skin not being removed from the carcass but scalded and dehaired.

Psychrotrophic organisms form only a small percentage of the initial microflora but come to predominate subsequently as the meat is held constantly at chill temperatures. An increase in microbial numbers is seen during cutting and boning, but this is due less to microbial growth, since the operation is usually completed within a few hours at temperatures below 10°C, than to the spreading of contamination to freshly exposed meat surfaces by equipment such as knives, saws and cutting tables.

The primary processing of poultry differs from red meat in a number of respects that have microbiological implications. First among these is the sheer scale of modern poultry operations where processing plants can have production rates up to 12000 birds per hour. This leave's little opportunity for effectively sanitising equipment and exacerbates problems associated with some of the procedures and equipment used which favour the spread of micro-organisms between carcasses.

During transport to the plant contamination can be spread between birds by faeces and feathers and from inadequately cleaned transport cages. Once at the plant, birds are hung by their feet on lines, electrically stunned and killed by cutting the carotid artery. The close proximity of the birds and the flapping wings further contribute to the spread of contamination.

This is followed by scalding where the birds are immersed in hot water at about 50°C to facilitate subsequent removal of the feathers. Each bird contributes large numbers of micro-organisms to the scald water and these will be spread between birds. This can be reduced to some extent by using a counter-current flow of birds and water so that the birds leaving the scalder are in contact with the cleanest water. Higher scald water temperatures will eliminate most vegetative bacteria but cause an unacceptable loosening of the skin cuticle.

After scalding, birds are mechanically defeathered by a system of rotating rubber fingers. A number of studies have demonstrated how these can pass organisms, for example *Salmonella*, from one carcass to others following it and when the fingers become worn or damaged they are liable to microbial colonisation. As the poultry carcass is not skinned, skin-associated organisms will not be removed.

The intestinal tract of poultry will contain high numbers of organisms including pathogens such as *Salmonella* and *Campylobacter*. Poultry evisceration therefore poses similar microbiological hazards to those with other animals but the size and structure of the carcass make it a much more difficult operation to execute hygienically.

To allow high processing rates, poultry evisceration is usually automated but this too leads to a high incidence of carcass contamination with gut contents. Since the carcasses are not split like those of sheep and cattle, effective washing of the gut cavity after evisceration is more difficult.

Poultry to be frozen is usually chilled in water and this offers a further opportunity for cross contamination. This is controlled by chlorination of the cooling water, use of a counter-current flow as in scalding, and a sufficient flow rate of water to avoid the build up of contamination.

SPOILAGE OF FRESH MEAT

Aerobic storage of chilled red meats, either unwrapped or covered with an oxygen permeable film, produces a high redox potential at the meat surface suitable for the growth of psychrotrophic aerobes. Non-fermentative Gram-negative rods grow most rapidly under these conditions and come to dominate the spoilage microflora that develops. Taxonomic description of these organisms has been somewhat unsettled over the years with some being described as *Moraxella* and *Moraxella*-like. Such terms have now been largely abandoned in favour of a concensus that has emerged from numerical taxonomy studies. In this, the principal genera are described as *Pseudomonas*, *Acinetobacter* and *Psychrobacter* with *Pseudomonas* species such as *P. fragi*, *P. lundensis* and *P. fluorescens* generally predominating. A dichotomous key describing the differential characteristics of these organisms and some of the names used previously to describe them is presented as Fig. 12.1. Other organisms are usually only a minor component of the spoilage microflora, but include psychrotrophic Enterobacteriaceae such as *Serratia liquefaciens* and *Enterobacter agglomerans*, lactic acid bacteria and the Gram-positive *Brochothrix thermosphacta*.

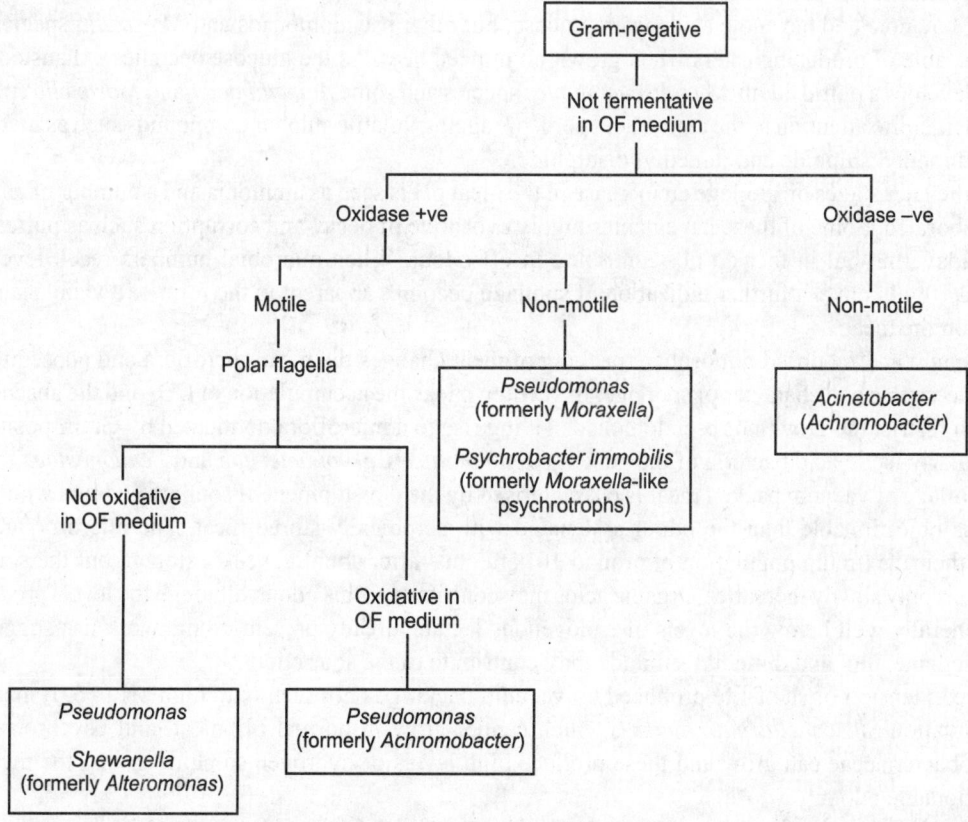

Fig. 12.1. Characteristics of some Gram-negatives associated with meat.

The first indication of spoilage in fresh meat is the production of off odours which become apparent when microbial numbers reach around 10^7 cfu cm^{-2}. At this point it is believed that the micro-organisms switch from the diminishing levels of glucose in the meat to amino acids as a substrate for growth. In meat with lower levels of residual glucose this stage is reached earlier (10^6 cfu cm^{-2}) and this accounts for the earlier onset of spoilage in high pH meat.

Bacterial metabolism produces a complex mixture of volatile esters, alcohols, ketones and sulphur-containing compounds which collectively comprise the off odours detected. Such mixtures can be analysed by a combination of gas chromatography and mass spectrometry and the origin of different compounds can be established by pure culture studies. These have confirmed the predominant role of pseudomonads in spoilage of aerobically stored chilled meat. Usually the different spoilage taints appear in a sequence reflecting the order in which components of the meat are metabolised. The first indication of spoilage is generally the buttery or cheesy odour associated with production of diacetyl (2,3-butanediune), acetoin (3-hydroxy-2-butanone), 3-methylbutanol and 2-methylpropanol. These compounds are produced from glucose by members of the Enterobacteriaceae, lactic acid bacteria and *Brochothrix thermosphacta*. Pseudomonads then begin to increase in importance and the meat develops a sweet or fruity odour. This is due to production of a range of esters by *Pseudomonas* and *Moraxella* species degrading glucose and amino acids and by esterification of acids and alcohols produced during the first phase of spoilage. Ester production is particularly associated with *Pseudomonas fragi* which can produce ethyl esters of acetic, butanoic and hexanoic acids from glucose, but other pseudomonads and *Moraxella* species are also capable of producing esters when grown on minced beef. As the glucose becomes exhausted, the meat develops a putrid odour when *Pseudomonas* species and some *Acinetobacter* and *Moraxella* species turn their entire attention to the amino acid pool, producing volatile sulphur compounds such as methane thiol, dimethyl sulphide and dimethyl disulphide.

In the later stages of spoilage an increase in the meat pH is seen as ammonia and a number of amines are elaborated. Some of these have names highly evocative of decay and corruption such as putrescine and cadaverine but in fact do not contribute to off odour. When microbial numbers reach levels of around 10^8 cfu cm^{-2}, a further indication of spoilage becomes apparent in the form of a visible surface slime on the meat.

Vacuum and modified-atmosphere packing of meat changes the meat microflora and consequently the time-course and character of spoilage. In vacuum packs the accumulation of CO_2 and the absence of oxygen restrict the growth of pseudomonads giving rise to a microflora dominated by Gram-positives, particularly lactic acid bacteria of the genera *Lactobacillus*, *Carnobacterium* and *Leuconostoc*.

Spoilage of vacuum packed meat is characterised by the development of sour acid odours which are far less objectionable than the odour associated with aerobically stored meat. The micro-organisms reach their maximum population of around 10^7 cfu cm^{-2} after about a week's storage but the souring develops only slowly thereafter. Organic acids may contribute to this odour, although the levels produced are generally well below the levels of endogenous lactate already present. Some work has suggested that methane thiol and dimethyl sulphide may contribute to the sour odour.

The extension of shelf-life produced by vacuum packing is not seen with high pH (>6.0) meat. In this situation *Shewanella putrefaciens*, which cannot grow in normal pH meat, and psychrotrophic Enterobacteriaceae can grow and these produce high levels of hydrogen sulphide giving the meat an objectionable odour.

In modified-atmospheres containing elevated levels of both CO_2 and O_2 growth of pseudomonads is restricted by the CO_2 while the high levels of O_2 maintain the bright red colour of oxygenated myoglobin in the meat. Here the microflora depends on the type of meat, its storage temperature, and whether it was vacuum packed or aerobically stored previously. In general terms though, the micro flora and spoilage tend to follow a similar pattern to that of vacuum packed meat. Heterofermentative lactic acid bacteria can be more numerous due to the stimulatory effect of oxygen on their growth and, under some circumstances, *Brochothrix thermosphacta*, Enterobacteriaceae and pseudomonads can be more important.

Meat can be processed in a number of different ways which affect its characteristics, shelf-life and microbiology. The variety of these is illustrated by Fig. 12.2.

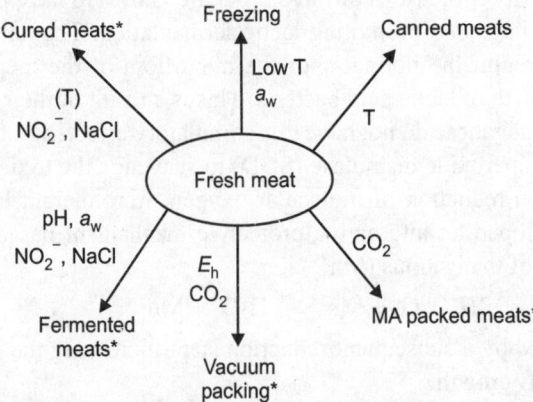

Fig. 12.2. Meat and meat products. T indicates elevated temperature; E_h, low redox potential; pH, reduced pH; a_w reduced a_w and *stored at chill temperatures.

FERMENTED MEATS

Fermented sausages are sometimes claimed to have originated in the Mediterranean region, although traditional products in China and Southeast Asia suggest that they probably developed independently in several locations. Like cheese-making, meat fermentation is a method for improving the keeping qualities of an otherwise highly perishable commodity. Key features in this are the combination of lactic fermentation with salting and drying which, in many cases, produces a product which is shelf-stable at ambient temperatures.

A further similarity to cheese is the bewildering variety of different types, 330 produced in Germany alone. In the United States fermented sausages are divided into two categories: dry, which have a moisture content of 35 per cent or less, and semi-dry typically containing about 50 per cent moisture. Spreadable fermented sausages, produced in Germany, such as Teewurst and Mellwurst are not dried during production and in this respect are similar to the Thai product *nam*.

The ingredients of a European-style fermented sausage may comprise:

Lean meat	55–70 per cent
Fat	25–40 per cent
Curing salts	3 per cent
Fermentable carbohydrate	0.4–2.0 per cent
Spices and flavouring	0.5 per cent
Starter, acidulant, ascorbic acid, etc.	0.5 per cent

Pork is most commonly used in southern Europe but elsewhere beef, mutton and turkey meat are also used. The meat should always be of high quality since the products are usually consumed without cooking and so are essentially a raw-meat product. Unlike fermented milk products, it is not possible to heat treat the meat before processing as this would destroy the sausage's textural characteristics, but some are given a final pasteurisation to ensure safety.

The curing salts added are a similar mixture of sodium chloride and sodium nitrate and/or nitrite to that used in the production of cured meats such as ham and bacon. Here too, they contribute to the taste, colour, safety, stability and texture of the product.

Spices are added primarily for reasons of flavour but are known to have potentially important roles in retarding microbial spoilage and promoting lactic fermentation. The antimicrobial effect of spice components, could help inhibit the normal spoilage microflora of the meat. Spices have also been shown to stimulate the growth of lactic acid bacteria. This is a result of their manganese content, spice extracts or spices low in manganese do not have this stimulatory effect. Most aerobes have micromolar quantities of the enzyme superoxide dismutase (SOD) to scavenge the toxic superoxide anion radical produced by a one-electron reduction of molecular oxygen. Aerotolerant lactic acid bacteria do not have SOD but have developed an alternative protective mechanism based on the accumulation of millimolar concentrations of manganous (Mn^{2+}) ion.

$$2H^+ + O_2^- + Mn^{2+} \rightarrow H_2O_2 + Mn^{3+} \qquad \ldots (12.1)$$

The Mn^{2+} is regenerated by a subsequent reduction step. Increasing the manganese content of the medium can stimulate LAB growth.

Other ingredients which may be included are glucono-δ-lactone which improves acidulation by slowly hydrolysing to produce gluconic acid, ascorbic acid to improve colour production and stability, and glucose to supplement the available fermentable sugar in the starting mix.

Ingredients are blended together in a bowlchopper at low temperature. When the ingredients have been blended together they are packed into casings of the appropriate diameter. Traditionally collagen from the gastrointestinal tract of animals has been used but nowadays fibrous cellulose and regenerated collagen produced from animal hides are more common. The packing material must have certain properties: it must adhere to the meat mix and must shrink with it during processing and must be permeable to moisture and smoke.

Fermented sausages are still often made by natural fermentations in which the selectivity of the starting mix determines which components of the heterogeneous microflora dominate. Starter cultures are however being increasingly used for the greater assurance of a satisfactory fermentation they provide. The principal components of commercial starters are lactic acid bacteria and nitrate-reducing bacteria. Some will also include yeasts and moulds such as *Debaryomyces hansenii* and *Candida famata*, and moulds, usually *Penicillium* spp. such as *P. nalgionense*. LAB included in early starters were mainly *Lactobacillus plantarum*, *Pediococcus acidilactici* and *Ped. pentosaceus*, not necessarily those most important in the natural fermentation. Surveys of naturally fermented products demonstrated that the dominant LAB were psychrotrophic, facultatively heterofermentative lactobacilli that were slightly less acid tolerant than usual (minimum pH 3.9 compared with 3.7–3.8). Most of these are now assigned to the species *Lactobacillus* sake and *Lactobacillus curvatus* and strains of these have been incorporated into commercial starters.

Members of the Micrococcaceae such as *Micrococcus varians* and *Staphylococcus carnosus* are important with respect to the reduction of nitrate to nitrite although this activity has also been demonstrated in some lactobacilli. Their presence would not be required in nitrite-cured products.

Sausage fermentations are conducted at temperatures ranging from 15°C up to in excess of 40°C, depending on the starter used, and last for 20–60 hours. The relative humidity is also controlled to ensure that a slow drying of the product commences. Acid production and the decrease of the pH to below 5.2 promote the coagulation of meat proteins and this aids moisture expulsion and development of the desired texture and flavour. It also contributes to the microbiological stability and safety of the product. North American and northern European sausages are often smoked. This confers a characteristic flavour but phenolic components of the wood smoke also have important anti-oxidative and antimicrobial properties which improve shelf-life. Fungal growth may occur on the surface of unsmoked sausages providing a particular character to these products as a result of fungal lipolytic, proteolytic and antioxidative activity.

In the final drying stage which can last up to 6 weeks, the moisture content is reduced further by storage at low temperatures, 7°–15°C, and at low relative humidity (65–85 per cent).

The combination of antimicrobial hurdles or barriers introduced during sausage fermentation is normally sufficient to ensure product safety. *Staphylococcus aureus* with its ability to tolerate reduced a_w and pH and grow anaerobically would seem well suited to growth in these products. Occasional outbreaks of *Staph. aureus* food poisoning have been reported from the United States where higher fermentation temperatures are used. However, studies suggest that *Staph. aureus* does not compete well with the LAB present, particularly if the latter have a large numerical superiority as a result of starter addition. The risk is also reduced since enterotoxin production appears to be more susceptible than growth to inhibition by adverse conditions.

Numbers of *Salmonella* and other Enterobacteriaceae have been shown to fall throughout fermentation and drying. It is, therefore, most important that only good quality raw materials are used so that undue reliance is not placed upon these factors.

Outbreaks of Verotoxin producing *E. coli* in the United States associated with fermented meats highlighted this problem and prompted the US Food Safety and Inspection Service to recommend that the procedures used in the production of ready-to-eat fermented products should achieve a 5 $\log_{10}$ cfu g^{-1} reduction in pathogen numbers.

One way of achieving this reliably would be to introduce a heating step. Following an outbreak of salmonellosis in the UK associated with a salami stick product imported from Germany, the production process was changed to incorporate a final pasteurisation step without adverse effects on sensory quality.

Nam, the Thai fermented sausage, differs in several respects from European fermented sausages. It is a low-fat product which is subjected to a short fermentation and is not dried. It is also wrapped in water-impermeable plastic material or, traditionally, banana leaves. As the fermentation proceeds and the pH drops the moisture is expelled but is trapped within the packaging giving the consumer an indication of the age of the product. It is not always stored chilled and its largely anecdotal association with food poisoning has prompted test marketing of irradiated *nam* in some areas of Thailand.

CONTAMINATION, PRESERVATION AND SPOILAGE OF MEAT AND MEAT PRODUCTS

Contamination

The healthy inner flesh of meats has been reported to contain few or no micro-organisms, although they have been found in lymph nodes, bone marrow and even flesh. The important contamination, however, comes from external sources during bleeding, handling and processing. During bleeding, skinning and cutting, the main sources of micro-organisms are the exterior of the animal (hide, hoofs and hair) and the intestinal tract. Recently approved 'humane' methods of slaughter, mechanical, chemical or electrical, have little effect on contamination, but each method is followed by sticking and bleeding, which can introduce contamination. As with the older methods of use of a knife on hogs and poultry, any contaminating bacteria on the knife soon will be found in meat in various parts of the carcass, carried there by blood and lymph. The exterior of the animal harbours large numbers and many kinds of micro-organisms from soil, water, feed and manure, as well as its natural surface flora, and the intestinal contents contain the intestinal organisms (Table 12.2). Knives, cloths, air and hands and clothing of the workers can serve as intermediate sources of contaminants. During the handling of the meat thereafter, contamination can come from carts, boxes or other containers, from other contaminated meat, from air and from personnel. Especially undesirable is the addition of psychrophilic bacteria from any source, e.g. from other meats that have been in chilling storage. Special equipment such as grinders, sausage stuffers and casings, and ingredients in special products, e.g. fillers and spices, may add undesirable organisms in appreciable numbers, and sawdust on floors of processing rooms may contaminate meat with mould spores. Growth of micro-organisms on surfaces contacting the meats and on the meats themselves increase their numbers. According to European workers, numbers of micro-organisms contaminating meats may be reduced by treatment of the surface with hot water.

Table 12.2. Average numbers of micro-organisms contaminating beef in packing-plant slaughter room.

Sample	Bacteria	Yeasts	Moulds
Beef, dressed, on floor	6400–830,000/cm^2		
Soil from animals (dry)	110,000,000/g	50,000/g	120,000/g
Animal feces (fresh)	90,000,000/g	200,000/g	60,000/g
Rumen content	2,000,000,000/g	180,000/g	1,600/g
Room air	140/cm^2 of plate		2/cm^2
Water, washing beef	20–10,000/ml		
Water, washing floor	1,000–16,000/ml		

Because of the varied sources, the kinds of micro-organisms likely to contaminate meats are many. Moulds of many genera may reach the surfaces of meats and grow there. Especially important are species of the genera *Cladosporium*, *Sporotrichum*, *Oöspora* (*Geotrichum*), *Thamnidium*, *Mucor*, *Penicillium*, *Alternaria* and *Monilia*. Yeasts, mostly asporogenous ones, often are present. Bacteria of many genera are found, among which some of the more important are *Pseudomonas*, *Achromobacter*, *Micrococcus*, *Streptococcus*, *Sarcina*, *Leuconostoc*, *Lactobacillus*, *Proteus*, *Flavobacterium*, *Bacillus*, *Clostridium*, *Escherichia*, *Salmonella*, and *Streptomyces*. Many of these bacteria can grow at chilling temperatures. There also is the possibility of the contamination of meat and meat products with human pathogens, especially those of the intestinal type.

In the retail market and in the home additional contamination usually takes place. In the market knives, saws, cleavers, slicers, grinders, chopping blocks, scales, sawdust, and containers, as well as the market operators, may be sources of organisms. In the home the refrigerator containers used previously to store meats can serve as sources of spoilage organisms.

Preservation

The preservation of meats, as of most perishable foods, usually is accomplished by a combination of preservative methods. The fact that most meats are very good culture media—high in moisture, nearly neutral in pH and high in nutrients—coupled with the facts that some organisms may be in the lymph nodes, bones and muscle and contamination with spoilage organisms is almost unavoidable, makes the preservation of meats more difficult than that of most kinds of food. Unless cooling is prompt and rapid after slaughter, meat may undergo undesirable changes in appearance and flavour and may support the growth of micro-organisms before being processed in some way for its preservation. Long storage at chilling temperatures may allow some increase in numbers of micro-organisms.

Asepsis

Asepsis or keeping micro-organisms away from meats as much as practicable during slaughtering and handling permits easier preservation by any method. Storage time under chilling conditions may be lengthened, ageing for tenderising becomes less of a risk, curing and smoking methods are more certain, and heating processes are more successful.

Asepsis begins with avoidance, as much as possible, of contamination from the exterior of the animal. Water spraying of the animal before slaughter has been recommended to remove as much gross dirt as possible from hair and hide, and a foot bath may be employed to remove dirt from the hoofs. Even so, the hide and hair of the animal are important sources of contamination of the surfaces of the carcass during skinning. The knife used to bleed animals after slaughter may contribute micro-organisms to the still circulating blood stream and also introduce organisms while penetrating the hide. Organisms may be added to hide and lungs of hogs during scalding. There is not only contamination from the hide during skinning but also from knives and from workers and their clothes. During evisceration, contamination may come from the animal's intestine, the air, the water for washing and rinsing the carcass, cloths and brushes employed on the carcass, the various knives, saws, etc. used, and the hands and clothing of the workmen; and some organisms may come from walls touched by the carcass or from splash or mist from the floors. Meat in the chill room may be subject to contamination from air, walls, floors and workers. Of special interest as a source of mould spores is the sawdust usually spread on the floor. Further contamination during cutting and trimming comes from knives, saws, conveyors, tables, air, water and workmen.

The fact that the micro-organisms added from the above-mentioned sources normally include practically all of the organisms involved in the spoilage of meats, many in appreciable numbers, emphasises the importance of aseptic methods. Once meat is contaminated with micro-organisms, their removal is difficult. Gross soil may be washed from surfaces, but the wash water may add organisms. Mouldy or otherwise spoiled surface areas of large pieces of meat, especially 'hung' or aged, meat, may be trimmed off, but this should not be considered effective as a preservative method.

Films used to wrap meats keep out bacteria and affect the growth of those already there. These films differ considerably in their penetrability to water, oxygen and carbon dioxide. Meats have been reported to have a shorter storage life in films less permeable to water. Fresh meats keep their red colour better in an oxygen-permeable film without evacuation. With a gastight film, more carbon dioxide from bacteria would be retained; this would result in a poorer colour, but would favour lactic acid bacteria over others. Cured meats preferably are packed in an oxygen tight film with evacuation. Evacuation helps restrict the growth of aerobes, especially moulds, reduces the rate of growth of staphylococci, and favours the growth of lactics, but apparently does not favour the growth of *Clostridium botulinum* any more than plain overwrapping does.

Use of heat

The canning of meat is a very specialised technique in that the procedure varies considerably with the meat product to be preserved. Most meat products are low-acid foods that are good culture media for any surviving bacteria. Rates of heat penetration range from fairly rapid in meat soups to very slow in tightly packed meats or in pastes. Chemicals added to meats, such as spices, salt, or nitrates and nitrites in curing processes, also affect the heat processing, usually making it more effective. Nitrates in meat aid in the killing of spores of anaerobic bacteria by heat and inhibit germination of surviving spores. Commercially canned meats may be divided into two groups on the basis of the heat processing used: (i) meats that are heat-processed in an attempt to make the can contents sterile or at least 'commercially sterile,' as for canned meats for shelf storage in retail stores, and (ii) meats that are heated enough to kill part of the spoilage organisms but must be kept refrigerated to prevent spoilage. Canned hams and loaves of luncheon meats are so handled.

Although the national canners association publishes minimal heat processes for vegetables and fruits, it does not do so for meats, but recommends that a research laboratory connected with the canning industry be consulted for directions. Processes that have been used for meat products in 1-1b cans at 250°F (121°C) are 45 minutes for boiled beef, 60 minutes for beef stew, 55 minutes for veal or beef loaf and corned-beef hash.

Use of a pressure cooker is mandatory, and the meats usually are precooked to facilitate packing. In Table 12.3 are examples of recommendations of process times at 240°F (115.5°C).

Table 12.3. Recommended process times for canned meat in a pressure cooker at 240°F (115.5°C).

Product	Container	Time, min.
Beef	Quart jars	90
Chicken	Quart jars	75
Chicken, boned	Quart jars	90
Pork	Pint jars	75
Pork	Quart jars	90

Heat may be applied to meat products in other ways than canning. Treatment of meat surfaces with hot water to lengthen the keeping time has been suggested, although this may lessen nutrients and damage colour. The cooking of wieners at the packing plant by steam or hot water reduces the numbers of micro-organisms and aids in the preservation. Heat applied during the smoking of meats and meat products helps reduce microbial numbers. The precooking or tenderising of hams reduces bacterial numbers somewhat but does not sterilise. Such products should be refrigerated, for they are perishable and they may support the growth of food-poisoning organisms if they are held at room temperatures. Similar considerations hold for cooked sausages like frankfurters and liver sausage, which also are spiced, but should be kept refrigerated. The cooking of meats for direct consumption greatly reduces the microbial content and hence lengthens the keeping time. Precooked frozen meats should contain few viable micro-organisms.

Use of low temperatures

More meat is preserved by the use of low temperatures than by any other method, and much more by chilling than by freezing.

Chilling

Modern packing-house methods involve chilling meat promptly and rapidly to temperatures near freezing, and chilling storage at only slightly above the freezing point. The more prompt and rapid this cooling, the less opportunity there will be for growth of mesophilic micro-organisms. The principles concerned in chilling storage, apply to meats as well as other foods. Storage temperatures vary from 29.5° to 36°F

(−1.4° to 2.2°C), with the lower temperatures favoured by most storage men. The time limit for chilling storage of beef is about 30 days, depending upon the numbers of micro-organisms present, the temperature, and the relative humidity; for pork, lamb and mutton 1 to 2 weeks; and for veal a still shorter period. Uncooked sausage, like uncured pork sausage in bulk or in links, must be preserved by refrigeration. It was emphasised that the relative humidity usually is lowered with an increase in storage temperature. Storage time can be lengthened by storage of meats in an atmosphere containing added carbon dioxide or ozone, or the temperature and relative humidity can be raised without shortening storage time. Although considerable experimental work has been done on the gas storage of meats, the method has not been used extensively. Increasing amounts of carbon dioxide in the atmosphere increasingly inhibit micro-organisms but also hasten the formation of metmyoglobin and methemoglobin and hence the loss of 'bloom', or natural colour (Fig. 12.3). The storage life of meat has been doubled, according to reports, by such gas storage. Experts do not agree upon the optimal concentration of carbon dioxide, recommendations varying from 10 to 30 per cent for most meats and up to 100 per cent for bacon.

Storage time also can be increased by the presence of 2.5 to 3 parts per million of ozone in the atmosphere. Storage up to 60 days at 36°F (2.2°C) and 92 per cent relative humidity without development of moulds or slime has been reported. Ozone is an active oxidising agent, however, that may give an oxidised or tallowy flavour to fats. It has been observed that while the levels of ozone cited will inhibit micro-organisms, much higher concentrations are necessary to stop growth that already has begun.

The micro-organisms that give trouble in the chilling storage of meats are the psychrophilic bacteria, chiefly of the genus *Pseudomonas*, although bacteria of the genera *Achromobacter*, *Micrococcus*, *Lactobacillus*, *Streptococcus*, *Leuconostoc*, *Pediococcus*, *Flavobacterium* and *Proteus*, and yeasts and moulds can grow in meats at low temperatures.

Freezing

Most meat sold in retail stores has not been frozen, but freezing often is used to preserve meats during shipment over long distances or for holding until times of shortage and, of course, considerable quantities of meat now are frozen in home freezers. Large pieces of meat, e.g. halves or quarters, are sharp-frozen, while hamburger and smaller, fancier cuts may be quick-frozen in wrapped packages. There is less drip from thawed mutton than from beef, and less from beef than from veal. The preservation of frozen meats is increasingly effective as the storage temperature drops from 10°F toward −20°F.

Meats for freezing are subject to the same risks of contamination by and growth of micro-organisms as meats for any other purpose. The freezing process kills about half the bacteria, and numbers decrease slowly during storage. The low-temperature bacteria that grow on meat during chilling, species of *Pseudomonas*, *Achromobacter*, *Micrococcus*, *Lactobacillus*, *Flavobacterium* and *Proteus*, can resume growth during the thawing of meat if this is done slowly. If directions are followed, packaged, quick-frozen meats are thawed too rapidly for appreciable growth of micro-organisms. At temperatures above 15°C (59°F) there is a possibility of growth and toxin production by Clostridium botulinum types A and B in thawed meat if enough time is allowed; and at temperatures as low as 3.3°C (38°F) by type E. Salmonellae survive freezing and may remain viable for months at low temperatures of storage. It has been reported that bacteria and spores dried in meat by freezing are more resistant to salt, curing ingredients and heat than their parent strains.

Use of irradiation

Irradiation with ultraviolet rays has been used in conjunction with chilling storage to lengthen the keeping time. It has been employed chiefly on large, hung pieces of meat in plant storage rooms but is used some in coolers in retail markets. The rays serve to reduce numbers of micro-organisms in the air and to inhibit or kill them on the surfaces of the meat reached directly by the rays. To be affected, the micro-organisms must be on the immediate surface, unprotected by fatty or opaque materials.

Irradiation also is used in the rapid ageing of meats that are 'hung' at higher than the usual chilling temperatures to reduce the growth of micro-organisms, especially moulds, on the surface. The ageing, or hanging, process is for the purpose of tenderising the meat by means of its own proteolytic enzymes and is used especially for obtaining tender steaks and other fancy cuts. Ordinary ageing is for several weeks at 36° to 38°F (2.2° to 3.3°C) with the relative humidity between 80 and 90 per cent and an air movement of 10 to 30 fpm, but with exposure to ultraviolet rays the time is reduced to 2 to 3 days at 60° to 65°F in a relative humidity of 85 to 90 per cent. Some oxidation, favoured by ultraviolet rays, and hydrolysis of fats may take place during ageing.

Electronic irradiation of meats still is in the experimental stage. When sterilisation is effected, undesirable changes in colour and flavour may appear.

Irradiation with cathode (beta) rays or gamma rays has been used experimentally in the preservation of small cuts or packages of meat. In February, 1963, the Food and Drug Administration approved irradiation of fresh canned bacon with a dose of 4.5 megarads and later gave permission for use of X-rays. Present interest is in irradiation of meats with ionising rays at levels lower than those needed for sterilisation, permitting a considerably lengthened storage life thereafter at chilling temperatures. This reduced dose of rays is made large enough to kill most of the important spoilage organisms on or near the surface of the meat, without noticeable harm to colour, odour or taste of the meat. Ham can be sterilised with rays, without marked changes.

Preservation by drying

Drying of meats for their preservation has been practiced for centuries. Jerky or sun-dried strips of beef, was a standard food of American pioneers. Some types of sausage are preserved primarily by their dryness. In dried beef, made mostly from cured, smoked beef hams, growth of micro-organisms may take place prior to processing and may develop in the 'pickle' during curing, but numbers of organisms are reduced by the smoking and drying process. Organisms may contaminate the dried ham during storage and the slices during cutting and packing.

Meat products like the dry sausages, dry salamis and dry cervelats, for example, are preserved chiefly by their low moisture content, for some varieties are not smoked. A dry outer surface on the casing of any sausage is protective.

Older methods of drying meats are usually combined with salting and smoking. During IInd World War pieces of freshly cooked beef and pork were dried by heat. Another method of drying pork involves a short nitrate-nitrite cure before drying and addition of lecithin as an antioxidant and stabiliser. Drying may be by vacuum, in trays, or by other methods. The final product keeps without refrigeration.

Freeze drying of meats is on the increase, with greater success with processed products such as meat patties, meat balls and stew, than with fresh meats. The US Armed Services, however, have been developing fresh-meat products, as have commercial plants here, in the British Isles and on the European Continent. The efficiency of the process is being improved enough to reduce costs to where production for retail sale has become practicable.

Meat for drying should be of good bacteriological quality, without previous development of appreciable numbers of micro-organisms or of undesirable flavour.

Use of preservatives

The utilisation of a controlled atmosphere containing added carbon dioxide or ozone in the chilling storage of meats has been discussed. The use of sulphur dioxide to give an unnaturally bright red colour to meats is prohibited. Preservation by heavy salting is an old method that usually results in an inferior product. Ordinarily salting is combined with curing and smoking in order to be effective.

Curing

The curing of meats is limited to beef and pork, either ground meat or certain cuts like hams, butts, jowls, sides, loins and bellies of hogs, and the hams, brisket and leg muscles of beef. Originally, curing of meats was for the purpose of preserving by salting without refrigeration, but most cured meats of the present day have other ingredients added and are refrigerated, and many also are smoked, and hence dried to some extent. The curing agents permitted are sodium chloride, sugar, sodium nitrate, sodium nitrite and vinegar, but only the first four are commonly used. The functions of the ingredients are as follows:

Sodium chloride or common salt, is used primarily as a preservative and flavouring agent. The cover pickle, used for immersing the meat, may contain about 15 per cent of salt, in contrast to the pumping pickle, injected into the meat, which has a higher concentration, approximating 24 per cent. Its primary purpose is to lower the a_w.

Sugar adds flavour and also serves as an energy source for nitrate-reducing bacteria in the curing solution or pickle. Sucrose is used chiefly, but glucose can be substituted if a short cure is employed or no sugar may be added. Sodium nitrate is indirectly a colour fixative and is mildly bacteriostatic in acid solution, especially against anaerobes. It also serves as a reservoir from which nitrite can be formed by bacterial reduction during the long cure.

Sodium nitrite is the source of nitric oxide, which is the real colour fixative (Fig. 12.3) and has some bacteriostatic effect in acid solution. The more spores of putrefactive clostridia there are in meats, the more sodium nitrite is needed to suppress them.

Most of the preservative effect of the curing agents, then, is attributed to the sodium chloride, with some bacteriostatic effect from the nitrite, and little effect from the nitrate. The salts, sugar and meat protein combine to lower the a_w value of the cured meats, e.g. of hams to about 0.95 to 0.97. Other preservative factors are the low curing temperature and smoking.

The purplish-red colour of meats (Fig. 12.3) is due to blood haemoglobin and muscle myoglobin, and oxygenation of these compounds produces oxyhaemoglobin and oxymyoglobin, which are bright red. Under acid and reducing conditions in the presence of nitrite, the red nitrosomyoglobin and nitrosohemoglobin are produced from myoglobin and haemoglobin (Fig. 12.3). The acid condition is produced by the meat itself, the reduced condition by the bacteria, and the nitric oxide for the reaction by reduction of the nitrite.

There are four methods for introducing the curing agents into meat: (i) the dry cure, in which dry ingredients are rubbed into the meat, as in curing belly bacon, (ii) the pickle cure, in which the meats are immersed in a solution of the ingredients, (iii) the injection cure, in which a concentrated solution of the ingredients is injected by needle into the arteries and veins of the meat via an artery or into the muscular tissue in various parts of the meat, as is done with pork hams, and (iv) direct-addition method, in which the curing agents are added directly to finely ground meats, such as sausage, and aid in their preservation.

The curing temperature, especially when a pickling solution is employed, usually is about 2.2° to 3.3°C (36° to 38°F), and the time of the cure varies with the methods used and the meats to be cured.

The older methods of curing in the pickle require several months, but the newer 'quick cure', in which the pickling solution is pumped into the meat, greatly shortens that time.

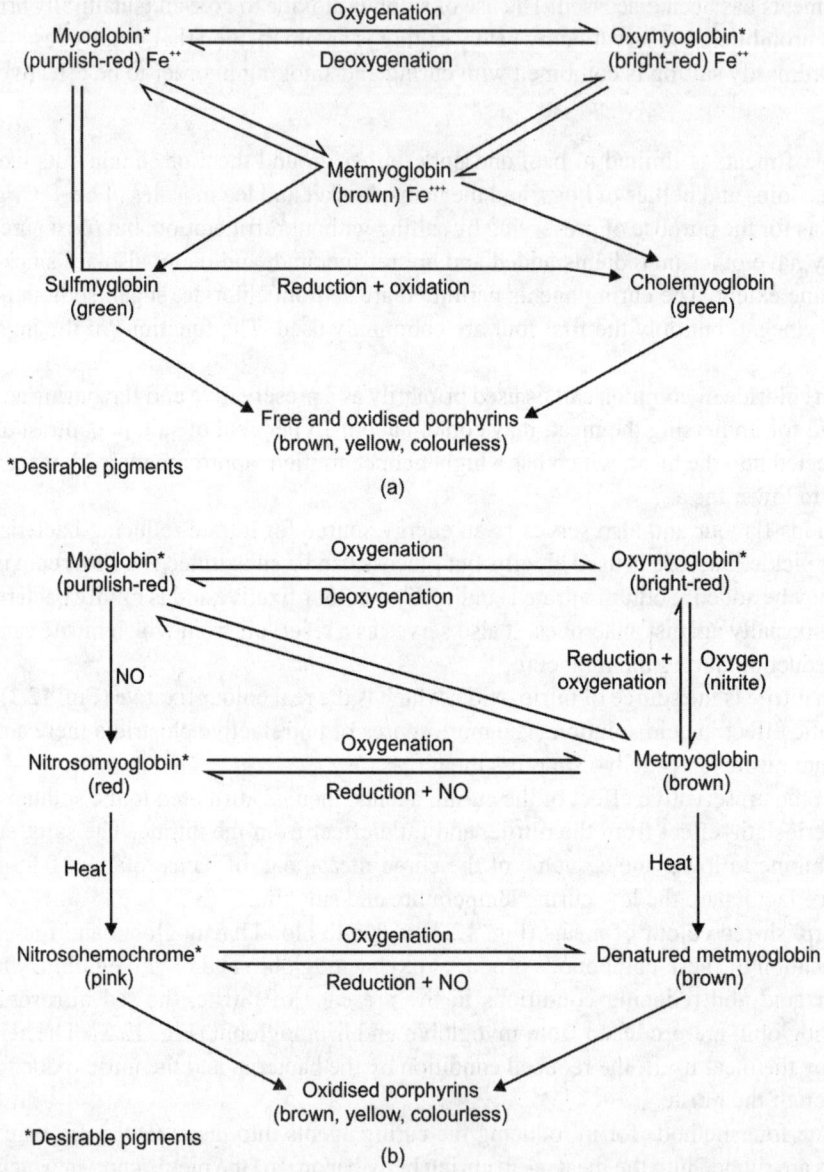

Fig. 12.3. Colour changes in meats. (a) Changes that may occur in raw meats, and (b) changes that may occur during the curing of meats. Similar changes take place in the blood pigment, hemoglobin.

Most meats are smoked after curing to aid their preservation; whereas others, like corned beef, are not smoked, but then must be refrigerated.

Some types of sausage, such as Thuringer, cervelat, Lebanon, bologna, the salamis and the dry and semidry summer sausages, undergo an acid fermentation, preferably of a mixed lactic acid kind, during their curing. This not only has a preservative effect, preventing undesirable fermentations, but also adds a desired tangy flavour. Many processors carry over the mixed lactic flora from a previous lot of sausage, but Niven has recommended inoculation with pure cultures of *Pediococcus cerevisiae* (not over 0.5 per cent of starter is permitted) to favour the desired lactic acid fermentation. A *Micrococcus* species also has been used. Kinds of micro-organisms that have been found in cured meats are shown in Table 12.4.

Table 12.4. Micro-organisms reported in cured meats.

Meat	Micro-organisms
Sausages	
Salami	Homofermentative lactobacilli
Big bologna	*Leuconostoc mesenteroides*, heterofermentative lactobacilli
Smoked links	*Leuconostoc mesenteroides*, heterofermentative lactobacilli
Frankfurters	Streptococci, pediococci, leuconostocs, lactobacilli, micrococci, spore-formers, yeasts
Fresh pork	Leuconostocs, microbacteria, lactobacilli
Bacon	
Sliced, packaged	Mostly lactobacilli; also micrococci, enterococci
Wiltshire	Micrococci, lactobacilli
Vacuum-wrapped	Streptococci, leuconostocs, pediococci, lactobacilli
Ham	
Raw	Lactobacilli, micrococci, microbacteria, enterococci, leuconostocs
Sliced, packaged	*Streptococcus faecium*, *Microbacterium* sp.
Pressed, spiced	Heterofermentative lactobacilli, leuconostocs
Canned	Enterococci, bacilli
Irradiated	Enterococci
Heated, irradiated	Bacilli, clostridia

Vinegar is added to the pickling solution in the preservation of foods like pickled pigs' feet, pickled spiced beef, and souses. Pigs' feet are cured in a solution of salt, sodium nitrate and sodium nitrite, cooked, and then held in a brine of salt and vinegar. Then they are packed into jars or other containers and covered with a fresh salt-vinegar brine, and the jar is sealed. Unless the acidity is unduly low, the product will not spoil.

Microbiology of meat-curing brines

The micro-organisms in curing brines and on immersed meats in them will vary with the initial condition of the meat and with the method of curing employed. The microbial content of the salt seems to have little significance except on salted meat, which after removal from brine or after dry salting sometimes develops red surface colonies of halophilic bacteria like those carried by the salt. In modern American short methods of curing meats, such as ham, bacteria in the brine apparently have little to do with changes that occur in the meat, for they do not reach high numbers and are killed mostly on the meat by the smoking that follows. Such brines contain principally lactic acid bacteria, except at the surface where micrococci and yeasts may develop. The lactics are chiefly lactobacilli and pediococci. In the old long cure, bacteria, especially micrococci, may function in reducing nitrate to nitrite, thus fixing the red colour in the meat.

Foreign methods of curing bacon usually involve immersion in fairly concentrated brines and use of these brines for a long period. The brines appear to build up, besides micrococci, a special mixture of cocci and Gram-positive and Gram-negative rods that, for the most part, form tiny colonies on agar media. They are halo tolerant to halophilic and reduce nitrates to nitrites. When hog bellies are treated with the dry curing mixture and compressed in boxes, growth of salt-tolerant, nitrate-reducing psychrophiles is permitted. Some beef-curing brines have been found to contain micrococci, lactobacilli, streptococci, *Achromobacter*, vibrios and perhaps pediococci, plus other bacteria in small numbers. Species of *Micrococcus* are active in many of the pickling solutions and have been found especially in those of high salt concentration used in curing British and Canadian bacons.

Smoking

In the use of wood smoke as a preservative it has been discussed that smoking has two main purposes, to add desired flavours and to aid in preservation. It was noted that the preservative substances added to the meat, together with the action of the heat during smoking, have a germicidal effect, and that the drying of the meat together with chemicals from the smoke inhibit microbial growth during storage.

Older methods of curing and smoking, where high salt concentrations were used in curing and greater drying and incorporation of preservative chemicals was accomplished in smoking, produced hams, dried beef, etc. that would keep without refrigeration. Many of the newer methods, however, yield a perishable product that must be refrigerated. Precooked or tenderised hams and sausages of high moisture content are examples.

Spices

Spices and condiments added to meat products like meat loaves and sausages are not in concentrations high enough to be preservative, but they may add their effect to those of the other preservative factors. Certainly products like bologna, Polish or frankfurter and other sausages owe their keeping quality to the combined effect of spicing, curing, smoking (drying), cooking and refrigerating.

Antibiotics

Although the only permitted use of antibiotics in flesh foods now is in poultry and fish, experiments have indicated that antibiotics can be used successfully in meats to prolong storage life at chilling or higher temperatures. The antibiotics most often recommended have been chlortetracycline, oxytetracycline and chloramphenicol. The antibiotics may be applied to meats in various ways: (i) the antibiotic may be fed the animal over a long period, (ii) it may be fed more intensively for a short period before slaughter, (iii) it may be infused into the carcass or into parts of it, and (iv) it may be applied to the surface of pieces of meat or mixed with comminuted meat. The feeding of an antibiotic brings about a selection of micro-organisms in the animal's intestinal tract, presumably reducing the numbers of spoilage bacteria there and therefore reducing the numbers that are likely to reach the meat from that source during slaughter and dressing. It has been suggested that injection of antibiotic before slaughter might be employed to prolong the keeping time of carcasses at atmospheric temperatures before they reach the refrigerator or to hold beef briefly at temperatures that will favour tenderisation of special cuts, as well as lengthen the keeping time of meats held at chilling temperatures. Infusion of an antibiotic into the carcass immediately after slaughter or into special parts would serve similar purposes. Storage life of meats could be lengthened by means of an antibiotic dip, such as that now permitted for poultry or by inclusion of antibiotic in ground meats.

Spoilage

Raw meat is subject to change by its own enzymes and by microbial action, and, in addition, its fat may be oxidised chemically. A moderate amount of autolysis is desired in the tenderising of beef and game by 'hanging' or ageing, but is not encouraged in most other raw meats. Autolytic changes include some proteolytic action on muscle and connective tissues and slight hydrolysis of fats. The defect caused by excessive autolysis has been called 'souring', an inexact term that, it will be noted, is applied to a variety of kinds of spoilage of food, and, in fact to almost any kind that gives a sour odour. 'Souring' due to autolysis is difficult to separate or distinguish from defects caused by microbial action, especially from simple proteolysis. However, this preliminary hydrolysis of proteins by the meat enzymes undoubtedly helps micro-organisms start growing in the meat by furnishing the simpler nitrogen compounds needed by many micro-organisms that cannot attack complete native proteins.

General principles underlying meat spoilage

It has been pointed out that during slaughter, dressing and cutting, micro-organisms come chiefly from the exterior of the animal and its intestinal tract, but that more are added from knives, cloths, air, workers, carts, boxes and equipment in general. A great variety of kinds of organisms are added, so that it can be assumed that under ordinary conditions most kinds of potential spoilage organisms are present and will be able to grow if favourable conditions present themselves.

Invasion of tissues by micro-organisms

Upon the death of the animal invasion of the tissues by contaminating micro-organisms takes place. Factors that influence that invasion are:

1. The load in the gut of the animal: The greater the load the greater will be the invasion of tissues. For that reason starvation for 24 hours before slaughter has been recommended.
2. The physiological condition of the animal immediately before slaughter: If the animal is excited, feverish or fatigued, bacteria are more likely to enter the tissues, bleeding is apt to be incomplete, thus encouraging the spread of bacteria, and chemical changes may take place more readily in the tissue, such as those due to better bacterial growth because of a higher pH, earlier release of juices from the meat fibres, and more rapid denaturation of proteins. Because glycogen is used up in fatigue, the pH will not drop from 7.2 to about 5.7, as it would normally.
3. The method of killing and bleeding: The better and more sanitary the bleeding, the better will be the keeping quality of the meat. Little has been reported on the effect of humane methods of slaughter on the keeping quality of meat, although it has been claimed that more greening was found in pork and bacon from electrically stunned animals than from those killed with carbon dioxide.
4. The rate of cooling: Rapid cooling will reduce the rate of invasion of the tissues by micro-organisms.

Micro-organisms are spread in the meat through the blood and lymph vessels and connective-tissue interspaces and, in ground meat, by grinding.

Growth of micro-organisms in meat

Meat is an ideal culture medium for many organisms because it is high in moisture, rich in nitrogenous foods of various degrees of complexity, plentifully supplied with minerals and accessory growth factors, usually has some fermentable carbohydrate (glycogen), and is at a favourable pH for most micro-organisms.

The factors that influence the growth of micro-organisms and hence the kind of spoilage are:

1. The kind and amount of contamination with micro-organisms and the spread of these organisms in the meat: For example, meat with a contaminating flora that is high in percentage of low temperature *Pseudomonas* (or *Achromobacter*) species would spoil at chilling temperatures more rapidly than meat with a low percentage of these psychrophiles.

2. The physical properties of the meat: The amount of exposed surface of the flesh has considerable influence on the rate of spoilage because the greatest load of organisms usually is there and air is available for aerobic organisms. Fat may protect some surfaces, but is subject to spoilage itself, chiefly enzymatic and chemical. The grinding of meat greatly increases the surface and encourages microbial growth for this reason and because it releases moisture and distributes bacteria throughout the meat. Skin on meat serves to protect the meat inside, although micro-organisms grow on it.

3. Chemical properties of the meat: It has been pointed out that meat in general is a fine culture medium for micro-organisms. The moisture content is important in determining whether organisms can grow and what kinds can grow, especially at the surface, where drying may take place. Thus the surface may be so dry as to permit no growth, a little moist to allow mould growth, still moister to encourage yeasts, and very moist to favour bacterial growth. The relative humidity of the storage atmosphere is important in this regard. Food for micro-organisms is plentiful, but the low content or absence of fermentable carbohydrate and the high protein content tend to favour the nonfermenting types of organisms, those that can utilise proteins and their decomposition products for nitrogen, carbon and energy.

   The pH of raw meat may vary from about 5.7 to over 7.2, depending upon the amount of glycogen present at slaughter and subsequent changes in the meat. A higher pH value favours microbial growth; a lower one usually makes it slower and may be selective for certain organisms, such as yeasts.

4. Availability of oxygen: Aerobic conditions at the surface of meat are favourable to moulds, yeasts and aerobic bacteria. Within the solid pieces of meat, conditions are anaerobic and tend to remain that way because the oxidation-reduction potential is strongly poised at a low level, although oxygen will diffuse slowly into ground meat and slowly raise the oxidation-reduction potential unless the casing or packaging material is impervious to oxygen. True putrefaction is favoured by anaerobic conditions.

5. Temperature: Meat should be stored at temperatures not far above freezing, where only low-temperature micro-organisms can grow. Moulds, yeasts, and psychrophilic bacteria grow slowly and produce characteristic defects to be discussed later. True putrefaction is rare at these low temperatures but is likely at room temperature. As for most foods, the temperature is most important in selecting the kinds of organisms to grow and the types of spoilage to result. At chilling temperatures, for example, psychrophiles are favoured and proteolysis is likely, caused by a dominating species of bacterium, followed by utilisation of peptides and amino acids by secondary species. At ordinary atmospheric temperatures, mesophiles would grow, such as coliform bacteria and species of *Bacillus* and *Clostridium*, with the production of moderate amounts of acid from the limited amounts of carbohydrates present.

General types of spoilage of meats

The common types of spoilage of meats can be classified on the basis of whether they occur under aerobic or anaerobic conditions and whether they are caused by bacteria, yeasts or moulds.

Spoilage under aerobic conditions

Under aerobic conditions bacteria may cause:

1. Surface slime: It may be caused by species of *Pseudomonas*, *Achromobacter*, *Streptococcus*, *Leuconostoc*, *Bacillus* and *Micrococcus*. Some species of *Lactobacillus* can produce slime. The temperature and the availability of moisture influence the kind of micro-organisms causing surface slime. At chilling temperatures, high moisture will favour the *Pseudomonas-Achromobacter* group; with less moisture, as on frankfurters, micrococci and yeasts will be encouraged; and with still less moisture moulds may grow. At higher temperatures, up to that of the room, micrococci and other mesophiles compete well with the pseudomonads and related bacteria. The numbers of micro-organisms necessary before detection of off-odour or slime in meats and other proteinaceous foods are shown in Table 12.5. Numbers in the millions per square centimetre or gram are required.

Table 12.5. Numbers of micro-organisms at time of appearance of odour and slime in proteinaceous foods (from numerous sources).

Food	Nos. when odour evident	Nos. when slime evident
Poultry meat	$2.5–100 \times 10^6/cm^2$	$10–60 \times 10^6/cm^2$
Beef	$1.2–100 \times 10^6/cm^2$	$3–300 \times 10^6/cm^2$
Frankfurters	$100–130 \times 10^6/cm^2$	$130 \times 10^6/cm^2$
Processed meats		$10–100 \times 10^6/cm^2$
Wiltshire bacon		$1.5–100 \times 10^6/cm^2$
Fish	$1–130 \times 10^6/cm^2$	
Shell or liquid eggs	$10 \times 10^6/g$	

2. Changes in colour of meat pigments (Fig. 12.3): The red colour of meat, called its 'bloom', may be changed to shades of green, brown or gray as the result of the production of oxidising compounds, e.g. peroxides or of hydrogen sulphide, by bacteria. Species of *Lactobacillus* (mostly heterofermentative) and *Leuconostoc* are reported to cause the greening of sausage.

3. Change in fats: The oxidation of unsaturated fats in meats takes place chemically in air and may be catalysed by light and copper. Lipolytic bacteria may cause some lipolysis and also may accelerate the oxidation of the fats. Some fats, like butterfat, become tallowy on oxidation and rancid on hydrolysis; but most animal fats develop 'oxidative rancidity' when oxidised, with off-odours due to aldehydes and acids. Hydrolysis adds the flavour of the released fatty acids. Rancidity of fats may be caused by lipolytic species of *Pseudomonas* and *Achromobacter* or by yeasts.

4. Phosphorescence: This rather uncommon defect is caused by phosphorescent or luminous bacteria, e.g. *Photobacterium* spp., growing on the surface of the meat.

5. Various surface colours due to pigmented bacteria: Thus 'red spot' may be caused by *Serratia morcescens* or other bacteria with red pigments. *Pseudomonas syncyanea* can impart a blue colour to the surface. Yellow discolourations are caused by bacteria with yellow pigments, usually species of *Micrococcus* or *Flavobacterium*. *Chromobacterium lividum* and other bacteria give greenish-blue to brownish-black spots on stored beef. The purple 'stamping-ink' discolouration of surface fat is caused by yellow-pigmented cocci and rods. When the fat becomes

rancid and peroxides appear, the yellow colour changes to a greenish shade and later becomes purplish to blue.

6. Off-odours and tastes: 'Taints', or undesirable odours and tastes, that appear in meat as the result of the growth of bacteria on the surface often are evident before other signs of spoilage. 'Souring' is the term applied to almost any defect that gives a sour odour that may be due to volatile acids, e.g. formic, acetic, butyric, and propionic, or even to growth of yeasts. 'Cold-storage flavour' or taint is an indefinite term for a stale flavour. Actinomycetes may be responsible for a musty or earthy flavour.

Under aerobic conditions yeasts may grow on the surface of meats causing sliminess, lipolysis, off-odours and tastes, and discolourations—white, cream, pink or brown-due to pigments in the yeasts.

Aerobic growth of moulds may cause:

1. Stickiness: Incipient growth of moulds makes the surface of the meat sticky to the touch.
2. Whiskers: When meat is stored at temperatures near freezing, a limited amount of mycelial growth may take place without sporulation. Such white, fuzzy growth can be caused by a number of moulds, including *Thamnidium chaetocladioides*, or *T. elegans*, *Mucor mucedo*, *M. lusitanicus*, or *M. racemosus*, *Rhizopus*, and others. Controlled growth of a special strain of *Thamnidium* has been recommended for improvement in flavour during ageing of beef.
3. Black spot: This usually is caused by *Cladosporium herbarum*, but other moulds with dark pigments may be responsible.
4. White spot: *Sporotrichum carnis* is the most common cause of white spot, although any mould with wet, yeast-like colonies, e.g. *Geotrichum*, could cause white spot.
5. Green patches: These are caused for the most part by the green spores of species of *Penicillium* such as *P. expansum*, *P. asperulum*, and *P. oxalicum*.
6. Decomposition of fats: Many moulds have lipases and hence cause hydrolysis of fats. Moulds also aid in the oxidation of fats.
7. Off-odours and tastes: Moulds give a musty flavour to meat in the vicinity of their growth. Sometimes the defect is given a name indicating the cause, e.g. 'thamnidium taint'.

Spots of surface spoilage by yeasts and moulds usually are localised to a great extent and can be trimmed off without harm to the rest of the meat. The time that has been allowed for diffusion of the products of decomposition into the meat and the rate of that diffusion will determine the depth to which the defect will appear. Extensive bacterial growth over the surface may bring fairly deep penetration. Then, too, facultative bacteria may grow inwards slowly.

Spoilage under anaerobic conditions

Facultative and anaerobic bacteria are able to grow within the meat under anaerobic conditions and cause spoilage. The terminology used in connection with this spoilage is inexact. Most used are the words 'souring', 'putrefaction' and 'taint', but these terms apparently mean different things to different people.

1. Souring: The term implies a sour odour and perhaps taste. This could be caused by formic, acetic, butyric, propionic and higher fatty acids or other organic acids such as lactic or succinic. Souring can result from: (i) action of the meat's own enzymes during ageing or ripening, (ii) anaerobic production of fatty acids or lactic acid by the bacterial action, and (iii) proteolysis without putrefaction, caused by facultative or anaerobic bacteria and sometimes called 'stinking sour fermentation'. Acid and gas formation accompany the action of the 'butyric' *Clostridium*

species and the coliform bacteria on carbohydrates. Vacuum-packed meats, especially those in gastight wrappers, commonly support the growth of lactic acid bacteria.

2. Putrefaction: True putrefaction is the anaerobic decomposition of protein with the production of foul-smelling compounds like hydrogen sulphide, mercaptans, indole, skatole, ammonia, amines, etc. It usually is caused by species of *Clostridium*, but facultative bacteria may cause putrefaction or assist in its production, as evidenced by the long list of species with the specific names 'putrefaciens', 'putrificus', 'putida', etc. chiefly in the genera *Pseudomonas* and *Achromobacter*. Also, some species of *Proteus* are putrefactive. The confusion in the use of the term putrefaction arises from the fact that any type of spoilage with foul odours, whether from the anaerobic decomposition of protein or the breakdown of other compounds, even non-nitrogenous ones, may erroneously be termed putrefaction. Thus, for example, trimethylamine in fish, or isovaleric acid in butter, are described as 'putrid' odours. Gas formation accompanies putrefaction by clostridia, the gases being hydrogen and carbon dioxide.

3. Taint: Taint is a still more inexact word applied to any off-taste or odour. The term 'bone taint' of meats refers to either souring or putrefaction next to the bones, especially in hams. Usually it means putrefaction.

Not only air but temperature has an important influence on the type of spoilage to be expected in meat. When meat is held at temperatures near 0°C (32°F), as recommended, microbial growth is limited to that of moulds, yeasts and bacteria able to grow at low temperatures. These include many of the types that produce sliminess, discolouration and spots of growth on the surface and many that can cause souring, such as *Pseudomonas*, *Achromobacter*, *Lactobacillus*, *Leuconostoc*, *Streptococcus* and *Flavobacterium* species. Most true putrefiers, like those in the genus *Clostridium*, require temperatures above those of the refrigerator.

Spoilage of different kinds of meats

The processing of meats by curing, smoking, drying or canning usually changes them and their microbial flora enough to encourage types of spoilage not undergone by fresh meats.

Spoilage of fresh meats

The spoilage of fresh meats has been covered in the preceding discussion of general types of spoilage. Little has been reported on the spoilage of fresh veal, pork, lamb or mutton, although presumably the spoilage would be similar to that of beef. Perhaps pork spoils more readily than other meats because of its high content of B vitamins.

Lactic acid bacteria, chiefly of the genera *Lactobacillus*, *Leuconostoc*, *Streptococcus*, *Brevibacterium* and *Pediococcus*, are present in most meats, fresh or cured, and can grow even at refrigerator temperatures. Ordinarily their limited growth does not detract from the quality of the meat; on the contrary, in certain types of sausage, such as salami, Lebanon and Thuringer, the lactic fermentation is encouraged. However, the lactic acid bacteria may be responsible for three types of spoilage: (i) slime formation at the surface or within, especially in the presence of sucrose, (ii) production of a green discoloration, and (iii) souring, when excessive amounts of lactic and other acids have been produced.

Fresh beef

Fresh beef undergoes the changes in colour mentioned: (i) changes in the haemoglobin and myoglobin, the red pigment in the blood and muscles, respectively, so as to cause loss of bloom and the production of reddish-brown methemoglobin and metmyoglobin and the green-gray-brown other oxidation pigments by action of oxygen and micro-organisms; (ii) white, green, yellow, greenish-blue to brown-black spots, and purple discolourations due to pigmented micro-organisms; (iii) phosphorescence; and (iv) spots due to various bacteria, yeasts and moulds. Beef also is subject to sliminess on the surface due to bacteria or yeasts, stickiness due to moulds, whiskers resulting from mycelial growth of moulds and souring and putrefaction by bacteria. Pseudomonads usually predominate in beef held at 10°C (50°F) or lower, but at 15°C (59°F) or above micrococci and pseudomonads grow in about equal numbers.

Hamburger

Hamburger held at room temperature usually putrefies, but at temperatures near freezing acquires a stale, sour odour. The sourness at low temperatures has been found to be caused chiefly by species of *Pseudomonas*, with help from lactic acid bacteria. *Achromobacter*, *Micrococcus* and *Flavobacterium* species may grow in some samples. A large number of kinds of micro-organisms have been found in hamburger held at higher temperatures, but no distinction has been made between mere presence and actual growth. Among the genera reported are *Bacillus*, *Clostridium*, *Escherichia*, *Aerobacter*, *Proteus*, *Pseudomonas*, *Achromobacter*, *Lactobacillus*, *Leuconostoc*, *Streptococcus*, *Micrococcus* and *Sarcina* of the bacteria, and *Penicillium* and *Mucor* of the moulds. A few yeasts also have been found. Ground beef packaged in polyvinylidene chloride and held refrigerated has been found to contain pseudomonads, lactic acid bacteria, micrococci and microbacteria.

Fresh pork sausage

Fresh sausage is made mostly of ground, fresh pork to which salt and spices have been added. It may be sold in bulk or in natural or artificial casings. Pork sausage is a perishable food that must be preserved by refrigeration and then can be kept only a relatively short time without spoilage. Souring, the most common type of spoilage at refrigerator temperatures of 0° to 11°C (32° to 51.8°F), has been attributed to growth and acid production by lactobacilli and leuconostocs, although *Microbacterium* and *Micrococcus* organisms may grow at higher storage temperatures. The encased pork sausages, and especially the 'little-pig' type, are subject to slime formation on the outside of the casing on long storage, or to variously coloured spots due to mould growth. Thus *Alternaria* has been found to cause small, dark spots on refrigerated links.

Spoilage of cured meats

Most of the cured meats are pork, although some cuts of beef may be cured. The inhibitory effect of nitrates against anaerobes has been mentioned previously. They hinder both growth and spore formation of anaerobes but favour aerobes. It is claimed that hydroxylamine and hydrogen peroxide produced from nitrates harm the anaerobes. Sodium nitrate is alleged to favour lactic acid bacteria in sausages like Thuringer or Essex that support a lactic fermentation. Curing salts make meats more favourable to growth of Gram-positive bacteria, yeasts and moulds than to the Gram-negative bacteria which usually spoil meats. They also reduce the thermal processing necessary to produce stable heated meat, foods, such as pork luncheon meats. Some meats, e.g. bulk chipped beef, are preserved by their high content of sodium chloride.

The load of micro-organisms on the piece of meat to be cured and any deterioration that has taken place will influence the success of the curing operation. Thus undesirable changes in the meat pigments will result in a discoloured cured product, incipient spoilage will give an inferior appearance and flavour to the product, and large numbers of spoilage bacteria may interfere with the cure.

Dried beef or beef hams

Beef hams are made spongy by species of *Bacillus*, sour by a variety of bacteria, red by *Halobacterium cutirubrum* or a red *Bacillus* species, and blue by *Pseudomonas syncyanea*, *Penicillium spinulosum* (purplish), and species of *Rhodotorula* yeasts.

Gas in jars of chipped dried beef has been attributed to a denitrifying, aerobic organism that resembles *Pseudomonas fluorescens*. The gases are oxides of nitrogen. *Bacillus* species have been known to produce carbon dioxide in the jars.

Sausage

In encased sausages, spoilage micro-organisms may grow on the outside of the casing, between the casing and meat, or in the interior. Growth of organisms can take place on the outside of the casings only if sufficient moisture is available. If moisture is available, micrococci and yeasts can form a slimy layer, as often occurs on frankfurters that have become moist because of removal from refrigerator to warmer temperatures. With less moisture, moulds may produce fuzziness and discolouration. Carbon dioxide, produced mostly by heterofermentative lactic acid bacteria, may swell packages of wieners or breakfast sausages when they are packaged in gastight, flexible film.

Growth between the casing and the meat is favoured by an accumulation of moisture there during cooking, if the casing is penetrable to water. Or, when two casings are employed, the inner casing may be wetted before the outer casing is applied, entrapping water between the casings. The slime at the surface of the meat or between the casings is formed chiefly by acid-producing micrococci. The penetrability of the inner casing to soluble nutrients favours the bacterial growth.

Various kinds of bacteria have been reported able to grow within sausages on long chilling storage or at storage temperatures above 10.5°C (51°F). Acid-forming micrococci, such as *Micrococcus candidus*, may grow in liver sausage and bologna, and species of *Bacillus* have been found growing in liver sausage. Low-temperature leuconostocs and lactobacilli also can grow and cause a souring that is not encouraged in most sausage but is favoured in certain varieties, such as Lebanon, Thuringer and Essex sausages. Fading of the red colour of sausage to a chalky gray has been attributed to oxygen and light and may be hastened by bacteria. Various causes have been suggested for 'chill rings', such as oxidation, the production of organic acids or reducing substances by bacteria, excessive water and undercooking. The greening of sausage may appear as a green ring not far from the casing, a green core, or a green surface. The cause of greening is probably the production of peroxides, e.g. hydrogen peroxide, by heterofermentative species of *Lactobacillus* and *Leuconostoc* or other catalase-negative bacteria, according to Niven. Jensen states that hydrogen sulphide also may be involved. Greening is favoured by a slightly acid pH and by the presence of small amounts of oxygen. The green ring below the surface of large sausages or green core in small sausages develops within 12 to 36 hours after the sausage has been processed, even under refrigeration; it is evident as soon as the sausage is cut and usually is not accompanied by surface slime. Bacterial growth and the production of heat-stable peroxide have taken place before smoking and cooking, and the peroxide continues to act to produce greening after the processing. Green cores in large sausage, e.g. big bologna, develop usually after 4 or more days of holding and within 1 to 12 hours after slicing, after large numbers of causative bacteria develop as a result of underprocessing and inadequate refrigeration. Greening of a cut surface indicates contamination with and growth of salt-tolerant, peroxide-forming bacteria (probably lactics) which can grow at low temperatures. Surface sliminess often accompanies the greening. The defect can be spread from sausage to sausage.

Production of nitric oxide gas in sausage by nitrate-reducing bacteria has been reported. Unless the casing or packaging material permits the passage of carbon dioxide, carbon dioxide may accumulate as the result of the action of heterofermentative lactics and cause swelling. This also can take place in packaged sliced, cured meats, in sandwich spreads, and in similar products in plastic casings or packages.

Bacon

Since the parts of the hog used for bacon and the curing processes vary in different parts of the world, the types of spoilage and the organisms concerned also vary. The bellies employed in the American process usually are subject to little change and are reported to emerge from the smokehouse comparatively free from moulds and yeasts and low in bacteria. Because of its salt tolerance and ability to grow at low temperatures, *Streptococcus faecalis* often is present. Moulds are the chief spoilage organisms on the cured bacon, especially on the sliced, packaged bacon when stored in the home refrigerator. Most trouble is encountered in late summer and early fall with species of *Aspergillus, Alternaria, Monilia, Oidium, Fusarium, Mucor, Rhizopus, Botrytis* and *Penicillium*. Few microbiological problems are encountered with dry-salt bellies and Oxford-style bellies. Any rancidity that develops usually is due to chemical changes. Sliced bacon may be deteriorated by oxidising and lipolytic bacteria on long storage, although chemical oxidation also may take place. Oxidising and sulphide forming bacteria also may be concerned in producing a poor colour in the flesh part of bacon, although wrong concentrations of nitrite are more often responsible, and chromogenic bacteria may cause discoloured areas. A yellowish-brown discolouration, showing the presence of tyrosine, has been blamed on proteolytic bacteria. Gumminess of pickle and bellies, now uncommon, results from the formation of gum by any of a large number of species of bacteria and yeasts.

An extensive study of the bacteriology of Wiltshire bacon has been made in Canada. In the manufacture of this bacon, the sides of the hog are cured in a very concentrated brine for a short period (6 to 8 days) at a low temperature (3.3° to 4.5°C or 37.9° to 40.1°F), permitting the growth of only psychrophilic, salt-tolerant bacteria. Little growth takes place in the curing pickle, but marked increases in bacteria take place on the sides of meat, sometimes enough to give sliminess to the surface. Visible growth or slime usually appears when the count is over 71,500,000 per square centimetre. Micrococci are most common in the brine, but other organisms, unable to grow in the cold brine, may grow before brining or during the storage of the pickled sides after baling.

Unopened, packaged, sliced bacon is spoiled mostly by lactobacilli, but micrococci and fecal streptococci may grow, especially if the wrapper is somewhat permeable to oxygen. Opened bacon may be spoiled by moulds. Vacuum-packed bacon supports the growth of coagulase-negative staphylococci at 37°C; at 20°C micrococci and lactobacilli grow. In canned bacon micrococci remove oxygen, then fecal streptococci grow, and finally lactobacilli predominate.

Ham

The term 'souring', as used for the spoilage of hams, covers all important types of spoilage, from a comparatively nonodourous proteolysis to genuine putrefaction with its very obnoxious odours of mercaptans, hydrogen sulphide, amines, indole, etc. and may be caused by a large variety of psychrophilic, salt-tolerant bacteria. Jensen lists a number of genera, species of which may cause souring: *Achromobacter, Bacillus, Pseudomonas, Lactobacillus, Proteus, Serratia, Bacterium, Micrococcus, Clostridium* and others, as well as some unnamed, hydrogen sulphide-producing streptobacilli that cause flesh-souring of ham. The types of souring are classified according to their location as sours of shank or tibial marrows, body or meat, aitchbone, stifle joint, body-bone or femur marrow and butt.

'Puffers', or gassy hams, are not encountered commercially but occur occasionally when inexpert curing is done.

When the long cure was used on hams, putrefaction by *Clostridium putrefaciens* was more common. This organism is able to grow at near-freezing temperatures and will begin growth even when the ideal rate of chilling of the ham is employed. Many of the bacteria causing souring cannot initiate growth under these conditions but must get started at higher temperatures to be able to grow at the low ones. Thus spoilage of southern country-style hams, chiefly loin or flesh sours, has been found to be proteolytic, putrefactive or even gassy, as the result of localised growth of various species of *Clostridium*. Presumably these bacteria grow before or after the curing process and are not inhibited much by the strengths of curing solutions employed.

The present method for curing hams by the quick-curing method, in which the curing solution is pumped into the ham by way of the veins, has reduced greatly the incidence of souring. The reduction of bacterial contamination and growth by proper slaughter and bleeding of hogs, adequate refrigeration, sealing of the marrows by sawing in the right places, prompt handling, use of bacteriologically satisfactory pickling solution and good overall sanitation, all have helped reduce the amount of souring.

Tenderised hams are really precooked and are given a mild cure. Such hams are perishable and should be protected from contamination and should be refrigerated during storage to prevent their deterioration by micro-organisms. Improperly handled tenderised hams may be spoiled by any of the common meat-spoilage bacteria, among which *Escherichia coli*, *Proteus* spp., and food-poisoning staphylococci (*Staphylococcus aureus*) have been reported.

Refrigerated packaged meats

Packaging films, permitting good penetration of oxygen and hence of carbon dioxide, favour the more aerobic bacteria, such as *Pseudomonas* and their production of off-flavours, slime and even putrefaction. This spoilage is much like that in the unwrapped meat. Films with poor gas penetration encourage lactic acid bacteria, especially when combined with vacuum packing. These bacteria in time cause souring, slime, and atypical flavours.

Curing solutions or pickles

Spoilage of the pickle or curing solution for ham and other cured meats is likely in the presence of available sugar and a pH well above 6.0. Spoilage of multiuse brines usually is putrefactive and is caused by *Vibrio*, *Achromobacter* or *Spirillum*. Souring can be caused by *Lactobacillus* and *Micrococcus* and slime by *Leuconostoc* or *Micrococcus lipolyticus*.

Turbid and ropy vinegar pickles about pigs' feet or sausages are caused chiefly by lactic acid bacteria from the meats, although yeasts may be responsible for cloudiness. Black spots on pickled pigs' feet may be caused by hydrogen sulphide-producing bacteria, and gas in vacuum-packed pickles may come from heterofermentative lactic acid bacteria or yeasts.

Chapter 13

Fish and Other Seafood

INTRODUCTION

A fish is any aquatic vertebrate animal that is typically ectothermic (or cold-blooded), covered with scales, and equipped with two sets of paired fins and several unpaired fins. Fish are abundant in the sea and in freshwater, with species being known from mountain streams (e.g. char and gudgeon) as well as in the deepest depths of the ocean (e.g. gulpers and anglerfish).

Fish are of tremendous importance as food for people around the world, either collected from the wild or farmed in much the same way as cattle or chickens. Fish are also exploited for recreation, through angling and fish-keeping, and are commonly exhibited in public aquaria.

Here we are mainly concerned with what most people think of as fish principally the free swimming teleosts and elasmobranchs. The same term can also encompass all seafoods including crustaceans with a chitinous exoskeleton such as lobsters, crabs and shrimp, and molluscs such as mussels, cockles, clams and oysters. Microbiologically these have many common features with free swimming fish.

Historically the extreme perishability of fish has restricted its consumption in a reasonably fresh state to the immediate vicinity of where the catch was landed. This has detracted only slightly from it playing a significant role in human nutrition as, throughout the world, traditional curing techniques based on combinations of salting, drying and smoking were developed which allowed more widespread fish consumption.

Poor keeping quality is a special feature of fish which sets it apart even from meat and milk. The biochemical and microbiological reasons for this are discussed later in this chapter.

STRUCTURE AND COMPOSITION

Although broadly similar in composition and structure to meat, fish has a number of distinctive features. Unlike meat, there are no visually obvious deposits of fat. Although the lipid content of fish can be up to 25 per cent, it is largely interspersed between the muscle fibres. A further feature which contributes to the good eating quality of fish is the very low content of connective tissue, approximately 3 per cent of total weight compared with around 15 per cent in meat. This, and the lower proportion of body mass contributed by the skeleton, reflect the greater buoyancy in water compared with that in air.

Muscle structure also differs. Inland animals it is composed of very long fibres while in fish they form relatively short segments known as myotomes separated by sheets of connective tissue known as myocommata. This gives fish flesh its characteristically flaky texture.

Fish flesh generally contains about 15–20 per cent protein and less than 1 per cent carbohydrate. In non-fatty fish such as the teleosts cod, haddock and whiting, fat levels are only about 0.5 per cent, while in fatty fish such as mackerel and herring, levels can vary between 3 and 25 per cent depending on factors such as the season and maturity.

MICROBIOLOGY OF PRIMARY PROCESSING

As with meat, the muscle and internal organs of healthy, freshly caught fish are usually sterile but the skin, gills and alimentary tract all carry substantial numbers of bacteria. Reported numbers on the skin have ranged from 10^2–10^7 cfu cm^{-2}, and from 10^3–10^9 cfu g^{-1} in the gills and the gut. These are mainly Gram-negatives of the genera *Pseudomonas*, *Shewanella*, *Psychrobacter*, *Vibrio*, *Flavobacterium* and *Cytophaga* and some gram-positives such as coryneforms and micrococci. Since fish are cold blooded, the temperature characteristics of the associated flora will reflect the water temperatures in which the fish live. The microflora of fish from northern temperate waters where the temperatures usually range between –2° and +12°C is predominantly psychrotrophic or psychrophilic. Most are psychrotrophs with an optimum growth temperature around 18°C. Far fewer psychrotrophs are associated with fish from warmer tropical waters and this is why most tropical fish keep far longer in ice than temperate fish. Bacteria associated with marine fish should be tolerant of the salt levels found in sea water. Though many do grow best at salt levels of 2–3 per cent, the most important organisms are those that are not strictly halophilic but euryhaline, i.e. they can grow over a range of salt concentrations. It is these that will survive and continue to grow as the salt levels associated with the fish decline, for example when the surface is washed by melting ice.

After capture at sea, fish are commonly stored in ice or refrigerated sea water until landfall is made. It is important that fresh, clean cooling agent is used as reuse will lead to a rapid build up or psychrotrophic contaminants and accelerated spoilage of the stored fish. Gutting the fish prior to chilling at sea is not a universal practice, particularly with small fish and where the time between harvest and landing is short. It does however remove a major reservoir of microbial contamination at the price of exposing freshly cut surfaces which will be liable to rapid spoilage. Similarly any damage to the fish from nets, hooks, etc. that breaches the fish's protective skin will provide a focus for spoilage. Subsequent processing operations such as filleting and mincing which increase the surface area to volume of the product also increase the rate of spoilage. Fish can be further contaminated by handling on board, at the dock and at markets after landing, particularly where they are exposed for sale and are subject to contamination with human pathogens by birds and flies. Generally though, fish have a far better safety record than mammalian meat. A number of types of foodborne illness are associated with fish (Table 13.1).

Table 13.1. Foodborne illness and pathogens associated with fish.

Vibrio cholerae
Vibrio parahaemolyticus
Vibrio vulnificus
Clostridium botulinum Type E
Enteric viruses
Scombroid fish poisoning
Paralytic shellfish poisoning

CRUSTACEANS AND MOLLUSCS

The propensity of crustaceans to spoil rapidly can be controlled in the case of crabs and lobsters by keeping them alive until immediately before cooking or freezing. This is not possible with shrimp or prawns, which are of far greater overall economic importance but die soon after capture. In addition to their endogenous microflora, shrimp are often contaminated with bacteria from the mud trawled up with them and are therefore subject to rapid microbiological deterioration following capture. Consequently they must be processed either by cooking or by freezing immediately on landing.

Some aspects of the production and processing of frozen cooked peeled prawns can pose public health risks. Increasingly prawns are grown commercially in farms where contamination of the ponds, and thence the product, with pathogenic bacteria can occur via bird droppings and fish feed. After cooking, which should be sufficient to eliminate vegetative bacterial contaminants derived from the ponds, the edible tail meat is separated from the chitinous exoskeleton. Peeling machines are used in some operations but large quantities are still peeled by hand, particularly in countries where labour is cheap. The handling involved gives an opportunity for the product to be contaminated with human pathogens after the bactericidal cooking step and prior to freezing.

The flesh of molluscs such as cockles, mussels, oysters and clams differs from that of crustaceans and free swimming fish by containing appreciable (3 per cent) carbohydrate in the form of glycogen. Though many of the same organisms are involved, spoilage is therefore glycolytic rather than proteolytic, leading to a pH decrease from around 6.5 to below 5.8. Molluscs are usually transported live to the point of sale or processing where the flesh can often be removed by hand. Although contamination may occur at this stage, the significant public health problems associated with shellfish arise more from their ability to concentrate viruses and bacteria from surrounding waters, the frequent pollution of these waters with sewage and the practice of consuming many shellfish raw or after relatively mild cooking.

SPOILAGE OF FRESH FISH

A number of factors contribute to the unique perishability of fish flesh. In the case of fatty fish, spoilage can be non-microbiological; fish lipids contain a high proportion of polyunsaturated fatty acids which are more reactive chemically than the largely saturated fats that occur in mammalian meat. This makes fish far more susceptible to the development of oxidative rancidity.

In most cases though, spoilage is microbiological in origin. Fish flesh naturally contains very low levels of carbohydrate and these are further depleted during the death struggle of the fish. This has two important consequences for spoilage. Firstly it limits the degree of post-mortem acidification of the tissues so that the ultimate pH of the muscle is 6.2–6.5 compared with around 5.5 in mammalian muscle. Fish which have a lower pH such as halibut (approx. 5.6) tend to have better keeping qualities. Secondly, the absence of carbohydrate means that bacteria present on the fish will immediately resort to using the soluble pool of readily assimilated nitrogenous materials, producing off-odours and flavours far sooner.

The composition of the nonprotein nitrogen fraction differs significantly from that in meat (Table 13.2). Trimethylamine oxide (TMAO) occurs in appreciable quantities in marine fish as part of the osmoregulatory system. TMAO is used as a terminal electron acceptor by non-fermentative bacteria such as *Shewanella putrefaciens* and this allows them to grow under microaerophilic and anaerobic conditions. The product of this reduction is trimethylamine which is an important component in the characteristic odour of fish (Fig. 13.1.) TMAO also contributes to a relatively high redox potential in the flesh since the E_h of the TMAO/TMA couple is +19 mV.

Table 13.2. Nitrogen-containing extractives in fish.

	Cod	Herring	Dogfish	Lobster
Total nitrogenous extractives g kg^{-1}	12	12	30	55
Free amino acids (mM l^{-1})	7	30	10	300
TMAO (mM l^{-1})	5	3	10	2
Urea (mM l^{-1})	0	0	33	0
Creatine (mM l^{-1})	3	3	2	0
Betaine (mM l^{-1})	0	0	2	1
Anserine	1	0	0	0

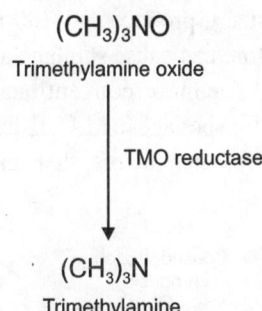

$$(CH_3)_3NO$$

Trimethylamine oxide

TMO reductase

$$(CH_3)_3N$$

Trimethylamine

Fig. 13.1. Reduction of trimethylamine oxide.

Elasmobranchs such as dogfish and shark contain high levels of urea. Bacterial urease activity in the flesh can produce ammonia very rapidly giving the product a pungent odour. Not only does this render the flesh itself uneatable but it can also taint the flesh of other fish stored nearby. It is for this reason that in many areas fishermen will discard all but the fins of shark when they catch them.

Shellfish such as lobster have a particularly large pool of nitrogenous extractives and are even more prone to rapid spoilage; a factor which accounts for the common practice of keeping them alive until immediately prior to consumption. Fish proteins are less stable than mammalian protein. As with meat, extensive proteolysis does not become apparent until the product is already well spoiled, but limited protein degradation may improve bacterial access to the nutrient pool of extractives.

The speed with which a product spoils is also related to the initial microbial load on the product: the higher the count the sooner spoilage occurs. Since fish from cold waters will have a larger proportion of psychrotrophs among their natural microflora, this can shorten the chill shelf-life appreciably. Spoilage of chilled fish is due principally to the activity of psychrotrophic gram-negative rods also encountered in meat spoilage, particularly *Shewanella putrefaciens* and *Pseudomonas* spp. The uniquely objectionable smell of decomposing fish is the result of a cocktail of chemicals, many of which also occur in spoiling meat. Sulphurous notes are provided by hydrogen sulphide, methyl mercaptan and dimethyl sulphide and esters contribute the 'fruity' component of the odour. A number of other amines in addition to TMA are produced by bacterial catabolism of amino acids. Skatole, a particularly unpleasant example produced by the degradation of tryptophan, also contributes to the smell of human faeces. The level of volatile bases in fish flesh has provided an index of spoilage, although this and other chemical indices used are often poor substitutes for the trained nose and eyes.

Figure 13.2 illustrates some of the different products made from fish, in terms of the general processing technologies. One interesting aspect that relates to some of the discussion above will be discussed here. The combination of a near neutral pH and availability of TMAO as an alternative electron acceptor means that vacuum and modified-atmosphere packing of fish does not produce the same dramatic extension of keeping quality seen with meat. Typically the shelf-life extension of vacuum and modified-atmosphere-packed cod will vary from less than 3 days to about 2 weeks. *Shewanella putrefaciens* can grow under these conditions producing TMA and hydrogen sulphide to spoil the product. Work in Denmark has also demonstrated that CO_2 tolerant marine vibrios like *Photobacterium phosphoreum* may be responsible for a non-sulphurous spoilage of these products in some instances.

This is a large (5 μm diameter), almost yeast-like, bacterium that has been isolated from the intestines of several different fish. Because of its size it produces 10–100 fold more TMA per cell than smaller organisms such as *Shewanella* and therefore can cause spoilage at lower populations, typically around 10^7 cfu g^{-1} compared with 10^8 cfu g^{-1} for more conventional bacteria. Whether *Shewanella* or *Photobacterium* is ultimately responsible for spoilage in MAP fish products probably depends on relative numbers present initially and whether any other factors, that might have differential affects on their growth rates, apply.

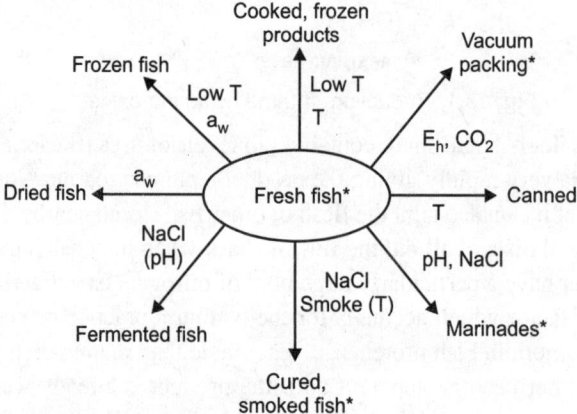

Fig. 13.2. Fish and fish products. T indicates elevated temperature; E_h, low redox potential; pH, reduced pH; a_w reduced a_w; and * stored at chill temperatures.

FERMENTED FISH

The term fermented fish is applied to two groups of product, mostly confined to East and Southeast Asia: the more widely known fish/salt formulations such as fish sauces and pastes, and fish/salt/carbohydrate blends. Strictly speaking, only in the latter case is the description 'fermented' fully justified. Microbial action in the production of fish sauces and pastes is slight if not insignificant and the term is being used in its looser, non-microbiological, sense to apply to any process where an organic material undergoes extensive transformation. In many areas where they are produced, fish sauces and pastes are the main flavour principle in the local cuisine and provide a valuable balanced source of amino acids. The names of some fish sauces and pastes and their countries of origin are given in Table 13.3.

Table 13.3. Fish sauces and pastes and their countries of origin.

Country	Name Sauce	Paste
	Amber/brown liquid, salty taste, cheese-like aroma	Red/brown salty paste
Burma	*ngapi*	*nga-ngapi*
Indonesia	*ketjap-ikan*	*trassi-ikan*
		trassi-udang (shrimps)
Kampuchea	*nuoc-mam*	*prahoc*
	nuoc-mam-gau-ca	*mam-ruoc* (shrimps)
	(livers only)	
Laos	*nam-pla* (pa)	*padec*
Malaysia	*budu*	*belachan* (shrimps)
Philippines	*patis*	*bagoong*
Thailand	*nam-pla*	*kapi*
Vietnam	*nuoc-mam*	*man-ca*
		man-tom (shrimps)

Fish sauces and pastes are usually made from a variety of small fish which are packed into tanks or jars with salt usually at a ratio of around three parts fish to one part salt. This is more than sufficient to saturate the aqueous phase, to produce an a_w below 0.75 and arrest the normal pattern of spoilage. The only organisms likely to be able to grow under such conditions are anaerobic extreme halophiles. Although there have been recent reports of isolations of organisms such as the proteolytic *Halobacterium salinarium* from fish sauce, their importance remains to be established since earlier work has shown that acceptable fish sauce could be made using fish sterilised by irradiation. The production process can take up to 18 months or more, during which the fish autolyse, largely through the action of enzymes in the gut and head of the uneviscerated fish, to produce a brown salty liquid rich in amino acids, soluble peptides and nucleotides. Products in which autolysis is less extensive are described as fish pastes.

Authentic lactic-fermented fish products have to include as an ingredient an exogenous source of fermentable carbohydrate. Considerable variation in recipes has been noted but production is governed by two general principles: the higher the salt content of the product, the longer the production process takes but the better the product's keeping qualities; and the higher the level of added carbohydrate, the faster the fermentation and the more acidic the flavour. Fish/salt/carbohydrate products (Table 13.4) are generally much less popular than the fish sauces and pastes and are produced on a smaller scale.

Table 13.4. Fermented fish/salt/carbohydrate products.

Country	Products
Japan	*I-shushi*, e.g. *ayu-sushi*, *funa-suchi*, *tai-suchi*
Kampuchea	*phaak*, *mam-chao*
Korea	*sikhae*
Laos	*som-kay-pa-eun*, *som-pa*, *mam-pa-kor*, *pa-chao*, *pa-khem*, *som-pa-keng*
Malaysia	*pekasam*, *cencalok*
Philippines	*burong-isda*, e.g. *burong-ayungi*, *burong-dalag*, *burong-bangus*
Thailand	*pla-ra*, *pla-som*, *pla-chao*, *som-fak*

Their production also tends to be more common away from the coast and to use freshwater fish. Though superficially their production appears similar to that of fermented meat sausages, they are quite distinctive.

In products such as *Burong-isda* (Philippines), *Pla-jao* and *Pla-som* (Thailand) and *I-shushi* (Japan), cleaned fish flesh is dry salted with about 10–20 per cent salt and left for a period of up to a day. The flesh is then usually removed from the brine that develops and may be subjected to further moisture reduction by sun-drying for a short period. Lactic fermentation is then initiated by addition of carbohydrate. This is usually in the form of rice although traditional saccharifying agents (*koji*, Japan; *look-pang*, Thailand; *ang-kak*, Philippines) employing mould enzymes may be added. These accelerate the fermentation, since most LAB are not amylolytic, and also increases the total acid produced. For example, *Burong-isda* containing *ang-kak* has a lower pH (3.0–3.9) than that produced with rice alone (4.1–4.5). Garlic is often added along with the rice as a flavouring ingredient and this may play a similar role in directing the fermentation as spices do in fermented sausage production. Garlic is also a source of the fermentable carbohydrate inulin. The product is normally ready for consumption after about two weeks of fermentation when the microflora is dominated by yeasts and LAB which are present at levels around 10^7 cfu g^{-1} and 10^8 cfu g^{-1} respectively.

With the exception of *I-shushi*, these products are usually cooked before consumption and this along with the low pH generally guarantees safety. However, the small, very often domestic-scale, production can lead to extreme variations in a product's character and failure to obtain a satisfactory rapid fermentation in *I-shushi* has led to outbreaks of botulism in Japan caused by *C. botulinum* type E.

CONTAMINATION, PRESERVATION AND SPOILAGE OF FISH AND OTHER SEAFOODS

Seafoods discussed in this section include fresh, frozen, dried, pickled and salted fish, as well as various shellfish. Freshwater fish also are considered.

Contamination

The flora of living fish depends upon the microbial content of the waters in which they live. The slime that covers the outer surface of fish has been found to contain bacteria of the genera *Pseudomonas*, *Achromobacter*, *Micrococcus*, *Flavobacterium*, *Corynebacterium*, *Sarcina*, *Serratia*, *Vibrio* and *Bacillus*. The bacteria on fish from northern waters are mostly psychrophiles, whereas fish from tropical waters carry more mesophiles. Freshwater fish carry freshwater bacteria, which include members of most genera found in salt water plus species of *Aeromonas*, *Lactobacillus*, *Brevibacterium*, *Alcaligenes* and *Streptococcus*. In the intestines of fish from both sources are found bacteria of the genera *Achromobacter*, *Pseudomonas*, *Flavobacterium*, *Vibrio*, *Bacillus*, *Clostridium* and *Escherichia*. Boats, boxes, bins, fish houses, and fishermen soon become heavily contaminated with these bacteria and transfer them to the fish during cleaning. The numbers of bacteria in slime and on the skin of newly caught ocean fish may be as low as 100 and as high as several million per square centimetre, and the intestinal fluid may contain from one thousand to 100 million per millilitre. Gill tissue may harbour a thousand to a million per gram. Washing reduces the surface count. Unopened fish or fish 'in the round', have been reported to keep better for a while than opened fish because contamination of the body cavity is avoided. Bacteria are supposed to spread through the fish flesh mostly via the gills.

Oysters and other shellfish that pass large amounts of water through their bodies pick up soil and water micro-organisms in this way, including pathogens if they are present. *Achromobacter* and *Flavobacterium* predominate. Shrimps, crabs, lobsters, and similar seafood have a bacteria-laden slime on their surfaces that probably resembles that of fish. Species of *Achromobacter*, *Bacillus*, *Micrococcus*, *Pseudomonas*, *Flavobacterium*, *Alcaligenes* and *Proteus* have been found on shrimp.

Since the surface flora of fish and other sea animals seems to consist chiefly of water bacteria, the icing of these foods would not be expected to add much in the way of contamination. Ices containing antiseptic or germicidal chemicals have been used; chlortetracycline may now be used as a dip or in ice for fish in many parts of the world and for scallops and unpeeled shrimp in the United States.

Preservation

Of all the flesh foods, fish is the most susceptible to autolysis, to oxidation and hydrolysis of fats, and to microbial spoilage. Its preservation, therefore, involves prompt treatment by preservative methods, and often these methods are rigorous compared to those used on meats. When fish are gathered far from the processing plant, preservative methods must be applied even on the fishing boat.

Rigor mortis is especially important in the preservation of fish, for it retards post-mortem autolysis and bacterial decomposition. Therefore any procedure that lengthens rigor mortis lengthens keeping time. It is longer if the fish have had less muscular activity before death and have not been handled roughly and bruised during catching and later processing, and is longer in some kinds of fish than in others. Reducing the holding temperature will lengthen the period. Aseptic methods to reduce the contamination of seafood are difficult to apply, but some of the gross contamination prior to processing can be avoided by general cleansing and sanitisation of boats, decks, holds, bins, or other containers and processing equipment in the plant and by use of ice of good bacteriological quality. The removal of soil from contaminating surfaces and from the fish by adequate cleansing methods, including effective detergent solutions, helps greatly to reduce the microbial 'load' on the fish. The removal of organisms is difficult, but the fact that most of the contamination is on the outer surface of the fish and other seafood permits the removal of many of the micro-organisms by washing off slime and dirt.

Use of heat

Canning has proved to be a successful method for preserving seafoods. Like meats they are low-acid foods and for the most part have a slow rate of heat penetration and hence are difficult to heat-process. Also some kinds of seafoods soften considerably or even fall apart when sterilisation in the can is attempted. Some seafoods, e.g. oysters, are packed into cans and are not heat processed, but are preserved by refrigeration. A few kinds are pasteurised, crab meat, for example, and refrigerated until use. Most canned seafoods, however, are heat-processed so as to be sterile, or at least 'commercially sterile'. The process varies with the product being canned and the size and shape of the container. In general, the heat processes are more severe than those used for meats, but some special products are lightly processed. A few recommendations for minimal processes for marine products given by the National Canners Association are shown in Table 13.5.

Table 13.5. Recommended heat processes for canned marine products.

Product	Can name	Initial temperature, °F	Time, min.	
			240°F	250°F
Crab meat (brine), no liner	½ tuna	70	35	20
Mackerel (brine)	8Z tall	70	75	60

(*Contd ...*)

Product	Can name	Initial temperature, °F	Time, min.	
			240°F	250°F
		130	70	50
Oysters, cove	No. 1	70	24	14
Salmon	½ flat	60	75	–
Shrimp (wet)	No. 1	70	26	14
		90	25	13
Tuna (oil)	½ tuna	70	75	55

The cooking of fish or other seafood for human consumption reduces their content of viable micro-organisms and lengthens their keeping time.

Use of low temperatures

It is only after death of the fish or other sea animal that autolysis gets underway with softening and production of off-flavour, and microbial growth becomes uncontrolled; as has been stated these changes are delayed by rigor mortis. Oysters in their shells, for example, will not decompose so long as they remain alive, and life is lengthened by chilling storage of shell oysters. Carp seined from Middle Western lakes have been kept alive and hence in good condition by shipment in tanks to the New York market. 'Feedy' fish, that is, those stuffed with food, seem to decompose faster than normal fish.

Chilling

Because fish flesh autolyses and the fats become oxidised at temperatures above freezing—rapidly at summer temperatures and more slowly as the temperature is dropped toward freezing—preservation by chilling temperatures is, at best, temporary. When fish or other seafood is obtained at some distance from the receiving plant, the necessity for chilling on the boat depends upon the kind of fish, whether it is dressed there or not, and the atmospheric temperature. In general, small fish are more perishable than large ones; and dressed fish autolyse more slowly than whole fish but are spoiled more readily by bacteria. When outside temperatures are warm and distances of transportation are great, it becomes necessary to chill the fish and related foods on the fishing boat by packing in crushed ice or by mechanical refrigeration in order, to slow down autolysis and microbial growth until the products are marketed or are processed for longer preservation. The incorporation of preservatives in the ice used for chilling fish will be discussed later. The time allowable for holding in ice or in chilling storage will vary considerably with the kind of fish or other seafood, but will not be long in most instances. In general, chilling storage on shore is useful only when retail markets are near at hand and turnover is rapid. Otherwise, some other method of preservation is applied, such as freezing, salting, drying, smoking or canning, or combinations of these methods.

Freezing

Most of the modern methods of freezing foods initially were developed for freezing fish. In olden days, ice with added salt was employed. With the advent of mechanical refrigeration, sharp freezing was employed and the fish were 'glazed', that is, a layer of ice was frozen around the outside. Whole fish, especially the larger ones, usually are sharp-frozen in air or in a salt brine. Quick freezing is applied to wrapped fillets or steaks, although whole smaller fish may be so frozen. As with meats, quick-frozen fish may thaw to more like their original condition than fish frozen more slowly. During storage the fats of frozen fish are subject to hydrolysis and oxidation. Fatty fish deteriorate more rapidly than lean ones, probably because of more hydrolysis.

Decapitated raw shrimp are frozen and glazed, and some cooked shrimp are frozen. Other seafoods preserved by freezing include scallops, clams, oysters, spiny lobster tails, and cooked crab and lobster meat. Most of these products are packaged before freezing.

As with meats, freezing kills part but not all of the micro-organisms present, and growth will take place after thawing if time permits. Fish carry a flora of psychrophilic bacteria, most of which survive freezing and are ready to grow on thawing, e.g. *Pseudomonas*, *Achromobacter* and *Flavobacterium* species. Spores of type E *Clostridium botulinum* will survive freezing and storage and may grow and produce toxin when temperatures reach 3.3°C (38°F) or above. Frozen raw seafoods contain few enterococci, coliforms or staphylococci. Numbers of these organisms may be increased in the processing plant by cutting, breading and battering operations. Precooking reduces only coliforms to any extent.

Use of irradiation

Preservation of fish by ultraviolet rays has been tried but not put into practice. Experiments have indicated that gamma or cathode irradiation of some kinds of fish may be successful.

Preservation by drying

The dry salting of fish or immersion in brine constitutes a method of drying, in that moisture is removed or tied up. Oxidation of fish oils is not retarded and may cause deterioration. Salting of fish is being done to a lesser extent in the United States than formerly but still is used widely throughout the world. Salt cod is prepared by a combination of salting and air drying. The flesh is then removed from bones and skin.

Sun drying of fish, either of small fish or of strips of flesh, is not practiced extensively in many countries. Part of the preservative effect of smoking is the result of the drying of the fish.

Use of preservatives

The salting or marination of fish by dry salt or in brine is effective not only because of the drying effect, mentioned in the preceding section, but also because of the effect of the sodium chloride as a chemical preservative. This method is used to a considerable extent in many countries of the world. The chemical and bacteriological qualities of the salt are important, for impurities such as calcium and magnesium salts may hinder the penetration of the sodium chloride, and halophilic or salt-tolerant bacteria that are introduced may cause discolourations of the fish.

Because of the great perishability of fish, investigators have tried numerous chemicals as preservatives, either applied directly to the fish or incorporated in the ice used in chilling them.

Preservatives used on fish

In the intensive search for chemical preservatives that could be applied directly to round fish or fillets or as dips, a large number of chemicals have been tried, ranging from those that most control agencies would approve to those whose use would be questionable. Sodium chloride, an acceptable preservative, has been discussed.

Fish may be dry-salted so as to contain 4 to 5 per cent of salt. The salt contributes halophiles which may discolour the fish (e.g. a red colour from *Serratia salinaria*). Species of *Micrococcus* usually grow on the fish, and there is a decrease in *Flavobacterium*, *Achromobacter*, *Pseudomonas* and others. Curing of fish may be 'mild', that is, with light salting, or may be in heavy brine or with solid salt, and may be followed by smoking. Benzoic acid and benzoates have been only moderately successful as preservatives. Sodium and potassium nitrites and nitrates have been reported to lengthen the keeping time and are permitted in some countries. Sorbic acid has been found to delay spoilage of smoked or salted fish. . Boric acid has been used in Europe with some improvement in the keeping quality, but its use is illegal here. Other chemicals for which claims of success have been made, but whose use is contraindicated, include formaldehyde, hypochlorites, hydrogen peroxide, sulphur dioxide, undecylenic acid, capric acid, p-oxybenzoic acid and chloroform.

Antibiotics also have been tried experimentally, usually in a dip or in ice. Of those tested, chlortetracycline and oxytetracycline seemed best, and now their use is permitted. Chloramphenicol is fairly effective and penicillin, streptomycin and subtilin are poor or useless.

Storage of fish in an atmosphere containing over 20 per cent of carbon dioxide has been found to lengthen the keeping time, but this method has not come into commercial use. Pickling of fish may mean salting or acidification with vinegar, wine or sour cream. Herring is treated in various ways: salted, spiced and acidified. Various combinations of these treatments, coupled with an airtight container, preserve the fish, although refrigeration also must be employed for some products.

Formerly, fish was smoked primarily for its preservation, and the smoking was heavy, but now that canning, chilling and freezing are available to lengthen keeping time, much of the smoking of fish is primarily for flavour and hence is light. The smoke treatment and other preservative methods combined with it vary with the kind of fish, size of pieces and keeping time desired. Fish to be smoked usually are eviscerated and decapitated, but may be in the round, split or cut into pieces. Commonly, salting, light or heavy, precedes smoking and serves not only to flavour the fish but also to improve its keeping quality by reducing the moisture content. Drying may be aided by air currents. The smoking may be done at comparatively low temperatures, 80° to 100°F (26.7° to 37.8°C) or at high temperatures like 150° to 200°F, which result in partial cooking of the fish.

Microbiology of fish brines

Numbers of bacteria in fish curing brines vary with the concentration of salt, temperature of the brine, the kind and amount of contamination from the fish introduced, and the duration of use of the brine, and range from 10,000 to 10,000,000 bacteria per millilitre. Salt concentrations usually are between 18 per cent and saturation, but may be lower, especially after fish are introduced. The higher the temperature of the brine, the more salt is necessary to prevent its spoilage. Contamination comes from the fish, which ordinarily introduce chiefly species of *Pseudomonas*, *Achromobacter* and *Flavobacterium*, from ice, which introduces these genera plus *Corynebacterium* and cocci and from mechanically introduced sources, e.g. dust, which add cocci. On continued use of the brine, numbers of organisms increase, because of addition from successive lots of fish and because of growth of salt-tolerant bacteria such as the micrococci. As the brine ages there is a decrease in numbers of *Achromobacter* and an increase chiefly in corynebacteria in low-salt brines and in micrococci in high-salt brines.

Preservatives incorporated in ice

So-called 'germicidal ices' are prepared by adding a chemical preservative to water prior to its freezing. These ices are eutectic when the added chemical is uniformly distributed throughout, as with sodium chloride or noneutectic, when distribution is not uniform, as with sodium benzoate. Noneutectic ice is finely crushed for use on fish so as to get the chemical evenly spread in it.

Many investigators have sought the ideal chemical to be incorporated in ice for icing fish and have tested with some success a large number of chemicals, including hypochlorites, chloramines, benzoic acid and benzoates, colloidal silver, hydrogen peroxide, ozone, sodium nitrite, sulphonamides, antibiotics, propionates, levulinic acid, and many others. Both the American and Canadian governments, and those of other nations, now permit the incorporation of chlortetracycline (Aureomycin) in ice to be used by fishermen to preserve fish on trawlers and during transportation. The purpose of the application of preservative chemicals to fish either directly or as dips or germicidal ices is to kill or inhibit micro-organisms on the surfaces of the fish where at first they are most numerous and active.

Antioxidants

Fats and oils of many kinds of fish, especially the fatter ones, such as herring, mackerel, mullet and salmon, are composed to a great extent of unsaturated fatty acids and hence are subject to oxidative changes producing oxidative rancidity and sometimes undesirable alterations in colour. To counteract these undesirable changes, antioxidants may be applied as dips, coatings, glazes or gases. Good results have been reported with nordihydroguaiaretic acid, ethyl gallate, ascorbic acid and other compounds and with storage in carbon dioxide.

Spoilage

Like meat, fish and other seafood may be spoiled by autolysis, oxidation or bacterial activity, or most commonly by combinations of these. Most fish flesh, however, is considered more perishable than meat because of more rapid autolysis by the fish enzymes and because of the less acid reaction of fish flesh that favours microbial growth. Also, many of the fish oils seem to be more susceptible to oxidative deterioration than most animal fats. The experts agree that the bacterial spoilage of fish does not begin until after rigor mortis, when juices are released from the flesh fibres. Therefore, the more this is delayed or protracted, the longer will be the keeping time of the fish. Rigor mortis is hastened by struggling of the fish, lack of oxygen and a warm temperature, and is delayed by a low pH and adequate cooling of the fish. The pH of the fish flesh has an important influence on its perishability, not only because of its effect on rigor mortis, but also because of its influence on the growth of bacteria. The lower the pH of the fish flesh, the slower in general will be bacterial decomposition. The lowering of the pH of the fish flesh results from the conversion of muscle glycogen to lactic acid.

Factors Influencing Kind and Rate of Spoilage

The kind and rate of spoilage of fish will vary with a number of factors:

1. The kind of fish: The various kinds of fish differ considerably in their perishability. Thus some flat fish spoil more readily than round fish because they pass through rigor mortis more rapidly, but a flat fish like the halibut keeps longer because of the low pH (5.5) of its flesh. Certain fatty fish deteriorate rapidly because of oxidation of the unsaturated fats of their oils. Fishes high in trimethylamine oxide soon yield appreciable amounts of the 'stale-fishy' trimethylamine.
2. The condition of the fish when caught: Fish that are exhausted as the result of struggling, lack of oxygen and excessive handling spoil more rapidly than those brought in with less ado, probably because of the exhaustion of glycogen and hence smaller drop in pH of the flesh. 'Feedy' fish, that is, those full of food when caught, are more perishable than those with an empty intestinal tract.
3. The kind and extent of contamination of the fish flesh with bacteria: These may come from mud, water, handlers, and the exterior slime and intestinal content of the fish and are supposed

to enter the gills of the fish, from which they pass through the vascular system and thus invade the flesh, or to penetrate the intestinal tract and thus enter the body cavity. Even then, growth probably is localised for the most part, but the products of bacterial decomposition penetrate the flesh fairly rapidly by diffusion. In general, the greater the load of bacteria on the fish, the more rapid will be the spoilage. This contamination may take place in the net (mud), in the fishing boat, on the docks or, later, in the plants. Fish in the 'round', that is, not gutted, have not had the flesh contaminated with intestinal organisms, but it may become odourous because of decay of food in the gut and diffusion of decomposition products into the flesh. This process is hastened by the digestive enzymes attacking and perforating the gut wall and the belly wall and viscera, which in themselves have a high rate of autolysis. Gutting the fish on the boat spreads intestinal and surface-slime bacteria over the flesh, but thorough washing will remove most of the organisms and adequate chilling will inhibit the growth of those left. Any damage to skin or mucous membranes will harm the keeping quality of the product.

4. Temperature: Chilling of the fish is the most commonly used method for preventing or delaying bacterial growth and hence spoilage until the fish is used or is otherwise processed. The cooling should be as rapid as possible to 32° to 30°F (0° to −1°C), and this low temperature should be maintained. Obviously, the warmer the temperature, the shorter will be the storage life of the fish. Prompt and rapid freezing of the fish is still more effective in its preservation.

5. Use of an antibiotic ice or dip.

Evidences of Spoilage

Since the change is gradual from a fresh condition to staleness and then to inedibility, it is difficult to determine or agree on the first appearance of spoilage. A practical test to determine the quality of fish has been sought for many years, but none has proved entirely satisfactory. A chemical test for trimethylamine is backed by most workers for use on saltwater fish, although some support other methods, such as an estimate of volatile acids or volatile bases, or a test for pH, hydrogen sulphide, ammonia, etc. Bacteriological tests are too slow to be useful. Reay and Shewan describe the succession of external changes in a fish as it spoils and finally becomes 'putrid'. The bright, characteristic colours of the fish fade and dirty, yellow or brown discolourations appear. The slime on the skin of the fish increases, especially at the flaps and gills. The eyes gradually sink and shrink, the pupil becoming cloudy and the cornea opaque. The gills turn a light-pink and finally grayish-yellow colour. Most marked is the softening of the flesh, so that it exudes juice when squeezed and becomes easily indented by the fingers. The flesh is easily stripped from along the backbone, where a reddish-brown discolouration develops toward the tail and is a result of the oxidation of haemoglobin.

Meanwhile a sequence of odours is evolved: first the normal, fresh, seaweedy odour, then a sickly sweet one, then a stale-fishy odour due to trimethylamine, followed by ammoniacal and final putrid odours, due to hydrogen sulphide, indole and other malodourous compounds. Fatty fish also may show rancid odours. Cooking will bring out the odours more strongly.

Bacteria Causing Spoilage

The bacteria most often involved in the spoilage of fish are part of the natural flora of the external slime of fishes and their intestinal contents. The predominant kinds of bacteria causing spoilage vary with the temperatures at which the fish are held, but at the chilling temperatures usually employed, species of *Pseudomonas* are most likely to predominate, with *Achromobacter* and *Flavobacterium* species next in order of importance. Appearing less often, and then at higher temperatures, are bacteria of the genera *Micrococcus* and *Bacillus*. Reports in the literature list other genera as having species involved in fish spoilage; such as *Escherichia*, *Proteus*, *Serratia*, *Sarcina* and *Clostridium*. Most of these would grow only at ordinary atmospheric temperatures and probably would do little at chilling temperatures.

Normally pseudomonads increase in numbers on chilled fish during holding, achromobacters decrease, and flavobacteria increase temporarily and then decrease. The bacteria grow first on the surfaces and later penetrate the flesh. Fish have a high content of nonprotein nitrogen, and autolytic changes caused by their enzymes increase the supply of nitrogenous foods (e.g. amino acids and amines) and glucose for bacterial growth. From these compounds the bacteria make trimethylamine, ammonia, amines (e.g. putrescine and cadaverine), lower fatty acids, and aldehydes, and eventually hydrogen and other sulphides, mercaptans and indole, which products are indicative of putrefaction. A musty or muddy odour and taste of fish has been attributed to the growth of *Streptomyces* species in the mud at the bottom of the body of water and the absorption of the flavour by the fish. As has been indicated, discolourations of the fish flesh may occur during spoilage; yellow to greenish-yellow colours caused by *Pseudomonas fluorescens*, yellow micrococci and others; red or pink colours from growth of *Sarcina*, *Micrococcus* or *Bacillus* species, or by moulds or yeasts; and a chocolate-brown colour by an asporogenous yeast. Pathogens parasitising the fish may produce discolourations or lesions.

Spoilage of Special Kinds of Fish and Seafoods

The previous discussion has been limited for the most part to the spoilage of fish preserved by chilling. Salt fish are spoiled by salt-tolerant or halophilic bacteria of the genera *Serratia*, *Micrococcus*, *Bacillus*, *Achromobacter*, *Pseudomonas* and others, which often cause discolourations, a red colour being common. Moulds are the chief spoilage organisms on smoked fish. Marinated (sour pickled) fish should present no spoilage problems unless the acid content is low enough to permit growth of lactic acid bacteria or the entrance of air permits mould growth. Frozen fish, too, should present no bacteriological problems after freezing, but, of course, their quality depends on what has happened to the fish prior to freezing. Japanese fish sausage is subject to souring caused by volatile-acid production by bacilli or to putrefaction, despite the addition of nitrite and permitted preservatives.

In general, shellfish are subject to types of microbial spoilage similar to those for fish. However, in chilled shrimp *Achromobacter* seems to increase the most and is chiefly responsible for spoilage, although there may be a temporary increase in pseudomonads and a decrease in *Flavobacterium*, *Micrococcus*, and *Bacillus*. Crab meat is deteriorated by *Pseudomonas* and *Achromobacter* at chilling temperatures, and mainly by *Proteus* at higher temperatures. Species of *Pseudomonas*, *Achromobacter*, *Flavobacterium*, and *Bacillus* have been incriminated in the spoilage of raw lobsters. Oysters remain in good condition as long as they are kept alive in the shell at chilling temperature, but they decompose rapidly when they are dead, as in shucked oysters. The type of spoilage of the shucked oysters depends upon the temperature at which they are stored. Oysters are not only high in protein but also contain sugars which result from the hydrolysis of glycogen. At temperatures near freezing, *Pseudomonas* or *Achromobacter* species are the most important spoilage bacteria, but *Flavobacterium* and *Micrococcus* species also may grow.

The spoilage is termed 'souring' although the changes are chiefly proteolytic. At higher temperatures the 'souring' may be the result of the fermentation of the sugars by coliform bacteria, streptococci, lactobacilli and yeasts to produce acids and a sour odour. Early growth of *Serratia*, *Pseudomonas*, *Proteus* and *Clostridium* may take place. An uncommon type of spoilage by an asporogenous yeast causes pink oysters.

Chapter 14

Vegetables and Fruits

INTRODUCTION

The plant kingdom provides a considerable part of human food requirements and, depending on the particular plant species, use is made of every part of the plant structure from root, tuber, stem, leaves, fruit and seeds. Plants have evolved many strategies to survive the predation of herbivores and omnivores, including humans, and these strategies include, not only protective mechanisms to protect vegetative parts such as leaves, stems and roots, but also the development of rich, succulent fruits to encourage animals to help in the dispersal of seeds.

As the human race settled down from the nomadic hunter-gatherer state to form increasingly large stable communities so a wider range of plants have been brought into cultivation. Plant products are grown on an ever larger scale and many are stored for significant periods after harvest and may be transported from one part of the world to another.

Microbiological problems may occur at all stages in the production of plant products. During growth in the field there is a wide range of plant pathogens to contend with and, although these are dominated by the fungi, there are a significant number of bacteria and viruses. A further range of micro-organisms may cause post-harvest spoilage although there cannot be an absolutely clear boundary between plant pathogens and spoilage organisms because many plant products are made up of living plant tissue even after harvest.

Plants have evolved many mechanisms to prevent microbial invasion of their tissues. The outer surface is usually protected by a tough, resistant cuticle although the need for gas exchange requires specialised openings in parts of the leaf surface, the stomata and lenticels, which may provide access by some micro-organisms to plant tissue. Plant tissues may contain antimicrobial agents which are frequently phenolic metabolites, indeed the complex polyphenolic polymer known as lignin is especially resistant to microbial degradation. Many plants produce a special group of antimicrobial agents, the phytoalexins, in response to the initiation of microbial invasion. The low pH of the tissues of many fruits provides considerable protection against bacteria and the spoilage of these commodities is almost entirely by fungi. In contrast, many vegetables have somewhat higher pH and may be susceptible to bacterial spoilage (Table 14.1).

Another physical factor influencing the pattern of spoilage is the availability of water. Cereals, pulses, nuts and oilseeds are usually dried post-harvest and the low water activity should restrict the spoilage flora to xerophilic and xerotolerant fungi. These two groups of plant products, i.e. fruits, vegetables, etc. are sufficiently distinct that they will now be considered separately.

Table 14.1. pH values of some fruits and vegetables.

Fruits	pH	Vegetables	pH
Apples	2.9–3.3	Asparagus	5.4–5.8
Apricots	3.3–4.4	Broccoli	5.2–6.5
Bananas	4.5–5.2	Cabbage	5.2–6.3
Cherries	3.2–4.7	Carrots	4.9–6.3
Grapefruit	3.0	Cauliflower	6.0–6.7
Grapes	3.4–4.5	Celery	5.6–6.0
Limes	2.0–2.4	Lettuce	6.0–6.4
Melons	6.2–6.7	Parsnip	5.3
Oranges	3.3–4.3	Rhubarb	3.1–3.4
Pears	3.4–4.7	Runner beans	4.6
Plums	2.8–4.6	Spinach	5.1–6.8
Raspberries	2.9–3.5	Sweet potato	5.3–5.6
Tomatoes	3.4–4.9	Turnips	5.2–5.6

FRUITS AND FRUIT PRODUCTS

Despite the high water activity of most fruits, the low pH leads to their spoilage being dominated by fungi, both yeasts and moulds but especially the latter. The degree of specificity shown by many species of moulds, active in the spoilage of harvested fruits in the market place or the domestic fruit bowl, reflects their possible role as pathogens or endophytes of the plant before harvest. Thus *Penicillium italicum* and *P. digitatum* show considerable specificity for citrus fruits, being the blue mould and green mould respectively of oranges, lemons and other citrus fruits. *Penicillium expansum* causes a soft rot of apples and, although the rot itself is typically soft and pale brown, the emergence of a ring of tightly packed conidiophores bearing enormous numbers of blue conidiospores, has led to this species being referred to as the blue mould of apples. This particular species has a special significance because of its ability to produce the mycotoxin patulin which has been detected as a contaminant in unfermented apple juices but not in cider.

Other common diseases of apples and pears include the black spot or scab, caused by the ascomycete *Venturia inaequalis* (anamorph *Spilocaea pomi* = *Fusicladium dendriticum*), and a brown rot caused by another ascomycete, *Monilinia fructigena* (= *Sclerotinia fructigena*, anamorph *Monilia fructigena*). Apple scab spoils the appearance of fruit, and would certainly reduce its commercial value, but does not cause extensive rotting of the tissue. The brown rot, however, can lead to extensive damage of fruit both on the tree and in storage.

The typical brown rot is usually associated with rings of brown powdery pustules of the imperfect, or anamorph, stage, however fruit which is infected, but apparently healthy when it goes into store, can be reduced to a shiny black mummified structure in which much of the fruit tissue has been replaced by fungal material and the whole apple has become a functional sclerotium, or over wintering resting body, of the fungus. Although rarely seen in the United Kingdom, it is this structure which may germinate in the spring to produce the stalked apothecia of the perfect, or teleomorph, stage.

An especially widespread mould on both fruits and vegetables is the grey mould *Botrytis cinerea*, which is the imperfect stage of another ascomycete, *Botryotinia fuckeliana* (= *Sclerotinia fuckeliana*).

Infection of grapes on the vine by this same mould can lead to drying out of the grape and an increase in sugar concentration and wines made from such contaminated fruit are considered to be very special. Under these circumstances the fungus has been referred to as *La Pourriture Noble*—the noble rot.

To avoid excessive mould spoilage of harvested fruit during storage and transport it is necessary to harvest at the right stage of maturity and avoid damage and bruising. Mouldy fruit should be removed and destroyed and good hygiene of containers and packaging equipment is essential to prevent a build-up of mould propagules. The development of international trade in many fruit species has led to the use of some biocides to prevent mould spoilage. Benomyl has proved useful where it can be applied to the surface of fruits, such as citrus and bananas, in which the skins would normally be discarded (this, of course, is not the case for citrus used for marmalade and other preserves). In some parts of the world moulds like *Penicillium digitatum* have developed increased resistance to benomyl. Biphenyl is quite an effective protectant when incorporated into the wrapping tissues of fruit such as oranges when they are individually wrapped. Captan has been used as a spray for strawberries in the field to control *Botrytis* but its use must be stopped well before harvest.

Reduced temperature and increased carbon dioxide concentration may also be useful in controlling mould spoilage during storage and transport but many fruits are themselves sensitive to low temperatures and enhanced CO_2 levels and appropriate conditions need to be established for each commodity.

Canned fruits are normally given a relatively low heat treatment because of their low pH and although most mould propagules would be killed the ascospores of some members of the Eurotiales are sufficiently heat resistant to survive. Species of *Byssochlamys* are the best known but the increasing use of more exotic fruits is providing cases where spoilage of canned fruits have been due to such organisms as *Neosartorya fischeri* (anamorph *Aspergillus fischerianus*) and *Talaromyces flavus* var. *macrosporus* (anamorph *Penicillium* sp.).

VEGETABLES AND VEGETABLE PRODUCTS

The higher pH values of the tissues of many vegetables makes them more susceptible to bacterial invasion than fruits although there are also a number of important spoilage fungi of stored vegetables. The bacteria involved are usually pectinolytic species of the Gram-negative genera *Erwinia*, *Pseudomonas* and *Xanthomonas*, although pectinolytic strains of *Clostridium* can also be important in the spoilage of potatoes under some circumstances, and the non-sporing Gram-positive organism *Corynebacterium sepedonicum* causes a ring rot of potatoes. Table 14.2 lists a range of micro-organisms which may cause spoilage of fresh vegetables.

The role of plant pathogens in subsequent spoilage post-harvest may be complex, thus *Phytophthora infestans* causes a severe field disease of the potato plant, frequently causing death of the plant, but it may also remain dormant within the tubers and either cause a rot of the tubers during storage, or a new cycle of disease in the next season's crop.

However, the most frequent agents of spoilage are not the plant pathogens themselves but opportunistic micro-organisms which gain access to plant tissue through wounds, cracks, insect damage or even the lesions caused by the plant pathogens. All freshly harvested vegetables have a natural surface flora, including low numbers of pectinolytic bacteria, and it is becoming increasingly evident that healthy tissue of the intact plant may also contain very low numbers of viable micro-organisms (endophytic).

The onset and rate of spoilage will depend on the interactions between the physiological changes occurring in the tissues after harvest and changes in microbial activity.

Harvesting itself will produce physiological stress, principally as a result of water loss and wilting, and cut surfaces may release nutrients for microbial growth. This stress may also allow growth of the otherwise quiescent endophytic flora.

Table 14.2. Some micro-organisms involved in the spoilage of fresh vegetables.

Micro-organism	Vegetable	Symptom
Bacteria		
Corynebacterium sepedonicum	Potato	Ring rot of tubers
Pseudomonas solanacearum	Potato	Soft rot
Erwinia carotovora var. atroseptica	Potato	Soft rot
Streptomyces scabies	Potato	Scab
Xanthomonas campestris	Brassicas	Black rot
Fungi		
Botrytis cinerea	Many	Grey mould
Botrytis allii	Onions	Neck rot
Mycocentrospora acerina	Carrots	Liquorice rot
Trichothecium roseum	Tomato Cucurbits	Pink rot
Fusarium coeruleum	Potato	Dry rot
Aspergillus alliaceus	Onion Garlic	Black rot

The most frequently observed form of spoilage is a softening of the tissue due to the pectinolytic activity of micro-organisms. Pectin, the methyl ester of α-1,4-poly-D-galacturonic acid, and other pectic substances are major components of the middle lamella between the cells making up plant tissue and once it is broken down the tissue loses its integrity and individual plant cells are more easily invaded and killed. Pectic substances may be quite complex and include unesterified pectic acid as well as having side chains of L-rhamnose, L-arabinose, D-galactose, D-glucose and D-xylose. Several distinct enzymes are involved in the degradation of pectin and their role is illustrated in Fig. 14.1. As described in the case of fruits, the prevention of spoilage during storage and transport of vegetables must involve a range of measures. The control of the relative humidity and the composition of the atmosphere in which vegetables are stored is important but there is a limit to the reduction of relative humidity because at values below 90–95 per cent, loss of water from vegetable tissues will lead to wilting. It is essential to avoid the presence of free water on the surfaces of vegetables and temperature control may be just as important to prevent condensation. The presence of a film of water on the surface will allow access of motile bacteria such as *Erwinia* and *pseudomonads* to cracks, wounds and natural openings such as stomata. A combination of constant low temperature, controlled relative humidity and a gas phase with reduced oxygen (ca. 2–3 per cent) and enhanced CO_2 (ca. 2–5 per cent) has made it possible to store the large hard cabbages used in coleslaw production for many months making the continuous production of this commodity virtually independent of the seasons. Vegetables should not normally be a cause of public health concern but the transmission of pathogenic bacteria such as *Salmonella* and *Shigella* is possible by direct contamination from faeces of birds and animals, the use of manure or sewage sludge as fertiliser, or the use of contaminated waters for irrigation. Celery, watercress, lettuce, endive, cabbage and beansprouts have all been associated with *Salmonella* infections, including typhoid and paratyphoid fevers, and an outbreak of shigellosis has been traced to commercial shredded lettuce.

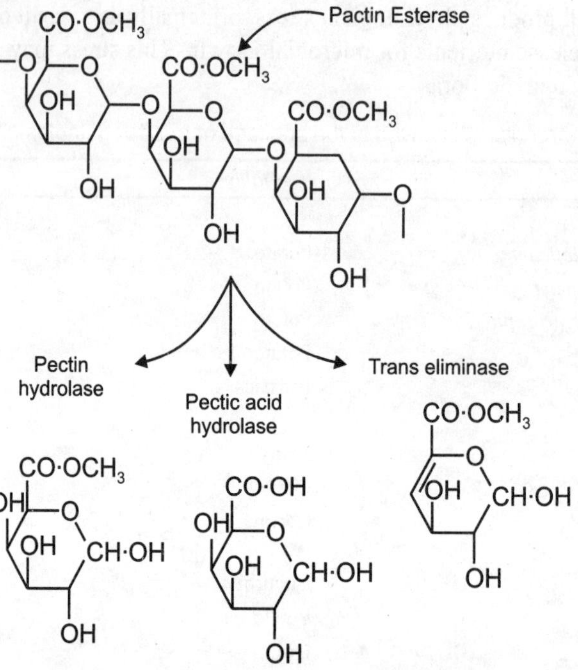

Fig. 14.1. Enzymic activities leading to the degradation of pectin.

Not all pathogens are necessarily transmitted to vegetables by direct or indirect faecal contamination. Organisms such as *Clostridium botulinum* have a natural reservoir in the soil and any products contaminated with soil can be assumed to be contaminated with spores of this organism, possibly in very low numbers. This would not normally present a problem unless processing or storage conditions were sufficiently selective to allow subsequent spore germination, growth and production of toxin. In the past, this has been seen mainly as a problem associated with underprocessed canned vegetables, but now it must be taken into consideration in the context of sealed, vacuum or modified atmosphere packs of prepared salads.

Those salads containing partly cooked ingredients, where spores may have been activated and potential competitors reduced in numbers, could pose particular problems. In 1987 a case of botulism caused by *Clostridium botulinum* type A was associated with a pre-packed rice and vegetable salad eaten as part of an airline meal. Similar risks may occur in foil-wrapped or vacuum packed cooked potatoes or film-wrapped mushrooms and in all these cases adequate refrigeration appears to be the most effective safety factor.

Another group of pathogens naturally associated with the environment includes the psychrotrophic species *Listeria monocytogenes* which is commonly associated with plant material, soil, animals, sewage and a wide range of other environmental sources. Raw celery, tomatoes and lettuce were implicated on epidemiological grounds as a possible cause of listeriosis which occurred in several hospitals in Boston, USA in 1979, although direct microbiological evidence was missing. An outbreak of listeriosis in Canada in 1981 was associated with coleslaw. Strains of *L. monocytogenes* can certainly grow on shredded cabbage and salad vegetables such as lettuce at temperatures as low as 5°C and modified-atmospheres seem to have no effect on this organism.

FERMENTED VEGETABLES

Sauerkraut and Kimchi

Most horticultural products can be preserved by a lactic acid fermentation. In the West the most important commercially are cabbage, cucumbers and olives, although smaller amounts of others such as carrots, cauliflower, celery, okra, onions, sweet and hot peppers, and green tomatoes are also fermented. In Korea fermented vegetables known as kimchi are an almost ubiquitous accompaniment to meals. More than 65 different types of kimchi have been identified on the basis of differences in raw materials and processing. Cabbages and radishes are the main substrates but garlic, peppers, onions and ginger are often also used. Surveys have shown its importance in the Korean diet, variously reporting kimchi to comprise 12.5 per cent of the total daily food intake or a daily adult consumption of 50–100 grams in summer increasing to 150–200 grams in winter.

Sauerkraut production is thought to have been brought to Europe from China by the Tartars. Like a number of other traditional fermentations, the commercial process is technologically simple (Fig. 14.2), but involves some interesting and complex chemistry and microbiology.

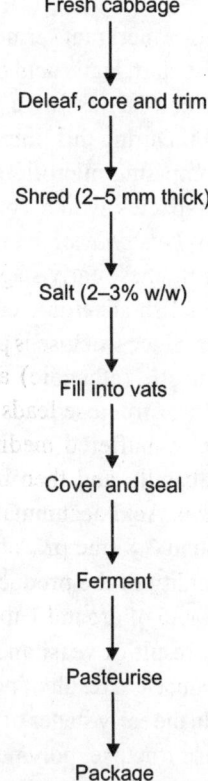

Fresh cabbage

Deleaf, core and trim

Shred (2–5 mm thick)

Salt (2–3% w/w)

Fill into vats

Cover and seal

Ferment

Pasteurise

Package

Fig. 14.2. Sauerkraut production.

Usually where sauerkraut is produced commercially special cabbage cultivars are grown. These tend to have a higher solids content than normal and so minimise production of liquid waste during processing. The outer leaves are removed mechanically and the cabbages decored before cutting into shreds about 1 mm thick. The shredded cabbage is then salted and packed into vats for the fermentation stage. The level of salting is critical to obtaining a satisfactory product, it must be within the range 2–3 per cent w/w and is normally about 2.25 per cent. Too little salt (<2 per cent) and the product softens unacceptably, too much salt (>3 per cent) and the correct microbial sequence is not obtained. The salt serves a number of purposes:

1. It extracts moisture from the shredded cabbage by osmosis to form the brine in which the fermentation will take place.
2. It helps to inhibit some of the natural microflora of the cabbage such as pseudomonads which would otherwise cause spoilage and helps to select for the lactic acid bacteria.
3. It helps maintain the crisp texture of the cabbage by withdrawing water and inhibiting endogenous pectolytic enzymes which cause the product to soften.
4. Finally, salt contributes to the flavour of the product.

Traditionally, fermentation vats have been made of wood but nowadays are more often of concrete with a synthetic polymer lining to protect from attack by the acid brine. The tanks are sealed by covering the salted cabbage with plastic sheeting. They are then filled with brine to press the sheeting on to the cabbage expelling the entrapped air.

Although commercial starter cultures for sauerkraut fermentation are available, they are used less often than in other food fermentations. At the start, lactic acid bacteria (LAB) comprise only about 1 per cent of the total microflora, but many of the non-lactics fail to grow and two days later LAB account for more than 90 per cent of the total microflora. During this time, they produce sufficient acid to decrease the pH to below 4 further inhibiting the competing microflora. Underlying this overall dominance by LAB is a natural succession of different species which contribute to the characteristic flavour of sauerkraut. The fermentation is initiated by *Leuconostoc mesenteroides* which is among the less acid and salt-tolerant LAB but grows fastest during these early stages. As a heterofermenter it produces CO_2 which replaces entrapped air and helps establish anaerobic conditions within the product and prevent the oxidation of vitamin C and loss of colour. Since fructose is present as an alternative electron acceptor, it also produces appreciable amounts of acetic (ethanoic) acid from acetyl-CoA which is a major contributor to sauerkraut flavour. Reduction of fructose leads to the accumulation of mannitol. As the pH drops due to acid production in a weakly buffered medium so the *Leuconostoc* is inhibited and replaced, first by heterofermentative lactobacilli, and then by more acid-tolerant homofermentative lactobacilli such as *Lactobacillus plantarum*. Acid accumulation continues in the form of lactic acid although the pH stabilises somewhere around 3.8 (the pK_a of lactic acid). At the end of fermentation which can last from 4–8 weeks the total acidity of the product is 1.7–2.3 per cent, expressed as lactic acid, with a ratio of volatile to nonvolatile acid of around 1 to 4.

Defects of sauerkraut arise mostly as a result of yeast and mould growth. These can produce off-odours, loss of acidity, a slimy, softened product as a result of pectolytic activity, or a pink discolouration due to the growth of the yeast *Rhodotorula*. In the early stages of fermentation, *Leuconostoc mesenteroides* fermenting sucrose will preferentially utilise fructose, polymerising the glucose moieties to produce a dextran slime. This is however transient and is later degraded and utilised by other LAB.

In some brined and fermented vegetables nutrients are not particularly well conserved. These tend to employ high salt levels which draw nutrients and moisture from the product into a high-strength brine which is often discarded and replaced before consumption. This is not the case with sauerkraut which uses a low-salt brine and is not desalted before use. As a result several vitamins are partially conserved, particularly ascorbic acid, vitamin C. Sauerkraut was used extensively as an antiscorbutic (for the prevention of scurvy) in the Dutch navy in the 18th century.

Some losses of vitamin C will occur during processing, a 50 per cent reduction was observed in the first five weeks of kimchi fermentation, but nutritional labels on commercial sauerkraut in the United States usually show an ascorbic acid content of 50 per cent of the recommended daily allowance per 100 g serving.

Kimchi is similar to sauerkraut in some respects since cabbage is a common ingredient and the level of salt used is low (<3 per cent). It differs principally in having a shorter fermentation time; the best taste is claimed after 3 days at 20°C when the acidity is 0.6 per cent and the pH around 4.2. Consequently *Leuconostoc mesenteroides* is the principal organism responsible for the fermentation and dominance of *Lactobacillus plantarum* is regarded as a defect which results in an excessively sour product.

FERMENTATION OF CUCUMBERS, CABBAGE AND OLIVES

The pickling of vegetables for purposes of preservation probably originated in China with the use of brines, and subsequently dry salting. The three vegetables of most commercial significance in this context are cabbage, cucumbers and olives, but others that may be fermented include artichokes, beet, carrots, cauliflower, celery, garlic, green beans, green tomatoes, peppers, turnip and a variety of Asian commodities.

Cucumbers

Whereas cucumbers (*Cucumis sativus*) retailed for their direct use are customarily bred to have tough skins, those targeted for pickling need to have a thin and relatively tender coating. They are harvested at a relatively immature stage, before the seeds have matured and before the area around the seeds has gone soft and starts to liquefy through the action of polygalacturonases on cell-wall hemicelluloses. The most valuable cucumbers are also the smaller ones. The cucumbers are sorted according to their diameter, and those that are too long are cut to a length that will readily fit into jars.

Other breeding criteria include disease resistance, yield, the growth locale and a relatively small seed area. Cucumbers should be straight and uniform with a length to diameter ratio of 3:1. They should be firm, green and free from internal defects. Chemical parameters include the level of cucurbitacins, which afford bitterness, sugars (which are the substrates for the fermentation), malic acid (relevant to the extent to which 'bloaters' are produced during fermentation) and the level of polygalacturonase. Opportunities for molecular biology in the optimisation of these parameters are being explored.

Cucumbers that are grown locally are processed within one day, whereas those grown further afield are refrigerated on shipping. If brined, they can be transported internationally.

Pickling cucumbers are preserved by one of three methods. Some two-fifths are preserved by fermentation, possibly accompanied by pasteurisation. Pasteurisation alone (reaching an internal temperature of 74°C for 15 min.) is applied to another 40 per cent, of the total, while the remainder rely solely on refrigeration. For pasteurised and refrigerated processing, acid (produced separately, i.e. not through *in situ* fermentation) is usually added, perhaps accompanied by sodium benzoate.

Most commercial cucumber fermentations rely on a natural microflora. Sometimes, however, the natural microflora is heavily depleted by hot water blanching (66°–80°C for 5 min.), in which case there may be seeding with *Lactobacillus plantarum*. The various stages of microbial growth are indicated in Table 14.3. When the flower has withered, it tends to have increased levels of micro-organisms and, furthermore, the flowers also contain polygalacturonase that plays a significant role in softening cucumbers by hydrolysing the polysaccharide matrix. The major fermentation sugars are glucose and fructose and these are metabolised to lactic acid, acetic acid, ethanol, mannitol and carbon dioxide. *Lb. plantarum* is normally the predominant organism in the natural microflora, mostly producing lactic acid. A malolactic fermentation is important in converting malate in the cucumbers to lactic acid.

Table 14.3. Stages of microbial involvement in vegetable fermentation.

Stage	Microbial events
Start	A range of Gram-positive and Gram-negative bacteria present
Primary fermentation	Most bacteria inhibited in the acid conditions created by the lactic acid bacteria. Lactic acid bacteria and yeast are able to thrive
Secondary fermentation	Lower pH now inhibiting lactic acid bacteria, but not yeasts growing fermentatively
Post-fermentation	Surface growth of oxidative bacteria, moulds and yeasts in open tanks. However, if in sealed anaerobic tanks, no growth if pH is low enough and salt concentration high enough

The fresh cucumbers are immersed in brine in bulk tanks. The control parameters are pH, temperature and the level of salt. The brine is typically lowered to a pH of around 4.5 with either vinegar or lactic acid. This facilitates the loss of carbon dioxide (by shifting the equilibrium from bicarbonate towards carbonic acid). Furthermore, it has a major impact on which organisms grow, for instance, the growth of Enterobacteriaceae is suppressed at the lower pH whereas lactic acid bacteria are able to thrive in the absence of competition from organisms not able to tolerate these acidic conditions. The optimum salt level is 5–8 per cent sodium chloride with the temperature in the range 15°–32°C. The species involved are listed in Table 14.4.

During fermentation, the brine is purged with either nitrogen or air to prevent bloater formation, and the cucumbers are maintained submerged. Whereas air is the cheaper option, nitrogen is preferable as there is then less yeast and fungal growth, fewer off flavours and less colour development. Potassium sorbate (0.035 per cent) is typically added to inhibit the growth of fungi. It is critical that the end product should possess a firm, crisp texture. Furthermore, as lactic acid is deemed too tart for products such as hamburger dill, a draining stage is employed with replacement of the brine by vinegar.

Pasteurised products typically contain 0.5–0.6 per cent acetic at a pH of 3.7. The relative content of acid and sugar is adjusted depending on the desired sourness/sweetness balance.

Table 14.4. Lactic acid bacteria involved in fermentation of vegetables.

Homofermentative
Enterococcus faecalis
Lactobacillus bavaricus
Lactococcus lactis
Pediococcus pentosaceus
Heterofermentative
Lactobacillus brevis
Leuconostoc mesemeroides
Mix
Lactobacillus plantarum[a]

[a] This organism uses hexoses homofermentatively but pentoses heterofermentatively.

Cabbage

Sauerkraut is pickled cabbage (*Brassica oleracea*). The cabbages of choice will have large heads (8–12 lb) that are compact (dense), contain few outer green leaves and have desirable flavour, colour and texture. They are bred for yield, pest resistance, storability and content of dry matter.

Cabbages are increasingly harvested mechanically and are graded, cored, trimmed, shredded and salted. Their water content is about 30 per cent and shredding is to a diameter of approximately 1 mm.

The shredded cabbage is soaked in brine in reinforced concrete tanks of capacity 20–180 tons and loosely covered with plastic sheeting. Alternatively, cabbage may be dry salted to about 2 per cent by weight and allowed to self-brine through its own moisture.

The cabbage is distributed to a slight concave surface and water put on top of the plastic cover to anchor it and ensure that anaerobic conditions can develop. Fermentation can take some 3 weeks, ideally at temperatures below 20°C.

Lactic acid bacteria constitute a relatively small proportion of the total bacterial count and comprise five major species: *Enterococcus faecalis*, *Leuconostoc mesenteroides*, *Lactobacillus brevis*, *Pediococcus cerevisiae* and *Lb. plantarum*. Despite their low levels, these organisms represent the most significant contributor to the fermentation. A low salt concentration (ca. 2 per cent) and the low temperature (18°C) favour heterofermentative organisms. Conversely, a high salt content (3.5 per cent) and high temperature (32°C) promote homofermentative fermentation. The normal sequence is heterofermentation first, followed by homofermentation. The main sugars in cabbage are glucose and fructose and, to a lesser extent, sucrose. They are converted to acetic acid, mannitol and ethanol in the first week, together with CO_2 which is important for establishing anaerobiosis. After a week or so, the brine becomes too acidic for the heterofermentative organisms and the fermentation is continued by the homofermenters, *Lb. plantarum*. Production of lactic acid continues until all the sugars are consumed and the pH has dropped from around 6 to 3.4.

The cabbage stays in the tanks until more than 1 per cent lactic acid has been produced (30 days or more). The material is then either stored in the same vessel or is processed at this stage to the finished product.

The sauerkraut is removed either manually or by mechanical fork and is packaged into can, glass or plastic. Sodium benzoate (0.1 per cent w/v) may be added as a preservative and the material stored at 4°C. If canned, the product is pasteurised and no preservative is added. Pasteurisation is at 74°–82°C for 3 minutes. Heating is by steam injection or immersion and the product hot filled into cans.

Sauerkraut can be spoiled by Clostridia if the latter proliferates in the early stages of the process. Other potential problem organisms are oxidative yeasts and moulds. Discolouration may arise not only from the oxidation of cabbage components but also from the action of Rhodotorula which generates a red hue.

Olives

Olives (*Olea europaea*) are primarily fermented in the Mediterranean countries of Greece, Italy, Morocco, and Spain. Part of the reason for the process is to eliminate the acute bitterness of the olive that is due to the glycoside oleuropin. Soaking the olive in brine or dilute caustic leads to the hydrolysis and removal of this material.

Nowadays olives are mostly fermented in plastic-clad tanks of fibreglass or stainless steel, perhaps buried underground in the interests of temperature regulation. There are basically two fermentation approaches.

Untreated naturally ripe black olives in brine

The olives are picked when completely ripened (turned from green to black or purple) and are not treated with lye (alkali solution) so that they retain bitterness and fruitiness. They are put into the tanks with 6–10 per cent sodium chloride solution and allowed to undergo spontaneous fermentation by an endogenous microflora comprising lactic acid bacteria and yeasts. The olives are subsequently sorted and graded before packaging.

Lye-treated green olives in brine

The olives are harvested when green or yellow and treated with a 1.3–3.5 per cent lye solution for up to 12 hours at 12°–20°C to remove most of the bitterness. After washing with cold water, they are taken in stages up to a concentration of 10–13 per cent sodium chloride, a gradual process so as to avoid shrivelling. Endogenous fermentation is allowed to progress for up to a month at 24°–27°C, prior to sorting and grading and packaging into glass jars.

In olive fermentations there is no use of starter cultures, although a proportion of brine from a previous fermentation may be used to supplement the new brine.

In the early stages of fermentation, there is activity of the aerobic organisms Citrobacter, Enterobacter, Escherichia, Flavobacterium, Klebsiella and Pseudomonas. These organisms will not grow when the salt is increased beyond 6–10 per cent. Stage two comprises the activity of the lactic acid bacteria (Lactobacillus, Lactococcus, Leuconostoc, Pediococcus), with the progressively dropping pH destroying the initial microflora. The onset of the third stage is once the pH reaches 4.5, with the predominant organism being *Lb. plantarum*, together with fermentative and oxidative yeasts (Candida, Hansenula, Saccharomyces).

CONTAMINATION, PRESERVATION AND SPOILAGE OF VEGETABLES AND FRUITS

It has been estimated that one-fourth of all produce harvested is spoiled before consumption. Spoilage of fresh fruits and vegetables usually occurs during storage and transport and while waiting to be processed. Unlike many other foods, fruits and vegetables after picking and before processing are 'alive' for an extended time. The resulting respiration of these products and the normal ripening process complicate an independent discussion of the microbiological spoilage of fruits and vegetables. Many of the microbiological spoilage problems discussed are really 'market diseases' of these products. Vegetables and fruits may be fresh, dried, frozen, fermented, pasteurised or canned.

Contamination

As soon as fruits and vegetables are gathered into boxes, lugs, baskets or trucks during harvesting, they are subject to contamination with spoilage organisms from each other and from the containers unless these have been adequately sanitised. During transportation to market or the processing plant, mechanical damage may increase susceptibility to decay and growth of micro-organisms may take place. Precooling of the product and refrigeration during transportation will slow such growth. Washing the fruit or vegetable may involve a preliminary soaking or may be achieved by agitation in water or, preferably, by a spray treatment. Soaking and washing by agitation tend to distribute spoilage organisms from damaged to whole foods. Recirculated or reused water is likely to add organisms, and the washing process may moisten surfaces enough to permit growth of organisms during a holding period. Washing with detergent or germicidal solutions will reduce numbers of micro-organisms on the foods.

Sorting spoiled fruits or vegetables or trimming spoiled parts removes micro-organisms, but additional handling may result in mechanical damage and therefore greater susceptibility to decay. When these products are sold in the retail market without processing, they are not ordinarily subjected to much further contamination, except for storage in the market in contaminated bins or other containers, possible contact with decaying products, handling by salespeople and customers, and perhaps spraying with water or packing with chipped ice. This spraying gives a fresh appearance to the vegetables and delays decomposition but also adds organisms, e.g. psychrotrophs, from water or ice and gives a moist surface to encourage their growth on longer storage.

In the processing plant the fruits or vegetables are subjected to further contamination and chances for growth of micro-organisms, or numbers and kinds of organisms may be reduced by some procedures. Adequate washing at the plant causes a reduction in numbers of micro-organisms on the food, as do peeling by steam, hot water, or lye and blanching (heating to inactivate enzymes, etc.). Sweating of products during handling increases numbers. Processes such as trimming, mechanical abrasion or peeling, cutting, pitting or coring, and various methods of disintegration may add contaminants from the equipment involved. In fact, every piece of equipment coming in contact with food can be a significant source of micro-organisms unless it has been cleaned and sanitised adequately. Modern metal equipment with smooth surfaces and without cracks, dead ends, etc. is made to facilitate such treatments. Examples of possible sources of contamination of foods with micro-organisms are trays, bins, tanks, pipes, flumes, tables, conveyor belts and aprons, fillers, blanchers, presses, screens and filters. Wooden surfaces are difficult to clean and sanitise and therefore are especially likely to be sources of contamination, as are cloth surfaces, e.g. on conveyor belts. Neglected parts of any food-handling system can build up numbers of micro-organisms to contaminate the food. Hot-water blanching, although it reduces total numbers of organisms on the food, may cause the buildup of spores of thermophilic bacteria, causing the spoilage of canned foods, e.g. flat sour spores in peas.

Buildup of populations of micro-organisms on equipment as the result of microbial growth in the exudates and residues from fruits and vegetables may greatly influence the amount of contamination of the foods and the growth of the contaminants. Not only is there the possibility of the addition of large numbers of organisms from this source, there is also the likelihood that these will be organisms in their logarithmic phase of growth and therefore able to continue rapid growth. This effect is especially evident on vegetables following blanching. This heat treatment reduces the bacterial content considerably, damages many of the surviving cells, and consequently lengthens their lag period. On the other hand, the actively growing contaminants from the equipment can attain large numbers if enough time is allowed before freezing, drying or canning; such growth is usually the cause of very high bacterial counts.

Inclusion of decayed parts of fruits increases the numbers of micro-organisms in fruit juices. Numbers in orange juice, for example, and numbers of coliforms are increased greatly by the inclusion of fruits with soft rots. Heating of grapes before extraction reduces numbers of organisms in the expressed juice, but pressing introduces contamination.

The kinds of micro-organisms from equipment will depend on the product being processed, for that product will constitute the culture medium for the organisms. Thus pea residues would encourage bacteria that grow well in a pea medium and in tomatoes those organisms which can develop in tomato juice. As the equipment is used throughout the day, the organisms can continue to build up. At the end of the run, however, when equipment is cleaned and sanitised, the total numbers of micro-organisms thereon are greatly reduced, and if the operation is efficient, only the resistant forms survive. Therefore, spores of bacteria are likely to survive, and if conditions for growth are present while the equipment is idle, these sporeformers may increase in numbers, especially in poorly cleaned parts. The thermophilic sporeformers so troublesome to canners of vegetables build up in this manner and add to the difficulty of giving the foods an adequate heat process. The numbers of such organisms on poorly cleaned and sanitised equipment may be high at the start of a day's run and decrease as the day progresses, but the reverse usually is true. A layoff during the run permits a renewed increase in numbers. It is obvious that the numbers of micro-organisms that enter foods from equipment depend on the opportunities given these organisms for growth and that these opportunities are the result of inadequacy of cleaning and sanitising combined with favourable conditions of moisture and temperature for an appreciable period of time. Added ingredients such as sugar and starch may add spoilage organisms, especially spores of thermophilic bacteria.

Preservation of Vegetables

Micro-organisms on the surfaces of freshly harvested fruits and vegetables include not only those of the normal surface flora but also those from soil and water and perhaps plant pathogens (Table 14.5). Any of a number of kinds of moulds also may be there, and sometimes a few yeasts. If the surfaces are moist or the outer surface has been damaged, growth of some micro-organisms may take place between harvesting and processing or consumption of the vegetables. Adequate control of temperature and humidity will reduce such growth.

Table 14.5. General microbiological profile of harvested fruits and vegetables*.

Product	Micro-organisms isolated	Approximate quantitative range
Vegetables	Bacteria	10^3–10^7/g
	Pseudomonas	
	Alcaligenes	
	Erwinia	
	Xanthomonas	
	Other Gram-negatives	
	Micrococci	
	Bacillus	
	Lactic acid bacteria	
	Coryneforms	
	Moulds	10^3–10^4/g
	Fusarium	
	Alternaria	
	Aureobasidium	
	Penicillium	
	Sclerotinia	
	Botrytis	
	Rhizopus	

(Contd ...)

Product	Micro-organisms isolated	Approximate quantitative range
Fruits	Bacteria: The inherent low pH of most fruits favours a predominance by moulds; however, gram-negative species as above can be isolated	Usually less than 10^8/g
	Moulds: As above plus *Cladosporium* *Phoma* *Trichoderma*	10^3–10^4/g

* There is considerable variation in the numbers and types of micro-organisms present on vegetables and fruits. The species, the amount of adhering dirt or soil, the location and the presence or absence of physical damage would all be significant variables.

Asepsis

While a limited amount of contamination of vegetables will take place between harvesting and processing or consumption, gross contamination can be avoided. Boxes, lugs, baskets and other containers should be practically free of the growth of micro-organisms, and some will need cleaning and sanitation between uses. Examples are the lugs or other containers used for transporting peas to the processing plant. These containers may support a considerable amount of growth of bacteria on their moist interior and be a source of high numbers of organisms on the peas. Contact of vegetables undergoing spoilage with healthy vegetables will add contamination and may lead to losses. Contamination from equipment at the processing plant can be reduced by adequate cleaning and sanitising. Especially feared is a buildup of heat-resistant spores of spoilage bacteria, e.g. the spores of flat sour bacteria, putrefactive anaerobes or *Clostridium thermosaccharolyticum*.

Bacterial counts on fresh vegetables to be processed, upon arrival at the plant, may range from 10^2 to 10^7 per gram depending on the species and condition.

Removal of micro-organisms

Thorough washing of vegetables removes most of the casual contaminants on the surface but leaves much of the natural microbial surface flora. Unless the wash water is of good bacteriological quality, it may add organisms, and subsequently growth may take place on the moist surface. Chlorinated water sometimes is used for washing, and detergents may be added to facilitate the removal of dirt and micro-organisms. Part of the mould growth on strawberries, for example, can be removed by washing with a nonionic detergent solution.

Use of heat

Vegetables to be dried or frozen, and some to be canned, are scalded or blanched to inactivate their enzymes. At the same time the numbers of micro-organisms are reduced appreciably, perhaps by 1000 to 10,000 folds.

Use of low temperatures

As has been indicated, a few kinds of vegetables that are relatively stable, such as root crops, potatoes, cabbage and celery, can be preserved, for a limited time by common or cellar storage.

Chilling

Most vegetables to be preserved without special processing are cooled promptly and kept at chilling temperatures. The chilling is accomplished by use of cold water, ice or mechanical refrigeration or by vacuum cooling (moistening plus evacuation), as used for lettuce. In many cases precooling, i.e. cooling before normal cold storage, is done immediately after harvesting by use of a cold water spray, a practice referred to as hydrocooling. Each kind of vegetable has its own optimal temperature and relative humidity for chilling storage. The 'freshening' of leafy vegetables (lettuce, spinach) by a water spray will cool the products if cold water is employed and will aid in their preservation.

Control of the composition of the atmosphere in the storage of vegetables has not been used as much as with fruits. The addition of carbon dioxide or ozone to the air has been recommended by some workers. Ultraviolet rays have not been successful because the rays do not hit all surfaces of the vegetables as they are packaged and handled.

Sweet potatoes are an example of a vegetable requiring special conditions of chilling storage. Ordinary potatoes turn sweet at temperatures below 2.2° to 4.4°C and are stored at higher temperatures if they are to be used for potato chips. Sweet potatoes and onions are subjected to special curing treatments before storage.

Freezing

The selection and preparation of vegetables, their blanching, their freezing, and the changes during these processes have been discussed already. On the surface of vegetables are the micro-organisms of the natural flora, plus contaminants from soil and water. If the surfaces are moist, growth of some of these organisms will take place before the vegetable reaches the freezing plant. There, washing reduces the numbers of some organisms and adds some organisms, and scalding or blanching (86° to 98°C) brings about a great reduction in numbers, as much as 90 to 99 per cent in some instances (Table 14.6). But during the cooling and handling before freezing there is an opportunity for recontamination from equipment and for growth of organisms, so that under .poor conditions 1 million or more organisms per gram of vegetable may be present at freezing. The freezing process reduces the number of organisms by a percentage that varies with the kinds and numbers originally present, but on the average about half of them are killed.

Table 14.6 illustrates the changes in numbers of organisms on snap beans as they pass through various operations in a freezing plant. During storage in the frozen condition there is a steady decrease in numbers of organisms, but there are at least some survivors of most kinds of organisms after the usual storage period.

Table 14.6. Numbers of organisms per gram on snap beans after passing through unit operations in a freezing plant.

Source of sample	Average plate count per gram*
Before cutter	7,40,000
After cutler and shaker	5,73,000
After blancher	1000
After shaker, before sorting belt	1,88,000
Final package	36,000

* Average of seventeen samples during 9 days. Plates incubated at 32°C.

The kind of bacteria most likely to grow on thawing will depend on the temperature and the elapsed time. Species of *Micrococcus* are predominant on thawing vegetables such as sweet corn and peas when the temperature of thawing is fairly low, although *Achromobacter* and *Enterobacter* spp. also are commonly present. Lactobacilli are also common on peas under such conditions. One species of *Micrococcus* may grow at first, followed by another species later. At higher temperatures, species of *Flavobacterium* also may multiply. As the small packages of quick-frozen vegetables usually are handled in the home, where the frozen food is placed directly into boiling water and cooked, there is no further opportunity for microbial growth. During freezing most vegetables wilt and become limp, and during storage frozen vegetables may undergo colour changes.

When thawed vegetables are held at room temperature for any considerable period, there is a chance that food-poisoning bacteria may grow and produce' toxin. Jones and Lochhead, for example, found enterotoxin-forming staphylococci in frozen corn. Sterilised corn inoculated with staphylococci of the food-poisoning type, then frozen and then thawed and held at a room temperature of 20°C for a total elapsed time of 1 day permitted growth of these cocci and the production of enough enterotoxin to cause symptoms of food poisoning, Enterotoxin produced in this way would not be entirely destroyed by the customary cooking of the vegetable. *Clostridium botulinum* has been found in frozen vegetables and can be assumed to be present often. Fortunately, the conditions for growth and toxin production would be unusual; power failure in freezers for several days during floods or hurricanes is an example of such conditions. Cooking frozen vegetables will not kill all spores of *Clostridium botulinum*, and such cooked food should not be allowed to stand at room temperature for any extended period of time.

Bacterial counts in frozen vegetables may range from a few to 10^5 per gram. Frequently, coliforms and enterococci can be recovered. The presence of *E. coli*, however, is unusual and can lead one to question sanitary practices.

Drying

As the methods of drying vegetables and vegetable products have improved, public acceptance has increased, so that now a number of dried food products have wide sale. Dried vegetables and vegetable products are used in dried soups, and dried spices and condiments are used as flavouring materials.

Many vegetables can be dried by a process called explosive puffing. Usually small pieces of the diced, partially dehydrated vegetables are placed in a closed rotating chamber. Heat is applied, and the chamber is pressurised to a predetermined level; then the pressure is released instantaneously. This results in an additional loss of water, but more important, a porous network of capillaries is formed in the product. The increased porosity simplifies further drying and imparts good reconstituting ability.

Growth of the micro-organisms surviving blanching may take place up to the time of drying and add to the count of the dried product. Drying by heat destroys yeasts and most bacteria, but spores of bacteria and moulds usually survive, as do the more heat-resistant vegetative cells. Microbial counts on dried vegetables, either after drying or as purchased in the retail market, usually are considerably higher than on dried fruits, because there are likely to be higher numbers before drying and a greater percentage survival afterward. Most vegetables are less acid than fruits, and consequently the killing effect of the heat is less. Samples of dried vegetables from retail markets contain micro-organisms in the hundreds of thousands or even millions per gram, although these dried foods can be produced so as to contain a much smaller number of organisms.

When dried vegetables are sulphured to preserve a light colour, their microbial content is reduced. If the vegetables are dried adequately and stored properly, there will be no growth of micro-organisms in them. During storage there is a slow decrease in the number of viable organisms, more rapid during the first few months and slower thereafter. The spores of bacteria and moulds, some of the micrococci and microbacteria are resistant to desiccation and will survive better than other micro-organisms and will constitute an increasingly large percentage of the survivors as the storage time lengthens.

Use of preservation

The addition of preservatives to vegetables is not common, although the surfaces of some vegetables may receive special treatment. Rutabagas and turnips sometimes are paraffined to lengthen their keeping time. Zinc carbonate has been reported to eliminate most mould growth on lettuce, beets and spinach. Biphenyl vapours will control *Fusarium* on potatoes. A controlled atmosphere of carbon dioxide or ozone about chilled vegetables has been tried experimentally but has had little practical use.

Added preservative

Sodium chloride is the only added chemical preservative in common use. The amount added to vegetables may vary from the 2.25 to 2.5 per cent in making sauerkraut up to saturation for cauliflower. The lower concentrations of salt permit an acid fermentation by bacteria to take place; as the percentage of salt is increased, the rate of acid production becomes slower until a level of salt is reached that will permit no growth or production of acid. Vegetables that are high in protein, such as green peas and lima beans, as well as some that soften readily, such as onions and cauliflower, are preserved by the addition of enough salt to prevent any fermentation: from 70° to 80°C salometer (18.6 to 21.2 per cent salt) up to saturation (26.5 per cent salt). It should be noted that upon the addition of brine or salt to vegetables, water is drawn from them and serves to decrease the salt concentration in the liquid.

The popularity of salad bars has resulted in an increased use of sulphites as salad fresheners, i.e. to prevent enzymatic browning of lettuce, cole slaw and other salad items. Sulphite residues in foods may be associated with asthmatic attacks and their levels in restaurant salads has been surveyed.

Developed preservatives

At room temperature an acid fermentation is normal for shredded, chopped or crushed vegetables containing sugar, but instead of a clean, acid flavour from the action of lactic acid bacteria, undesirable flavours and changes in body may result from growth of coliform bacteria, bacilli, anaerobes, proteolytic bacteria and others. The addition of salt to such materials serves to reduce competition from undesirable organisms and hence to encourage the lactic fermentation. The salt also serves to draw the juice from the vegetables and bring about better distribution of the lactic acid bacteria. The amount of sugar in the vegetable affects the acidity that can be produced, while the amount of salt and the temperature determine the rate of acid production and the kinds of bacteria involved in it. In general, as the salt content is increased, the rate of acid formation becomes slower and the numbers of kinds of bacteria concerned become fewer. Some recipes call for a comparatively low salt content at the start, increasing amounts as the fermentation continues, and finally enough salt to prevent further growth of bacteria. This method is employed in the brining of vegetables such as string beans and corn.

Preservation by irradiation

Experimental treatment with gamma rays to inactivate micro-organisms causing decay, followed by storage, has resulted in discolouration, softening, or other deterioration of most vegetables. However, irradiation has been used successfully to delay sprouting of potatoes, onions and garlic and to kill insect reproduction on some vegetables.

Preservation of Fruits and Fruit Products

In general, principles similar to those for both vegetables and vegetable products are involved in the preservation of fruits and fruit products. The surfaces of healthy fruits include the natural flora plus contaminating micro-organisms from soil and water and therefore have a surface flora much like that listed for vegetables; however, yeasts and moulds will predominate. In addition, some fruits will contain plant pathogens or saprophytic spoilage organisms which may grow subsequent to harvesting. Such defective fruits should be sorted, and spoiled portions may be trimmed out. A few micro-organisms are present in the interior of occasional healthy fruits.

Asepsis

Fruits, like vegetables, may be subject to contamination between harvesting and processing from containers and from spoiling fruits, and care should be taken to avoid such contamination as much as possible. Before harvest, fruits are usually exposed to insecticides and fungicides and may have their flora altered by such treatments.

Removal of micro-organisms

Thorough washing of fruits serves to remove not only dirt and hence casual contaminating micro-organisms but also poisonous sprays. Washing may be with water, detergent solutions or even bactericidal solutions such as chlorinated water. Trimming also removes micro-organisms. Clear fruit juices may be sterilised by filtration.

Use of heat

Fruits seldom are blanched before other processing because blanching causes excessive physical damage.

Note that the fruits are in one of two groups on the, basis of their pH: the acid foods, such as tomatoes, pears and pineapples, or the high-add foods, such as berries. A steam-pressure steriliser is not required for most fruits, since heating at about 100°C is sufficient and can be accomplished by flowing steam or boiling water. In general, the more acid the fruit, the less heat required for its preservation. Similar principles are involved in canning fruit juices.

Use of low temperatures

A few fruits, such as apples, can be preserved for a limited time in common or cellar storage, but controlled lower temperatures usually are employed during most of the storage period of fruits.

Chilling

Each fruit has its own optimal temperature and relative humidity for chilling storage; even varieties of the same fruit may differ in their requirements. Fruits have been treated with various chemicals before or during storage to aid in their preservation. Thus hypochlorites, sodium bicarbonate, borax, propionates, biphenyl, o-phenylphenols, sulphur dioxide, thiourea, thiabendazole, dibromotetrachloroethane and other chemicals have been recommended. Fruit also has been enclosed in wrappers treated with chemicals, e.g. sulphite paper on grapes, iodine paper on grapes and tomatoes or borax paper on oranges. Waxed wraps, paraffin oil, paraffin, waxes and mineral oil have been applied for mechanical protection.

There has been considerable research on the combination of the chilling storage of fruits with control of the atmosphere of the storage room. This control may consist merely of regulation of the concentrations of oxygen and carbon dioxide in the atmosphere or may involve the addition or removal of carbon dioxide or oxygen or the addition of ozone.

Controlled-atmosphere (CA) storage implies the altering of various gases from normal atmospheric concentrations. Usually this is done by increasing the CO_2 concentration and decreasing the O_2 concentration. A related term, modified atmosphere (MA), is defined similarly, but MA storage is usually used to describe CA conditions which are not accurately maintained or conditions where the air is initially replaced with gas but no further measures are taken to keep the gas atmosphere constant. 'Gas storage' means CA or MA storage. Under certain circumstances only one gas is used, e.g. packaging a product in 100 per cent N_2; this type of storage would more precisely be referred to as nitrogen gas storage. Several conditions of CA storage are compiled in Table 14.7. The optimal concentration of carbon dioxide and oxygen and proportion of these gases varies with the kind of fruit and even with the variety of fruit.

Table 14.7. Conditions of controlled-atmosphere storage for several fruits and vegetables.

Item	CO_2, %	O_2, %
Apples	1.5–10.0	2.5
Lettuce	2.5	2.5
Cabbage	2.5	5.0
Onions	5–10.0	3.0
Peaches	5.0	0

Although carbon dioxide storage has been employed chiefly with apples, it can be used successfully with pears, bananas, citrus fruits, plums, peaches, grapes and other fruits.

Ozone in concentrations of 2 to 3 ppm in the atmosphere has been reported to double the storage time of loosely packed small fresh fruits, such as strawberries, raspberries, currants and grapes, and of delicate varieties of apples.

Ethylene in the atmosphere is used to hasten ripening or produce a desired colour change and is not considered preservative, although a combination of this gas and activated hydrocarbons has been suggested for the preservation of fruits.

Freezing

The surfaces of fruits contain the natural surface flora plus contaminants from soil and water. Any spoiled parts that are present will add moulds or yeasts. During preparation of fruits for freezing, undesirable changes may take place, such as darkening, deterioration in flavour and spoilage by micro-organisms, especially moulds. Washing the fruit removes most of the soil micro-organisms, and adequate selection and trimming will reduce many of the moulds and yeasts involved in spoilage. With proper handling there should be little growth of micro-organisms before freezing. Some fruits are frozen in large drums (up to 50 lb); it would be mandatory to cool the fruit before filling the container to ensure that the product is frozen quickly. The freezing process reduces the numbers of micro-organisms but also usually causes some damage to the fruit tissues, resulting in flabbiness and release of some juice. During storage in the frozen condition the physical changes described already occur as well as a slow but regular decrease in numbers of micro-organisms. Yeasts (*Saccharomyces, Cryptococcus*) and moulds (*Aspergillus, Penicillium, Mucor, Rhizopus, Botrytis, Fusarium, Alternaria*, etc.) have been reported to be the predominant organisms in frozen fruits, although small numbers of soil organisms, e.g. species of *Bacillus, Pseudomonas, Achromobacter*, etc. survive freezing. Yeasts are most likely to grow during slow thawing. Numbers of viable micro-organisms in frozen fruits are considerably lower than in frozen vegetables. Large numbers of mould hyphae may be indicative of the freezing of inferior fruit that included rotten parts.

The numbers of micro-organisms in frozen fruit juices depend on the condition of the fruit, the washing process, the method of filtration and the opportunities for contamination and growth before freezing. There may be from a few hundred to over 1 million organisms per millilitre present in the juice at the time of freezing. The inclusion of rotten parts of the fruit increases the numbers of organisms markedly. The washing process, especially the kind of solution used for washing, has a considerable influence on the numbers of organisms, since those on the surface of fruits are difficult to remove. Numbers can build up in the washing solution, on moist surfaces of the washed fruit, and in the juice itself before freezing. In the plant, too, there is an opportunity for the addition of organisms from the equipment. The freezing process markedly reduces numbers, but added sugar or increased concentration of the juice has a protective effect against killing. The decrease in numbers of organisms during storage in the frozen condition is slow but is faster than in most neutral foods. The kind of organisms are chiefly those of soil, water and rots, together with the natural surface flora of the fruit. Prominent usually are coliforms, enterococci, lactics, e.g. *Leuconostoc* and *Lactobacillus* species, *Alcaligenes* and yeasts.

Since coliform bacteria, mostly of the *Enterobacter aerogenes* type, form part of the natural flora of fruits, they are present in both fresh and frozen fruit juices. The use of decayed fruit for the juice increases the numbers of coliforms, but these organisms decrease during storage. Because coliforms normally are present, there are objections to the use of the presumptive test for coliforms to indicate sanitary quality of the juice. It has been suggested that tests be made for the fecal coliform, *Escherichia coli* or *Streptococcus faecalis*.

Drying

It was noted that the numbers of micro-organisms in dried fruits are comparatively low and that spores of bacteria and moulds are likely to be the most numerous. An occasional sample may contain high numbers of mould spores, indicating that growth and sporulation of moulds has taken place on the fruit before or after dehydration. Alkali treatment, sulphuring, blanching and pasteurisation reduce numbers of micro-organisms.

Use of preservatives

The use of chemical preservatives to lengthen the keeping time of fruits has been discussed already, where it was noted that chemicals have been applied to fruits chiefly as a dip or spray or impregnated in wrappers for the fruits. Among substances that have been applied to the outer surfaces of fruit are waxes, hypochlorites, biphenyl and alkaline sodium *o*-phenylphenate. Wrappers for fruits have been impregnated with a variety of chemicals including iodine, sulphite, biphenyl, *o*-phenylphenol plus hexamine and others. As a gas or fog about the fruit, carbon dioxide, ozone and ethylene plus chlorinated hydrocarbons have been tried. Sulphur dioxide and sodium benzoate are preservatives that have been added directly to fruits or fruit products. Most of the chemical preservatives mentioned have been primarily antifungal in purpose.

Green olives are the only fruits which are preserved on a commercial scale with assistance from an acid fermentation. Locally, other fermented fruits sometimes are prepared, such as fermented green tomatoes and Rumanian preserved apples. In all these products the lactic acid fermentation is of chief importance.

Spoilage

The deterioration of raw vegetables and fruits may result from physical factors, action of their own enzymes, microbial action or combinations of these agencies. Mechanical damage resulting from action of animals, birds or insects or from bruising, wounding, bursting, cutting, freezing, desiccation or other mishandling may predispose toward increased enzymatic action or the entrance and growth of micro-organisms. Previous damage by plant pathogens may make the part of the plant used as food unfit for consumption or may open the way for growth of saprophytes and spoilage by them. Contact with spoiling fruits and vegetables may bring about transfer of organisms, causing spoilage and increasing the wastage. Improper environmental conditions during harvesting, transit, storage and marketing may favour spoilage. Most of the discussion to follow will be concerned with microbial spoilage, but it always should be kept in mind that the plant enzymes continue their activity in raw plant foods. If oxygen is available, the plant cells will respire as long as they are alive and hydrolytic enzymes can continue their action after death of the cell.

The fitness of foods for consumption is judged partly on the basis of their maturity. If the desired stage of maturity is greatly exceeded, the food may be considered inedible or even spoiled. An example is an overripe banana, with its black skin and brown, mushy interior.

Diseases of vegetables and fruits may result from the growth of an organism that obtains its food from the host and usually damages it or from adverse environmental conditions that cause abnormalities in functions and structures of the vegetable or fruit. The diseases caused by pathogens and the decompositions caused by saprophytic organisms will be of chief interest in the following discussion, although clear distinction between these types of organisms is not possible. However, diseases not caused by organisms should be mentioned because they may sometimes be confused with those caused by organisms in that they may be rather similar in appearance. Examples of nonpathogenic diseases are brown heart of apples and pears, blackheart of potatoes black leaf speck of cabbage, and red heart of cabbage.

General types of microbial spoilage

The most common or predominant type of spoilage varies not only with the kind of fruit or vegetable but also to some extent with the variety. Microbial spoilage may be due to: (i) plant pathogens acting on the stems, leaves, flowers, or roots of the plant, on the fruits or other special parts used as foods, e.g. roots or tubers, or on several of these locations, and (ii) saprophytic organisms, which may be secondary invaders after action of a plant pathogen or may enter a healthy fruit or vegetable, as in the case of various 'rots', or grow on its surface, as when bacteria multiply on moist, piled vegetables. At times a saprophyte may succeed a pathogen or a succession of saprophytes may be involved in the spoilage. Thus, for example, coliform bacteria may grow as secondary invaders and be present in appreciable numbers in fruit and vegetable juices if rotten products have been included.

Although each fruit or vegetable has certain types of decomposition and kinds of micro-organisms predominant in its spoilage, some general types of microbial spoilage are found more often than the rest in vegetables and fruits. The most commonly occurring types of spoilage are as follows:

1. Bacterial soft rot, caused by *Erwinia carotovora* and related species, which are fermenters of pectins. *Pseudomonas marginalis* and *Clostridium* and *Bacillus* spp. have also been isolated from these rots. It results in a water soaked appearance, a soft, mushy consistency and often a bad odour.
2. Gray mould rot, caused by species of *Botrytis*, e.g. *B. cinerea*, a name derived from the gray mycelium of the mould. It is favoured by high humidity and a warm temperature.

3. Rhizopus soft rot, caused by species of *Rhizopus*, e.g. *R. stolonifer*. A rot results that often is soft and mushy. The cottony growth of the mould with small, black dots of sporangia often covers masses of the foods.

4. Anthracnose, usually caused by *Colletotrichum lindemuthianum*, *C. coccodes* and other species. The defect is a spotting of leaves and fruit or seedpods.

5. Alternaria rot, caused by *Alternaria tenuis* and other species. Areas become greenish-brown early in the growth of the mould and later turn to brown or black spots.

6. Blue mould rot, caused by species of *Penicillium digitatum* and other species. The bluish-green colour that gives the rot its name results from the masses of spores of the mould.

7. Downy mildew, caused by species of *Phytophthora*, *Bremia* and other genera. The moulds grow in white, woolly masses.

8. Watery soft rot, caused chiefly by *Sclerotinia sclerotiorum*, is found mostly in vegetables.

9. Stem-end rots, caused by species of moulds of several genera, e.g. *Diplodia*, *Alternaria*, *Phomopsis*, *Fusarium* and others, involve the stem ends of fruits.

10. Black mould rot, caused by *Aspergillus niger*. The rot gets its name from the dark-brown to black masses of spores of the mould, termed 'smut' by the layperson.

11. Black rot, often caused by species of *Alternaria* but sometimes of *Ceratostomella*, *Physalospora* and other genera.

12. Pink mould rot, caused by pink-spored *Trichothecium roseum*.

13. Fusarium rots, a variety of types of rots caused by species of *Fusarium*.

14. Green mould rot, caused usually by species of *Cladosporium* but sometimes by other green-spored moulds, e.g. *Trichoderma*.

15. Brown rot, caused chiefly by *Sclerotinia* (*Monilinia fructicola*) species.

16. Sliminess or souring, caused by saprophytic bacteria in piled, wet, heating vegetables.

Fungal spoilage of vegetables often results in water soaked, mushy areas, while fungal rots of fleshy fruits such as apples and peaches frequently show brown or cream coloured areas in which mould mycelia are growing in the tissue below the skin and aerial hyphae and spores may appear later. Some types of fungal spoilage appear as 'dry rots', where the infected area is dry and hard and often discoloured. Rots of juicy fruits may result in leakage. The composition of the fruit or vegetable influences the likely type of spoilage. Thus, bacterial soft rot is widespread for the most part among the vegetables which are not very acid, and among the fruits is limited to those which are not highly acid (Table 14.8). Because most fruits and vegetables are somewhat acid, are fairly dry at the surface and are deficient in B vitamins, moulds are the most common causes of spoilage. The composition, too, must determine the particular kinds of moulds most likely to grow; thus some kinds of fruits or vegetables support a large variety of spoilage organisms and other kinds comparatively few.

Table 14.8. The chief market diseases of several vegetables and fruits.

Item	Market disease
Lily family	
Asparagus	Bacterial soft rot, fusarium rot, gray mould rot, phytophthera rot
Onions	Bacterial soft rot, black mould rot, gray mould rot
Garlic	Bacterial soft rot, black mould rot

(Contd ...)

Item	Market disease
Pulse or legume family	
Green beans	Bacterial soft rot, gray mould rot, rhizopus soft rot
Wax beans	
Lima beans	
Parsley family	
Carrots	Bacterial soft rot, black rot, fusarium rot, gray mould rot, watery soft rot
Parsnips	Bacterial soft rot, watery soft rot, gray mould rot
Celery	Bacterial soft rot, watery soft rot, gray mould rot
Parsley	Bacterial soft rot, watery soft rot
Beets	Bacterial soft rot, black rot, blue mould rot, fusarium rot
Endive	Bacterial soft rot, watery soft rot, downy mildew, gray mould rot
Globe artichokes	Gray mould rot
Lettuce	Bacterial soft rot
Rhubarb	Bacterial soft rot, gray mould rot
Small fruits	
Blackberries	Blue mould rot, gray mould rot, rhizopus rot
Grapes	Black mould rot, gray mould rot, rhizopus rot, blue mould rot
Strawberries	Gray mould rot, leather rot (*Phytophthera cactorum*), rhizopus rot
Citrus fruits	
Lemons	Alternaria rot, anthracnose, blue mould rots, stem-end rots
Limes	
Oranges	
Grapefruit	
Subtropical fruits	
Avocados	Anthracnose, rhizopus rot
Bananas	Anthracnose, *Fusarium, Gleoporium, Pestalozzia*
Figs	Alternaria rot, blue mould rot, cladosporium rot
Dates	Yeasts, various moulds
Stone fruits	
Peaches	Alternaria (or green mould rot), gray mould rot, black mould rot; blue mould rot, brown
Apricots	rot, cladosporium rot, rhizopus rot
Plums	
Cherries	
Pomes	
Apples	Numerous moulds
Pears	Black rot, blue mould rot, brown rot, gray mould, rhizopus rot
Spinach	Bacterial soft rot, gray mould rot
Sweet potatoes	Alternaria rot, black rot (*Ceratostornella fimbriata*), rhizopus soft rot
Potatoes	Fusarium tuber rots, bacterial ring rot, bacterial soft rot

(Contd ...)

Item	Market disease
Crucifers	
Cabbage	Bacterial soft rot, gray mould rot, black rot, watery soft rot
Brussel sprouts	Bacterial soft rot, gray mould rot, black rot, watery soft rot
Cauliflower	Bacterial soft rot, gray mould rot, black rot, watery soft rot
Broccoli	Bacterial soft rot
Radishes	Bacterial soft rot, clubroot rot, rhizoctonia rot (*Rhizoctonia carotae*)
Turnips	Bacterial soft rot, clubroot rot, rhizoctonia rot
Rutabagas	Bacterial soft rot: gray mould rot, black rot, watery soft rot
Cucurbits	
Cucumber	Rhizopus soft rot, bacterial soft rot, blue mould rot, gray mould rot
Cantaloupe	Rhizopus soft rot, diplodia rot, bacterial soft rot, pink mould rot, fusarium rot
Pumpkin	Rhizopus soft rot, diplodia rot, phytophthera rot, gray mould rot
Squash	Rhizopus soft rot, gray mould rot
Watermelon	Rhizopus soft rot, gray mould rot, phytophthera rot, bacterial soft rot
Tomatoes	Alternaria rot, bacterial canker, bacterial spot, gray mould rot, green mould rot, rhizopus rot
Peppers	Alternaria rot, gray mould rot
Eggplant	Fruit rot (phomopsis rot)

The likelihood of the entrance of spoilage organisms also is important in influencing the possibility of spoilage and the kind that takes place. Damage by mechanical means, plant pathogens, or bad handling will favour entrance. The location of the plant part used also is important; thus underground parts such as roots, tubers or bulbs as in radishes, beets, carrots and potatoes are in direct contact with moist soil and become infected from that source. Fruits such as strawberries, cucumbers, peppers and melons may be in direct contact with the surface of the soil. Leaves, stems and flowers, as in lettuce, the greens, cabbage, asparagus, rhubarb and broccoli, are especially exposed to contamination by plant pathogens or damage by birds and insects, as are most fruits, whether ordinarily classified as vegetables or 'fruits'.

The character of the spoilage will depend on the product attacked and the attacking organism. When the food is soft and juicy, the rot is apt to be soft and mushy and some leakage may result. There are, however, some kinds of spoilage organisms that have a drying effect so that dry or leathery rots or discoloured surface areas may result. In some instances most of the mycelial growth of the mould is subsurface and only a rotten spot shows, as in most rotting of apples. In other types of spoilage the growth of the mould mycelium on the outside is apparent and may be coloured by spores.

The identification of a type of spoilage of a fruit or vegetable makes possible the application of available methods for the prevention of such decay.

Spoilage of fruit and vegetable juices

Juices may be squeezed directly from fruits or vegetables, may be squeezed from macerated or crushed material so as to include a considerable amount of pulp or may be extracted by water, e.g. prune juice. These juices may be used in their natural concentrations or may be concentrated by evaporation or freezing, and may be preserved by canning, freezing or drying.

Juices squeezed or extracted from fruits are more or less acid, depending on the product, the pH ranging from about 2.4 for lemon or cranberry juice up to 4.2 for tomato juice and all contain sugars, the amounts varying from about 2 per cent in lemon juice up to almost 17 per cent in some samples of grape juice. Although moulds can and do grow on the surface of such juices if the juices are exposed to air, the high moisture content favours the faster-growing yeasts and bacteria. Which of the latter will predominate in juices low in sugar and acid will depend more on the temperature than on the composition. The removal of solids from the juices by extraction and sieving raises the oxidation-reduction potential and favours the growth of yeasts.

Most fruit juices are acid enough and have sufficient sugar to favour the growth of yeasts within the range of temperature that favours them, namely, from 15.6° to 35°C. The deficiency of B vitamins discourages some bacteria.

Therefore, the normal change to be expected in raw fruit juices at room temperatures is an alcoholic fermentation by yeasts, followed by the oxidation of alcohol and fruit acids by film yeasts or moulds growing on the surface if it is exposed to air or the oxidation of the alcohol to acetic acid if acetic acid bacteria are present. The types of yeasts growing depend on the kinds predominant in the juice and on the temperature, but usually wild yeasts, such as the apiculate ones, producing only moderate amounts of alcohol and considerable amounts of volatile acid will carry out the first fermentation. At temperatures near the extremes of the range indicated (15.6° to 35°C), the undesirable yeasts are more likely to grow than those producing desirable flavours.

At temperatures above 32.2° to 35°C lactobacilli would be likely to grow and form lactic and some volatile acids because these temperatures are too high for most yeasts. At temperatures below 15.6°C wild yeasts may grow, but the more the temperature drops toward freezing, the more likely the growth of bacteria and moulds rather than yeasts. The acidity may be reduced by film yeasts and moulds growing on the surface.

In addition to the usual alcoholic fermentation, fruit juices may undergo other changes caused by micro-organisms: (i) the lactic acid fermentation of sugars, mostly by heterofermentative lactic acid bacteria such as *Lactobacillus pastorianus*, *L. brevis* and *Leuconostoc mesenteroides* in apple or pear juice and by homofermentative lactic acid bacteria such as *Lactobacillus arabinosus*, *L. leichmanii* and *Microbacterium*, (ii) the fermentation of organic acids of the juice by lactic acid bacteria, e.g. *Lactobacillus pastorianus*, malic acid to lactic and succinic acids, quinic acid to dehydroshikimic acid and citric acid to lactic and acetic acids, and (iii) slime production by *Leuconostoc mesenteroides*, *Lactobacillus brevis* and *L. plantarum* in apple juice and by *L. plantarum* and streptococci in grape juice.

Vegetable juices contain sugars but are less acid than fruit juices, having pH values in the range of 5.0 to 5.8 for the most part. Vegetable juices also contain a plentiful supply of accessory growth factors for micro-organisms and hence support good growth of the fastidious lactic acid bacteria. Acid fermentation of the raw juice by these and other acid-forming bacteria would be a likely cause of spoilage, although yeasts and moulds can grow.

Concentrates of fruit and vegetable juices, because of their increased acidity and sugar concentration, favour the growth of yeasts and of acid- and sugar- tolerant *Leuconostoc* and *Lactobacillus* species. Such concentrates usually are canned and then heat treated or frozen. Heat processing kills the important micro-organisms that could cause spoilage and freezing prevents the growth of such organisms.

Chapter 15

Sugar and Sugar Products

INTRODUCTION

Sugar products discussed in this chapter include sucrose (cane and beet sugar), molasses, syrups, maple sap and sugar, honey, and candy.

Sugar is a class of edible crystalline substances, mainly sucrose, lactose and fructose. Human taste buds interpret its flavour as sweet. Sugar as a basic food carbohydrate primarily comes from sugar cane and from sugar beet, but also appears in fruit, honey, sorghum, sugar maple (in maple syrup), and in many other sources. It forms the main ingredient in much candy. Excessive consumption of sugar has been associated with increased incidences of diabetes, obesity and tooth decay.

Sucrose (common name: table sugar, also called saccharose) is a disaccharide of glucose and fructose with an α (alpha) 1,2-glycosidic linkage. It is best known for its role in human nutrition and is formed by plants but not by other organisms including animals.

Molasses is a thick by-product from the processing of the sugar beet or sugar cane into sugar. The quality of molasses depends on the maturity of the sugar cane or beet, the amount of sugar extracted and the method of extraction.

Syrup is a thick, viscous liquid, containing a large amount of dissolved sugars, but showing little tendency to deposit crystals. The viscosity arises from the multiple hydrogen bonds between the dissolved sugar, which has many hydroxyl (OH) groups and the water. Technically and scientifically, the term syrup is also employed to denote viscous, generally residual, liquids, containing substances other than sugars in solution. Artificial maple syrup is made with water and an extremely large amount of dissolved sugar. The solution is heated so more sugar can be put in than normally possible. The solution becomes super-saturated.

Maple syrup is a sweetener made from the sap of maple trees. It is sometimes used as an ingredient in baking, the making of candy, preparing desserts, or as a sugar source and flavouring agent in making beer. Sucrose is the most prevalent sugar in maple syrup.

Honey is a sweet fluid produced by honey bees (and some other species) and derived from the nectar of flowers. Honey gets its sweetness from the monosaccharides fructose and glucose and has approximately the same relative sweetness as that of granulated sugar (97 per cent of the sweetness of sucrose, a disaccharide). Honey has attractive chemical properties for baking and a distinctive flavour which leads some people to prefer it over sugar and other sweeteners.

Candy, specifically sugar candy, is a confection made from a concentrated solution of sugar in water, to which flavourings and colourants are added. Candies come in numerous colours and varieties and have a long history in popular culture.

ALTERNATIVES TO SUGAR

Trends in sugar consumption seem to be changing in developed countries and particularly in the USA. Increasing number of diabetics, growing health consciousness among people and availability of a multitude of alternative sweeteners are some of the reasons behind this change. One often hears that sugar gives calories and that it is fattening; and so a search starts for a substitute that will give sweetness, but no calories.

It is occasionally feared that sugar production may slowly become a thing of the past, as more and more people switch over from sugar to substitute sweeteners. How seriously is such an apprehension be taken? Can sugar be totally replaced from our diet? Is there any real substitute for it?

Before seeking answers to questions like these, one must first understand what sugar does and how it acts once it is added to foodstuff. Many chemicals are now known that occur in nature, are sweet in taste and can be grouped together as simple sugars. Glucose, fructose, maltose, lactose, etc. are some such compounds. Sucrose or the common household sugar familiar to every one, is also one of them.

Sucrose occurs as a natural constituent in fruit, honey, milk and vegetables. It is an essential ingredient of such prepared foods as cakes, jams, chocolates and sweetmeats; however, it is optional in items like tea, coffee, soup, salad, rayata, etc. Irrespective of its source, sucrose provides prompt satisfaction of hunger and bestows a feeling of freshness. It fulfils several roles in foods. Indeed, the physical and chemical properties of any sugar-containing food are, at least in part, due to their sugar (sucrose) content.

Sucrose (referred to as sugar hereafter) offers the opportunity of preparing foods and drinks appropriate to occasion. Variety and acceptability of foods can be increased by changing their sugar content. Sugar not only confers sweet taste, but also bulk and texture to foods. It promotes secretion of saliva once a mouthful of food is taken. If used in adequate quantity, sugar delays the process of staling and helps preserve the food. However, under certain conditions, it may hasten its spoilage.

The proportion of sugar used in any food—homemade or factory-made—is determined by what the product is intended to be. For example, by varying the proportion of the two main ingredients, viz. milk and sugar and after appropriate processing, products like ice cream, chocolate, burfi of rabdi can be obtained.

If the range is possible, the quantity of sugar to be used is decided on the basis of consumers' preference, particularly in manufactured food. It is interesting to note how one or more of the aforementioned functions of sugar are of importance in a particular food in which it is used.

Sweetness

Sugar imparts sweetness to food and enhances its palatability. This, in turn, may encourage one's (real or false) appetite and lead to over-eating. The intensity of sweetness considered ideal is the combined effect of the nature of food, the situation in which it is eaten and individual preferences.

Flavour

Sugars, after water, are major constituent in foods, e.g. fresh fruit and vegetables. Sugar, whether naturally present or added, contributes to the flavour of certain foods, which in themselves are not sweet, e.g. milk, fresh vegetables, breakfast cereals, soups, etc. Here, sugar contributes to the total perceived flavour without sweetness predominating.

Consumers are often unaware that a little sugar is added even to savoury products (e.g. certain biscuits, bhujiya or chivda) because they do not expect it to be present in these items. Added sugar enhances the flavour of even sweet foods. For example, mango pulp with a little added sugar tastes better than plain pulp, even if it is sweet. Also, in most soft drinks, the characteristic flavour would not be experienced in the absence of a little natural or added sugar.

Development of flavour is a key function of sugar in foods that contain starch and sugars and that are heated prior to use. Thus, bread, cake, (roasted) potato, peanuts, coffee-beans, etc. possess typical generated flavour that cannot be perceived in them when raw. Simultaneously, browning takes place in these products and often it is desirable. Pale golden potato chips or faint reddish brown peanuts appear more appealing.

But strong heating leads to undesirable browning, which renders the product unattractive and also spoils its flavour. On mild heating, pure sugar turns brown. This reaction is known as caramelisation. But the heat induced reaction between sugar and amino acids (emanated from proteins in the food) is known as Maillard reaction. It changes amino acids (nutrients) into flavour compounds (non-nutrients). Hence Maillard reaction is disadvantageous from the nutritional point of view. The loss of amino acids is small though and there should be no undue concern about its safety in as much as man has preferred to roast, bake or boil much of his food ever since he discovered fire.

Bulk

Sugar enlarges the bulk of many food products. In cakes, jams, chocolates and sweetmeats of different types, sugar constitutes a substantial and essential part in that the products could not exist without it, or retain its traditional characteristics. Without the bulk provided by sugar, many foods, as we know them, cannot be made. Sugar, in such products, cannot be replaced to any significant extent if they are to remain on the market.

Mouth-feel

Texture or mouth-feel is a qualitative aspect of bulk and an intrinsic component of the characteristic textures of certain foods. In some sweetmeats and cakes, the physical state and the proportion of sugar largely determine their texture. Thus, the soft, light and spongy texture of cake, the crunchy texture of certain biscuits or the chewy texture of *chikki* is largely attributable to sugar. Soft drinks (e.g. nimbu shikanji) made with intense sweeteners (e.g. saccharin) are less viscous and less soothing and have a different mouth-feel *vis-à-vis* a similar product made with sugar.

Preservation

Large quantity of sugar in water-containing foods helps prevent the growth of microbes, e.g. bacteria and mould. These microbes require water to grow. If the food contains enough dissolved sugar the latter holds back water in it which is no longer available to the microbes. If, however, only a small quantity of sugar is used in these foods, the microbes may utilise it as their nutrient, thrive and thus hasten the process of fermentation and staling. Hence durable sweetmeats (e.g. burfi, laddoo, etc.) and fruit jams usually contain high proportion of sugar.

Substitutes for Sugar

While selecting the substitutes for sugar, two of its qualitative aspects, viz. sweetness and bulk prove decisive. On the basis of these two, the said substitutes can be classified into three groups:

1. Bulk sweeteners that provide bulk, as well as sweetness.
2. Intense sweeteners that provide sweetness without bulk.
3. Bulking agents that supply bulk without sweetness.

The bulking agents can be regarded as true substitutes for sucrose only when they are appropriately combined with intense sweeteners. Erythritol, xylitol, mannitol, sorbitol, maltitol and hydrogenated glucose syrup are some of the bulk sweeteners in use today. Chemically, these are closely related to sugar; yet they differ from it in terms of intensity of sweetness, solubility in water and stability to heat.

These differences *per se* are not objectionable, but are sufficient to prevent their use as simple substitutes for sugar. Moreover, all these compounds are laxative to varying degree and should be used with discretion and a warning label. Some of these compounds occur in nature, but not as significant constituents of natural foods.

They can be made by chemical and/or enzymatic transformations of components of plant matter. Intense sweeteners, being much sweeter than sugar, provide sweetness with negligible bulk.

They provide (if at all) only a small number of calories. They can replace sugar in foods where bulk is unimportant, e.g. tea, coffee, soft drinks, etc. Many intensely sweet compounds are known today. But only a few of them are in use. Saccharin is, by far, the most well-known among these. Discovered in 1878, it is 550 times sweeter than sugar. Being a non-proprietary chemical, it is supplied under different commercial names in different countries.

Aspartame (aspartylphenylalanine methyl ester) sold under the names Candarel, Nutrasweet (Monsanto) and Sugarfree (Cadila) is 160 times sweeter than sugar. Being unstable to heat, it is unsuitable for foods that undergo prolonged or intense cooking. However, it is incorporated in soft drinks, e.g. Pepsi and Coca-Cola. Patients of phenylketonurea, who need a diet containing very low quantity of phenylalanine, should use it under medical supervision.

Two other artificial sweeteners are Acesulphame-K and Thaumatin. The former is 130 times sweeter than sugar and supplied by Hoechst under the name Sunnet. The latter, a protein isolated from certain West African berries, is 1600 times sweeter than sucrose and available under the name Talin (Cultor Food Science). Its sweet taste lingers on in the mouth for a long time.

It is noteworthy that the aforesaid artificial sweeteners are in no way related to sugar. A sweetener launched recently by McNeil Nutritionals (a subsidiary of Johnson and Johnson), however, is a direct descendant of sugar. The active ingredient of this new product called Splenda is sucralose, a trichloro derivative of sucrose. Sucralose possesses all properties desirable in an ideal sweetener.

Thus, it is 650 times sweeter than sucrose, tastes like its parent, dissolves in water and is stable to heat as and a wide range of acidity. It is neither metabolised in the human body, nor the mouth bacteria can use it. It is non-toxic.

By and large, artificial sweeteners are expensive and not every one can afford to use them daily. These chemicals are given the status of food additive only after rigorous safety evaluation. Nevertheless, some doubt remains about effects of their long-term use.

Bulking agents confer body or bulk on food without adding significantly to its calorific value. Their excessive use may lead to disorders of the digestive-system. Alpha-cellulose and polydextrose are the two relatively well-known bulking agents. The former is a type of cellulose that is neither metabolised in, nor absorbed by, the human body. The latter is an artificial polymer of glucose that is only partly metabolised. It provides 25 per cent of calories as provided by most edible carbohydrates. Water holding ability of these products helps create a feeling of fullness in the stomach. Taste and the general physical properties of these products limit the extent to which these can replace sugar.

Starch (used in soup and sauce), pectin (jam and jelly) and edible gum (confectionery and ice-cream), which are employed primarily for their thickening and gelling properties, are the other products that can serve as useful substitutes for sugar albeit in a limited way.

Legally, it is desirable to restrict, as far as practicable, the use of substances with no nutritional value as ingredients of food. According to one broad estimate, 98 per cent of the world sugar production is used to sweeten something somewhere. Moreover, sugar fulfils 85 per cent of the demand of the world sweetener market. The remaining 15 per cent is satisfied by high fructose syrup (7 per cent), artificial sweeteners (4 per cent) and others (4 per cent). From the foregoing discussion and considering the ever increasing population, abundant supply of sugar, its low cost and wide applications in foods and the fact that it is replenishable it can be argued that there is no alternative to sugar. The utility of its substitutes mentioned above is bound to remain limited. Even if their consumption goes up over a period of time, the consumption of sugar is unlikely to be affected adversely.

CONTAMINATION

Sucrose

The raw juice expressed from sugarcane may become high in microbial content unless processing is prompt. The relevant micro-organisms are those from the sugarcane and the soil contaminating it and therefore comprise slime producers, such as species of *Leuconostoc* and *Bacillus*; representatives of the genera *Micrococcus*, *Flavobacterium*, *Alcaligenes*, *Xanthomonas*, *Pseudomonas*, *Erwinia* and *Enterobacter*; a variety of yeasts, chiefly in the genera *Saccharomyces*, *Candida* and *Pichia*; and a few moulds (Table 15.1). Much contamination may come from debris or fine particles on the sides or joints of troughs at the plant. If organisms grow to any extent, inversion of sucrose or even destruction of sugar may take place. Activity of the organisms continues from cutting of the cane through extraction to clarification of the juice, a process which kills yeasts and vegetative cells of bacteria. Bacterial spores are present from then on, through sedimentation, filtration, evaporation, crystallisation and centrifugation, but may be reduced in numbers by these processes, although spores of thermophiles may be added from equipment. Bagging of the raw sugar also may add some micro-organisms. During the refining of the raw sugar, contamination may come from equipment and organisms are added during bagging.

Table 15.1. Microbiological profile of sugarcane, cane juice, raw sugar and sucrose.

Product	Micro-organisms present	Approximate quantitative range
Sugarcane	Bacteria	$10^2–10^8$/g
	Enterobacter	
	Leuconostoc	
	Flavobacterium	
	Xanthomonas	
	Bacillus	
	Erwinia	
	Pseudomonas	
	Moulds	$10^2–10^4$/g
	Yeast	$10^2–10^4$/g
Raw cane juice	Bacteria	$10^4–10^8$/ml
	as above plus *Micrococcus*	

(Contd ...)

Product	Micro-organisms present	Approximate quantitative range
	Lactobacillus	
	Actinomyces	
	Moulds	
	Aspergillus	
	Cladosporium	
	Monilia	
	Penicillium	
	Yeast	
	Saccharomyces	
	Candida	
	Pichia	
	Torulopsis	
Raw sugar	Bacteria	10^2–10^4/g
	Bacillus	
	Clostridium	
	Desulphotomaculum	
	Osmophilic yeast	
	Aspergillus	
	Penicillium	
	Osmophilic moulds	
	Hansenula	
	Pichia	
	Saccharomyces	
Sucrose	Bacteria	10^1–10^2/g
	Mostly sporeformers, if any, and minimal yeast and moulds	

In the manufacture or beet sugar, cleaned beets are sliced into thin slices and the sugar is removed by a diffusion process at 60° to 85°C. Sources of contamination are flume waters and diffusion-battery waters. Thermophiles may grow in the latter up to 70°C. Contamination also may take place during refining and bagging of the sugar. Granulated sugar now on the market is very low in microbial content for the most part, containing from a few to several hundred organisms per gram, mostly bacterial spores.

Maple Syrup

Sap of the sugar maple in the vascular bundles is sterile or practically so but becomes contaminated from outside sources in the tapholes and by the spout, plastic tubing and buckets of other collection vessels. If a period of unusual warmth occurs before the sap is collected, considerable growth of yeasts and bacteria may take place in the sap.

Micro-organisms entering sap between its flow from the tree and being boiled and concentrated are mostly psychrotrophic, gram-negative rods of *Pseudomonas*, *Alcaligenes* and *Flavobacterium*, plus yeasts and moulds. Paraformaldehyde taphole pellets are inserted into the drilled hole to prevent microbial growth from blocking the flow. In sugar-bush locations that are exposed to unusual dust and air contamination, collection of sap by a series of plastic tubes results in lower bacterial contamination. However, in a well-controlled sugar bush the microbial content of sap collected by tubing is not significantly different from that obtained by using individual pails. Sap-gathering tanks, usually mobile, must be sanitised regularly to prevent development of high numbers of bacteria in the sap when it reaches the evaporator. Bacterial counts in sap are usually less than 10,000 per millilitre, but higher numbers can develop as a result of warmer temperatures near the end of the season and poor sanitation.

Honey

The chief sources of micro-organisms in honey are the nectar of flowers and the honeybee. Yeasts have been shown to come from the nectar and from the intestinal content of the bee; bacteria also come from the latter source. Honey rarely contains staphylococci or enteric bacteria. Common isolates are usually acidophilic and glycolytic yeasts, which can damage the product. Honey has been found to contain lysozyme, an enzyme with a bacteriostatic as well as a lytic effect on most gram-positive bacteria. The use of antibiotics such as neomycin and streptomycin is widespread in beekeeping, and these antibiotics have been found in the honey obtained from treated larvae and bees. Traces of these antibiotics in the honey would, of course, have an effect on its microbial flora. Honey is one of the suspected food vehicles for the source of *C. botulinum* spores in cases of infant botulism. About 10 per cent of the suspected honey samples contained viable spores.

A study by Ruiz-Argueso and Rodriguez-Navarro suggested that *Gluconobacter* and *Lactobacillus* are the two main groups of bacteria present during maturation of nectar to honey.

Candy

Candies from retail markets contain from 0 to 2 million bacteria per piece, but most pieces harbour no more than a few hundred. Few coliform bacteria are found. The candies receive most of their contamination from their ingredients, although some contamination may be added to unwrapped pieces by air, dust and handling. The several thousand types of candies and confections can be divided into two categories for microbiological consideration: (i) cold-processed, and (ii) hot-processed confections. Moulded chocolate and chocolate coatings for creamed centres fall into the first category. Temperatures during processing may only approach pasteurisation temperature. Examples of the second category include hard candy, jellies, caramels and fudges. Processing temperatures for these items vary, but they all are exposed to a more severe heat treatment than are items in the first category.

Candies are infrequently associated with food-poisoning outbreaks, but chocolate candies have been incriminated in cases of salmonellosis. The problem appears to be one of cross contamination in the plant between raw and roasted cocoa beans, with the raw beans or environmental isolates serving as the source of contamination. Although temperatures of 60°C for 10 hours. are not uncommon during processing and blending of milk chocolate, the low moisture content or the dryness of the chocolate apparently protects the salmonellae from heat.

PRESERVATION

Like cereals, sugars normally have a_w's so low that micro-organisms cannot grow. Only when moisture has been absorbed is there any chance for microbial spoilage. Storage conditions should be such that vermin are kept out and the sugar remains dry. The recommended storage temperature is similar to that for cereals.

Cane or sugar beets may be stored in a controlled atmosphere. Fungal growth is inhibited by 6 per cent carbon dioxide and 5 per cent oxygen.

During the manufacture of raw sugar and the subsequent refining process the numbers of micro-organisms present, which may have been large during extraction from cane or sugar beet, are reduced by most subsequent processes, e.g. clarification, evaporation, crystallisation, centrifugation and filtration. Chemical preservatives are effective in reducing microbial numbers during sugar refining. Special treatments to reduce numbers and kinds of organisms may be given during refining when the sugar is to be used for a special purpose, e.g. for soft drinks or canning. Care is taken to avoid buildup of organisms and their spores during processing, and numbers may be reduced by irradiation with ultraviolet rays or combined action of heat and hydrogen peroxide.

Because of their high sugar concentration and low a_w, most candies are not subject to microbial spoilage, although soft fillings of chocolate-covered candies may support the growth of micro-organisms. The bursting of chocolates is prevented by a uniform and fairly heavy chocolate coating and use of a fondant or other filling that will not permit the growth of gas formers.

Sirups and molasses usually have undergone enough heating to destroy most micro-organisms but should be stored at cool temperatures to prevent or slow chemical changes and microbial growth. Some molasses may contain enough sulphur dioxide to inhibit micro-organisms, but most sirups and molasses contain no added preservatives and prevent microbial growth because of the high osmotic pressure of the sugar solution.

The osmotic pressure increases with the extent of inversion (hydrolysis) of the sucrose. Mould growth on the surface is prevented by a complete fill of the container and is reduced by periodic mixing of the sirup or molasses.

The boiling process during evaporation of maple sap to maple sirup kills the important spoilage organisms. Such sirup, bottled hot and in a completely filled container, usually keeps well.

Honey distributed locally on a small scale usually is not pasteurised and therefore may be subject to crystallisation and to possible spoilage in time by osmophilic yeasts. Commercially distributed honey usually is pasteurised at 71° to 77°C for a few minutes. A recommended treatment is to heat fairly rapidly to at least 71°C, hold there for 5 minutes, and cool promptly to 32.2° to 38°C.

SPOILAGE

The spoilage of sugars or concentrated solutions of sugars is limited to that caused by osmophilic or xerotolerant micro-organisms. Certain yeasts, especially those of the genus *Saccharomyces* and certain moulds would be the principal spoilage flora. Some species of bacteria have also been suggested as possible spoilage problems, including species of *Bacillus* and *Leuconostoc*. As the sugar concentrations decrease, increasing numbers of kinds of organisms can grow, so that sap from a maple tree would show types of spoilage that maple sirup could not.

Sucrose

During the manufacture of sugar, the original cane or beet juice becomes more and more purified toward sucrose and the concentration of sugar in solution becomes greater and greater until finally crystalline sugar is attained plus molasses that is high in sugar. The purer the product, the poorer it becomes as a culture medium for micro-organisms; the more concentrated it gets, the fewer kinds of organisms can grow in it.

Raw juice

The raw cane or beet juice is not high in sugar and contains a good supply of accessory foods for micro-organisms; it therefore is readily deteriorated by the numerous organisms present if sufficient time is allowed. Until clarification, gum and slime may be formed, e.g. dextran by *Leuconostoc mesenteroides* or *L. dextranicum* and levan by *Bacillus* spp. or, less commonly, by yeasts or moulds.

Sugar in storage

Liquid sugar with sugar content as high as 67° to 72°brix will support the growth of yeasts (*Saccharomyces, Candida, Rhodotorula*) and moulds which may enter from the air. Dilution by absorption of moisture at the surface may result in growth of micro-organisms and hence deterioration of the product. This can be prevented by circulation of filtered sterile air across the top of the storage tank or exposure to ultraviolet lamps.

Molasses and syrups

Microbial spoilage of molasses is not common, although it is difficult to sterilise by heat because of the protective effect of the sugar. Canned molasses or syrup may be subject to spoilage by osmophilic yeasts that survive the heat process. Molasses or syrup exposed to air will mould, in time, on the surface, and this also may occur at the surface of a bottled or canned syrup if air is left there and contamination has taken place prior to sealing. Some kinds of molasses are acid enough to cause hydrogen swells upon long storage.

Maple Sap and Syrup

As previously stated, sap from the sugar maple becomes contaminated when drawn. Although a moderate amount of growth may improve flavour and colour, the sap often stands under conditions that favour excessive growth of micro-organisms and hence spoilage. Five chief types of spoilage are recognised: (i) ropy or stringy sap, usually caused by *Enterobacter aerogenes*, although *Leuconostoc* spp. may be responsible, (ii) cloudy, sometimes greenish sap resulting from the growth of *Pseudomonas fluorescens*, with species of *Alcaligenes* and *Flavobacterium* sometimes contributing to cloudiness, (iii) red sap, coloured by pigments of red bacteria, e.g. *Micrococcus roseus* or of yeasts or yeast like fungi, (iv) sour sap, a catchall grouping for types of spoilage not showing a marked change in colour but having a sour odour and caused by any of a variety of kinds of bacteria or yeasts, and (v) mouldy sap, spoiled by moulds.

Maple syrup can be ropy because of *Enterobacter aerogenes*, yeasty as the result of growth of species of *Saccharomyces* yeasts, pink from the pigment of *Micrococcus roseus* or mouldy at the surface, where species of *Aspergillus, Penicillium* or other genera may grow. The sirup may become dark because of alkalinity produced by bacteria growing in the sap and inversion of sucrose. Maple sugar keeps well unless moistened, at which time moulds may grow.

Honey

Honey is variable in composition but must contain no more than 25 per cent moisture. Because of its high sugar content, 70 to 80 per cent, mostly glucose and levulose and its acidity, pH 3.2 to 4.2, the chief cause of its spoilage is osmophilic yeasts: species of *Zygosaccharomyces*, such as *Z. mellis, richteri* or *nussbaumeri* or *Torula (Cryptococcus) mellis*. Most moulds do not grow well on honey, although species of *Penicillium* and *Mucor* have developed slowly.

Most honey yeasts do not grow in the laboratory in sugar concentrations as high as those usually found in honey. Therefore, special theories for the initiation of growth of yeasts in honey have been advanced: (i) honey, being hygroscopic, becomes diluted at the surface, where yeasts begin to multiply and soon become adapted to the high sugar concentrations, (ii) crystallisation of glucose hydrate from honey leaves a lowered concentration of sugars in solution, and (iii) on long-standing, yeasts gradually become adapted to the high sugar concentrations. The critical moisture content for the initiation of yeast growth has been placed at 21 per cent. The degree of inversion of sucrose to glucose and levulose by the bees and the content of available nitrogen also are listed as factors determining the likelihood of growth. The fermentation process usually is slow, lasting for months, and the chief products are carbon dioxide, alcohol, and nonvolatile acids which give an off-flavour to the honey. Darkening and crystallisation usually accompany the fermentation.

Candy

Most candies are not subject to microbial spoilage because of the comparatively high sugar and low moisture content. Exceptions are chocolates with soft centres of fondant or of inverted sugar, which, under certain conditions, burst or explode. Yeasts growing in these candies develop a gas pressure which may disrupt the entire candy or more often will push out some of the syrup or fondant through a weak spot in the chocolate coating. Often this weak spot is on the poorly covered bottom of the chocolate, where a cylinder of fondant squeezes out. The defect is prevented by using a filling that will not support growth of the gas formers and by coating the candy with a uniformly thick and strong layer of chocolate. The microbial spoilage flora of many confectionery products is summarised in Fig. 15.1.

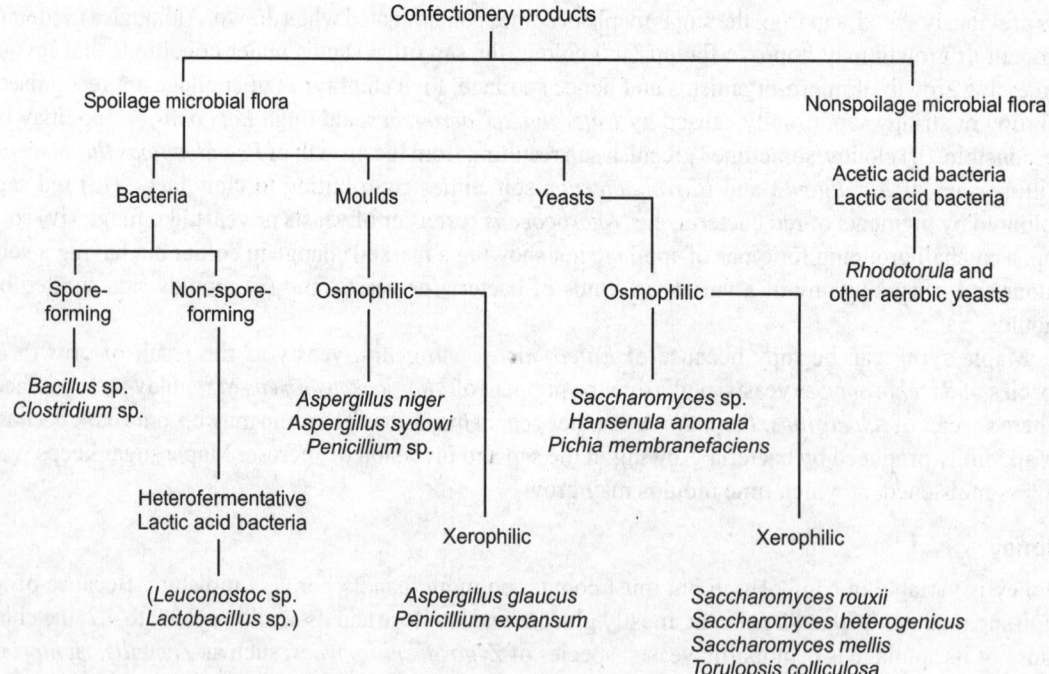

Fig. 15.1. Spoilage flora of confectionery products.

Chapter 16

Cocoa, Tea, Coffee, Soya Sauce and Allied Products

INTRODUCTION

The starting material for cocoa and chocolate is the seed of *Theobroma cacao* which was first cultivated by the Aztec and Mayan civilisations more than 2500 years ago and imported by the Spanish in 1528. Processing is in the tropics where the cocoa is grown, with ensuing manufacturing in the countries where the end products are consumed.

There are two major types of *T. cacao*. Criollo affords cocoas that have a refined flavour but low yield. Forastero affords much higher yields and is therefore the predominant type used, accounting for approximately 95 per cent of the cocoa beans used in the manufacture of chocolate and cocoa products.

Cocoa pods develop on the trunks and branches of the tree and are harvested throughout the year. They comprise an embryo and shell. There are between 35 and 45 seeds (or beans or cotyledons) encased in a mucilaginous pulp known as the endocarp and composed of sugars (mainly sucrose), pectins, polysaccharides, proteins, organic acids and salts (Table 16.1). The plant contains alkaloids, notably the methylxanthines theobromine (1–2 per cent of the dry weight) and caffeine (0–2 per cent) (Fig. 16.1) The former affords bitterness to cocoa. The embryo of the seed comprises two folded cotyledons that are covered with a rudimentary endosperm. It is these cotyledons that are used for making cocoa and chocolate (Fig. 16.2).

Table 16.1. The composition of the cocoa cotyledon.

Component	Percentage by weight
Water	32–39
Cocoa butter (lipid)	30–32
Protein	8–10
Polyphenols	5–6
Starch	4–6
Pentosans	4–6
Cellulose	2–3
Theobromine	2–3
Salts	2–3
Sucrose	2–3
Caffeine	1
Acids	1

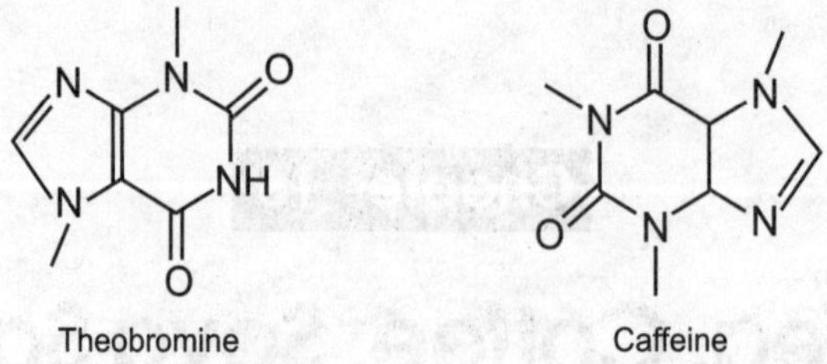

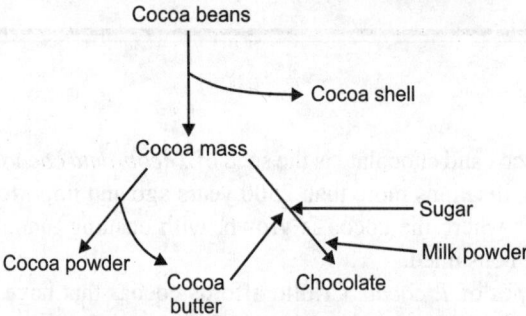

Theobromine   Caffeine

Fig. 16.1. Methylxanthines in cocoa.

Cocoa beans

→ Cocoa shell

Cocoa mass

Sugar

Cocoa powder

Milk powder

Cocoa
butter   Chocolate

Fig. 16.2. An overview of cocoa processing.

The ripe pods are harvested and their husks broken using sharp objects or wooden billets. The wet beans are removed from the husk and heaped (50–80 cm deep) on the ground or in boxes (100 cm deep) to allow 'sweatings' to drain from the bottom. The beans are covered mainly with banana leaves and left for 5–7 days with one or more turnings to allow for a more even fermentation. The temperature will rise to around 50°C and must be maintained below 60°C to avoid over fermentation and excessive growth of fungi.

FERMENTATION OF COCOA

During fermentation, the pulp becomes infected with diverse micro-organisms from the environment. At the start of fermentation, the low pH and high sugar in the surrounding pulp favour anaerobic fermentation by yeasts and also the growth of lactic acid bacteria. The ethanol produced represents a substrate for the acetic acid bacteria, which predominate when the sugars are exhausted. Pectinolytic activity is supplied by *Kluyveromyces marxianus,* but Saccharomyces, Torulopsis and Candida are other yeasts that have significant roles to play. The pectinolysis leads to the draining of the pulp off the beans as 'sweatings'. This allows air into the spaces between the beans and so, late in fermentation, aerophiles develop, including *Bacillus*, as well as filamentous fungi, such as *Aspergillus fumigatus*, *Penicillium* and *Mucor* spp. The increasing concentration of ethanol and acetic acid, together with a rise in heat, eventually leads to the death of the bean. Once this occurs, the biological barriers within the cotyledon are broken down, permitting the release of several types of enzymes.

Initially the anaerobic conditions inside the cotyledon favour hydrolytic enzymatic reactions but, later, aerobic conditions prevail, which favour oxidative reactions, especially of the polyphenols.

Invertase hydrolyses sucrose to the reducing sugars glucose and fructose. These will later combine with peptides and amino acids. During roasting of the beans (discussed later), these compounds enter into the Maillard reaction, and the resultant flavoursome substances are highly significant for the flavour of chocolate.

Glycosidases release polyphenols from their attachment to sugars. The anthocyanidins released polymerise to leucocyanidins, which in turn complex with some of the protein, lessening their astringency and bitterness, as well as reducing the levels of unpleasant flavours and odours sometimes associated with roasted proteins.

After fermentation, the beans are exposed to drying, either by sun or by a forced hot-air source. Drying is an important continuation of the fermentation process and, consequently, flavour-precursor development. During drying, aerobic conditions prevail, favouring oxidative reactions, especially of the polyphenols through the action of PPOs. Since fermentation is a gradual process spread over a 5–7 days period, the action of PPO commences towards the end of the anaerobic phase of fermentation. Quinones are also formed by the oxidative changes brought by the action of the PPO on the polyphenols. These complex with free amino and imino groups of proteins, the tanning of the protein leading to a colour change in the beans and a reduction of astringency.

There appears to be a fine balance between the fermentation and drying that must be adhered to if a consistent flavour is to be achieved in the bean. It is barely credible that the crude and sometimes haphazard methods employed allow this balance to be maintained. Care must be taken not to dry the beans too rapidly, which can lead to case hardening of the bean, thus entrapping more of the unwanted volatile acetic acid.

Whichever method is used, it is essential that the beans are dried down to 5–7 per cent moisture to inhibit the development of mould during storage. The ensuing mouldy taste in the chocolate is almost impossible to eradicate by further processing.

The extent to which the biochemical changes have progressed during fermentation and drying is assessed from the colour change of the cotyledons, resulting from the oxidation of the polyphenolic constituents. A brown colour in the bean is indicative of complete fermentation, purple/brown suggests partial fermentation, purple signifies under-fermented and slate-colouration indicates that the bean has not been fermented. Chocolate made from slate-coloured beans is bitter, astringent and almost devoid of chocolate flavour.

Acetic acid is a by-product of the fermentation of the sugars occurring in the surrounding pulp and significant diffusion into the cotyledon during fermentation causes a decrease in the pH of the beans. For some types of Forastero beans, pH is used as a secondary measurement of the degree of fermentation.

Levels of theobromine and caffeine decline during fermentation, as is also the case for the lipid component of the bean, cocoa butter.

Cocoa butter is fully saturated, hence it is one of the most stable fats in nature and resistant to oxidation. Depending on its polymorph, cocoa butter has a melting temperature of approximately 34.5°C, some 2.5°C lower than normal body temperature. Its melting profile is sharp, so that the chocolate made from it melts cleanly in the mouth with no residual, waxy aftertaste. However, sufficient unmelted solids remain to give body to the chocolate at regular distribution temperatures.

The melt temperature of cocoa butter varies according to the genetics and geographical source of the cocoa. Malaysian cocoa butter has the highest melt temperature and is the hardest in texture. Depending on the season, Brazilian cocoa butter, produced from the winter crop, is the softest and has the lowest melting temperature.

The starch remains virtually chemically unchanged during the fermentation process.

Roasting

Roasting results in the reduction of moisture in the beans from 7 per cent to approximately 1.5 per cent. Much of the volatile acidity, mainly acetic, is evaporated. Non-enzymatic browning and Strecker reactions occur, leading to a diversity of molecules that represent the main part of the chocolate flavour and aroma. These include several types of pyrazines, aldehydes, ketones, esters and oxazoles. Some 400–500 compounds form the basis of chocolate flavour.

Depending on the geographical origin of the beans, roasting temperatures will vary between 110°C and 220°C. The lower temperatures are used for the more fragile and subtly flavoured beans.

Production of Cocoa Mass or Chocolate Liquor

At the beginning of the process of converting the dried cocoa beans into chocolate liquor, the beans are first passed over magnets and vibrating screens to remove any unwanted debris. The beans are then roasted whole, then winnowed or passed over infrared heaters to pop the outer shell. This shell is then removed by a winnowing process which separates the non-usable shell from the nib (raw cotyledon).

The roasted, de-shelled bean and/or nibs are ground to a fine particle size of about 100–120 μm by different types of grinding machines, such as stone, ball, pin mills, etc.

Cocoa Butter

This is extracted from the milled chocolate liquor by mechanical pressing through mesh metal screens by hydraulic presses operating at high pressure at about 90°C. The resulting-cocoa butter has a distinct chocolate flavour, which some companies deem too strong for milk chocolate. They prefer to use a more odourless steam-deodourised cocoa butter.

A by-product of pressing the chocolate liquor is cocoa press cake and this is pulverised to cocoa powder.

Depending on the pressure that the chocolate liquor has been exposed to, the residual cocoa butter content of the cocoa powder ranges from 10 to 20 per cent. Defatted cocoas are processed either by expeller press or solvent extraction.

Production of Chocolate

Sugar (usually pre-pulverised), chocolate liquor and whole milk powder are first mixed to form a paste that can be passed through a five-roll refiner. The paste is ground to an average particle size, which for regular commercial chocolate is about 10–15 μm.

This paste is filled into a machine known as a conche, within which there is dry mixing and aeration on a massive scale. During the conching process, which can take between 6 and 72 hours, the moisture and volatile acids are evaporated which results in a reduction of the viscosity of the chocolate. For milk chocolate, conching is performed at 50°–65°C, but for dark chocolate it is in the range 60°–90°C.

Due to the high shearing forces for long periods in the conching process, major changes occur in the texture. The finished chocolate is more cohesive, less crumbly when set, and the taste is much more mellow and less harsh and bitter. The loss of acetic acid ensures a reduction in acid taste. Chocolate receiving high-shearing action and, therefore, better aeration, shows a reduction in astringency, which would suggest that further oxidation of polyphenols is occurring.

During lengthy shearing, there is a better distribution of fat over the dry particles, especially the highly flavoured 'spikey' particles. This may result in a smoother, less bitter astringent taste in the finished chocolate.

The final step in the conching process is the addition of lecithin to reduce the viscosity of chocolate to a workable rheological mass. The chocolate is now ready for use in either a coating or moulding operation. Cocoa butter has five distinct polymorphs and, before it can be used in coating or moulding, it must be put through a cooling, mixing regime to achieve the correct stable form V polymorph. This process is called tempering. There are literally dozens of ways to achieve the correct stable cocoa butter crystallisation.

Tempering involves first cooling the chocolate with agitation, taking the temperature from 45°–50°C to approximately 27°–28°C. At this point, the chocolate is quite viscous and will contain the unstable form IV polymorph. The temperature is then raised to a working temperature of between 29° and 32.5°C, which will vary depending on the source of cocoa butter and the presence of anhydrous dairy butter fat. After coating and moulding, the chocolate must be carefully cooled to avoid the reintroduction of form IV crystals. The chocolate is now ready for packing and is preferably held at a constant 18°C during the distribution cycle.

TEA

Tea refers to the agricultural products of the leaves, leaf buds and internodes of the *Camellia sinensis* plant, prepared and cured by various methods. Tea also refers to the aromatic beverage prepared from the cured leaves by combination with hot or boiling water, and is the colloquial name for the *Camellia sinensis* plant itself.

After water, tea is the most widely-consumed beverage in the world. It has a cooling, slightly bitter, astringent flavour.

The four types of tea most commonly found on the market are black tea, oolong tea, green tea and white tea, all of which can be made from the same bushes, processed differently, and in the case of fine white tea grown differently. Pu-erh tea, a double-fermented black tea, is also often classified as amongst the most popular types of tea.

The term 'herbal tea' usually refers to an infusion or tisane of leaves, flowers, fruit, herbs or other plant material that contains no *Camellia sinensis*. The term 'red tea' either refers to an infusion made from the South African rooibos plant, also containing no *Camellia sinensis*, or, in Chinese, Korean, Japanese and other East Asian languages, refers to black tea.

Leaf size is the chief criterion for the classification of tea plants: tea is classified into: (i) Assam type, characterised by the largest leaves; (ii) China type, characterised by the smallest leaves; and (iii) Cambod, characterised by leaves of intermediate size.

Processing and Classification

A tea's type is determined by the processing through which it goes. Leaves of *Camellia sinensis* soon begin to wilt and oxidise if not dried quickly after picking. The leaves turn progressively darker as their chlorophyll breaks down and tannins are released. This process, enzymatic oxidation, is called fermentation in the tea industry, although it is not a true fermentation: it is not caused by micro-organisms, and is not an anaerobic process. The next step in processing is to stop the oxidation process at a predetermined stage by heating, which deactivates the enzymes responsible. With black tea this is done simultaneously with drying.

Without careful moisture and temperature control during manufacture and packaging, the tea will grow fungi. The fungus causes real fermentation that will contaminate the tea with toxic and sometimes carcinogenic substances, as well as off-flavours, rendering the tea unfit for consumption.

Tea is traditionally classified based on the techniques with which it is produced and processed:

1. White tea: Unwilted and unoxidised.
2. Yellow tea: Unwilted and unoxidised but allowed to yellow.
3. Green tea: Wilted and unoxidised.
4. Oolong: Wilted, bruised and partially oxidised.
5. Black tea: Wilted, sometimes crushed and fully oxidised.
6. Post-fermented tea: Green Tea that has been allowed to ferment/compost.

Blending and Additives

Almost all teas in bags and most other teas sold in the West are blends. Blending may occur in the tea-planting area (as in the case of Assam), or teas from many areas may be blended. The aim is to obtain better taste, higher price, or both, as a more expensive, better-tasting tea may cover the inferior taste of cheaper varieties.

Some teas are not pure varieties, but have been enhanced through additives or special processing. Tea is highly receptive to inclusion of various aromas; this may cause problems in processing, transportation and storage, but also allows for the design of an almost endless range of scented and flavoured variants, such as vanilla, caramel and many others.

Content

Tea contains catechins, a type of antioxidant. In a fresh tea leaf, catechins can compose up to 30 per cent of the dry weight. Catechins are highest in concentration in white and green teas, while black tea has substantially fewer due to its oxidative preparation. Tea also contains theanine and the stimulant caffeine at about 3 per cent of its dry weight, translating to between 30 mg and 90 mg per 8 oz (250 ml) cup depending on type, brand and brewing method. Tea also contains small amounts of theobromine and theophylline, as well as fluoride, with certain types of brick tea made from old leaves and stems having the highest levels.

Dry tea has more caffeine by weight than coffee; nevertheless, more dried coffee is used than dry tea in preparing the beverage, which mean that a cup of brewed tea contains significantly less caffeine than a cup of coffee of the same size. Tea has no carbohydrates, fat or protein.

Preparation

The traditional method of making a cup of tea is to place loose tea leaves, either directly, or in a tea infuser, into a tea pot or teacup and pour hot water over the leaves. After a couple of minutes the leaves are usually removed again, either by removing the infuser or by straining the tea while serving.

Most green teas should be allowed to steep for about three minutes, although some types of tea require as much as ten minutes. The strength of the tea should be varied by changing the amount of tea leaves used, not by changing the steeping time. The amount of tea to be used per amount of water differs from tea to tea but one basic recipe may be one slightly heaped teaspoon of tea (about 5 ml) for each teacup of water (200 ml) (8 oz) prepared as above. Stronger teas, such as Assam, to be drunk with milk are often prepared with more leaves, and more delicate high grown teas such as a Darjeeling are prepared with a little less (as the stronger mid-flavours can overwhelm the champagne notes). The best temperature for brewing tea depends on its type. Teas that have little or no oxidation period, such as a green or white tea, are best brewed at lower temperatures between 60° and 85°C (140°–185°F), while teas with longer oxidation periods should be brewed at higher temperatures around 100°C (212°F). The higher temperatures are required to extract the large, complex, flavourful phenolic molecules found in fermented tea, although boiling the water reduces the amount of dissolved oxygen in the water.

Some tea sorts are often brewed several times using the same tea leaves. Historically, in China, tea is divided into a number of infusions. The first infusion is immediately poured out to wash the tea, and then the second and further infusions are drunk. The third through fifth are nearly always considered the best infusions of tea, although different teas open up differently and may require more infusions of hot water to bring them to life.

One way to taste a tea, throughout its entire process, is to add hot water to a cup containing the leaves and after about 30 seconds to taste the tea. As the tea leaves unfold (known as 'The Agony of the Leaves') they give up various parts of themselves to the water and thus the taste evolves. Continuing this from the very first flavours to the time beyond which the tea is quite stewed will allow an appreciation of the tea throughout its entire length.

Black tea

The water for black teas should be added at boiling point (100° or 212°F). Many of the active substances in black tea do not develop at temperatures lower than 90°C. For some more delicate teas lower temperatures are recommended. The temperature will have as large an effect on the final flavour as the type of tea used. The most common fault when making black tea is to use water at too low a temperature. Since boiling point drops with increasing altitude, this makes it difficult to brew black tea properly in mountainous areas. It is also recommended that the teapot be warmed before preparing tea, easily done by adding a small amount of boiling water to the pot, swirling briefly, before discarding. Black teas are usually brewed for about 4 minutes and should not be allowed to steep for less than 30 seconds or more than about five minutes (a process known as brewing or mashing in the UK, specifically in Yorkshire). Longer steeping times make the tea bitter (at this point it is referred to as being *stewed* in the UK). When the tea has brewed long enough to suit the tastes of the drinker, it should be strained while serving. The popular varieties of black tea include the Assam tea, the Darjeeling tea and the black Ceylon tea.

Green tea

Water for green tea, according to most accounts, should be around 80° to 85°C (176° to 185°F); the higher the quality of the leaves, the lower the temperature. Hotter water will burn green-tea leaves, producing a bitter taste. Preferably, the container in which the tea is steeped, the mug, or teapot should also be warmed beforehand so that the tea does not immediately cool down. High-quality green and white teas can have new water added as many as five or more times, depending on variety, at increasingly high temperatures. Recently, green tea (as well as some black teas) have been shown to significantly increase interferon levels in tea consumers, which lends credence to the theory that some teas help boost the immune system.

Oolong tea (or Wulong)

Oolong teas should be brewed around 90° to 100°C (194° to 212°F), and again the brewing vessel should be warmed before pouring in the water. Yixing purple clay teapots are the traditional brewing vessel for oolong tea. For best results use spring water, as the minerals in spring water tend to bring out more flavour in the tea. High quality oolong can be brewed multiple times from the same leaves, and unlike green tea it improves with reuse. It is common to brew the same leaves three to five times, the third steeping usually being the best.

Premium or delicate tea

Some teas, especially green teas and delicate Oolong teas, are steeped for shorter periods, sometimes less than 30 seconds. Using a tea strainer separates the leaves from the water at the end of the brewing time if a tea bag is not being used. However, black Darjeeling tea, the premium Indian tea, needs a longer than average steeping time. Elevation and time of harvest offer varying taste profiles, proper storage and water quality also have a large impact on taste.

Pu-erh tea (or Pu'er)

Pu-erh teas require boiling water for infusion. Some prefer to quickly rinse pu-erh for several seconds with boiling water to remove tea dust which accumulates from the ageing process. Infuse pu-erh at the boiling point (100°C or 212°F), and allow to steep for 30 seconds or up to five minutes.

Serving

In order to preserve the pre-tannin tea without requiring it all to be poured into cups, a second teapot may be employed. The steeping pot is best unglazed earthenware; Yixing pots are the best known of these, famed for the high quality clay from which they are made. The serving pot is generally porcelain, which retains the heat better. Larger teapots are a post-19th century invention, as tea before this time was very rare and very expensive. Experienced tea-drinkers often insist that the tea should not be stirred around while it is steeping (sometimes called winding in the UK). This, they say, will do little to strengthen the tea, but is likely to bring the tannins out in the same way that brewing too long will do. For the same reason one should not squeeze the last drops out of a teabag; if stronger tea is desired, more tea leaves should be used.

Adding milk to tea

The addition of milk to tea was first mentioned in 1680 by the epistolist Madame de Sévigné. Many teas are traditionally drank with milk. These include Indian masala chai and British tea blends. These teas tend to be very hearty varieties which can be tasted through the milk, such as Assams or the East Friesian blend. Milk is thought to neutralise remaining tannins and reduce acidity. The Chinese do not usually drink milk with tea (or indeed use milk at all) but the Manchurians do, and the elite of the Manchu Dynasty continued to do so. Hong Kong-style milk tea is based on British colonial habits.

The order of steps in preparing a cup of tea is a much-debated topic. Some say that it is preferable to add the milk before the tea, as the high temperature of freshly brewed tea can denature the proteins found in fresh milk, similar to the change in taste of UHT milk, resulting in an inferior tasting beverage. Others insist that it is better to add the milk after brewing the tea, as most teas need to be brewed as close to boiling as possible. The addition of milk chills the beverage during the crucial brewing phase, meaning that the delicate flavour of a good tea cannot be fully appreciated. By adding the milk afterwards, it is easier to dissolve sugar in the tea and also to ensure that the desired amount of milk is added, as the colour of the tea can be observed.

Additives and Flavours

Many flavourings are added to varieties of tea during processing. Among the best known are Chinese Jasmine tea, with jasmine oil or flowers, the spices in Indian Masala chai and Earl Grey tea, which contains oil of bergamot. A great range of modern flavours have been added to these traditional ones.

Other popular additives to tea by the tea-brewer or drinker include sugar, honey, lemon (traditional in Russia and Italy), fruit jams and mint. In China sweetening tea was traditionally regarded as a feminine practice. In colder regions such as Mongolia, Tibet and Nepal, butter is added to provide necessary calories. Tibetan butter tea contains rock salt and dre (yak) butter, which is then churned vigorously in a cylindrical vessel closely resembling a butter churn. The same may be said for salt tea, which is consumed in some cultures in the Hindu Kush region of northern Pakistan.

Tea can also be fortified by the addition of alcohol, such as whisky or brandy.

The flavour of the tea can also be altered by pouring it from different heights, resulting in varying degrees of oxidisation. The art of high-altitude pouring is used principally by people in Northern Africa (e.g. Morocco), but also in West Africa (e.g. Guinea, Mali, Senegal) and can positively alter the flavour of the tea, but it is more likely a technique to cool the beverage destined to be consumed immediately. In certain cultures the tea is given different names depending on the height it is poured from. In Mali, gunpowder tea is served in series of three, starting with the highest oxidisation or strongest, unsweetened tea (cooked from fresh leaves), locally referred to as 'bitter as death'. Follows a second serving, where the same tea leaves are boiled again with some sugar added ('pleasant as life'), and a third one, where the same tea leaves are boiled for the third time with yet more sugar added ('sweet as love'). Green tea is the central ingredient of a distinctly Malian custom, the 'Grin', informal social gathering that cuts across social and economic lines, starting in front of family compound gates in the afternoons, extending late in the night, and widely popular in Bamako and other large urban areas.

In Southeast Asia, particularly in Malaysia, the practice of pouring tea from a height has been refined further using black tea to which condensed milk is added, poured from a height from one cup to another several times in alternating fashion and in quick succession, to create a tea with entrapped air bubbles creating a frothy 'head' in the cup. This beverage, teh tarik, literally, 'pulled tea', has a creamier taste than flat milk tea and is extremely popular in the region. Tea pouring in Malaysia has been further developed into an art form in which a dance is done by people pouring tea from one container to another, which in any case takes skill and precision. The participants, each holding two containers, one full of tea, pour it from one to another. They stand in lines and squares and pour the tea into each others' pots. The dance must be choreographed to allow anyone who has both pots full to empty them and refill whoever has no tea at any one point.

Economics of Tea

Tea is easily the most popular drink in the world in terms of consumption. It easily equals all other manufactured drinks in the world — including coffee, chocolate, soft drinks, and alcohol — put together. Most tea consumed outside East Asia is produced on large plantations in India or Sri Lanka, and is destined to be sold to large businesses. Opposite this large-scale industrial production there are many small 'gardens', sometimes minuscule plantations, that produce highly sought-after teas prized by gourmets. These teas are both rare and expensive, and can be compared to some of the most expensive wines in this respect.

India is the world's largest tea-drinking nation although the per capita consumption of tea remains a modest 750 grams per person every year.

Packaging

Tea bags

In 1907, American tea merchant Thomas Sullivan began distributing samples of his tea in small bags of Chinese silk with a drawstring. Consumers noticed that they could simply leave the tea in the bag, and better still re-use it with fresh tea. However, the potential of this distribution/packaging method would not be fully realised until later on. During World War II, tea was rationed. In 1953 (after rationing in the UK ended), Tetley launched the *tea bag* to the UK and it was an immediate success.

Tea leaves are packed into a small (usually paper) tea bag. It is easy and convenient, making tea bags popular for many people today. However, the tea used in tea bags has an industry name — it is called fannings or 'dust' and is the waste product produced from the sorting of higher quality loose leaf tea. It is commonly held among tea aficionados that this method provides an inferior taste and experience. The paper used for the bag can also be tasted by many, which can detract from the tea's flavour. Because fannings and dust are a lower quality of the tea to begin with, the tea found in tea bags is less finicky when it comes to brewing time and temperature.

Additional reasons why bag tea is considered less well-flavoured include:

Dried tea loses its flavour quickly on exposure to air. Most bag teas (although not all) contain leaves broken into small pieces; the great surface area to volume ratio of the leaves in tea bags exposes them to more air, and therefore causes them to go stale faster. Loose tea leaves are likely to be in larger pieces, or to be entirely intact. Breaking up the leaves for bags extracts flavoured oils.

The small size of the bag does not allow leaves to diffuse and steep properly.

Loose tea

The tea leaves are packaged loosely in a canister or other container. Rolled gunpowder tea leaves, which resist crumbling, are commonly vacuum packed for freshness in aluminised packaging for storage and retail. The portions must be individually measured by the consumer for use in a cup, mug or teapot. This allows greater flexibility, letting the consumer brew weaker or stronger tea as desired, but convenience is sacrificed. Strainers, 'tea presses', filtered teapots and infusion bags are available commercially to avoid having to drink the floating loose leaves and to prevent over-brewing. A more traditional, yet perhaps more effective way around this problem is to use a three-piece lidded teacup, called a gaiwan. The lid of the gaiwan can be tilted to decant the leaves while pouring the tea into a different cup for consumption.

Compressed tea

Some teas (particularly Pu-erh tea) are still compressed for transport, storage and ageing convenience. The tea brick remains in use in the Himalayan countries. The tea is prepared and steeped by first loosening leaves off the compressed cake using a small knife. Compressed teas can usually be stored for longer periods of time without spoilage when compared with loose leaf tea.

Instant tea

In recent times, 'instant teas' are becoming popular, similar to freeze dried instant coffee. Instant tea was developed in the 1930s, but not commercialised until the late 1950s, and is only more recently becoming popular. These products often come with added flavours, such as vanilla, honey or fruit, and may also contain powdered milk. Similar products also exist for instant iced tea, due to the convenience of not requiring boiling water. Tea connoisseurs tend to criticise these products for sacrificing the delicacies of tea flavour in exchange for convenience.

Storage

Tea has a shelf-life that varies with storage conditions and type of tea. Black tea has a longer shelf-life than green tea. Some teas such as flower teas may go bad in a month or so. An exception, Pu-erh tea improves with age. Tea stays freshest when stored in a dry, cool, dark place in an air-tight container. Black tea stored in a bag inside a sealed opaque canister may keep for two years. Green tea loses its freshness more quickly, usually in less than a year. Gunpowder tea, its leaves being tightly rolled, keeps longer than the more open-leafed Chun Mee tea. Storage life for all teas can be extended by using desiccant packets or oxygen absorbing packets, and by vacuum sealing.

When storing green tea, discreet use of refrigeration or freezing is recommended. In particular, drinkers need to take precautions against temperature variation.

Improperly stored tea may lose flavour, acquire disagreeable flavours or odours from other foods, or become moldy.

Tea and Health

The possible beneficial effects of tea consumption in the prevention of cancer and cardiovascular diseases have been demonstrated in animal models and suggested by studies *in vitro*. Similar beneficial effects, however, have not been convincingly demonstrated in humans: beneficial effects have been demonstrated in some studies but not in others. If such beneficial effects do exist in humans, they are likely to be mild, depending on many other lifestyle-related factors, and could be masked by confounding factors in certain populations. Another concern is that the amounts of tea consumed by humans are lower than the doses required for demonstrating the disease-prevention effects in animal models. Caution should be applied, however, in the use of high concentrations of tea for disease prevention. Ingestion of large amounts of tea may cause nutritional and other problems because of the caffeine content and the strong binding activities of tea polyphenols, although there are no solid data on the harmful effects of tea consumption. More research is needed to elucidate the biologic activities of green and black tea and to determine the optimal amount of tea consumption for possible health-beneficial effects.

In abstract, the health benefits of tea have been shown in animal studies, but at doses much higher than regularly consumed by humans, at which dosage levels may prove to be harmful to health. Several of the potential health benefits proposed for tea are outlined in this excerpt from Mondal as following:

Tea leaves contain more than 700 chemicals, among which the compounds closely related to human health are flavanoides, amino acids, vitamins (C, E and K), caffeine and polysaccharides. Moreover, tea drinking has recently proven to be associated with cell-mediated immune function of the human body. Tea plays an important role in improving beneficial intestinal microflora, as well as providing immunity against intestinal disorders and in protecting cell membranes from oxidative damage. Tea also prevents dental caries due to the presence of fluorine. The role of tea is well established in normalising blood pressure, lipid depressing activity, prevention of coronary heart diseases and diabetes by reducing the blood-glucose activity. Tea also possesses germicidal and germistatic activities against various gram-positive and gram-negative human pathogenic bacteria. Both green and black tea infusions contain a number of antioxidants, mainly catechins that have anti-carcinogenic, anti-mutagenic and anti-tumoric properties.

In a large study of over 11,000 men and women completed in 1993 and published in the 1999 *Journal* of *Epidemiology* and *Community Health*, there was actually shown an increase in the risk of coronary disease with the regular consumption of tea.

Ecological effects

Originally, coffee farming was done in the shade of trees, which provided habitat for many animals and insects. This method is commonly referred to as the traditional shaded method or 'shade-grown'. Many farmers have decided to switch their production method to sun cultivation, a method in which coffee is grown in rows under full-sun with little or no forest canopy. This causes berries to ripen more rapidly and bushes to produce higher yields, but requires the clearing of trees and increased use of fertiliser and pesticides. When compared to the sun cultivation method, traditional coffee production causes berries to ripen more slowly and produce lower yields, but the quality of the coffee is allegedly superior. In addition, the traditional shaded method is environmentally friendly and serves as a habitat for many species. Opponents of sun cultivation say environmental problems such as deforestation, pesticide pollution, habitat destruction, and soil and water degradation are the side effects of these practices. The American Birding Association has led a campaign for 'shade-grown' and organic coffees, which it says are sustainably harvested. However, while certain types of shaded coffee cultivation systems show greater biodiversity than full-sun systems, they still compare poorly to native forest in terms of habitat value.

Processing

Roasting

Coffee berries and their seeds undergo several processes before they become the familiar roasted coffee. First, coffee berries are picked, generally by hand. Then they are sorted by ripeness and colour and the flesh of the berry is removed, usually by machine and the seeds—usually called beans—are fermented to remove the slimy layer of mucilage still present on the bean. When the fermentation is finished, the beans are washed with large quantities of freshwater to remove the fermentation residue, which generates massive amounts of highly polluted coffee waste-water. Finally, the seeds are dried; the best, but least utilised method of drying coffee is by using drying tables. In this method the pulped and fermented coffee is spread thinly on raised beds, which allows the air to pass on all sides of the coffee. The coffee is then mixed by hand. and the drying that takes place is more uniform, and fermentation is less likely. Most coffee from Africa is dried in this manner and certain coffee farms around the world are starting to utilise this traditional method as well. Next, the coffee is sorted, and labelled as green coffee. Another way to let the coffee beans dry is to let them sit on a cement patio and rake over them in the sunlight. Some companies use cylinders to pump in heated air to dry the coffee beans, though this is generally in places where the humidity is too high to correctly get the moisture out.

The next step in the process is the roasting of the green coffee. Coffee is usually sold in a roasted state, and all coffee is roasted before it is consumed. It can be sold roasted by the supplier, or it can be home roasted. The roasting process influences the taste of the beverage by changing the coffee bean both physically and chemically. The bean decreases in weight as moisture is lost and increases in volume, causing it to become less dense. The density of the bean also influences the strength of the coffee and requirements for packaging. The actual roasting begins when the temperature inside the bean reaches 200°C, though different varieties of beans differ in moisture and density and therefore roast at different rates. During roasting, caramelisation occurs as intense heat breaks down starches in the bean, changing them to simple sugars that begin to brown, changing the colour of the bean. Sucrose is rapidly lost during the roasting process and may disappear entirely in darker roasts. During roasting, aromatic oils, acids and caffeine weaken, changing the flavour; at 205°C, other oils start to develop. One of these oils is *caffeol*, created at about 200°C, which is largely responsible for coffee's aroma and flavour.

Depending on the colour of the roasted beans as perceived by the human eye, they will be labelled as light, medium light, medium, medium dark, dark or very dark. A more accurate method of discerning the degree of roast involves measuring the reflected light from roasted beans illuminated with a light source in the near infrared spectrum. This elaborate light metre uses a process known as spectroscopy to return a number that consistently indicates the roasted coffee's relative degree of roast or flavour development. Such devices are routinely used for quality assurance by coffee-roasting businesses.

Darker roasts are generally smoother, because they have less fibre content and a more sugary flavour. Lighter roasts have more caffeine, resulting in a slight bitterness and a stronger flavour from aromatic oils and acids otherwise destroyed by longer roasting times. A small amount of chaff is produced during roasting from the skin left on the bean after processing. Chaff is usually removed from the beans by air movement, though a small amount is added to dark roast coffees to soak up oils on the beans. Decaffeination may also be part of the processing that coffee seeds undergo. Seeds are decaffeinated when they are still green. Many methods can remove caffeine from coffee, but all involve either soaking beans in hot water or steaming them, then using a solvent to dissolve caffeine-containing oils. Decaffeination is often done by processing companies, and the extracted caffeine is usually sold to the pharmaceutical industry.

Storage

Once roasted, coffee beans must be stored properly to preserve the fresh taste of the bean. Ideally, the container must be airtight and kept cool. In order of importance, air, moisture, heat and light are the environmental factors responsible for deteriorating flavour in coffee beans.

Folded-over bags, a common way consumers often purchase coffee, are generally not ideal for long-term storage because they allow air to enter. A better package contains a one-way valve, which prevents air from entering.

Preparation

Coffee beans must be ground and brewed in order to create a beverage. Grinding the roasted coffee beans is done at a roastery, in a grocery store or in the home. They are most commonly ground at a roastery and then packaged and sold to the consumer, though 'whole bean' coffee can be ground at home. Coffee beans may be ground in several ways. A burr mill uses revolving elements to shear the bean; an electric grinder smashes the beans with blunt blades moving at high speed; and a mortar and pestle crushes the beans.

The type of grind is often named after the brewing method for which it is generally used. Turkish grind is the finest grind, while coffee percolator or French press are the coarsest grinds. The most common grinds are between the extremes; a medium grind is used in most common home coffee brewing machines.

Coffee may be brewed by several methods: boiled, steeped or pressured. Brewing coffee by boiling was the earliest method, and Turkish coffee is an example of this method. It is prepared by powdering the beans with a mortar and pestle, then adding the powder to water and bringing it to a boil in a pot called a cezve or, in Greek, a briki. This produces a strong coffee with a layer of foam on the surface.

Machines such as percolators or automatic coffeemakers brew coffee by gravity. In an automatic coffeemaker, hot water drips onto coffee grounds held in a coffee filter made of paper or perforated metal, allowing the water to seep through the ground coffee while absorbing its oils and essences. Gravity causes the liquid to pass into a carafe or pot while the used coffee grounds are retained in the filter. In a percolator, boiling water is forced into a chamber above a filter by steam pressure created by boiling. The water then passes downward through the grounds due to gravity, repeating the process until shut off by an internal timer or, more commonly, a thermostat that turns off the heater when the entire pot reaches a certain temperature. This thermostat also serves to keep the coffee warm (it turns on when the pot cools), but requires the removal of the basket holding the grounds after the initial brewing to avoid additional brewing as the pot reheats. Purists do not feel that this repeated boiling is conducive to achieving the best-flavoured coffee. There is a measuring convention adopted for automatic coffeemakers, that is unique to coffee preparation, namely, using 'cup' to mean 6 ounces instead of 8 ounces of fluid. The increments labelled on the pot and water reservoir of an automatic coffeemaker usually correspond to this convention. This is because, typically, one uses about 1 rounded tablespoon of ground coffee per 6 ounces of water.

Coffee may also be brewed by steeping in a device such as a French press (also known as a *cafetière* or coffee press). Ground coffee and hot water are combined in a coffee press and left to brew for a few minutes. A plunger is then depressed to separate the coffee grounds, which remain at the bottom of the container. Because the coffee grounds are in direct contact with the water, all the coffee oils remain in the beverage, making it stronger and leaving more sediment than in coffee made by an automatic coffee machine.

The espresso method forces hot (but not boiling) pressurised water through ground coffee. As a result of brewing under high pressure (ideally between 9–10 atm), the espresso beverage is more concentrated (as much as 10 to 15 times the amount of coffee to water as gravity-brewing methods can produce) and has a more complex physical and chemical constitution. A well-prepared espresso has a reddish-brown foam called *crema* that floats on the surface.

Coffee may also be produced via a cold brew process, in which the water used is not heated beforehand. This preparation typically involves steeping coarsely ground beans in cold water for several hours, then removing the grounds with a filter.

Presentation

Once brewed, coffee may be presented in a variety of ways. Drip-brewed, percolated, or French-pressed/cafetière coffee may be served with no additives or sugar (colloquially known as black) or with milk, cream or both. When served cold, it is called iced coffee.

Espresso-based coffee has a wide variety of possible presentations. In its most basic form, it is served alone as a shot or in the more watered-down style café américano—a shot or two of espresso with hot water. The Americano should be served with the espresso shots on top of the hot water to preserve the crema. Milk can be added in various forms to espresso: steamed milk makes a cafè latte, equal parts steamed milk and milk froth make a cappuccino, and a dollop of hot foamed milk on top creates a caffè macchiato. The use of steamed milk to form patterns such as hearts or maple leaves is referred to as latte art.

Health and Pharmacology

Scientific studies have examined the relationship between coffee consumption and an array of medical conditions. Findings are contradictory as to whether coffee has any specific health benefits, and results are similarly conflicting regarding the negative effects of coffee consumption.

Coffee consumption has been shown to have minimal or no impact, positive or negative, on cancer development; however, researchers involved in an ongoing 22-year study by the Harvard School of Public Health state that 'the overall balance of risks and benefits (of coffee consumption) are on the side of benefits'. Various other studies have shown apparent reductions in the risks of Alzheimer's disease,

Parkinson's disease, heart disease, diabetes mellitus type 2, cirrhosis of the liver and gout. A longitudinal study in 2009 showed that moderate drinkers of coffee (3–5 cups per day) had lower chances of developing dementia, in addition to Alzheimer's disease. It increases the risk of acid reflux and associated diseases. Some health effects of coffee are due to its caffeine content, as the benefits are only observed in those who drink caffeinated coffee while others appear to be due to other components. For example, the antioxidants in coffee prevent free radicals from causing cell damage.

Caffeine is the major coffee constituent which the coffee tolerance or intolerance depends on. In a healthy liver, the majority of caffeine is degraded by the hepatic microsomal enzymatic system. Caffeine is mostly degraded to paraxanthine substances, partially to theobromine and theophylline, and a small amount of unchanged caffeine is excreted by urine. Therefore, the metabolism of caffeine depends on the state of this enzymatic system of the liver. Elderly individuals with a depleted enzymatic system do not tolerate coffee with caffeine. They are recommended to take decaffeinated coffee, and this only if their stomach is healthy, because both decaffeinated coffee and coffee with caffeine cause heartburn. Moderate amounts of coffee (50–100 mg of caffeine or 5–10 g of coffee powder a day) are well tolerated by a majority of elderly people, who enjoy to meet and chat over a cup of coffee. Excessive amounts of coffee, however, can in many individuals cause very unpleasant, exceptionally even life-threatening side effects.

Coffee consumption can lead to iron deficiency anemia in mothers and infants. Coffee also interferes with the absorption of supplemental iron.

American scientist Yaser Dorri has suggested that the smell of coffee can restore appetite and refresh olfactory receptors. He suggests that people can regain their appetite after cooking by smelling coffee beans, and that this method can also be used for research animals. Many high end perfume shops now offer coffee beans to refresh the receptors between perfume tests.

Over 1000 chemicals have been reported in roasted coffee; more than half of those tested are rodent carcinogens. Coffee's negative health effects are often blamed on its caffeine content. Research suggests that drinking caffeinated coffee can cause a temporary increase in the stiffening of arterial walls. Coffee is no longer thought to be a risk factor for coronary heart disease. Some studies suggest that it may have a mixed effect on short-term memory, by improving it when the information to be recalled is related to the current train of thought but making it more difficult to recall unrelated information. About 10 per cent of people with a moderate daily intake (235 mg per day) reported increased depression and anxiety when caffeine was withdrawn, and about 15 per cent of the general population report having stopped caffeine use completely, citing concern about health and unpleasant side effects.

Caffeine Content

Depending on the type of coffee and method of preparation, the caffeine content of a single serving can vary greatly. On average, a single cup of coffee (about 200 ml) or a single shot of espresso (about 30 ml) can be expected to contain the following amounts of caffeine:

1. Drip coffee: 115–175 mg (560–850 mg/l).
2. Espresso: 60 mg (2000 mg/l).
3. Brewed/Pressed: 80–135 mg (390–650 mg/l).
4. Instant: 65–100 mg (310–480 mg/l).
5. Decaf, brewed: 3–4 mg.
6. Decaf, instant: 2–3 mg.

CITRON

The citron is a fragrant fruit with the botanical name *Citrus medica*, which applies to both the Swingle and Tanaka systems. It is a prominent member in the genus *Citrus*, belonging to the Rutaceae or Rue family, sub-family *Aurantioideae*. The designation *Medica* is apparently derived from the similar ancient names *Media*, *Median Apple*, etc. which were influenced by Theophrastus, who believed the citron was native to Media, Persia or Assyria.

Uses

The citron is unlike the more common citrus species like the lemon or orange. While the most popular fruits are peeled in order to consume its pulpy and juicy segments, the citron's pulp is very dry containing only little insipid juice. Moreover, the main content of a citron is the thick white rind, which is very adherent to the segments, and cannot be separated from them easily.

Thus, from ancient through medieval times, the citron was used mainly for medical purposes: to combat against seasickness, pulmonary troubles, intestinal ailments and other disorders. The essential oil of the flavedo was also regarded as an antibiotic. Citron juice with wine was considered an effective antidote to poison.

Today, the citron is used for the fragrance or zest of its outer peel, but the most important part is still the albedo, and is widely employed in the food industry as succade. Today there is a rising market for the citron in the United States for the soluble fibre which is found in its thick albedo.

The citron is also used by Jews for a religious ritual during the Feast of Tabernacles, by whom it is called Etrog. Therefore, the citron was always considered as a Jewish symbol and is found on various Hebrew antiques and archeological findings. In Svenska the citron is named *Suckatcitron*, the citron of Succoth. In Iran, the citron's thick white rind is used to make jam. In South Indian cuisine, especially Tamil cuisine, citron is widely used in pickles and preserves. In Tamil, the unripe fruit is referred to as 'narthangai', which is usually salted and dried to make a preserve. The tender leaves of the plant are often used in conjunction with chili powder and other spices to make a powder, called 'narthellai podi', literally translating to 'powder of citron leaves'. Both narthangai and narthellai podi are usually consumed with thayir sadam.

In Korea, it is used to create Yujacha, a type of Korean tea. The fruit is thinly sliced (peel, pith and pulp) and soaked or cooked in honey or sugar to create a chunky syrup. This syrupy candied fruit is mixed with hot water as a fragrant tea, where the fruit at the bottom of the cup is eaten as well. Often preserved in the syrup for the cold months, Yujacha is served as a source of fruit in winter. It is also popular in Taiwan.

Description and Variation

The citron fruit is usually ovate or oblong, narrowing up till the stylar end. However, the citron's fruit shape is highly variable, due to the big quantity of albedo which forms independently according to the fruits' position on the tree, twig orientation, and many other factors. The pulp is usually acidic, but also sweet and even pulpless varieties are found.

Most citron varieties contain a large number of seeds. The monoembryonic seeds are white coloured; with dark innercoat and red-purplish chalazal spot for the acidic varieties and colourless for the sweet ones. Some citron varieties are also distinct with their persistent style, which is highly appreciated by the Jewish community.

Fingered citron

Citrons could be of very special beauty. The nicer ones are those with medium sized oil bubbles at the outer surface, which are medially distant each to another. Some of them are ribbed and faintly warted in outer surface, adding life and attraction to its beauty. There is also a fingered citron variety called Buddha's Hand. The colour varies from green, when unripe, to a yellow-orange when overripe. The citron would never fall off the tree and could reach 8–10 pounds (4–5 kg) if not picked off timely or even early. However, they should be picked off before the winter as the branches might break, or bend to the ground and may cause numerous fungal diseases for the tree.

Despite the variation among the cultivars, authorities agree that the citron species is a very old one. There is molecular evidence that all other cultivated citrus species only arose by hybridisation among the ancestral types, which are the citron, pummelo, mandarin and papedas.

The citron is believed to be the purest of them all, since it is usually fertilised by self-pollination, it hardly accepts foreign pollen, and is therefore considered to be the male parent rather than a female one.

Tempe bongkrèk

Tempe bongkrèk is a variety of tempeh from Central Java, notably Banyumas regency, that is prepared with coconut. This type of tempeh occasionally gets contaminated with the bacterium *Burkholderia cocovenenans*, and the unwanted organism produces toxins (Bongkrèk acid and toxoflavin) from the coconut, besides killing off the *Rhizopus* fungus due to the antibiotic activity of bongkrèk acid.

Fatalities from contaminated tempe bongkrèk were once common in the area where it was produced. Thus, the sale of tempeh bongkrèk is prohibited by law nowadays; clandestine manufacture continues however due to the superior culinary value. The problem of contamination is not encountered with bean or grain tempeh, which have a different composition of fatty acids that is not favourable for the growth of *B. cocovenenans* but encourages growth of *Rhizopus* instead. When bean or grain tempeh has the proper colour, texture and smell, it is a very strong indication that the product is safe. Tempe bongkrèk which is yellow is always highly toxic due to toxoflavin, but tempe bongkrèk with a normal colouration may still contain lethal amounts of bongkrèk acid.

Tempe Mendoan

A variation of tempeh cooking method, often found in Purwokerto. The origin of the word 'Mendoan' is from Banyumas regional dialect, which means 'to cook instantly in very hot oil', that results in raw and limp cooking.

ORIENTAL FERMENTED FOODS

Most of the oriental fermented foods mentioned below have moulds involved in their preparation. In the starter, termed koji by the Japanese and chou by the Chinese, moulds serve as sources of hydrolytic enzymes, such as amylases to hydrolyse the starch in the grains, proteinases, lipases and many others. For the most part the starters are mixtures of moulds, yeasts and bacteria, but for a few products pure cultures have been employed.

Soya Sauce

The chief oriental fermented food soya sauce is a brown, salty, tangy sauce used on dishes such as chop suey or as a constituent of other sauces. The methods of preparation of the starter and of manufacture of soya sauce have many variations and may result in different types of products.

Starter

The starters (koji or chou) may be mixed cultures carried over from previous lots or pure cultures grown separately. The substrate on which the starter is grown varies, although most often it is an autoclaved mixture of soyabeans, cracked wheat and wheat bran; a mixture of wheat bran and soyabean flour; or rice. This moistened material is inoculated with spores of *Aspergillus oryzae* (*A. soyae*), spread in small boxes or trays, and held at 25° to 30°C until the mould growth on the surfaces of the mash is judged to have attained a maximal content of enzymes (usually after about 3 days).

Miso

There are various fermented soyabean pastes in Asia, including Miso in Japan, Chiang in China, Jiang in Korea, Tauco in Indonesia, Taochieo in Thailand and Taosi in the Philippines.

Miso, nowadays made commercially, is for the most part used as the base for soups, with the remainder being employed in the seasoning of other foods. There are four basic steps, two of which are concurrent, namely the preparation of koji and of soyabeans.

Koji is made on polished rice and represents a source of enzymes that will hydrolyse soyabean components. Waxy components in the outer layers of unpolished rice inhibit the penetration by the Aspergillus mycelium. The rice is washed and soaked overnight at 15°C to a moisture content of 35 per cent. Excess water is removed and the material is steamed for 40–60 minutes. The rice is then spread on large trays and cooled to 35°C. Seed koji is added at 1 gram per kg rice.

The trays in koji rooms tend nowadays to be replaced by rotary drum fermenters that facilitate control of temperature, air circulation and relative humidity, as well as avoiding agglomeration of the rice. The temperature is held to 30°–35°C over a period of 40–50 hours. In this time, the rice becomes covered with white mycelium. Harvesting occurs before the occurrence of sporulation and pigment development. The material has a sweet aroma and flavour.

Salt is added as the material is removed from the fermenter so as to prevent further microbial growth.

The whole soyabeans employed for miso are large and selected for their ability to absorb water and cook rapidly. They are washed before soaking for 18–22 hours. The water is changed regularly especially during summer months in order to prevent bacterial spoilage. The beans swell to almost 2.5 times their volume. After draining, the beans are steamed at 115°C for 20 minutes when they become compressible.

The beans are mixed with salted koji. Starter cultures may be introduced, including osmophilic yeasts and bacteria. The micro flora includes Z. *rouxii*, Torulopsis, Pediococcus, Halophilus and *Streptococcus faecalis*.

The mixture, known as 'green miso', is packed into vats and anaerobic fermentation and ageing are allowed to proceed at 25°–30°C for various periods depending on the character required. Transfer occurs between vessels at least twice. White miso takes 1 week, salty miso 1–3 months and soyabean miso over 1 year. The miso is blended, mashed, pasteurised and packaged.

The characteristics of different miso are listed in Table 16.2. Amino acids represent a significant source of miso flavour, and they are generated from soyabean protein by the action of proteinases (which may be supplemented from exogenous sources). Miso contains 0.6–1.5 per cent acids (lactic, succinic and acetic) as a result of sugar fermentation. Esters produced from the reaction of alcohols with some fatty acids from the soyabean lipid are also important flavour contributors.

Table 16.2. Types of miso.

Base material	Colour	Taste	Time of fermentation/ageing
Rice	Yellow-white	Sweet	5–20 days
Rice	Red-brown	Sweet	5–20 days
Rice	Light yellow	Semi-sweet	5–20 days
Rice	Red-brown	Semi-sweet	3–6 months
Rice	Light yellow	Salty	2–6 months
Rice	Red-brown	Salty	3–12 months
Soyabeans	Dark red-brown	Salty	5–20 months
Barley	Yellow-red-brown	Semi-sweet	1–3 months
Barley	Red-brown	Salty	3–12 months

Natto

Natto is a Japanese product based on fermented whole soyabeans. Generally the product is dark with a pungent and harsh character. It is eaten with boiled rice, as a seasoning or as a table condiment in the way of mustard.

There are three types of natto is Japan. *Itohiki-natto* from Eastern Japan is produced by soaking washed soyabean overnight to double its weight, steaming for 15 minutes and inoculating with *Bacillus natto*, which is a variant of *Bacillus subtilis*. Fermentation is allowed to proceed for 18–20 hours at 40°–45°C. Polymers of glutamic acid are produced which afford a viscous surface and texture in the final product.

Yuki-wari-natto is produced by mixing itohiki-natto with salt and rice koji and leaving at 25°–35°C for 2 weeks.

For *hama-natto*, soyabeans are soaked in water for 4 hours and steamed for 1 hour, before inoculating with koji from roasted wheat and barley. After 20 hours (or when covered with green mycelium of *A. oryzae*), the material is either sundried or dried by warm air to about 12 per cent moisture. The beans are submerged in salt brine containing strips of ginger and allowed to age under pressure for up to 1 year. The surface microflora contributing to enzymolysis and flavour development includes Pediococci, Streptococci and Micrococci.

MOULD FERMENTATIONS

Mould fermentations are an aspect of fermented foods that, up until now, we have mentioned only briefly. Failure to remedy this neglect would give a seriously unbalanced view for, in the East particularly, moulds play a key role in a number of food fermentations.

Tempeh

Tempeh, or tempe in Javanese, is made by a natural culturing and controlled fermentation process that binds soybeans into a cake form. It is especially popular on the island of Java, where it is a staple source of protein. Like tofu, tempeh is made from soyabeans, but tempeh is a whole soybean product with different nutritional characteristics and textural qualities. Tempeh's fermentation process and its retention of the whole bean give it a higher content of protein, dietary fibre and vitamins compared to tofu, as well as firmer texture and stronger flavour. Tofu, by contrast, is said to be more versatile in dishes. Because of its nutritional value, tempeh is used worldwide in vegetarian cuisine; some consider it to be a meat analogue. Even long before Westerners found and realised its rich nutritional value, tempeh was referred to as 'Javanese meat'.

Production

Tempeh begins with whole soyabeans, which are softened by soaking and dehulled, then partly cooked. Speciality tempehs may be made from other types of beans, wheat, or may include a mixture of beans and whole grains.

A mild acidulent, usually vinegar, may be added in order to lower the pH and create a selective environment that favours the growth of the tempeh mold over competitors. A fermentation starter containing the spores of fungus *Rhizopus oligosporus* is mixed in. The beans are spread into a thin layer and are allowed to ferment for 24 to 36 hours at a temperature around 30°C (86°F). In good tempeh, the beans are knitted together by a mat of white mycelia.

Under conditions of lower temperature, or higher ventilation, gray or black patches of spores may form on the surface — this is not harmful, and should not affect the flavour or quality of the tempeh. This sporulation is normal on fully mature tempeh. A mild ammonia smell may accompany good tempeh as it ferments, but it should not be overpowering. In Indonesia, ripe tempeh (two or more days old) is considered a delicacy.

Nutrition

The soya protein in tempeh becomes more digestible as a result of the fermentation process. In particular, the oligosaccharides that are associated with gas and indigestion are greatly reduced by the *Rhizopus* culture. In traditional tempeh making shops, the starter culture often contains beneficial bacteria that produce vitamins such as B12 (though it is uncertain whether this B12 is always present and 'bioavailable'). In western countries, it is more common to use a pure culture containing only *Rhizopus oligosporus* which makes very little B12 and could be missing *Klebsiella pneumoniae* which has been shown to produce significant levels of B12 in tempeh when present.

Preparation

In the kitchen, tempeh is often prepared by cutting it into pieces, soaking in brine or salty sauce, and then frying. Cooked tempeh can be eaten alone, or used in chili, stir frys, soups, salads, sandwiches and stews. Recent popular vegan cookbooks have come up with more creative ways of cooking tempeh, using it as a vegetarian substitution for breakfast meats, such as sausage and bacon. Tempeh has a complex flavour that has been described as nutty, meaty and mushroom-like. Tempeh freezes well, and is now commonly available in many western supermarkets as well as in ethnic markets and health food stores. Tempeh performs well in a cheese grater, after which it may be used in the place of ground beef (as in tacos). When thin sliced and deep fried in oil, tempeh obtains a crispy golden crust while maintaining a soft interior—its sponge-like consistency make it suitable for marinades. Dried tempeh (whether cooked or raw) provides an excellent stew base for backpackers.

Types

Name	Description
tempe bongkrèk	made from or with coconut press cake
tempe bosok (busuk)	rotten tempeh, used in small amounts as a flavouring

tempe gembus	made from okara
tempe gódhóng	tempeh made in banana leaves
tempe goreng	deep-fried tempeh
tempe mendoan	raw-fried tempeh
tempe kedelai	simply tempeh, made from soyabeans
tempe murni	tempeh made in plastic wrap (lit. pure soyabean cake)
tempe oncom	also *onchom*; made from peanut press cake; orange colour; *Neurospora sitophila*

A new form of tempeh based on barley and oats instead of soya was developed by scientists at the Swedish Department of Food Science in 2008. It can be produced in climate regions where it is not possible to grow soyabeans.

Tempeh is a traditional mould-fermented food in Indonesia, though it has also attracted interest in the Netherlands and United States. The most popular type of tempeh is produced from soyabeans and is also known as tempeh kedele. The process of tempeh production is outlined in Fig. 16.3. Whole clean soyabeans are soaked overnight in water to hydrate the beans. A bacterial fermentation occurs during this stage decreasing the pH to 4.5–5.3.

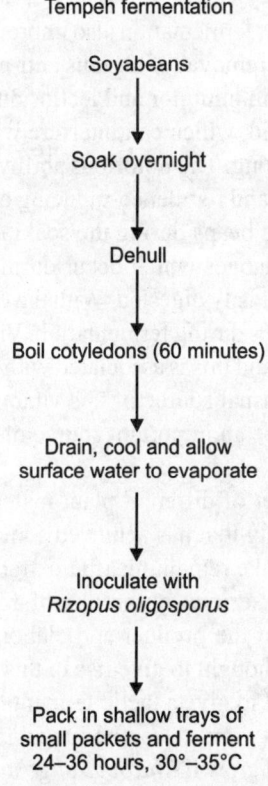

Tempeh fermentation

Soyabeans

Soak overnight

Dehull

Boil cotyledons (60 minutes)

Drain, cool and allow
surface water to evaporate

Inoculate with
Rizopus oligosporus

Pack in shallow trays of
small packets and ferment
24–36 hours, 30°–35°C

Fig. 16.3. Tempeh production.

The hydrated beans are dehulled and the moist cotyledons cooked; a process which pasteurises the substrate, destroys the trypsin inhibitor and lectins contained in the bean and releases some of the nutrients required for fungal growth. After cooking, the beans are drained and may be pressed lightly to remove excess moisture before spreading into shallow bamboo trays and allowing to cool. Starter culture is added either by mixing some tempeh in with the cooked soyabeans prior to packing in the trays or by sprinkling a spore inoculum, prepared by extended incubation of a piece of tempeh, on to the beans.

The fermentation is invariably a mixed culture of moulds, yeasts and bacteria but the most important component appears to be *Rhizopus oligosporus,* although other *Rhizopus* and *Mucor* species are often isolated. Over two days incubation at ambient temperature (30°–35°C), the mycelium develops throughout the mass of beans knitting it together. During fermentation the pH rises to around 7, fungal proteases increase the free amino acid content of the product and lipases hydrolyse over a third of the neutral fat present to free fatty acids.

Unlike many fermented foods, tempeh production is not a means of improving the shelf-life of its raw material which is in any case inherently quite stable. Tempeh contains antioxidants which retard the development of rancidity but will keep for only one to two days as sporulation of the mould discolours the product and a rich ammoniacal odour develops as proteolysis proceeds.

Tempeh production does however improve the acceptability of an otherwise rather unappealing food. Fresh tempeh has a pleasant nutty odour and flavour and can be consumed in a variety of ways, usually after frying in oil.

In addition to improving acceptability, fermentation also improves the nutritional quality of soyabeans. In part this stems from the reduction or removal of various anti-nutritional factors at different stages in the processing. Destruction of the trypsin inhibitor and lectins during cooking of the beans has already been mentioned and levels of phytic acid, which can interfere with mineral nutrition, are also reduced by about a third in the course of processing. The notorious ability of beans to produce flatulence is also regarded as an anti-nutritional property and flatulence-inducing oligosaccharides such as stachyose and raffinose are partially leached out of the beans during the soaking stage.

Despite the extensive proteolytic changes which occur during fermentation, studies have failed to show that the protein in tempeh is more easily digested. With the exception of thiamine which decreases, other vitamins increase to varying degrees during fermentation. Vitamin B_{12}, the anti-pernicious anaemia factor, shows the most marked increase and this is associated with the growth of the bacterium *Klebsiella pneumoniae* during fermentation. The usual source of this vitamin in the diet is animal products and it has been suggested that tempeh could be an important source of B_{12} for people subsisting on a largely vegetarian diet.

Tempeh can be made from a number of different plant materials including other legumes, cereals and agricultural by-products. One variety that has achieved some notoriety is tempeh bongkrek which is made in central Java using the presscake remaining after extraction of coconut oil. Tempeh bongkrek has been associated with occasional serious outbreaks of food poisoning due to the bacterium *Burkholderia cocovenenans* growing in the product and elaborating the toxins bongkrekic acid and toxoflavin (Fig. 16.4). Two factors are thought to give rise to this problem. Reduction or omission of an initial soaking of the presscake may fail to give a lactic fermentation sufficient to reduce the pH below 6, a level at which the bacterium cannot grow. Also, the fungal inoculum may be too small since it has been shown that *B. cocovenenans* cannot grow if *Rhizopus oligosporus* has more than a tenfold numerical superiority (estimated by plate counts). Ontjom is a tempeh-like product produced in Indonesia from peanut presscake which normally has a fruity/mincemeat character. It can be produced using the tempeh mould but *Neurospora intermedia* is also often used. This mould has strong α-galactosidase activity which can further contribute to the reduction of flatulence-inducing oligosaccharides.

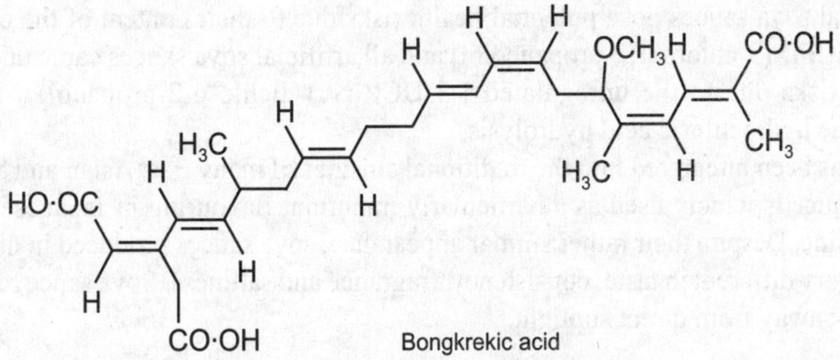

Fig. 16.4. Toxoflavin and bongkrekic acid.

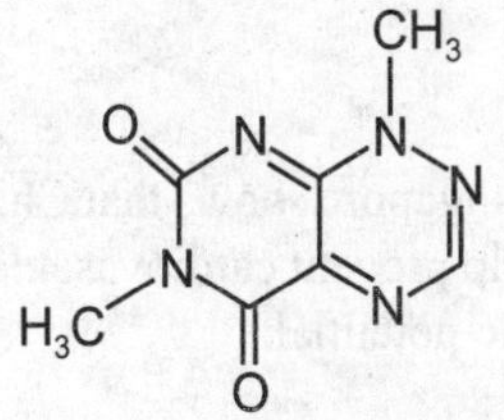

SOYA SAUCE

Soya sauce, soya sauce (Commonwealth) is a fermented sauce made from soyabeans (soyabeans), roasted grain, water and salt. Soya sauce was invented in China, where it has been used as a condiment for close to 2500 years. In its various forms, it is widely used in East and Southeast Asian cuisines and increasingly appears in Western cuisine and prepared foods.

Soya sauce is made from soyabeans.

Authentic soya sauces are made by mixing the grain and/or soyabeans with yeast or *koji* the mould *Aspergillus oryzae* or *A. sojae*) and other related micro-organisms. Traditionally soya sauces were fermented under natural conditions, such as in giant urns and under the sun, which was believed to contribute to additional flavours. Today, most of the commercially-produced counterparts are instead fermented under machine-controlled environments.

Although there are many types of soya sauce, all are salty and 'earthy'-tasting brownish liquids used to season food while cooking or at the table. Soya sauce has a distinct basic taste called umami by the Japanese (literally 'delicious taste'). Umami was first identified as a basic taste in 1908 by Kikunae Ikeda of the Tokyo Imperial University. The free glutamates which naturally occur in soya sauce are what give it this taste quality.

Artificially Hydrolysed

Many cheaper brands of soya sauces are made from hydrolysed soya protein instead of brewed from natural bacterial and fungal cultures. These soya sauces do not have the natural colour of authentic soya sauces and are typically coloured with caramel colouring, and are popular in Southeast Asia and China, and are exported to Asian markets around the globe. They are derogatorily called Chemical Soya Sauce, but despite this name are the most widely used type because they are cheap. Similar products are also sold as 'liquid aminos' in the US and Canada.

Some artificial soya sauces pose potential health risks due to their content of the chloropropanols carcinogens 3-MCPD (3-chloro-1,2-propanediol) and all artificial soya sauces came under scrutiny for possible health risks due to the unregulated 1,3-DCP (1,3-dichloro-2-propanol) which are minor by-products of the hydrochloric acid hydrolysis.

Soya sauce has been integrated into the traditional cuisines of many East Asian and Southeast Asian cultures. Soya sauce is widely used as a particularly important flavouring in Japanese, Thai, Korean, and Chinese cuisine. Despite their rather similar appearance, soya sauces produced in different cultures and regions are very different in taste, consistency, fragrance and saltiness. Soya sauce retains its quality longer when kept away from direct sunlight.

Health

Positive

A study by National University of Singapore shows that Chinese dark soya sauce contains 10 times the antioxidants of red wine, and can help prevent cardiovascular diseases. Soya sauce is rich in lactic acid bacteria and of excellent anti-allergic potential.

Negative

Soya sauce does not contain a level of the beneficial isoflavones associated with other soya products such as tofu or edamame. It can also be very salty, having a salt content of between 17–19 per cent so it may not be a suitable condiment for people on a low sodium diet. Low-sodium soya sauces are produced, but it is impossible to make soya sauce without using some quantity of salt.

Carcinogens in artificial soya sauces

In 2001 the United Kingdom Food Standards Agency found in tests of various low-grade soya sauces (those made from hydrolysed soya protein, rather than being naturally fermented) that some 22 per cent of samples contained a chemical called 3-MCPD (3-monochloropropane-1,2-diol) at levels considerably higher than those deemed safe by the European Union. About two-thirds of these samples also contained a second chemical called 1,3-DCP (1,3-dichloropropane-2-ol) which experts advise should not be present at any levels in food. Both chemicals have the potential to cause cancer and the Agency recommended that the affected products be withdrawn from shelves and avoided. Furthermore, the latter unregulated chemical can cause genetic damage to be passed on to offspring who never consumed the sauces.

Britain's Food Standards Agency (FSA) issued a Public Health Advice leaflet in June 2001 to warn against a small number of soya sauce products having been shown to contain high levels of potentially cancer-causing chemicals.

In Vietnam, 3-MCPD was found in toxic levels (In 2004, the HCM City Institute of Hygiene and Public Health found 33 of 41 sample of soya sauce with high rates of 3-MCPD, including six samples with up to 11,000 to 18,000 times more 3-MCPD than permitted, an increase over 23 to 5644 times in 2001) in soya sauces there in 2007, along with formaldehyde in the national dish Pho, and banned pesticides in vegetables and fruits. In March 2008, some Australian soya sauces were found to contain carcinogens and consumers were advised to avoid consumption.

Soya sauce and allergies

Most varieties of soya sauce also contain wheat. Individuals with a wheat allergy, Celiac disease, or a gluten intolerance should avoid this condiment and dishes seasoned with soya sauce.

A healthy organic alternative to soya sauce is a soya-based product which contains no added salt, vegetable protein from soyabeans and purified water. Such products may be labelled 'liquid aminos'.

Soya Sauce and Rice Wine

Though they are markedly different in character, rice wine and soya sauce share sufficient common features in their production to warrant discussing them together. Both are representatives of products which involve mould activity in a two-stage fermentation process. The mould starter used is often known as koji, a Japanese term derived from the Chinese character for mouldy grains. In the koji stage, aerobic conditions allow moulds to grow on the substrate producing a range of hydrolytic enzymes necessary for utilising the macromolecular material present. In the case of soya sauce (Fig. 16.5), soaked and cooked soyabeans are mixed with roasted cracked wheat in about equal proportions and inoculated with tane koji or seed koji. This has been previously grown-up on a similar mixture of substrates and contains a mixture of strains of *Aspergillus oryzae*. The moulds are then allowed to grow throughout the mass of material spread as layers about 5 cm deep for 2–3 days at 25°–30°C.

In the second, mash or *moromi* stage, conditions are made anaerobic so no further mould growth can occur. In soya sauce production, this is achieved by mixing the *koji* with an approximately equal volume of brine to give a final salt concentration of 17–20 per cent. Although the moulds can no longer grow, the activity of a whole battery of hydrolytic enzymes continues breaking down proteins, polysaccharides and nucleic acids to produce a liquid rich in soluble nutrients. Yeasts and lactic acid bacteria dominate the microflora producing a number of flavour components and converting roughly half of the soluble sugars to lactic acid and ethanol so that the final soya sauce normally has a pH of 4.5–4.9 and ethanol and lactic acid contents of 2–3 per cent and 1 per cent respectively. The halophilic lactic acid bacterium *Tetragenococcus halophilus* (formerly *Pediococcus halophilus*) and the yeasts *Zygosaccharomyces rauxii* and *Torulopsis* have been identified as being important in this stage.

The *moromi* stage can be quite protracted, lasting up to a year or more, at the end of which the mash is pressed to remove the solid residues which may then be mixed with brine to undergo a second fermentation and produce a lower grade product. The liquid is pasteurised and filtered, possibly after a period of maturation, and then bottled. Rather similar steps are involved in the production of soyabean pastes known as *miso* in Japan and *chiang* in China. These include up to 40 per cent of a grain such as rice or barley, use dry salt rather than brine and employ a shorter fermentation so the product has the consistency of a paste rather than a liquid.

In the brewing of the Japanese rice wine, sake, a koji prepared on steamed rice is used. Although the mould used is the same species as in soya sauce production, *Aspergillus oryzae,* the strains used in *sake* production are particularly noted for their ability to produce amylolytic enzymes. In the *moromi* stage, water is added along with strains of the yeast *Saccharomyces cerevisiae* specially adapted to the *sake* fermentation. During this stage amylolytic enzymes from the mould continue to break down the starch in the rice to produce fermentable sugars which are then converted to ethanol by the yeast. The high alcohol content of around 20 per cent v/v achieved in such fermentations is thought to be due to a combination of factors.

Particularly important is the slow rate of fermentation which results from the relatively low fermentation temperature (13°–18°C) and the slow release of fermentable sugars. The high solids content in the *moromi* is also thought to help in keeping the yeast in suspension and active at such high alcohol concentrations. At the end of fermentation which typically lasts for three weeks, the product is settled, filtered and blended before being pasteurised and bottled.

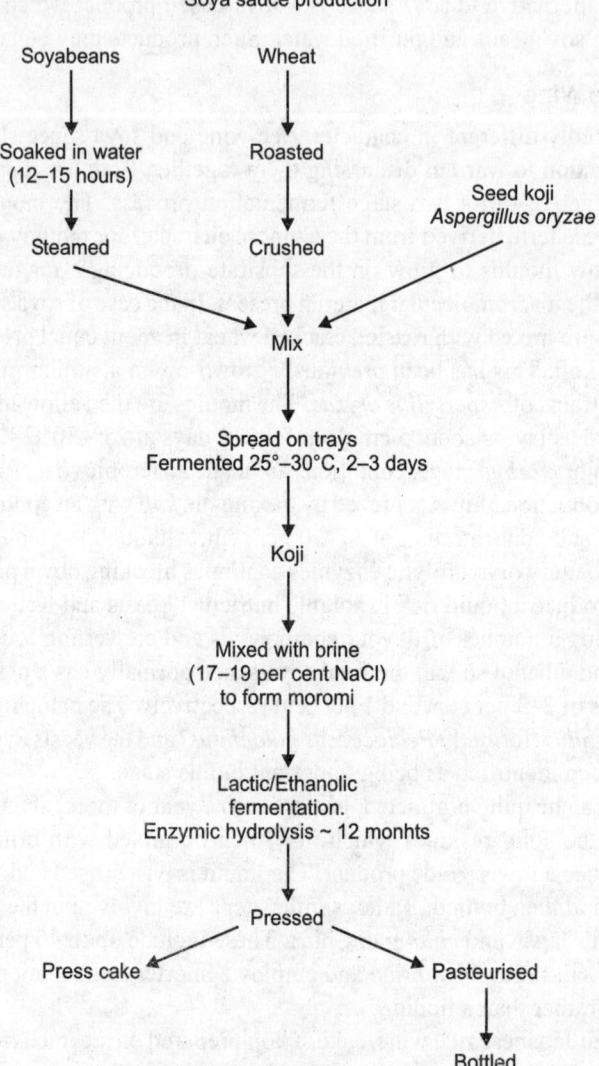

Soya sauce production

Fig. 16.5. Soya sauce production.

A number of other rice-based mould starters are used in the countries of East and Southeast Asia to fulfil a similar role to koji (Table 16.3). They are used to produce sweetened rice products which can be consumed fresh or added to other products or can be used as a base for the production of rice wine and rice vinegar.

Table 16.3. Amylolytic mould preparations.

koji	Japan
look pang	Thailand
ang-kak	Philippines

(Contd ...)

ragi-tapai	Malaysia/Indonesia
nuruk	Korea
peh-yueh	China
bakhar	India

The microbiological composition of these generally differs from that of koji and comprises primarily *Rhizopus* and *Mucor* species and amylolytic yeasts. Some of the compounds that contribute to the flavour of soya sauce are given in Table 16.4.

Table 16.4. Some of the compounds that contribute to the flavour of soya sauce.

Acetaldehyde	*Furfural*
Acetic acid	Furfuryl acetate
Acetoin	Furfuryl alcohol
Acetone	Guaiacol
2-Acetyl furan	2,3-Hexanedione
2-Acetyl pyrrole	2-Hexanone
Benzaldehyde	4-Hydroxy-2-ethyl-5-methyl-3(2H)-furanone
Benzoic acid	4-Hydroxy-5-ethyl-2-methyl-3(2H)-furanone
Benzyl alcohol	4-Hydroxy-5-methyl-3(2H)-furanone
Borneol	Maltol
Bornyl acetate	Methional
Butanoic acid	3-Methylbutanal
1-Butanol	3-Methylbutanoic acid
Diethyl succinate	3-Methyl-1-butanol
2,6-Dimethoxyphenol	3-Methylbutyl acetate
2,3-Dimethylpyrazine	2-Methylpropanal
2,6-Dimethylpyrazine	2-Methylpropanoic acid
Ethanol	2-Methyl-1-propanol
Ethyl acetate	3-Methylpyrazine 3-methyl-3-tetrahydrofuranone
Ethyl benzoate	4-Pentanolide
3-Ethyl-2,5-dimethylpyrazin	Phenylacetaldehyde
4-Ethylguaiacol	2-Phenylethanol
Ethyl lactate	2-Phenylethylacetate
2-Ethyl-6-methylpyrazine	Propanal
Ethyl myristate	2-Propanol
4-Ethylphenol	
Ethyl phenylacetate	

MYCOPROTEIN

Although less high profile than it was 25–30 years ago, there is still interest in the cultivation of microbes specifically as foodstuffs, rather than as agents in the production of other products. The term 'single cell protein' was coined to describe these products, which were based on diverse bacteria and yeasts, growing on a range of carbon sources (Table 16.5).

Table 16.5. Some single cell protein processes.

Substrate	Organism
Cellulose	*Alcaligenes, Cellulomonas*
Ethanol	*Candida utilis, Acinetobacter calcoaceticus*
Glucose	*Fusarium venenatum*
Hydrocarbons	*Candida tropicalis, Yarrowia lipolytica*
Methane	*Methylococcus capsulatus*
Methanol	*Methylomonas clara, Methylophilus methylotrophus, Pichia pastoris*
Molasses	*Candida utilis*
Starch	*Saccharomyces cerevisiae, Saccharomycopsis fibuligeral, Candida utilis*
Sucrose	*Candida utilis*
Sulphite waste liquor	*Candida utilis*
Whey	*Candida intermedia, Candida krusei, Candida pintolepesii, Candida utilis, Kluyveromyces lactis, Kluyveromyces marxianus, Lactobacillus bulgaricus*

Only one product has survived in substantial quantity to this day, Quorn™. It is a joint venture between two major British companies and has been marketed as a meat substitute since 1984.

The organism, *Fusarium venenatum*, is grown at 30°C in rigorously sterile conditions in air lift (pressure cycle) fermenters. The liquid medium flows continuously into the fermenter (the residence time is 5–6 hours), and the conditions are highly aerobic, with the compressed air serving both as nutrient and as the vehicle for agitation.

Carbon source is glucose produced by the hydrolysis of corn starch, and ammonium salts are included as the nitrogen source. The pH is maintained at 4.5–7.0 and iron, manganese, potassium, calcium, magnesium, cobalt, copper and biotin are added. Unlike the other products, the cells themselves are really all that impact on the properties of the finished product in the present instance. The medium composition is relevant only insofar as it impacts the yield and properties of the organism *per se* and has no role to play, for instance, in determining final product flavour or appearance.

The continuous fermentation system will be re-established every 1000 hours. After fermentation, the cell suspension is heat-shocked to reduce the extent of development of RNA degradation products, the presence of which will otherwise elevate the risk of gout in those partaking of the foodstuff. Heating is at 64°C to eliminate the enzymes that convert RNA to nucleotides.

The cell suspension is harvested by centrifugation and the hyphae mixed with binding agents and flavourants and heated to cause a gelling of the binder and a linking of the hyphae. The product is some 45 per cent protein, 14 per cent fat and 26 per cent fibre by dry weight. It is 11 per cent protein, 3 per cent available carbohydrate, 6 per cent fibre, 3 per cent fat, 2 per cent ash and 75 per cent water by wet weight. It is sold in a variety of commercial forms, for example, pieces and minced.

Nutritionally, it stacks up very well against other foods. It possesses a complete complement of essential amino acids and is a particularly good source of threonine, which tends to be the limiting amino acids in meat. Quorn has little saturated fat and has a favourable ratio of polyunsaturated to saturated fatty acids when compared with beef and chicken. It is devoid of cholesterol and is low in calories. It possesses significant levels of fibre in the form of chitin and β-glucan from the Fusarium cell walls. It contains the breadth of B vitamins, with the exception of B_{12}. Finally it is devoid of phytic acid, and so tends not to interfere with metal uptake from the diet.

Chapter 17

Miscellaneous Foods

INTRODUCTION

In this chapter: fatty foods, salad dressings, essential oils, bottled soft drinks, spices and other condiments, salt and nutmeats are discussed.

Food products compounded from combinations of the different groups of foods also would combine their microbial contents, and the new product may furnish a good culture medium for micro-organisms that previously had little chance to grow. Thus, yeasts from sugar added to bottled soft drinks may spoil the product. The bottlers of carbonated beverages have bacteriological standards for sugar: not over 200 mesophilic bacteria per 10 grams and not more than 10 yeasts or moulds. The water and flavouring materials also are potential sources of contamination. Spices and other condiments added to foods may be important sources of micro-organisms, although spices may be treated with propylene oxide gas or may be irradiated to give them a low microbial content. Micro-organisms are added to salad dressings by ingredients such as spices, condiments, eggs and pickles. Salt (sodium chloride), especially solar salt, may add halophilic and salt-tolerant bacteria to salted fish and other salted or brined products.

FATTY FOODS

Fats and Oils

Vegetable fats and oils are lipid materials derived from plants. Physically, oils are liquid at room temperature, and fats are solid. Chemically, both fats and oils are composed of triglycerides, as contrasted with waxes which lack glycerine in their structure. Although many different parts of plants may yield oil, in commercial practice, oil is extracted primarily from seeds.

The melting temperature distinction between oils and fats is imprecise, since definitions of room temperature vary, and typically natural oils have a melting range instead of a single melting point.

Vegetable fats and oils may be edible or inedible. Examples of inedible vegetable fats and oils include processed linseed oil, tung oil and castor oil used in lubricants, paints, cosmetics, pharmaceuticals and other industrial purposes. Although thought of as esters of glycerine and a varying blend of fatty acids, fats and oils also typically contain free fatty acids, monoglycerides and diglycerides.

Many vegetable oils are consumed directly or used directly as ingredients in food — a role that they share with some animal fats, including butter and ghee. The oils serve a number of purposes in this role:

1. Shortening: to give pastry a crumbly texture.
2. Texture: oils can serve to make other ingredients stick together less.

3. Flavour: while less-flavourful oils command premium prices, oils such as olive oil or almond oil may be chosen specifically for the flavour they impart.

4. Flavour base: oils can also 'carry' flavours of other ingredients, since many flavours are present in chemicals that are soluble in oil.

Secondly, oils can be heated, and used to cook other foods. Oils that are suitable for this purpose must have a high flash point. Such oils include the major cooking oils—canola, sunflower, safflower, peanut, etc. Some oils, including rice bran oil, are particularly valued in Asian cultures for high temperature cooking, because of their unusually high flash point.

Unsaturated vegetable fats and oils can be transformed through partial or complete hydrogenation into fats and oils of higher melting point. The hydrogenation process involves 'sparging' the oil at high temperature and pressure with hydrogen in the presence of a catalyst, typically a powdered nickel compound. As each double-bond is broken, two hydrogen atoms each form single bonds with the two carbon atoms. The elimination of double-bonds by adding hydrogen atoms is called saturation; as the degree of saturation increases, the oil progresses towards being fully hydrogenated. An oil may be hydrogenated to increase resistance to rancidity (oxidation) or to change its physical characteristics. As the degree of saturation increases, the oil's viscosity and melting point increase.

The use of hydrogenated oils in foods has never been completely satisfactory. Because the centre arm of the triglyceride is shielded somewhat by the end fatty acids, most of the hydrogenation occurs on the end fatty acids. This makes the resulting fat more brittle. A margarine made from naturally more saturated oils will be more plastic (more 'spreadable') than a margarine made from, say, hydrogenated soya oil. In addition, partial hydrogenation results in the formation of large amounts trans fats in the oil mixture, which, since the 1970s, have increasingly been viewed as unhealthy.

Vegetable-based oils, like castor oil, have been used as medicine and as lubricants for a long time. Castor oil has numerous industrial uses, primarily due to the presence of hydroxyl groups on the fatty acid chains. Castor oil and other vegetable oils which have been chemically modified to contain hydroxyl groups, are becoming increasingly important in the production of polyurethane plastic for many applications. These modified vegetable oils are known as natural oil polyols.

Extraction

The 'modern' way of processing vegetable oil is by chemical extraction, using solvent extracts, which produces higher yields and is quicker and less expensive. The most common solvent is petroleum-derived hexane. This technique is used for most of the 'newer' industrial oils such as soyabean and corn oils. Another way is physical extraction, which does not use solvent extracts. It is made the 'traditional' way using several different types of mechanical extraction. This method is typically used to produce the more traditional oils (e.g. olive), and it is preferred by most 'health-food' customers in the USA and in Europe. Expeller-pressed extraction is one type, and there are two other types that are both oil presses: the screw press and the ram press. Oil seed presses are commonly used in developing countries, among people for whom other extraction methods would be prohibitively expensive.

The fatty parts of foods, the foods made up chiefly of fats and oils, and the fats and oils themselves are subject more often to chemical than to microbial spoilage. Besides the fatty glycerides, natural fats and oils usually contain small amounts of fatty acids, glycerol or other liquid alcohols, sterols, hydrocarbons, proteins and other nitrogenous compounds, phosphatides and carotenoid pigments. The chief types of spoilage result from hydrolysis, oxidation or combinations of the two processes. The terms applied to the different types of spoilage often are used rather loosely, although when applied to the deterioration of a specific kind of fat or oil they may have a definite meaning. The term rancidity sometimes is used for the result of any change in fats or oils that is accompanied by undesirable flavours, regardless of the cause. The spoilage due to oxidation, chemical or microbial, is termed oxidative rancidity, as distinguished from changes resulting from hydrolysis, by lipases originally present or by those from micro-organisms, causing hydrolytic rancidity. Extensive oxidation, usually following hydrolysis and the release of fatty acids, can result in ketonic rancidity. Flavour reversion is defined as the appearance of objectionable flavours from less oxidation than is needed to produce rancidity. Oils that contain linolenic acid, fish oils and vegetable oils, for example, are subject to flavour reversion.

The oxidation of fats and oils may be catalysed by various metals and rays and by moisture as well as by micro-organisms; such oxidation is prevented or delayed by natural or added antioxidants. Hydrolysis by lipases results in fatty acids and glycerol or other alcohols. Fats subjected to either or both of these types of changes may contain fatty oxy and hydroxy acids, glycerol and other alcohols, aldehydes, ketones and lactones; in the presence of lecithin, they may include trimethylamine, with its fishy odour.

Butterfat and meat fats become 'tallowy' as the result of oxidation, but butterfat is called rancid when only hydrolysis to fatty acids and glycerol has taken place.

Some of the pigments produced by micro-organisms are fat-soluble and, therefore, can diffuse into fat, producing discolourations ranging through yellow, red, purple and brown. Best known is the 'stamping-ink' discolouration of meat fat that Jenson and others have shown to be caused by yellow pigmented micrococci and bacilli. The fat-soluble pigment is an O-R indicator that changes from yellow to green to blue and finally to purple as the fat becomes more oxidised by the peroxides formed by the bacteria. Yellow, pink and fed fat-soluble pigments may be produced by various bacteria, yeasts and moulds.

Bacteriostatic and bactericidal properties have been claimed for many of the fixed vegetable and animal oils, but most of them, like the fats, can be hydrolysed and oxidised by micro-organisms. These fatty materials ordinarily are very low in moisture, a condition that favours moulds more than other micro-organisms. Moulds cause both oxidative and hydrolytic decomposition that results in rancidity. Bacteria causing rancidity of butter cause a similar defect in olive oil. Among the bacteria that can decompose fats are species of *Pseudomonas, Micrococcus, Bacillus, Serratia, Achromobacter* and *Proteus*; and among the moulds, species of *Geotrichum, Penicillium, Aspergillus, Cladosporium* and *Monilia*. Some yeasts, especially film yeasts, are lipolytic. Copra and cocoa butter may be spoiled by moulds.

Negative health effects

A high consumption of omega-6 polyunsaturated fatty acids (PUFAs), which are found in most types of vegetable oil (e.g. soyabean oil, corn oil — the most consumed in USA, sunflower oil, etc.), may increase the likelihood that postmenopausal women will develop breast cancer. Similar effect was observed on prostate cancer in mice. Other analysis suggested an inverse association between total polyunsaturated fatty acids and breast cancer risk.

ESSENTIAL OILS

An essential oil is a concentrated, hydrophobic liquid containing volatile aroma compounds from plants. They are also known as volatile or ethereal oils, or simply as the 'oil of' the plant material from which they were extracted, such as oil of clove. An oil is 'essential' in the sense that it carries a distinctive scent or essence, of the plant. Essential oils do not as a group need to have any specific chemical properties in common, beyond conveying characteristic fragrances. They are not to be confused with essential fatty acids. Essential oils are generally extracted by distillation. Other processes include expression or solvent extraction. They are used in perfumes, cosmetics and bath products, for flavouring food and drink, and for scenting incense and household cleaning products.

Various essential oils have been used medicinally at different periods in history. Medical applications proposed by those who sell medicinal oils range from skin treatments to remedies for cancer, and are often based on historical use of these oils for these purposes. Such claims are now subject to regulation in most countries, and have grown correspondingly more vague, to stay within these regulations.

Interest in essential oils has revived in recent decades, with the popularity of aromatherapy, a branch of alternative medicine which claims that the specific aromas carried by essential oils have curative effects. Oils are volatilised or diluted in a carrier oil and used in massage, diffused in the air by a nebuliser or by heating over a candle flame, or burned as incense, for example.

Essential oils or volatile oils are products obtained from the plant kingdom in which the odouriferous and flavouring characteristics are concentrated. These present no spoilage problems but on the contrary may have some preservative effect as ingredients of foods, e.g. mustard, cinnamon, garlic and onion oils. Most of them do not affect the heat resistance of micro-organisms.

Salad Dressings

Salad is any of a wide variety of dishes including: green salads; vegetable salads; salads of pasta, legumes, or grains; mixed salads incorporating meat, poultry or seafood; and fruit salads. They include a mixture of cold or hot foods, often including vegetables and/or fruits. Green salads include leaf lettuce and vegetables with a dressing. Other salads are based on pasta, noodles, jelly or even Cool Whip. Most salads are traditionally served cold, although some, such as German potato salad, are served hot.

The word 'salad' comes from the French salad of the same meaning, which in turn is from the Latin salata, 'salty', from sal, 'salt'. Vegetables seasoned with brine was a popular Roman dish.

Green salads including leaf lettuces are generally served with a dressing, as well as various toppings such as nuts or croutons, and sometimes with the addition of meat, fish, pasta, cheese, eggs or whole grains. Salad is often served as an appetiser before a larger meal, but can also be a side dish, or a main course. The 'green salad' or 'garden salad' is most often composed of leafy vegetables such as lettuce varieties, spinach or rocket (arugula). Due to their low calorie density, green salads are a common diet food. The salad leaves are cut or torn into bite-sized fragments and tossed together (called a tossed salad), or may be placed in a predetermined arrangement.

Other common vegetable additions in a green salad include cucumbers, peppers, mushrooms, onions, spring onions, red onions, avocado, carrots, celery and radishes. Other ingredients such as tomatoes, pasta, olive, hard boiled egg, artichoke hearts, heart of palm, roasted red bell peppers, cooked potatoes, rice, sweet corn, green beans, black beans, croutons, cheeses, meat (e.g. bacon, chicken), or fish (e.g. tuna, shrimp) are sometimes added to salads.

The concept of salad dressing varies across cultures. There are many commonly used salad dressings in North America. Traditional dressings in southern Europe are vinaigrettes, while mayonnaise is predominant in eastern European countries and Russia. In Denmark dressings are often based on crème fraîche. In China, where Western salad is a recent adoption from Western cuisine, the term salad dressing refers to mayonnaise or mayonnaise-based dressings. Many light edible oils are used as salad dressings, including olive oil, corn oil, soyabean oil, safflower oil, etc.

Salad dressings contain oil, which may become oxidised or hydrolysed, and enough moisture to permit microbial growth. For the most part, however, their acidity (about pH 3 to 4) is too great for most bacteria but favourable for yeasts or moulds. Egg or egg products, pickles, relish, pimientos, sugar, starch, gums, gelatine, spices and other ingredients may add micro-organisms, sometimes in appreciable numbers, and may make the dressings better media for microbial growth. The three types of spoilage of mayonnaise and similar dressings are: (i) separation of the oil or water from the emulsion, (ii) oxidation and hydrolysis of the oils by chemical or biological action, and (iii) growth of micro-organisms to produce gas, off-flavours, or other defects. Darkening often takes place.

The decomposition of salad dressings and related products can be caused by bacteria, yeasts or moulds. The acidity, coupled with the sugar content about 4.5 per cent on the average in the water phase of mayonnaise, is most favourable to yeasts, which have been reported to cause gassiness. Species of *Zygosaccharomyces* and *Saccharomyces* have spoiled mayonnaise, salad dressing and French dressing. Bacteria would have to be acid-tolerant to spoil most types of dressing. Therefore, it is not unexpected to learn of a heterofermentative lactobacillus resembling *Lactobacillus brevis* causing gas in a salad dressing. More surprising is the report of species of *Bacillus*, e.g. *B. subtilis* and *B. megaterium*, as organisms causing gas, rancidity and separation, since they are not acid-tolerant. Yeasts growing with *B. megaterium* could account for the gas. Darkening and separation of thousand Island dressing with a pH of 4.2 to 4.4 by *B. vulgatus* from the pepper and paprika have been reported. Moulds can grow on salad dressings if air is available and are favoured by the addition of starch or pectin to the dressing.

Salad recipes

Salad recipes are: (i) balsamic vinegar, (ii) caesar dressing, (iii) blue cheese, (iv) louis dressing, (v) ranch dressing, (vi) Russian dressing, (vii) honey dijon, (viii) thousand Island dressing, (ix) French dressing, (x) Italian dressing, (xi) vinaigrette, (xii) wafu dressing, (xiii) tahini, and (xiv) hummus.

Toppings and garnishes

Popular salad garnishes are anchovies, bacon bits (real or imitation), garden beet, bell peppers, shredded carrots, diced celery, cress, croutons, sliced cucumber, parsley, sliced mushrooms, sliced red onion, radish, sunflower seeds (shelled), real or artificial crab meat (surimi) and cherry tomatoes. Various cheeses, nuts, berries, seeds and other ingredients can also be added to green salads. Blue cheese, parmesan cheese and feta cheese are often used. Colour considerations are sometimes highlighted by using edible flowers, red radishes and other colourful ingredients.

Entree salads

Entree salads or 'dinner salads' may contain grilled or fried chicken pieces, seafood such as grilled or fried shrimp or a fish steak such as tuna, mahi-mahi or salmon. Sliced steak, such as sirloin or skirt, can be placed upon the salad. Caesar salad, Chef salad, Cobb salad, Greek salad and Michigan salad are types of dinner salad.

Barbecue and picnic salads

Pasta salads, potato salads and egg salads are often served at barbecues and picnics. These salads can be made ahead of time and refrigerated.

Fruit salads

Fruit salads are made of fruit and include the fruit cocktail that can be made fresh or from canned fruit.

Dessert salads

Dessert salads are made with jello and or cool whip and often include no leafy greens. These salads include jello salad, pistachio salad and ambrosia. There are also regional versions such as snickers salad, glorified rice and cookie salad popular in parts the Midwestern United States and Minnesota.

BOTTLED BEVERAGES

A drink, or beverage, is a liquid specifically prepared for human consumption. In addition to basic needs, beverages form part of the culture of human society.

Despite the fact that most beverages, including juice, soft drinks and carbonated drinks, have some form of water in them; water itself is often not classified as a beverage, and the word beverage has been recurrently defined as not referring to water.

Essential to the survival of all organisms, water has historically been an important and life-sustaining drink to humans. Excluding fat, water composes approximately 70 per cent of the human body by mass. It is a crucial component of metabolic processes and serves as a solvent for many bodily solutes. Health authorities have historically suggested at least eight glasses, eight fluid ounces each, of water per day (64 fluid ounces or 1.89 litres), and the British dietetic association recommends 1.8 litres. The United States environmental protection agency has determined that the average adult actually ingests 2.0 litres per day. Distilled (pure) water is rarely found in nature. Spring water, a natural resource from which much bottled water comes, is generally imbued with minerals. Tap water, delivered by domestic water systems in developed nations, refers to water piped to homes through a tap. All of these forms of water are commonly drunk, often purified through filtration.

Alcoholic beverages: An alcoholic beverage is a drink that contains ethanol, commonly known as alcohol (although in chemistry the definition of 'alcohol' includes many other compounds). Beer has been a part of human culture for 8000 years.

Non-alcoholic beverages: Non-alcoholic beverages are drinks that would normally contain alcohol, such as beer and wine but are made with less than 0.5 per cent alcohol by volume. The category includes drinks that have undergone an alcohol removal process such as non-alcoholic beers and dealcoholised wines.

Soft drinks: The name 'soft drink' specifies a lack of alcohol by way of contrast to the term 'hard drink' and the term 'drink', the latter of which is nominally neutral but often carries connotations of alcoholic content. Beverages like colas, sparkling water, iced tea, lemonade, squash and fruit punch are among the most common types of soft drinks, while hot chocolate, hot tea, coffee, milk, tap water, alcohol and milkshakes do not fall into this classification. Many carbonated soft drinks are optionally available in versions sweetened with sugars or with non-caloric sweeteners.

The ease with which the nonalcoholic beverages spoil and the type of spoilage depend on the composition of the soft drink. Carbonation is inhibitory or even germicidal to some micro-organisms, and the acidity resulting from carbonation and the addition of acids, e.g. citric, lactic, phosphoric, tartaric and malic, inhibits the growth of organisms not tolerant to acidity. Also benzoic acid (75 mg/kg) may be added as a preservative. Nonacid drinks such as root beer are better culture media for spoilage organisms than are acid drinks such as the cola drinks, ginger ale and fruit-flavoured drinks. The ingredients of soft drinks not only affect the suitability for microbial growth but also can affect the kinds and numbers of micro-organisms present and hence the likelihood of spoilage organisms being added. In addition, the bottles and closures are possible sources of contamination. The water for soft drinks is purified in regard to carbonate and mineral content and is filtered.

The filtration process may remove micro-organisms or, if the filter is badly contaminated, add them. Ultraviolet irradiation sometimes is used to destroy micro-organisms in the water. Discolouration of water and a flocculent precipitate may be caused by growth of algae. Treatment with chlorine or chlorine dioxide has been recommended to kill the algae and filtration, e.g. through diatomaceous earth, to remove the flocculent dead cells.

Yeasts, chiefly *Torulopsis* and *Candida*, are the most likely causes of poilage of soft drinks, for most such beverages are acid and contain sugar. One worker found that 85 per cent of 1500 spoiled samples of carbonated beverages had been spoiled by yeasts. Since the sugars are a possible source of yeasts, the American bottlers of carbonated beverages have set a standard of not more than ten yeasts per 10 grams of dry sugar. Fruit concentrates are another possible source of yeasts.

Cloudiness and ropiness are types of spoilage of soft drinks. Cloudiness results from marked growth of various yeasts or bacteria and ropiness from the development of capsulated bacteria, most of which seem to be of the genus *Bacillus*. Bacteria may enter from ingredients, bottles or closures. Occasionally, *Gluconobacter*, *Lactobacillus* or *Leuconostoc* may be isolated from spoiled soft drinks. An *Achromobacter* species was found responsible for a musty odour and taste in root beer.

Since moulds must have air, they cannot grow on carbonated beverages but may develop at the surface of uncarbonated ones containing air above the liquid. They may come from sugar, colouring materials or flavouring materials, from the air or from bottles or closures.

SPICES AND OTHER CONDIMENTS

A spice is a dried seed, fruit, root, bark, leaf or vegetative substance used in nutritionally insignificant quantities as a food additive for the purpose of flavour, colour or as a preservative that kills harmful bacteria or prevents their growth.

Many of these substances are also used for other purposes, such as medicine, religious rituals, cosmetics, perfumery or eating as vegetables. For example, turmeric is also used as a preservative; licorice as a medicine; garlic as a vegetable. In some cases they are referred to by different terms.

In the kitchen, spices are distinguished from herbs, which are leafy, green plant parts used for flavouring purposes. Herbs, such as basil or oregano, may be used fresh, and are commonly chopped into smaller pieces. Spices, however, are dried and often ground or grated into a powder. Small seeds, such as fennel and mustard seeds, are used both whole and in powder form.

Salt, sugar and ground black pepper corns are commonly available on Western restaurant tables; however, they are not always considered to be condiments.

A condiment is a relish, sauce or seasoning added to food to impart a particular flavour or to complement the dish. Often pungent in flavour and therefore added in fairly small quantities, popular condiments include salt, pepper, ketchup, mustard, olive oil and vinegar.

Usually applied by the diner at the table, condiments generally have the consistency of a thick liquid or paste and are served from a bottle, jar or bowl. They may also be dry, such as a mixture of herbs and seasonings. Many condiments are available packaged in single-serving sachets, particularly when supplied with take-out and fast foods.

Condiments are sometimes added prior to serving, for example a sandwich made with ketchup or mustard. Some condiments are used during cooking to add flavour or texture to the food; for example, barbecue sauce, teriyaki sauce and soya sauce all have flavours that can enhance the tastes of a variety of different meats and vegetables. There are some overlaps between condiments and seasonings.

The dry spices are not normally subject to spoilage, although mould growth during their drying may give them a heavy load of mould spores. Chip dips flavoured with vegetables or spices usually have much higher total, coliform and mould counts than those flavoured with cheese. As has been mentioned, treatment of the spices with propylene oxide greatly reduces their content of micro-organisms. Other treatments to reduce the initial flora would include irradiation, steam, hot ethanol vapours and acid treatments followed by neutralisation. Spices can be purchased with guaranteed low numbers of organisms. Prepared mustard can be spoiled by yeasts and by species of *Proteus* and *Bacillus*, usually with a gassy fermentation. Horseradish seldom spoils but on the contrary is bacteriostatic to bactericidal.

SALT

Salt is a dietary mineral composed primarily of sodium chloride that is essential for animal life, but toxic to most land plants. Salt flavour is one of the basic tastes, an important preservative and a popular food seasoning.

The three kinds of salt used in foods are: (i) solar salt from the evaporation of surface salt water, (ii) mined or rock salt, and (ii) welled salt from salt dissolved from subterranean salt deposits. Solar salt contains halophiles, such as *Halobacterium salinarium*. About three-fourths of the bacteria are *Bacillus* organisms, and the rest are mainly *Micrococcus* and *Sarcina*. Mined salt has been found to contain about 70 per cent *Micrococcus*, 20 per cent coryneforms and 4 per cent *Bacillus*; putrefactive anaerobes also have been found. Wet salt used on fish averages about 10 to 1000 organisms per gram. Most purified salt, however, adds few organisms to foods. Chloride and sodium ions, the two major components of salt, are necessary for the survival of all known living creatures, including humans. Salt is involved in regulating the water content (fluid balance) of the body. Salt cravings may be caused by trace mineral deficiencies as well as by a deficiency of sodium chloride itself. Conversely, over-consumption of salt increases the risk of health problems, including high blood pressure.

Table salt is refined salt, 99 per cent sodium chloride. It usually contains substances that make it free-flowing (anti-caking agents) such as sodium silicoaluminate or magnesium carbonate. It is common practice to put a desiccant, such as a few grains of uncooked rice, in salt shakers to absorb extra moisture and help break up clumps when anti-caking agents are not enough. Table salt has a particle density of 2.165 g/cm^3, and a bulk density (dry, ASTM D 632 gradation) of about 1.154 g/cm^3.

Health Effects

Sodium is one of the primary electrolytes in the body. All four cationic electrolytes (sodium, potassium, magnesium and calcium) are available in unrefined salt, as are other vital minerals needed for optimal bodily function. Too much or too little salt in the diet can lead to muscle cramps, dizziness or even an electrolyte disturbance, which can cause severe, even fatal, neurological problems. Drinking too much water, with insufficient salt intake, puts a person at risk of water intoxication (hyponatremia). Salt is even sometimes used as a health aid, such as in treatment of dysautonomia. The risk for disease due to insufficient or excessive salt intake varies because of biochemical individuality. Some have asserted that while the risks of consuming too much salt are real, the risks have been exaggerated for most people, or that the studies done on the consumption of salt can be interpreted in many different ways.

NUTMEATS

Nutmeats in the shell are usually sterile or nearly so. Shelled nuts to be used as ingredients of foods, e.g. in frozen desserts, may be contaminated with bacteria, yeasts and moulds. The test for coliform bacteria is used most often to indicate possible contamination with fecal matter during handling. Roasting and heating in oil or sugar solution reduce the load of micro-organisms. Moulds may produce mycotoxins on nuts, such as aflatoxin production in peanuts.

CEREAL

Cereals, grains or cereal grains, are grasses (members of the monocot families *Poaceae* or *Gramineae*) cultivated for the edible components of their fruit seeds (botanically, a type of fruit called a caryopsis) the endocarp, germ and bran. Cereal grains are grown in greater quantities and provide more food energy worldwide than any other type of crop; they are therefore staple crops. In their natural form (as in whole grain), they are a rich source of vitamins, minerals, carbohydrates, fats and oils, and protein. However, when refined by the removal of the bran and germ, the remaining endocarp is mostly carbohydrate and lacks the majority of the other nutrients. In some developing nations, grain in the form of rice, wheat or maize (in American terminology, corn) constitutes a majority of daily sustenance. In developed nations, cereal consumption is more moderate and varied but still substantial. The word cereal derives from Ceres, the name of the Roman goddess of harvest and agriculture.

The cereals, which all belong to the Gramineae or the grass family, are one of the most important sources of carbohydrates in the human diet. Some of the more important cereal crops are listed in Table 17.1. Wheat, rice and maize are by far the most important cereal crops on the basis of worldwide tonnage. However, each cereal species is adapted to grow in a particular range of climatic conditions although plant breeding programmes have extended the ranges of several of them. The common wheat is the major cereal of temperate parts of the world, and is grown extensively in both northern and southern hemispheres, whereas the durum wheat is grown extensively in the Mediterranean region and in the warmer, drier parts of Asia, North and South America. Rye can be grown in colder parts of the world and is an important crop in central Europe and Russia. Maize, which originated from the New World, is now grown extensively throughout the tropics and subtropical regions of both northern and southern hemispheres. Similarly, although rice was originally of Asian origin, it is also grown in many parts of the world. Although sorghum and some of the millets are not very important in terms of world tonnage, they are especially well adapted to growing in warm, dry climates and may be locally the most important cereals in such regions as those bordering the southern edge of the Sahara desert.

Table 17.1. Some of the more important cereal crops.

Botanical name	Common name
Triticum aestivum	Common wheat (bread wheat)
Triticum durum	Durum wheat (pasta wheat)
Hordeum spp.	Barley
Avena sativa	Oats
Secale cereale	Rye
Zea mays	Maize (American corn)
Oryza sativa	Rice
Sorghum vulgare	Sorghum
Panicum miliaceum	Millet
Pennisetum typhoideum	Bulrush millet

The microbiology of cereals, during growth, harvest and storage is dominated by the moulds and it is convenient to consider two groups of fungi. The field fungi are well adapted to the sometimes rapidly changing conditions on the surfaces of senescing plant material in the field. Although they require relatively high water activities for optimum growth, genera such as *Cladosporium*, *Alternaria* and *Epicoccum* are able to survive the rapid changes that can occur from the desiccation of a hot sunny day to the cool damp conditions of the night. The genus *Fusarium* includes species which have both pathogenic and saprophytic activities. Thus *F. culmorum* and *F. graminearum* can cause both stem rot and head blight of wheat and barley in the field and these field infections may lead to more extensive post-harvest spoilage of these commodities if they are stored at too high a water activity. By contrast the so-called storage fungi seem to be well adapted to the more constant conditions of cereals in storage, and generally grow at lower water activities (Table 17.2). The most important genera of the storage fungi are *Penicillium* and *Aspergillus*, although species of *Fusarium* may also be involved in spoilage when grain is stored under moist conditions.

Table 17.2. Minimum water activity requirements of some common field and storage fungi.

Species	Minimum
Field fungi	
Fusarium culmorum	0.89
Fusarium graminearum	0.89
Alternaria alternata	0.88
Cladosporium herbarum	0.85
Storage fungi	
Penicillium aurantiogriseum	0.82
Penicillium brevicompactum	0.80
Aspergillus flavus	0.78
Aspergillus candidus	0.75
Eurotium amstelodami	0.71
Wallemia sebi	0.69

Water activity and temperature are the most important environmental factors influencing the mould spoilage of cereals and the possible production of mycotoxins, and Table 17.3 shows the relationship between water content and water activity for barley, oats and sorghum. Although xerophilic moulds such as *Eurotium* spp. and *Aspergillus restrictus* may grow very slowly at the lower limit of their water activity range (0.71 corresponding to about 14 per cent water content in wheat at 25°C) once they start growing and metabolising they will produce water of respiration and the local water activity will steadily rise allowing more rapid growth. Indeed it could increase sufficiently to allow mesophilic mould spores to germinate and grow; the process being, in a sense, autocatalytic. There is a sequence of observable consequences of the process of mould growth on cereals starting with a decrease in germinability of the grain. This is followed by discolouration, the production of mould metabolites including mycotoxins, demonstrable increase in temperature (self-heating), the production of musty odours, caking and a rapid increase in water activity leading finally to the complete decay with the growth of a wide range of micro-organisms.

Table 17.3. Equilibrium relative humidity, water activity and moisture content (as % wet weight) of cereals at 25°C.

Equilibrium relative humidity (%)	Water activity a_w	Water potential (MPa)	Water content (% wet weight)		
			Barley	Oats	Sorghum
15	0.15	−261	6.0	5.7	6.4
30	0.30	−166	8.4	8.0	8.6
45	0.45	−110	10.0	9.6	10.5
60	0.60	−70	12.1	11.8	12.0
75	0.75	−39	14.4	13.8	15.2
90	0.90	−14.5	19.5	18.5	18.8
100	1.00	0.0	26.8	24.1	21.9

Preservation of High-moisture Cereals

Although not directly relevant to human foods, the availability of high-moisture cereals, such as barley, provides a highly nutritious winter feed for cattle. Long-term storage of such material can be achieved by a lactic acid fermentation comparable to the making of silage, or by the careful addition of fatty acids such as propionic acid. If this process is not carried out carefully then it may be possible to have sufficient propionic acid to inhibit the normal spoilage moulds associated with cereals in a temperate climate, but not enough to inhibit *Aspergillus flavus*. It has been shown that, even though partially inhibited in its growth, this mould can produce aflatoxin B_1 at enhanced levels under these conditions. If such material is fed to dairy cattle there is the possibility of aflatoxin M_1 being secreted in the milk and it then becomes a problem in human foods and not just a problem of animal feeds.

Pulses, Nuts and Oilseeds

The pulses are members of the huge legume family of plants, the Fabaceae also known as the Papilionaceae and Leguminosae, which form a major source of vegetable proteins and include such important crops as peas, beans, soya, groundnuts and lentils. Although many species of peas and beans are familiar to us as fresh vegetables, millions of tons of the mature seeds of soya beans and groundnuts are harvested for longer term storage every year and may be susceptible to mould spoilage if not stored under appropriate conditions. Several of the leguminous seeds, such as groundnuts and soyabeans, are also valuable sources of vegetable oils but there are plants from many other diverse families which are now used to provide food quality vegetable oils, rapeseed from the crucifers, sunflower seed from the daisy family, oil palm and olives to mention just a few. Edible nuts may also come from a botanically wide range of tree species and many of them are rich in oil and give similar microbiological problems as oilseeds.

Seeds rich in oil, such as groundnuts, have a much lower water content at a particular water activity than cereals, thus groundnuts with a 7.2 per cent water content have a water activity of about 0.65–0.7 at 25°C. Apart from the problem of mycotoxin formation in moulded oilseeds, several mould species have strong lipolytic activity leading to the contamination of the extracted oils with free fatty acids which may in turn undergo oxidation to form products contributing to rancidity. The most important lipolytic moulds are species of *Aspergillus*, such as *A. niger* and *A. tamarii*, *Penicillium* and *Paecilomyces*, while at higher water activities species of *Rhizopus* may also be important. Figure 17.1 shows the influence of moisture content and damage on the formation of free fatty acids (FFA) in groundnuts stored for 4 months. It can be seen that in wholesome nuts there is a steady increase in FFA formation with an increase in moisture content and this is due to the plants own lipolytic enzymes. However, damaged groundnuts show a more rapid rise at low moisture contents, presumably due to increased contact of enzymes and substrate as a result of damage, but they also show an especially rapid rise in FFA at moisture contents greater than 7.2 per cent corresponding to the active growth of lipolytic moulds.

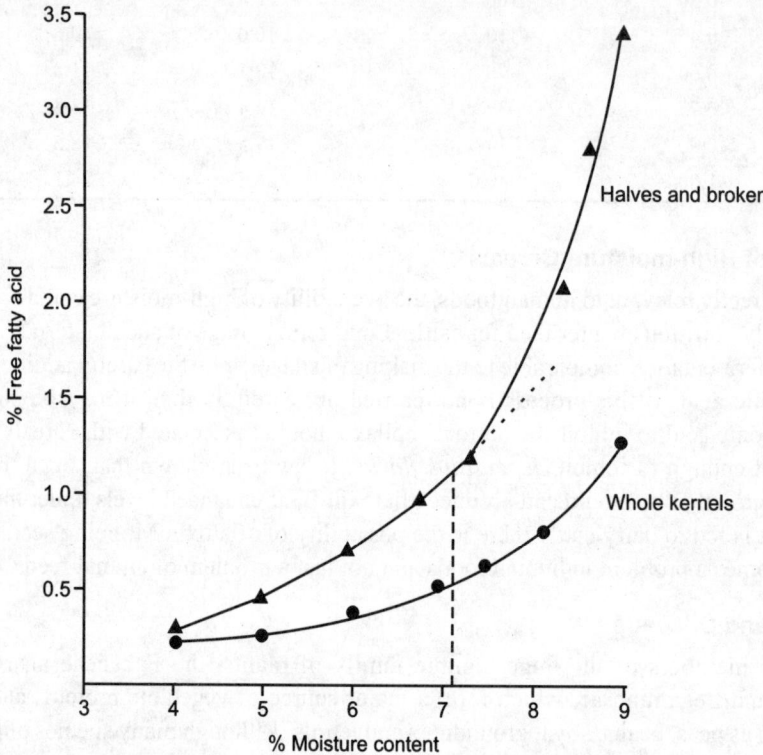

Fig. 17.1. The influence of moisture content on free fatty acid formation in groundnuts stored for four months. 7.2 per cent moisture content corresponds to a_w 0.65–0.70 at 25°C so fungal growth may occur.

If cereals, pulses, oilseeds and tree nuts are harvested with as little damage as possible and dried to an appropriate water content it should be possible to store them for considerable periods of time so long as they are not exposed to excessive temperature abuse during storage. The problems which may arise when large storage facilities, such as silos, are not carefully designed to avoid temperature differentials arising within the stored commodity. The migration of water in these circumstances can result in the germination of fungal spores and the growth of mycelium creating a localised region of fungal activity releasing further water of respiration into the region. In this way, despite the commodity initially going into store at what was judged to be a safe water content, it may nevertheless go mouldy over a period of time. It should be noted that, although a commodity may be dry enough to avoid direct microbiological spoilage, it may not be secure against the ravages of pests such as insects and rodents and their activity may lead to secondary invasion and mould spoilage.

Chapter 18

Microbial Biomass, Single Cell Protein and Other Microbial Products

INTRODUCTION

The term biomass applies to the mass of substance generated by the growth of living organisms, be they micro-organisms, plants or animals. Sugarcane, grain, tubers and wood are a few of the examples. The term also includes agricultural produces, as well as by-products of agriculture or by-products of crop processing such as straw, corn stovers, sugarcane bagasse, etc. Biomass may be generated deliberately as single cell protein, which refers to yeast, moulds or bacteria grown primarily for their protein content, which are used for animal feed or human food.

Biomass from by-products of crop processing such as corn stovers, straw, sugarcane bagasse, etc. are available in abundance and not utilised in a big way, except burning of bagasse as fuel in sugar mills. Still there is surplus bagasse available for other use. The basic reaction involved in biomass formation is photosynthesis, which is a process of fixation of carbon by living plants from atmospheric carbon dioxide with water by chloroplasts in presence of sunlight, releasing oxygen back to atmosphere. Biomass is nothing but recycled carbon dioxide with solar energy in the most versatile form. The biomass is a complex mixture of carbohydrate polymers known as cellulose and hemicellulose, with lignin and small amount of other compounds known as extractives.

While 'Biotechnology' has been defined in many forms, in essence it implies the use of microbial, animal or plant cell or enzymes to synthesise, breakdown or transform materials. The European Federation of Biotechnology considers biotechnology as 'the integration of natural sciences and organisms, cells, parts thereof, and molecular analogues for products and services'. Biotechnologies are transformation of renewable raw materials.

This is as such applied to processes as ancient as fermentation and modern as recombinant DNA genetic engineering. Biotechnology is defined as 'the application of biological organisms, systems or processes to manufacturing and service industries'. Figure 18.1 illustrates the broad scope and application of biotechnology.

Bioconversion is the transformation of one substance to another by means of living organisms, or by enzymes or other products derived from a living organism. Yeast, for example, converts sugar to carbon dioxide and alcohol, and lactobacilli converts alcohol to acetic acid. The sweetener used in soft drinks and processed foods these days, is made by enzymatic conversion of the glucose of corn syrup to fructose. Biotechnology and bioconversion are synonymous.

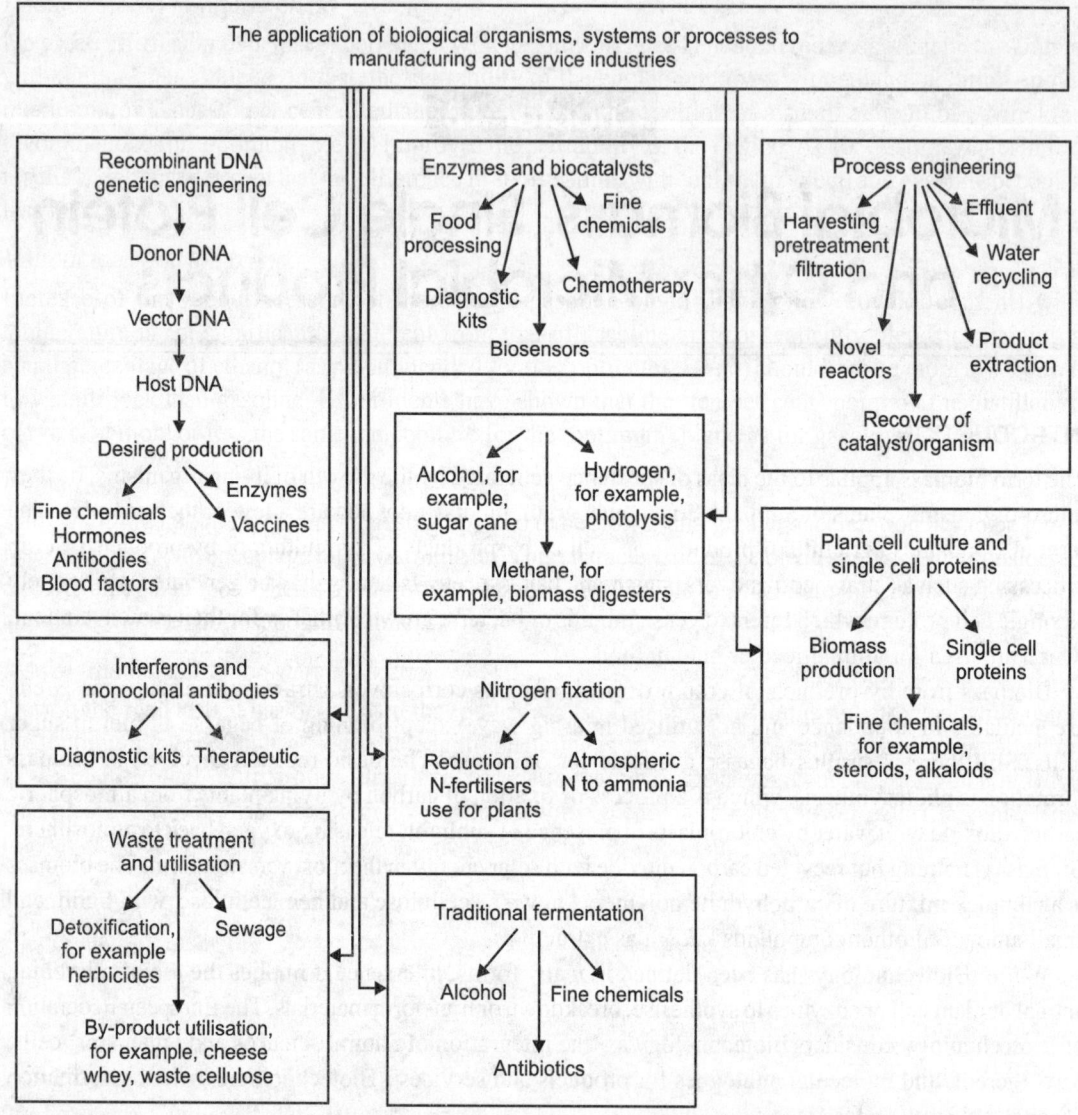

Fig. 18.1. The scope of biotechnology.

Energy is a key input not only for daily household needs, but also in all developmental activities. As on today, the main primary source of energy is out of fossil fuels, which are rapidly dwindling. The main player, petroleum, will be exhausted completely in the not too distant future. But the demand of energy is ever increasing due to industrialisation, economic development and population growth. In this backdrop, renewable energy sources are a must if the economy of the world is to be carried forward.

The basic reaction involved in biomass is photosynthesis, which is a process of fixation of carbon by living plants from atmospheric carbon dioxide with water by chloroplasts in presence of sunlight, releasing oxygen back to the atmosphere. Biomass is nothing but recycled carbon dioxide with solar energy in the most versatile form.

Plant photosynthesis alone fixes about 2×10^{11} tonnes of carbon each year with an energy content of 2×10^{21} joules, which represent about 10 times the world's annual energy consumption and 200 times our food energy consumption.

The actual efficiency of capturing solar energy by green plants may be around 3–4 per cent, the more effective photosynthetic plants like maize, sorghum and specially sugarcane being the most productive. Photosynthetically derived biomass, which exists in many available forms, can be transformed into storable fuels and chemical feedstocks such as ethanol and methane gas. Biomass, the renewable source of energy, can be converted into either direct energy or energy-carrier compounds by:

1. Direct combustion.
2. Anaerobic digestion systems.
3. Destructive distillation.
4. Gasification.
5. Chemical or biochemical hydrolysis.

The ways of converting biomass to usable fuels has been summarised in Fig. 18.2.

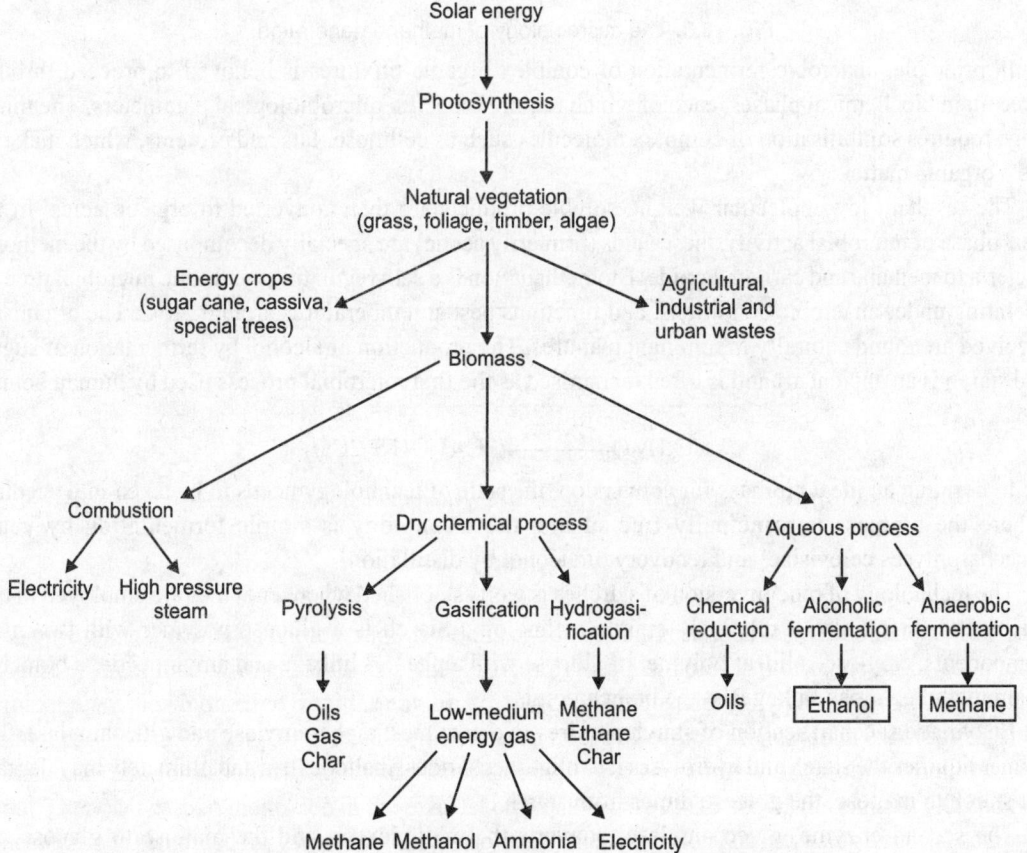

Fig. 18.2. Options for the conversion of biomass to energy.

The micro-biology of methane generation is complex, involving mixtures of anaerobic micro-organisms, which has been summarised in Fig. 18.3.

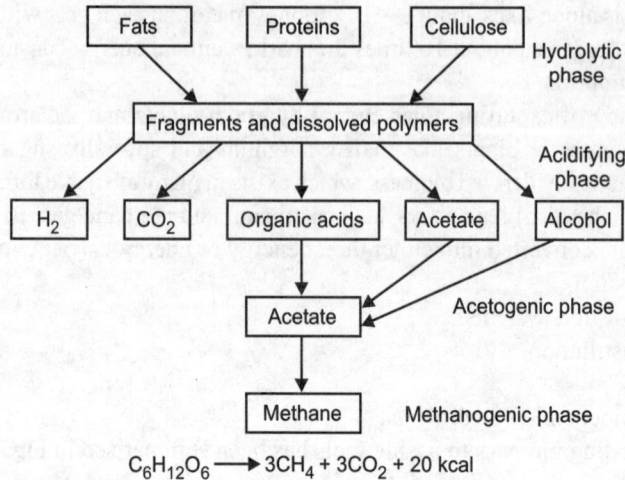

$$C_6H_{12}O_6 \longrightarrow 3CH_4 + 3CO_2 + 20 \text{ kcal}$$

Fig. 18.3. The microbiology of methane generation.

In principle, anaerobic fermentation of complex organic mixtures is believed to proceed through three main biochemical phases, each of which requires specific microbiological parameters. The initial stage requires solubilisation of complex molecules such as cellulose, fats and proteins, which make up most organic matter.

The resultant low molecular weight, soluble products are then converted to organic acids. In the final phase of microbial activity, these acids (primarily acetic) are specially decomposed by the methonic bacteria to methane and carbon dioxide. Biomethanation is a self-regulating symbiotic microbial process operating under anaerobic conditions, and functions best at temperatures around 30°C. The organisms involved are found naturally in ruminant manures. The production of alcohol by fermentation of sugars and starch is an ancient art and is often recognised as the first microbial process used by human beings.

$$C_6H_{12}O_6 \xrightarrow{\text{Zymase}} 2C_2H_5OH + 2CO_2$$

In defining an ideal biomass for conversion, the state of technology needs to be taken into account. Where the biomass is principally free sugars, the technology is simple fermentation by yeast, 'Saccharomyces cerevisiae' and recovery of alcohol by distillation.

The technology of bioconversion of starches is well established where enzymes are employed in two stages and this is also a relatively simple technology. Starch is a glucose polymer with two main components: amylose, a linear polymer of glucose with alpha-1,4 linkage and amylopectin, a branched chain including alpha linkages at the branch points.

Enzymatic saccharification of starch requires two enzymes, alpha-amylase and glucoamylase. The former liquifies the starch and hydrolyses it to oligosaccharides, maltodextrin and ultimately may degrade the starch to maltose, the glucose dimer from starch.

The second enzyme, gluco amylase, converts the maltodextrin and the maltose to glucose, the fermentable sugar. By contrast, the conversion of wood and other lignocellulosics involves several stages and the processing is complex. A flow diagram of ethyl alcohol distillery from molasses or cane juice has been shown in Fig. 18.4. The process of manufacture of starch by wet milling of corn and further to alcohol may be seen in Fig. 18.5.

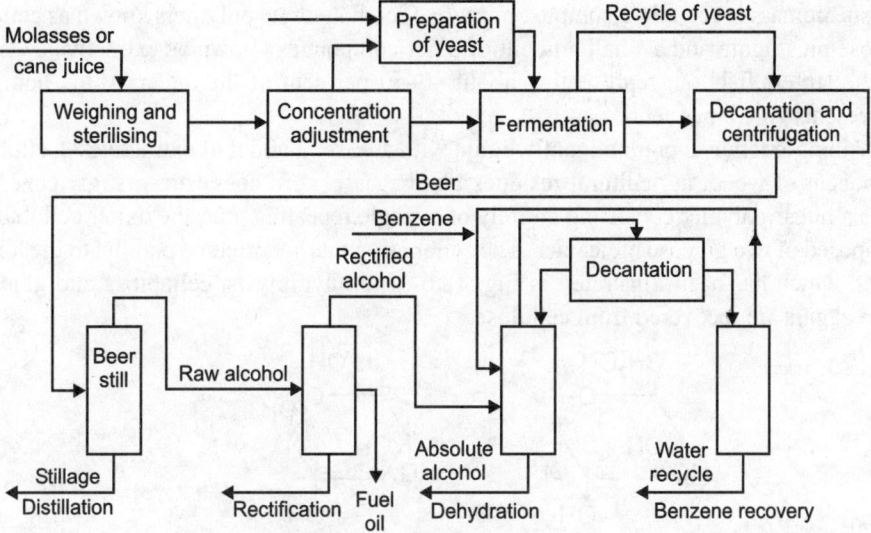

Fig. 18.4. Ethyl alcohol distillery.

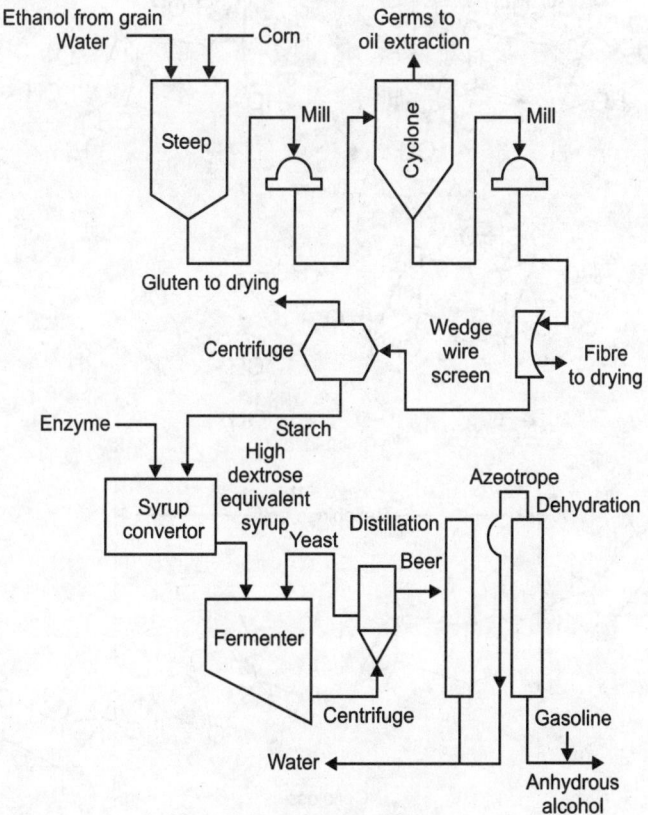

Fig. 18.5. Wet milling of corn.

Cellulosic biomass is actually a complex mixture of carbohydrate polymers known as cellulose and hemicellulose plus lignin and a small amount of other compounds known as extractives. Cellulose is generally the largest fraction, representing about 40–50 per cent of the material; the hemicellulose portion represents 20–40 per cent.

The remaining fraction is predominantly lignin with a lesser amount of extractives. Cellulose is the main component of wood, agricultural residues like bagasse, corn cobs, straw, sugar cane tops, etc. Cellulose is a linear polymer consisting entirely of a single repeating unit, the dimer cellobiose which in turn composed of two glucose molecules. The cellobiose units are oriented parallel to the long axis of the polymer, which has been illustrated in Fig. 18.6. Upon hydrolysis, cellobiose and glucose, both fermentable sugars are recovered from cellulose.

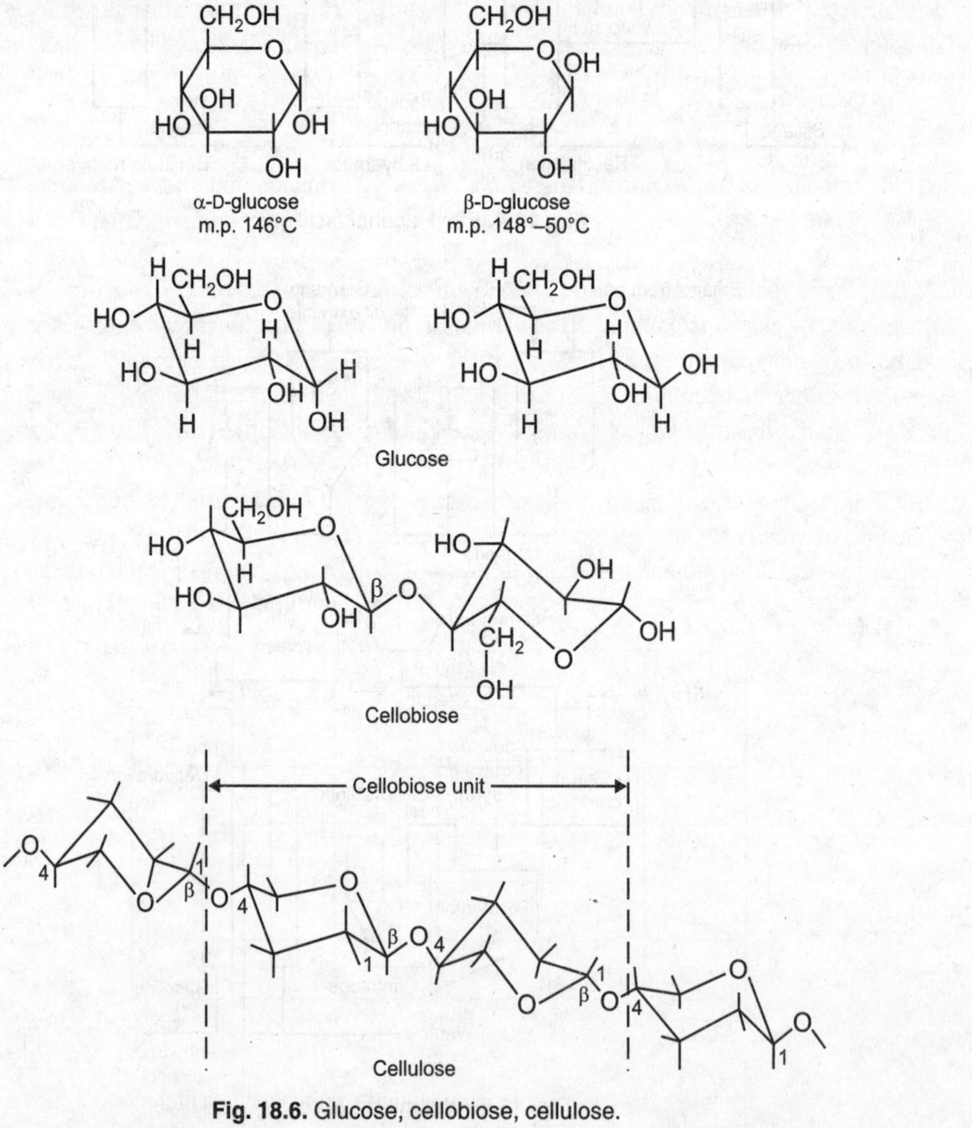

α-D-glucose
m.p. 146°C

β-D-glucose
m.p. 148°–50°C

Glucose

Cellobiose

Cellobiose unit

Cellulose

Fig. 18.6. Glucose, cellobiose, cellulose.

The fermentation of cane juice, molasses or the glucose obtained by saccharification of corn and other grains to alcohol is a long-established and mature technology practised in hundreds of industrial plants throughout the world. The conversion of cellulose to alcohol is not. In cellulosics, fermentation to alcohol is difficult because of generation of powerful inhibitors during acid treatment.

This section deals with fermentation processes involved in the production of microbial cells as major fermentation end-products. Microbial cells are produced for two main application—as a source of protein for animal or human food single cell protein (SCP) or for use as a commercial inoculum in food fermentations and for agriculture, waste treatment and other applications. As a commodity, single-cell protein must be competitive with commercial animal and plant proteins in terms of price and nutritional value and must conform with human or animal food safety requirements. Productivity, yield and selling price are the major factors affecting the economics of SCP production. Microbial inoculants, which are used as a process aid, generally have a higher value. In this case the objective of the production process is to optimise yield of viable cells of defined biological activity and with good shelf-life characteristics. These two major product categories are considered separately below. *Saccharomyces cerevisiae* yeast is categorised primarily as a microbial inoculant. Inactive dried brewer's or baker's yeast is also used as a dietary source of vitamins and trace minerals in specific medical conditions. Considerable amounts of yeast extract are produced from baker's yeast as a source of flavour and vitamins.

SINGLE CELL PROTEIN (SCP) PRODUCTION

Substrates

The major substrates which have been used in SCP production are alkanes, alcohols and carbohydrates.

Candida utilis has been produced as a protein supplement by fermentation of sulphite waste liquor in Germany during both World Wars and by growth on molasses in Jamaica at the end of World War II. Subsequently a number of companies in the USA and one in Finland produced Candida as a fodder yeast on sulphite waste liquor using the German open-top Waldhof fermenter. However, due to an over-abundance of plant protein material, these processes eventually became uneconomical. More recently, a Finnish company developed a fungal SCP production process, the Pekilo process, to grow *Paecilomyces varioti* for animal feed using spent sulphite waste liquor as substrate.

Cellulose from natural sources and waste wood is an attractive starting material for SCP production because of its abundance. The association of cellulose with lignin in wood makes it somewhat intractible to microbial degradation and thermal or chemical pretreatment, used in combination with enzymatic hydrolysis, is usually required. Systems using cellulolytic organisms appear to have promise, but economic viability has yet to be achieved.

Cellulose from natural sources and waste wood is an attractive starting material for SCP production because of its abundance. The association of cellulose with lignin in wood makes it somewhat intractible to microbial degradation and thermal or chemical pretreatment, used in combination with enzymatic hydrolysis, is usually required. Systems using cellulolytic organisms appear to have promise, but economic viability has yet to be achieved.

Whole milk whey or deproteinised whey is a carbohydrate source which creates disposal problems. The major problems with whey for SCP production are usually insufficient substrate, seasonal supply variations and its high water content (> 90 per cent) which makes transport prohibitively expensive. While most organisms do not utilise lactose as a carbon source, strains of the yeast *Kluyveromyces fragilis* readily grow on lactose and a number of fermentation plants have been built to produce animal or human food-grade SCP using this organism. Some of these plants are designed to switch from SCP production to ethanol production depending on market forces.

The Symba process was developed in Sweden to produce SCP from potato starch using two yeast strains. *Saccharomycopsis fibuligera* produces the enzymes necessary for starch degradation enabling co-growth of *Candida utilis*. The production process, intended for animal feed production was designed to handle potato-processing waste but suffered from problems of lack of substrate supply continuity. Food-grade glucose was the substrate chosen by Rank Hovis McDougall for production of fungal SCP using *Fusarium graminearum*. The strategy adopted was to additionally take advantage of mycelial fibre content to produce a range of high added value products including meat analogues for human consumption.

The original alkane SCP fermentation process, developed at the Laverna Refinery in France, used 10–20 per cent wax contained in gas-oil. Substrate costs were very low but, because of its crude nature, exhaustive extractive processing was required to recover the yeast free of gas-oil flavour taint and possible gas-oil carcinogens. There was also a microbial contamination tendency due to the nonaseptic nature of the process. These drawbacks led to the closure of the plant in 1975. The disadvantages associated with use of crude gas-oil and non-asepsis were taken into account by Italproteine, a joint venture between BP and ANIC. The process used purified *n*-paraffins which were fully utilised by the cells, simplifying SCP recovery. Japanese companies, Dainippon and Kanegufuchi, working along similar lines to Italproteine, gained clearance in Japan to have their products accepted for animal feed but the decision was reversed by strong consumer campaign based on fears of the presence of carcinogenic residues. The Kanegufuchi process was licensed to Liquichimica in Italy, who built a 1,00,000 T/year capacity plant which was then subjected to an embargo similar to the Sardinia plant. A plant, designed by Dainippon, in Romania using *Candida pichia* was reported to have been commissioned.

Methane was initially considered as an SCP raw material because, as a gas product, purification problems after fermentation would be minimal. Disadvantages associated with methane-based processes are related to the greater oxygen requirement necessary to fully oxidise methane compared to paraffins, the low solubility of methane in water and the requirement that the fermentation plant be flame-proof as methane-oxygen mixtures are highly explosive. Methane is, however, easily converted to methanol with requires less oxygen, less fermenter cooling, is highly water-soluble and has minimal explosion risks. ICI, which manufactures bulk methanol, chose this substrate for bacterial SCP production for animal feed. The company designed a non-mechanical 'pressure cycle fermenter', which uses air for both agitation and aeration, in the world's largest single aerobic aseptic fermenter of 3000 m^3 capacity. The process, which produces 50–60000 T/year SCP, using the organism *Methylophilus methylotrophus*, was commissioned in 1992–1993 but has suffered from dramatic increases in methanol prices. The economic difficulties encountered by ICI with the animal-feed process and the greater commercial promise of the RHM *Fusarium* process led to a joint venture between these companies in 1999 with the objective of producing *Fusarium* SCP in the large ICI fermentation plant. Ethanol, which has similar advantages as a substrate to methanol, was used as substrate by Pure Culture Products for production of food-grade protein from food-grade ethanol using *Candida utilis*. Process economics likewise suffered as a result of increases in ethanol costs.

ECONOMICS OF SCP PRODUCTION

The initial reasoning by companies such as ICI and others to enter SCP production was to produce, at low cost, high-value SCP from petroleum, for addition to animal feed, thereby replacing imported protein additives such as soyabean meal. Factors which contributed to the failure of hydrocarbon SCP to make a major commercial impact include the 1993 dramatic oil price increases which raised feedstock and energy costs, parallel increases in plant construction costs and the lower price increases achieved by agricultural products including soyabean relative to industrial products. When one considers that crude oil prices increased by a factor of six in 1993 and that the cost of substrate for SCP processes represents 40–60 per cent or total manufacturing cost, the negative impact on hydrocarbon-based SCP processes may be understood. Agricultural crops, the major competitor to SCP for animal feed, manifest a remarkable ability to respond to market forces and maintain price stability. In addition to the more conventional animal-feed crops such as soya, high-protein crops such as ground nut, rape seed, cotton seed and winged bean are now gaining a market share in this business and expansion of maize gasohol production has provided new sources of animal-feed by-products. Consequently, the economics of animal-feed SCP have so far appeared unattractive and higher value products are being sought. Rank Hovis McDougall (RHM) and Pure Culture Products have adopted a different strategy and aimed their products at the human food market. RHM in particular have taken advantage of the fibre component of the fungus to produce high added value meat analogues containing high dietary fibre, 50 per cent protein and having other desirable advantages such as low sodium and low fat.

The main economic factors in SCP production are productivity, yield and selling price. Table 18.1 summarises productivity and yield factors for SCP production using various organism/substrate combinations. Cell dry weight and dilution factors are usually 15–30 kg m^{-3} and 0.1–0.4 hr^{-1} respectively giving productivity (weight of cells produced per unit volume per unit time) of 1.5–12 kg m^{-3} hr^{-1}. Since productivity is often limited by oxygen-transfer rates and effectiveness of fermenter cooling due to exothermic metabolism, values in the range 3–5 kg m^{-3} hr^{-1} are more normal. Because substrate cost is such a large proportion of manufacturing cost of most SCP products, high cell yield (weight of cells produced per unit weight of substrate utilised) and minimal formation of by-products is essential.

Table 18.1. Productivity and yield factors of SCP biomass, exfermenter, achieved in pilot or production scale plants.

Substrate	Organism	Yield (Y) (kg cell wt/kg substrate utilised)	Cell dry wt (x) (kg m^{-3})	Dilution rate (hr^{-1})	Productivity (kg m^{-3} hr^{-1})
n-Paraffin	Yeast	0.95	15–20	0.11	ca. 2
n-Paraffin	Yeast	1.2	–	–	3
Methanol	Bacteria	0.4	–	–	2
Ethanol	Yeast	0.8	–	–	4.5
Molasses	Yeast	0.85	–	–	5.2
Methanol	Bacteria	0.5	20–25	0.4	8–10
Sulphite waste liquor	Fungus	ca. 0.5	17	0.2	2.8–3.4
Methanol	Bacteria	ca. 0.5	30	0.16–0.19	4.8–5.7

Choice of Micro-organism

Key criteria used in selecting suitable strains for SCP production should take into account the following:
1. The substrates to be used as carbon, energy and nitrogen source and the need for nutrient supplement.
2. High specific growth rates, productivity and yields on a given substrate.
3. pH and temperature tolerance.
4. Aeration requirements and foaming characteristics.

5. Growth morphology in the fermenter.
6. Safety and acceptability—non-pathogenic, absence of toxin products.
7. Ease of SCP recovery.
8. Protein, RNA and nutritional composition of product.
9. Structural properties of the final product.

In general, fungi have the capacity to degrade a wider range of complex plant materials, particularly plant polysaccharides. They can tolerate low pH which contributes to reducing fermenter infections. Growth of fungi as short highly-branched filaments rather than in pelleted form is essential in order to optimise growth rate. However, this filamentous morphology produces rheologically more complex fermentation broths which are difficult to aerate.

Bacteria in general have faster growth rates than fungi and grow at higher temperatures, thereby reducing fermenter cooling requirements. Bacterial and yeast fermentations are easier to aerate. In contrast to fungi, which are easily recovered by filtration, bacterial and yeasts require use of sedimentation techniques including centrifugation.

Bacterial in general produce a more favourable protein composition than yeasts or fungi. Protein content in bacteria can range from 60 to 65 per cent whereas fungi selected for biomass production and yeasts have protein contents in the range 33 to 45 per cent. However, associated with the higher bacterial protein levels is a much higher level of nutritionally undesirable RNA of 15 to 25 per cent.

Micro-organisms involved in SCP production must be safe and acceptable for use in food or feed. They should be non-pathogenic and non-toxin forming. Organisms should be stable genetically so that the strain with optimal biochemical and physiological characteristics may be maintained in the process through many hundreds of generations. In addition, regulatory bodies are concerned that strain degeneration could result in production of a strain with undesirable nutritional characteristics.

Fermenter Design

Economics dictates that production should be carried out in the minimum number of large-scale fermenters. Key parameters in the achievement of high biomass productivity on a large scale are high oxygen-transfer rates, promoting high respiration rates which in turn increase metabolic heat production and the need for an efficient cooling system. Assuming a mass balance of biomass-producing organisms of

$$C_6H_{12}O_6 + O_2 + NPKMgS \longrightarrow Biomass + CO_2 + H_2O$$
$$(2.0) \quad (0.7) \quad (0.1) \qquad (1.0) \quad (1.1) \quad (0.7)$$

and a heat evolution of 3–4 kcal g^{-1} cell mass, a cell-mass productivity of 4 kg m^{-3} hr^{-1} requires an OTR of 2.8 kg m^{-3} hr^{-1} and produces 14,000 kcal m^3 hr^{-1} heat. In order to maximise fermentation productivity it is essential to operate continuous fermentation processes, thereby maintaining high microbial growth rates and minimising fermenter down-time.

Some of the fermenter designs used in SCP production are illustrated in Fig. 18.7. Mechanically agitated fully-baffled bioreactors (Fig. 18.7a) with turbine mixers and with air introduction through a sparger have been used by ICI for the n-alkane pilot-scale process developed in Scotland and for the three 1800 m^3 fermenters in Sardinia. Conventional turbine systems are not considered to be very satisfactory for very large fermenters and number of large scale SCP processes have used air-agitated vessels. For gas-oil substances, ICI used a draft tube air lift design (Fig. 18.7b). A correlation existed between the rising speed of air bubbles in the draft tube and fermenter productivity and the draft tube was optimised relative to biomass while minimising energy requirements. A Kanegufuchi-designed, modified air-lift fermenter, in which the fermentation medium is driven by the force of inflowing air from a large vessel through an external circulatrory loop, was used for the Liquichimica alkane plant (Fig. 18.7c).

The ICI pressure cycle pilot fermenter, used in SCP production from methanol, is likewise a combination of an air-lift and loop reactor consisting of an air-lift column, a down-flow tube with heat removal and a gas-release space (Fig. 18.7d). The production fermenter no longer contained the external down-flow tube (Fig. 18.7e). This fermenter is equipped with a complex air sparger containing 3000 outlets, which facilitates aeration, agitation and effective distribution of methanol substrate, which is toxic in high concentrations.

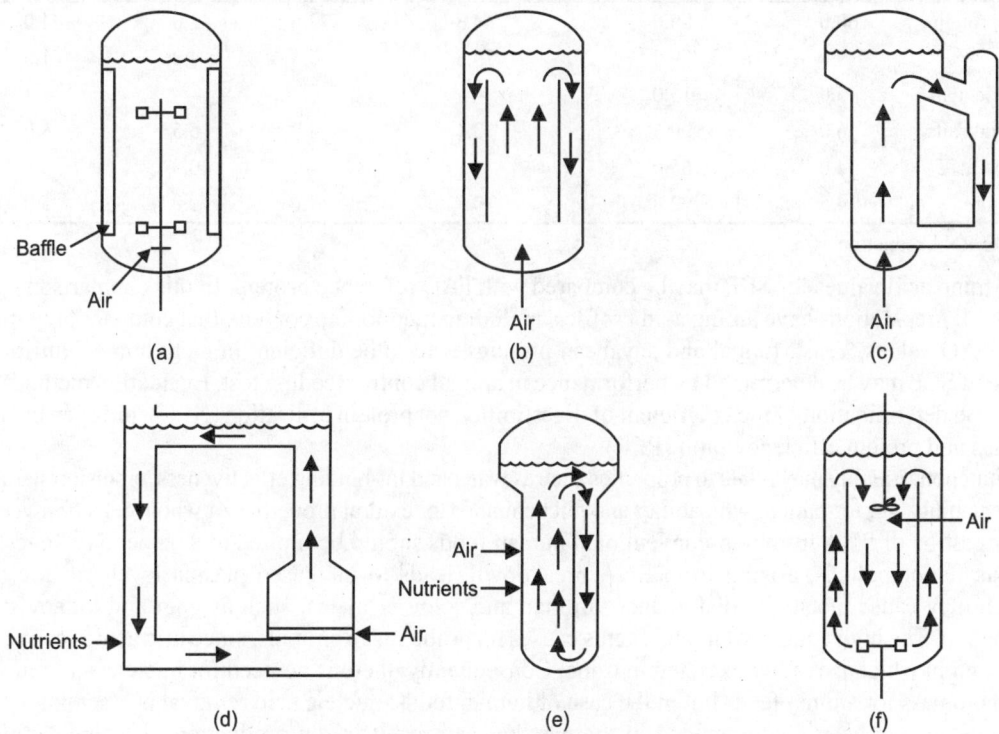

Fig. 18.7. Fermenter designs used in SCP production.

While air-lift fermenter designs may be used for fungal pelleted growth, only filamentous growth is appropriate for fungal SCP production. Long and/or highly branched filamentous mycelia, even at low cell densities (< 10 kg m^{-3}) tend to develop high pseudoplastic viscosities resulting in inefficient oxygen transfer. Pellets also have 'inefficient' internal oxygen transfer. In addition there is a complex relationship between impeller shear and cell morphology. Low shear rates induce long unbranched mycelia, having few growth tips and low growth rates. In order to optimise mass transfer in fungal biomass fermentations involving *fusarium graminearum*, a fermenter was designed, which separates these function, with two impellers each driven by separate shaft and run at optimum speeds (Fig. 18.7f). Following the development of a joint venture between RHM and ICI, the ICI pilot SCP fermenter was modified to produce the RHM 'Mycoprotein' but difficulties were encountered in scaling up the *Fusarium* process in the ICI production fermenter. Nevertheless, the outlook for the process is optimistic.

Product Quality and Safety

SCP has potential applications in animal feed, human food and as functional protein concentrates. Nutritional characteristics are important in the case of feed and food and safety considerations are relevant to all these applications. The overall composition of selected single-cell protein preparations is illustrated in Table 18.2.

Table 18.2. Composition (%) of single-cell protein compared with soya meal and milk powder.

Component	Alkane yeast	Methanol bacterium	Fusarium graminearum*	Alga	Soya meal	Milk powder
Raw protein	60.0	80.0	44.3	72.6	42.0	34.0
Fat	9.0	9.5	13.8	7.3	4.0	1.0
Nucleic acid	5.0	15.0	–	–	–	–
Mineral salts	6.0	9.5	3.1	4.7	6.5	8.0
Amino acid	54.0	65.0	–	–	40.0	–
Moisture	4.5	2.8	0	3.6	10.0	5.0

* After RNA reduction

Amino acid values for SCP may be compared with FAO reference protein. In this comparison some bacterial preparations have amino acid profiles, including methionine content, that compare favourable with FAO values. Yeast, fungal and soyabean proteins tend to be deficient in methionine. Nutritional value of SCP may be determined by performance in animal control feeding test. Evaluation methods are based on determination of the coefficient of digestibility, net protein utilisation (NPU), nitrogen balance studies and protein efficiency ratio (PER).

Functional quality may relate to properties such as water and fat-binding effectiveness, emulsion stability, dispersability, gel formation, whipability and thickening or to textural properties of whole cells or mycelia.

Ingestion of RNA from non-conventional human foods should be limited to 2 oz per day. Ingestion of purine compounds, arising from RNA breakdown, leads to increased plasma levels of uric acid which may cause metabolic disturbances in man and some primates, such as gout and kidney stone formation. The high content of nucleic acids causes no problems to animals, since uric acid is converted to allantoin which is readily excreted in urine. Consequently, there is no need for nucleic acid removal from biomass for animal feeds but in the case of human foods, nucleic acid removal is essential. Alkali treatments have been recommended in the past but can result in the production of lysinoalanine, a nephrotoxic factor. More recent methods rely on temperature hold around 64°C, with inactivates fungal proteases and allows endogenous RNA-ases to hydrolyse RNA with release of nucleotides from cell to culture broth. A 30-minute stand in a continuous stirred tank reactor at 64°C reduces RNA levels in *F. graminearum* cells from about 80 mg g^{-1} to 2 mg g^{-1}.

SCP Fermentation Processes

In this section fermentation processes for production of SCP by *Candida* species grown on alkanes, by *Methylophilus methylotrophus* grown on methanol, by *Kluyveromyces fragilis* grown on whey and by *Fusarium graminearum* grown on glucose, will be discussed.

The *Candida* BP *n*-paraffin process flow sheet is illustrated in Fig. 18.8. The fermentation is operated under sterile conditions. Approximate nutrient requirements to produce 1 kg of SCP included 1–1.2 kg paraffin, 0.14 kg gaseous NH_3, 0.05 kg PO_4^{-3} plus other salts. Gaseous ammonia was fed, with air, both as nitrogen source and to control pH. Oxygen requirement per unit biomass produced by aerobic micro-organisms grown on *n*-hexadecane is 2.5 times higher than that required for growth on glucose and amounts to 2.2 kg O_2 per kg biomass. Heat produced was 6600 kcal/kg biomass. Consequently fermenters require substantial agitation. Because of the insoluble nature of alkanes, they exist in agitated fermenter broths as suspensions of alkane drops 1–100 μm is size. Hydrocarbon assimilation into cells appears to involve cell contact with tiny hydrocarbon droplets, 0.01–0.5 μm diameter. Creation of a micro-emulsion at the interface of the tiny droplets by a surface-active agent, which may be produced by the cells, seems to facilitate droplet adherence to the cell. The chief mechanism of alkane degradation in *Candida* is terminal oxidation with sequential production of primary alcohol, aldehyde and acid, followed by β-oxidation of the fatty acid to acetate. Cell recovery is by centrifugation, producing 15 per cent dry solids, evaporation to 25 per cent dry solids and spray-drying.

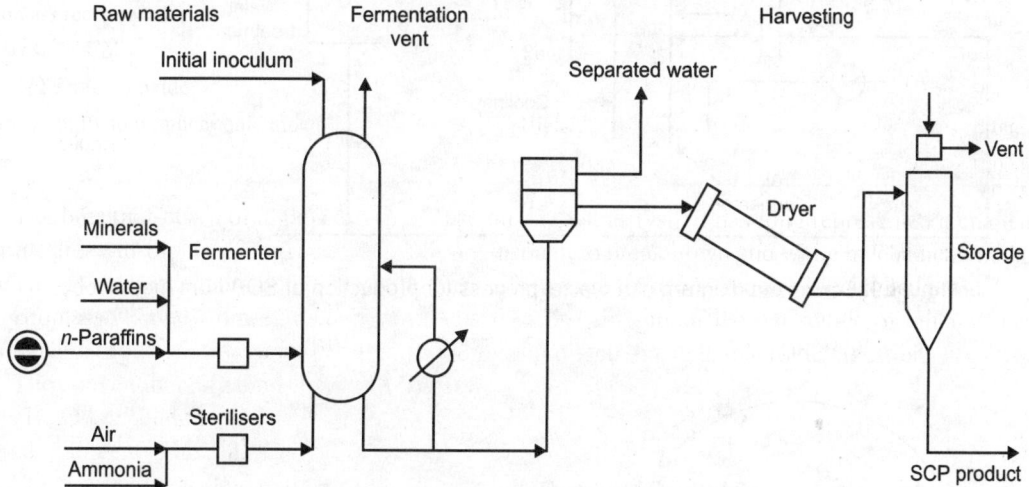

Fig. 18.8. BP *n*-paraffin SCP process.

The process outline for production of SCP from methanol by *Methylophilus methylotrophus* is illustrated in Fig. 18.9. The fermentation is run aseptically in the ICI pressure cycle fermenter. The nitrogen source is ammonia gas and pH is controlled between 6.0 and 7.0. Cell-specific growth rate is approximately 0.5 hr^{-1} and cell yield 0.5. Methanol is oxidised via dehydrogenation to formaldehyde which can either be assimilated for conversion to cell mass or further oxidised to CO_2 with concomitant energy production. In *Methylophilus*, formaldehyde is assimilated by the ribulose monophosphate pathway with ultimate conversion to fructose-6-phosphate (Fig. 18.10). Cells are recovered by agglomeration followed by centrifugation, flash-dried and ground. A feature of the process is the recycle of fermenter water.

The process outline for production of biomass or alcohol by *K. fragilis* grown on whey is illustrated in Fig. 18.11. Whey, which contains about 5 per cent lactose, 0.8 per cent protein, 0.7 minerals and 0.2–0.6 per cent lactic and, may require supplementation, with biotin. Biomass production requires and aerobic fermentation whereas aeration is minimal for ethanol production. For feed-grade biomass, the entire fermentation containing yeast, residual whey proteins, minerals and lactic acid may be recovered. For preparation of food-grade material, cells are harvested by centrifugation, washed and dried. Cell yield is 0.45–0.55 based on lactose consumed.

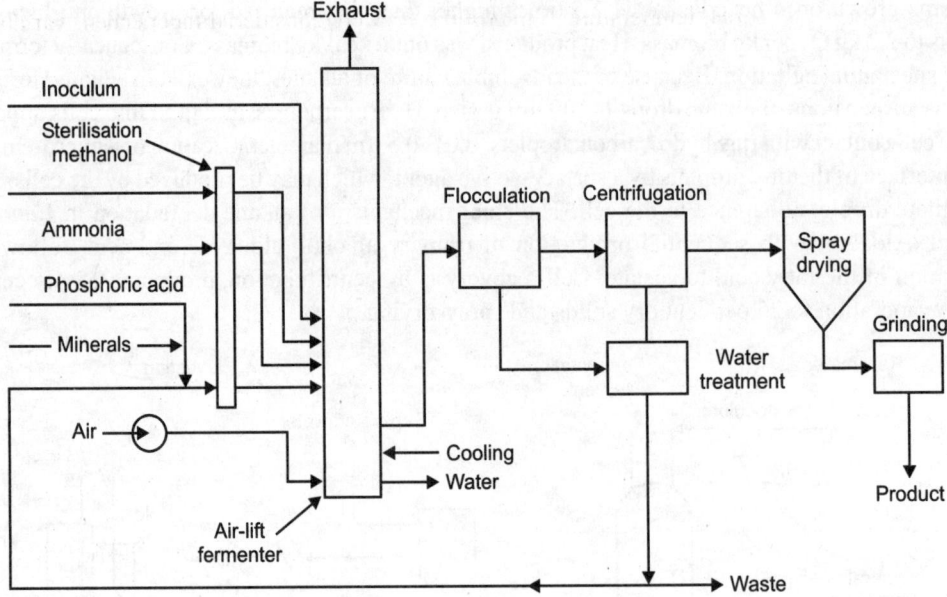

Fig. 18.9. Schematic diagram of a typical process for production of SCP from methanol.

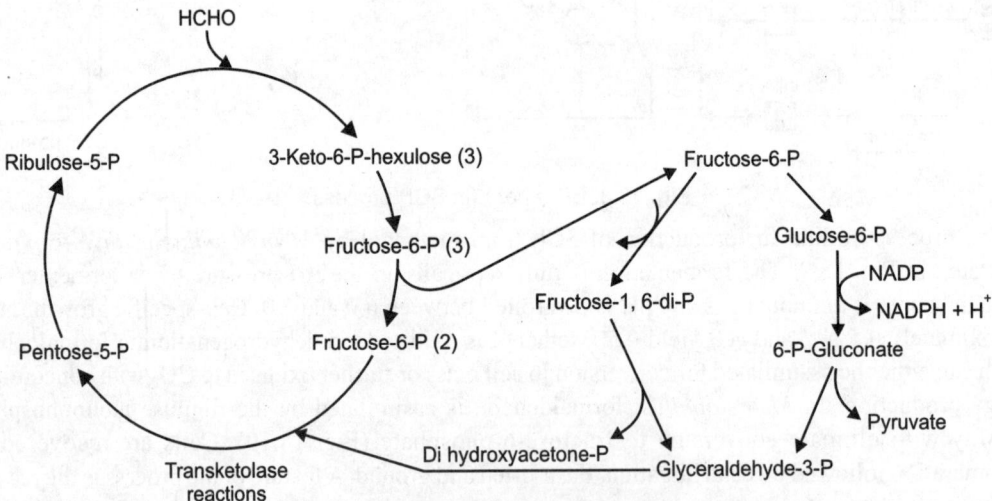

Fig. 18.10. Ribulose monophosphate cycle.

The RHM Mycoprotein fermentation process flow diagram is illustrated in Fig. 18.12. Medium constituents include food-grade glucose syrup, gaseous ammonia, salts and biotin. Fermentation pH is controlled at 6.0 by gaseous ammonia addition, fed into the air inlet stream. Cell concentrations are 15–20 kg m^{-3} and a specific growth rate of up to 0.2 hr^{-1} is achieved. Following cyclone separation and an RNA reduction step, cells are recovered by rotary vacuum filtration and formulated into a range of products.

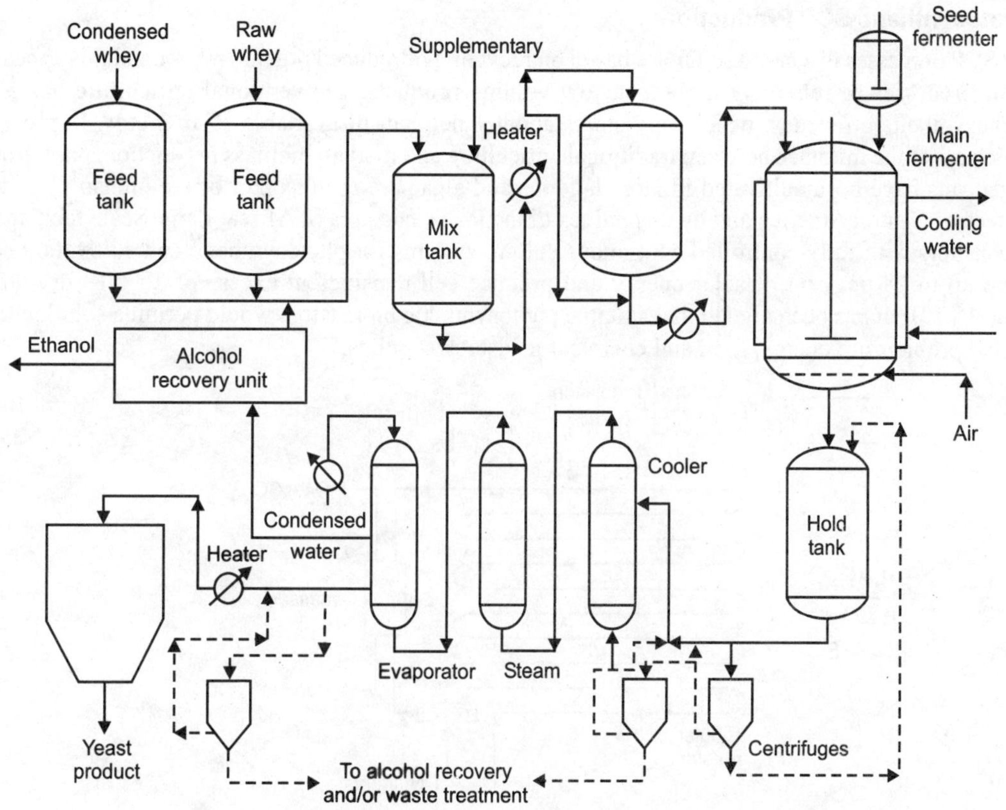

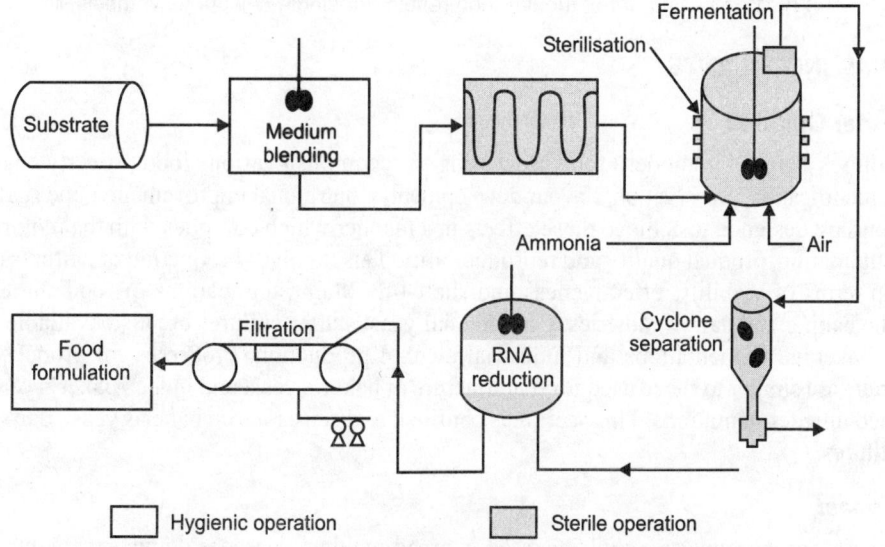

Fig. 18.11. Schematic diagram for production of alcohol and yeast from whey.

Fig. 18.12. The Rank Hovis McDougall Mycoprotein process.

Photosynthetic SCP Production

All SCP processes discussed so far are based on recycling of reduced organic matter and this appears to limit processes to relatively high-cost, low-volume products. Conventional agriculture has a low photosynthetic efficiency, which only stores about 1 per cent of available solar energy. In processes which are at the interface between traditional agriculture and modern biomass production, phototrophic organisms have been cultivated in large lagoons and algae are used as part of the human diet by the Aztecs of Central America and by the natives of the lake Chad area of Africa. Large-scale tubular loop bioreactors with fully-controlled continuous culture systems for photosynthetic cell cultivation could store up to 18 per cent of solar energy and produce cell densities in excess of 20 g l^{-1} dry weight (Fig. 18.13.). It has been argued that suitable photosynthetic bioreactors would permit a solution to the global problems of energy, food and chemical feedstock supplies.

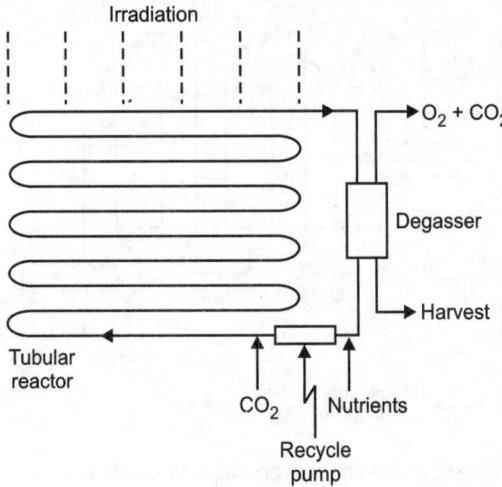

Fig. 18.13. Diagram of tubular-loop reactor for single-cell photosynthesis.

MICROBIAL INOCULANTS

Food Starter Cultures

Starter cultures are used in modern food processing to accomplish various food property changes such as texture modification, preservation, flavour development or nutritional improvement. Food starter culture applications are designed to achieve these effects in a manner which complies with the requirements of process automation, product quality and reproducibility. This involves production of cultures of defined activity in terms of viability, effectiveness and shelf-life. Major applications of food starter cultures exist in the baking and dairy industries. Commercial yeast starter cultures are also available for use in alcoholic beverage fermentations and industrial alcohol production. Processes for production of the latter starters are similar to those used for manufacture of baker's yeast and indeed baker's yeast is often used in alcoholic fermentations. This section is confined to discussions on baker's yeast, dairy and meat starter cultures.

Baker's yeast

Baker's yeast, *Saccharomyces cerevisiae*, used in bread-making, degrades dough sugars into a mixture of alcohol and carbon dioxide gas bubbles which become fixed in the dough. By excretion of compounds such as cysteine and glutathione, which breaks intramolecular disulphide bonds and by gas evolution, yeast acts to chemically modify and mechanically stretch gluten, the main protein of wheat.

Depending on environmental conditions, baker's yeast fermentations can be manipulated to favour alcohol production is optimised. Maximum theoretical biomass yield coefficient under these conditions is $\gamma_s = 0.075$. Under aerobic conditions in the presence of high sugar concentrations, a substantial level of alcohol is also formed due to the Crabtree effect. Maintenance of low sugar concentrations in aerated yeast fermentations by continuous sugar feeding favours biomass production.

Maximum theoretical biomass yield coefficient $\gamma_s = 0.54$. When excess oxygen is present, a yeast culture growing in 1.1 mM glucose (0.2 g l^{-1}) exhibits a maximum respiration rate (Q_{O_2}), a specific growth rate of $\mu = 0.2$–0.25 and negligible ethanol production. Under these conditions the respiratory quotient $(RQ = Q_{CO_2}/Q_{O_2})$ value is about 1.0. At increased glucose levels, respiration or oxygen transfer diminishes, ethanol is produced and the RQ value increases.

Molasses is the most widely used substrate for baker's yeast production. Molasses is generally deficient in nitrogen and phosphorus with respect to yeast nutritional requirements and needs to be supplemented with ammonium salts, orthophosphoric acid or other suitable phosphate forms. Biotin, which is required for growth of baker's yeast, is present in sufficient amounts in cane molasses but has to be added to beet molasses. Alternatively, a blend of beet with at least 20 per cent cane molasses may be used. Urea may replace ammonium salts as nitrogen source provided sufficient biotin, which is also required for urea hydrolysis, is incorporated in the medium.

Yeast production is a batch process involving up to eight scale-up stages. Typical production fermenter volumes are 50–350 m^3 or more. The first two inoculum stages usually involve aseptic fermentations. Later inoculum and production stages are usually not aseptic and do not involve pressure vessels. The final inoculum development stage and the main biomass production stage involve incremental molasses feeding. The principal objective of the main production stage is to achieve a high viable yield of yeast with an optimal balance of properties, high fermenting activity and good storage quality. Storage quality is improved by allowing some aeration to continue after molasses feeding is stopped which improves yeast uniformity and reduces RNA and protein synthesis.

In the production fermenter the aerobic fermentation is carried out at 28°–30°C and requires cooling since 3.5 kcal are generated per gram of yeast solids produced. The pH values range from 4.1 to 5.0. The pH values in the lower end of this range reduce bacterial contamination but tend to increase adsorption of molasses-colouring material. Most commercial fermentation processes start at lower pH value (4.0–4.4) and end at a higher pH range (4.8–5.0). Yeast concentrations of 40–60 g l^{-1} (dry) are obtained.

The amount of oxygen required for yeast growth is approximately 1 gram or 31 mM per gram of yeast solids. At the later stages of a yeast batch fermentation, yeast may be produced at a rate of up to 5 grams yeast solids per litre per hour, so that the fermenter aeration system must have an oxygen-transfer capability of approximately 150 mM per litre per hour. In general, efficient gas-sparged systems are used without impellers.

Solid-liquid separation is by continuous centrifugation (nozzle-type) to produce a yeast cream of 18–20 per cent, which is further concentrated to 27–28 per cent solids by rotary vacuum filtration during which starch may be used as a filter aid. Higher solids levels may be achieved by salting the cream prior to filtration, which reduces cellular moisture content osmotically. The crumbly cake produced by filtration is a widely marketed final product. Emulsifiers may be blended with the yeast cake to facilitate extrusion. Active dried yeast is usually produced using fluidised bed driers, whereby heated air is blown upwards through yeast particles at velocities capable of suspending the yeast in a fluid bed.

For rapid drying cycles of 10 and 30 minutes, air temperature of 100°–150°C are used at the start of the cycle while keeping the yeast temperature at 24°–40°C. The final moisture content is 7 per cent.

Starter cultures for the dairy industry

Micro-organisms are used in the manufacture of fermented dairy products to produce lactic acid, to secrete metabolites of characteristic flavour and to achieve other desirable chemical changes. The most important bacterial species involved as cheese-starter cultures are the mesophilic species *Streptococcus cremoris* and *Streptococcus lactis*, which are homofermentative, producing only lactic acid. For yoghurt manufacture the inoculum consist mainly of two thermophilic homofermentative starters, *Streptococcus thermophilus* and *Lactobacillus bulgaricus*, sometimes with *Lactobacillus acidophilus* incorporated at low levels. White moulds, *Penicillium camemberti* and its biotypes, *Penicillium candidum* and *Penicillium caseioculum*, are used in manufacture of surface mould-ripened cheese like Brie and Camembert and blue moulds such as *Penicillium roqueforti* are used in internal mould ripened cheeses such as Gorgonzola and Stilton.

Technology for fungal-spore production is relatively straightforward involving small-scale surface-culture methods. Spores are produced in powdered form by commercial culture firms.

Both bacterial mesophilic starter species are susceptible to invasion by bacteriophages, the major cause of starter failure in cheese-making and consequently the major thrust of starter-culture development is directed at overcoming problems related to bacteriophage infection. During the 1930s and 1940s crude mixed cheese-starter cultures were maintained by sub-culturing for years. Intensification of cheese-making through accelerated demand increased susceptibility of these crude cultivation practices to failure caused by bacteriophage. Single starter strains were introduced into commercial cheese-making and variability in starter activity became a serious problem. Measures taken to control bacteriophage contamination include aseptic starter propagation, sanitation of cheese-making equipment, use of enclosed cheese-making vats and shortening of ripening times. These practices were all insufficient to resolve the bacteriophage problem. From the 1950s; commercial culture suppliers provided freeze-dried and later frozen defined or undefined starter culture mixtures to cheese factories for both 'mother' or bulk starter preparation. Most of the *S. cremoris* and *S. lactis* strains were only sensitiye to specific number of phage type, and since sensitivity and resistance patterns differed among strains of an individual species, phage levels could be controlled by frequent rotation of phage-unrelated strains. Introduction of phage inhibitory media, containing phosphate salts to chelate the calcium required for bacteriophage propagation, minimised phage build-up during bulk starter preparation. Commercial concentrated cultures were introduced for direct inoculation of bulk starter tanks and later for direct cheese vat inoculation. Acceptable commercial dairy starter strains must be effective in acid and flavour production. Since the beginning of the 1980s, bacteriophage-insensitive strains have been successfully developed.

A flow diagram for large-scale production of lactic starter cultures is illustrated in Fig. 18.14. The objective of the fermentation and recovery process is to achieve a high yield of bacteriophage-free starter culture product. Fermentation media usually contain complex nutrients such as milk, whey, yeast extract, peptones, mono- or di-saccharides, vitamins, buffers, salts and phage-inhibiting constituents. Media may be sterilised by UHT processes. Optimum temperature for growth will vary depending on strain but is generally in the region 25°–30°C for streptococci and 30°–37°C for lactobacilli. pH control is desirable and generally in the range pH 5.4–6.3, with pH 6.0 preferred, using ammonia gas, other alkalis or internal buffering. The fermentation is usually agitated by gentle stirring. After the fermentation is complete, the broth is cooled and may be concentrated aseptically by filtration to yield a culture concentrate for direct inoculation or for storage by freezing or freeze-drying.

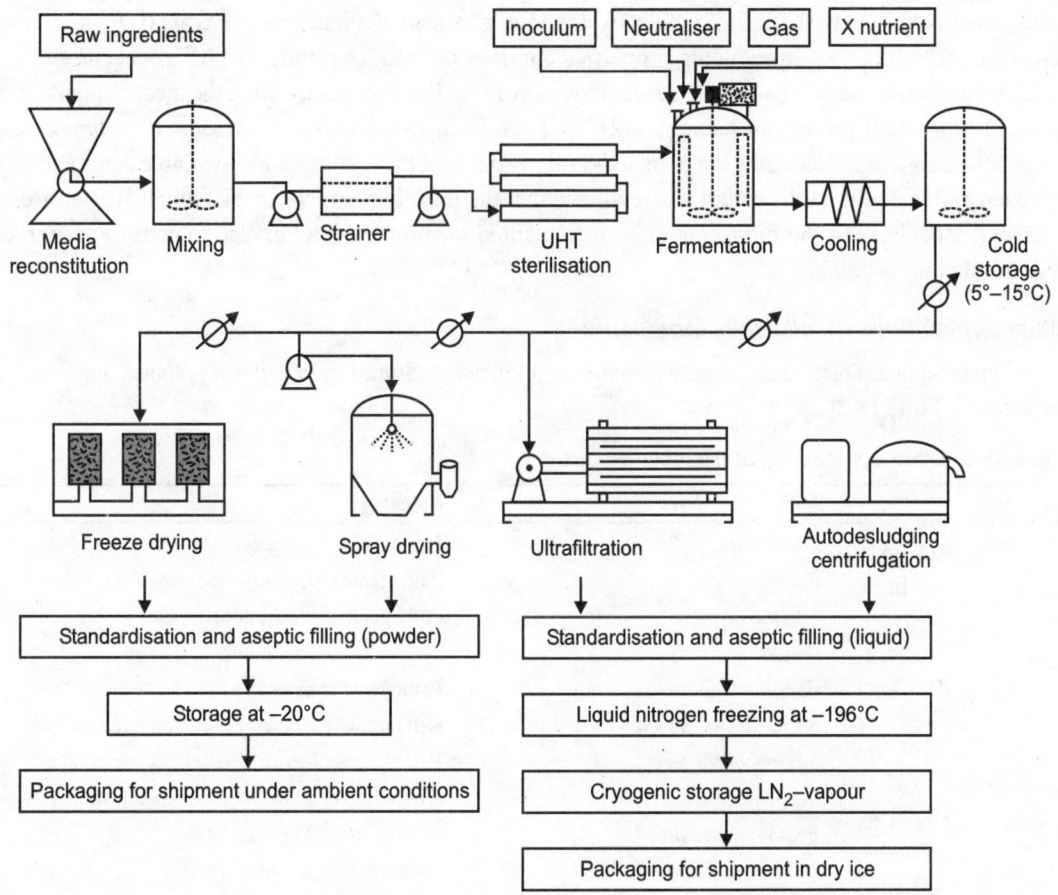

Fig. 18.14. Flow scheme for large-scale production of lactic starter cultures.

Meat starter cultures

The primary objective of fermenting meats is for preservation purposes. A microbial fermentation results in acid development which causes moisture removal, provides a desirable safety margin, improves stability and produces quality-related properties such as flavours and aromas which have not been duplicated solely by use of chemical additives. The majority of fermented meat products consist of dry and semi-dry sausages. Technical improvements in sausage-making were achieved by use of added sugar, to encourage rapid production of lactic acid, and the use of nitrate, which lowers the oxidation reduction potential of the meat as nitrate is converted to nitrite. This results is stabilisation of meat colour by preventing haemoglobin oxidation, provides an environment which favours micro-aerophilic lactic acid producers and suppresses development of undesirable bacteria. Desirable characteristics of meat starter cultures are (i) their ability to produce lactic acid, (ii) their tolerance to salts, spices, nitrate and nitrite and (iii) their capacity to reduce nitrate. More recently, the industry has moved towards using nitrite rather than nitrate, thereby eliminating the requirement for nitrate-reducing starters in some meat fermentations.

Organisms which have been successfully exploited as meat starter culture inoculants are (i) *Pediococcus cerevisiae*, which has acid-producing properties but does not reduce nitrate, (ii) *Micrococcus* species which reduce nitrate and contain catalase to remove any peroxides produced during the meat fermentation, and (iii) other acid-producing bacteria such as *Lactobacillus plantarum*, *Lactobacillus brevis* and *Leuconostoc mesenteroides*. Single and mixed-strain variants of these cultures are available commercially in frozen and freeze-dried form and it is predicted that the meat industry will make much greater use of microbial inoculants in the future not only in fermented meat processes but also to control growth of undesirable micro-organisms.

Other applications of microbial inoculants

Microbial inoculants are used in a variety of non-food application. Some key existing or potential applications are listed in Table 18.3.

Table 18.3. Other applications of microbial inoculants.

Application	Microbial species	Function
Insecticides	*Bacillus thuringiensis*	Pathogenic to lepidoptera larvae
	Bacillus popilliae	Pathogenic to Japanese beetle
	Bacillus alvei	Pathogenic to mosquitoes
	Bacillus circulans	Pathogenic to mosquitoes
	Bacillus sphaericus	Pathogenic to mosquitoes
	Serratia piscatorum	Kill butterfly larvae by reducing intestinal pH
	Streptococcus faecalis	Kill butterfly larvae by reducing intestinal pH
	Aerobacter aerogenes	Kill butterfly larvae by reducing intestinal pH
	Beauveria tenella	Pathogenic to May bug larvae
	Veticillium lecanii	Controls aphids and white flies
	Hirsutella thompsonii	Controls mites on citrus plants
	Metarrhizium sp.	Controls lepidoptera species
Mineral cycling	*Thiobacillus* spp.	Sulphur oxidation
	Beggiatoa spp.	Oxidises H_2S in rice soils
	Bacillus megaterium	Phosphate mineralisation and phosphorus
	Bacillus, pseudomonas	dissolution
	Chromobacterium spp.	
Nitrogen fixation	Free-living and symbiotic nitrogen-fixing prokaryotes	Emphasis on production of legume inoculants of *Rhizobium* species to increase nitrogen fixation
Plant growth acceleration using mycorrhizal fungi	Endomycorrhizae of the family Endogonaceae, phylum Zygomycota (vesicular-arbuscular fungi). Ectomycorrhizae of the phylum Dikaryomycota-majority are Basidiomycetes	Increased root nutrient and water uptake, protection against disease

(Contd...)

Application	Microbial species	Function
Silage-making	*Streptococcus faecium, Lactobacillus plantarum*, other acid-producing bacteria	pH reduction to accelerate ensilation
Probiotics	*Lactobacillus acidophilus, Streptococcus faecium*, rumen bacteria	Increase digestibility of animal feeds
Waste treatment	Methanogens	Anaerobic digestion
	Pseudomonas spp. *Acinetobacter* spp. and *Nocardia* spp.	Degrade alkanes and recalcitrant waste compounds
	Extracellular enzyme-producing bacteria	Hydrolyse waste proteins, carbohydrates and fats

Chapter 19

Production of Baker's Yeast

HISTORICAL INTRODUCTION

It is not known when yeast was first used to bake bread. The first records that show this use came from Ancient Egypt. Researchers speculate that a mixture of flour meal and water was left longer than usual on a warm day and the yeasts that occur in natural contaminants of the flour caused it to ferment before baking. The resulting bread would have been lighter and more tasty than the normal flat, hard cake. It is generally assumed that the earliest forms of leavening were likely very similar to modern sourdough; the leavening action of yeast would have been discovered from its action on flatbread doughs, and would either have been cultivated separately or transferred from batch to batch by means of previously mixed ('old') dough. Alternately, the development of leavened bread seems to have developed in close proximity to the development of beer brewing, and barm from the beer fermentation process can also be used in bread making.

Without a full understanding of microbiology, early bakers would have had little ability to directly control yeast cultures, but still kept locally interesting cultures by reusing doughs and starters to leaven later batches. However, it became possible to isolate and propagate favoured yeast strains in the same manner as was done in the beer industry, and it eventually became practical to propagate yeast in a slurry with a composition similar to beer wort, usually including barley malt and wheat flour. Such cultures (sometimes referred to in old American cookery as 'emptins', from their origins as the dregs of beer or cider fermentation) would become the ancestors of modern baker's yeast, as they generally were carefully maintained to avoid what would later be discovered to be bacterial contamination, including using preservatives such as hops as well as boiling the growth medium.

Later refinements in microbiology following the work of Louis Pasteur led to more advanced methods of culturing pure strains, making modern commercial yeast possible, and turning yeast production into a major industrial endeavour. The slurry yeast made by small bakers and grocery shops became cream yeast, a suspension of live yeast cells in growth medium, and then compressed yeast, the fresh cake yeast that became the standard leaven for bread bakers in much of the Westernised world during the early 20th century.

Today there are several retailers of baker's yeast; the biggest producers are Fleischmann's yeast and Lesaffre (who also owns the popular American label red star yeast). During World War II Fleischmann's developed a granulated active dry yeast for the United States armed forces, which did not require refrigeration and had a longer shelf life and better temperature tolerance than fresh yeast; it is still the standard yeast for US military recipes. The company created yeast that would rise twice as fast, cutting down on baking time. Lesaffre would later create instant yeast in the 1970s, which has gained considerable use and market share at the expense of both fresh and dry yeast in their various applications.

OUTLINE OF PRODUCTION OF BAKER'S YEAST

Baker's yeast is a major raw material in the baking process.

Product requires good bake activity (rapid fermentation in doughs of high osmotic pressure) along with good shelf-life, after storage at low moisture levels. Bakers yeast is an example of a relatively low value product produced on a large scale.

Sucrose hydrolysed externally using sucrase secreted by the cell. The resultant monosaccharides diffuse into the yeast where it is degraded to pyruvate via glycolysis or converted to storage carbohydrates via anabolic pathways.

A Respiratory bottleneck exists in pyruvate transfer to the mitochondrion (TCA cycle). If rate of pyruvate production via glycolysis exceeds the rate of pyruvate transfer to the mitochondrion, a pool of excess pyruvate is maintained. Excess pyruvate leads to rapid conversion of the excess to ethanol via acetaldehyde. This is energy inefficient as a catabolic proces—lower energy generation means lower biomass yields.

Storage carbohydates very important, resuscitation of organism dependant on acceptable levels of storage carbohydrates in the yeast. Their presence and quantity totally dependant on the organisms growth rate. *S. cerevisiae* regulates budding using storage carbohydrates—this means that the organism can maintain a consistent doubling time irrespective of oscillating environmental conditions.

High growth rate—large fraction of cells budding, low levels of storage carbohydrates. Low growth rate—small fraction of cells budding, better levels of storage carbohydrates. Therefore, we need to control this metabolic phenomenon using process technology possibilities to consider for fermentation process. Aerobic batch culture—no control of metabolism. Large levels of fermentation (ethanol production). Continuous culturing—no down time, no cleaning time, continuous production of product, control of growth rate through dilution rate, accumulation of storage carbohydrates at low growth rates. Let's consider the product requirements.

Product when inoculated into the dough does not require several doublings (2.75×10^8 cells ml^{-1} at the start, 3.00×10^8 cells ml^{-1} at the end)—just rapidly ferments based on the original innoculum size.

This means that trace contamination is acceptable as it will not establish itself in the bread quickly enough. If trace contamination is acceptable, requirement for clean not sterile conditions. Clean conditions drastically reduce process overheads and downstream processing overheads. However, it is difficult to operate continuous culture under clean conditions (non-sterile) trace contaminants rapidly establish themselves in continuous culture, becoming a significant proportion of the biomass over long periods of time.

Fed Batch culture has all the advantages of batch and continuous culture. Controllability of continuous culture ($D = F/V$).

Batch nature of batch culture (periodical shutdown prevents the establishment of trace contaminants).

Another feature of fed batch—at fixed F gradual slowing down in V—allows the accumulation of storage carbohydrates, trehalose and glycogen.

Media formulation and preparation molasses (by-product of sugar manufacturing industry) is received by the plant at approximately 80°Brix (55 per cent sucrose).

The molasses is diluted to 40°Brix and clarified for fermentation. Molasses is not an adequate media: nitrogen (ammonia, ammonium sulphate and urea), phosphorous sources (orthophosphates or phosphoric acid), vitamin (biotin and thiamin) and mineral supplements (magnesium and others) are added. The main characteristics of commercial products are given in Table 19.1.

Table 19.1. Main characteristics of commercial products.

Product	Form	Method of drying	Dry matter (%)	Protein (%)[a]	Gas evolution (ml)[b]
Compressed yeast	Blocks or granules		27–34	42–56	300–400
Active dry yeast	Irregular spheres	Rotolouver	92–94	40–43	160–185
	Irregular particles	Belt	92–94	40–43	140–160
Instant dry yeast	Small rods	Fluidised bed	94–96	42–52	230–340

[a]Defined 85 Kjeldshl-6.25 on dry weight basis.
[b]Defined as millilitres of CO_2 produced in 165 minutes per 285 mg of yeast dry matter in a standard dough consisting of flour, water yeast and salt at 28°C.

Process Considerations

Low value product—need to produce on a large scale using low cost substrate source. Fermentation process—fed batch, aerobic process, effective mixing required for product consistency. Fermentation performed at 30°C for 24 hours.

Process Technology

Large vessels cylindroconical in nature 100–200 m^3 in size. Two approaches to mixing—aeration only or conventional stirred tank bioreactors (aeration and agitation). Agitation provides more extensive mixing and more efficient power input for turbulent flow. Aeration—no moving parts, less mechanical failure, easier to clean. Typical system, horizontal tube with several orifices, result—lots of small bubbles, better interfacial area for mass transfer. Reported system, 30,000 holes, 1.5 mm diameter.

Proprietary aeration systems—result: good mixing without mechanical agitation.

Vogelbusch system: Airflow is self priming, a vacuum in the head space pulls air through a sparger mechanism located just below the top surface of the broth. The high velocity of the sparger dispersed air, results in penetration by the gas flow to the bottom of the bioreactor. This results in extremely turbulent flow. This is accompanied by the injection of fine bubbles into the base of the reactor. These bubbles are further dispersed as they rise into the turbulent regions of the bioreactor.

Types of Baker's Yeast

Active dried yeast, a granulated form in which yeast is commercially sold. Baker's yeast is available in a number of different forms. Though each version has certain advantages over the others, the choice of which form to use is largely a question of the requirements of the recipe at hand and the training of the cook preparing it. With occasional allowances for liquid content and temperature, the different forms of commercial yeast are generally considered interchangeable.

1. Cream yeast is the closest form to the yeast slurries of the 19th century, being essentially a suspension of yeast cells in liquid, siphoned off from the growth medium. Its primary use is in industrial bakeries with special high-volume dispensing and mixing equipment, and it is not readily available to small bakeries or home cooks.

2. Compressed yeast is essentially cream yeast with most of the liquid removed. It is best known in the form of cake yeast, which is essentially a soft solid, beige in colour, but is also available in crumbled form for bulk usage. It is highly perishable; though formerly widely available for the consumer market, it has become less common in supermarkets in some countries due to its poor keeping properties, having been obsoleted in some such markets by active dry and instant yeast. It is still widely available for commercial use, and is somewhat more tolerant of low temperatures than other forms of commercial yeast; however, even there, instant yeast has made significant market inroads.

3. Active dry yeast is the form of yeast most commonly available to noncommercial bakers, as well as the yeast of choice for situations where long travel or uncontrolled storage conditions are likely. It consists of coarse oblong granules of yeast, with live yeast cells encapsulated in a thick jacket of dry, dead cells with some growth medium. Under most conditions, active dry yeast must be proofed or rehydrated first and, despite its better keeping qualities than other forms, is generally considered more sensitive than other forms to thermal shock when actually used in recipes. Active dry yeast also provides an alternative to butter and salt for seasoning pop corn.

4. Instant yeast appears similar to active dry yeast, but has smaller granules with substantially higher percentages of live cells. It is more perishable than active dry yeast, but also does not require rehydration, and can usually be added directly to all but the driest doughs. Instant yeast generally has a small amount of ascorbic acid added as a preservative. Some producers provide two or more forms of instant yeast in their product portfolio; for example, LeSaffre's 'SAF instant Gol' is designed specifically for doughs with high sugar contents.

5. Rapid-rise yeast is a variety of yeast (usually a form of instant yeast) designed to provide greater carbon dioxide output to allow faster rising at the expense of shortened fermentation times. There is considerable debate as to the value of such a product; while most baking experts believe it reduces the flavour potential of the finished product. Rapid-rise yeast is often marketed specifically for use in bread machines.

6. Flake yeast is dead yeast, sold primarily as a nutritional supplement. It has little to no leavening power.

For most commercial uses, yeast of any form is packaged in bulk (blocks or freezer bags for fresh yeast; vacuum-packed brick bags for dry or instant); however, yeast for home use is often packaged in premeasured doses, either small squares for compressed yeast or sealed packets for dry or instant. A single dose (reckoned for the average bread recipe of between 500 g and 1000 g of dough) is generally about 2.5 tsp or about 7 g, though comparatively lesser amounts are used when the yeast is used in a preferment.

Baking

Baking is the technique of prolonged cooking of food by dry heat acting by convection, and not by radiation, normally in an oven, but also in hot ashes, or on hot stones. It is primarily used for the preparation of bread, cakes, pastries and pies, tarts, quiches and cookies. Such items are sometimes referred to as 'baked goods', and are sold at a bakery. A person who prepares baked goods as a profession is called a baker. It is also used for the preparation of baked potatoes, baked apples, baked beans, some pasta dishes such as lasagne, and various other foods, such as the pretzel.

Many commercial ovens are provided with two heating elements: one for baking, using convection and conduction to heat the food, and one for broiling or grilling, heating mainly by radiation. Meat may be baked, but is more often roasted, a similar process, using higher temperatures and shorter cooking times.

The baking process does not add any fat to the product, and producers of snack products such as potato chips are also beginning to replace the process of deep-frying with baking in order to reduce the fat content of their products.

The dry heat of baking changes the form of starches in the food and causes its outer surfaces to brown, giving it an attractive appearance and taste, while partially sealing in the food's moisture. The browning is caused by caramelisation of sugars and the Maillard reaction. Moisture is never really entirely 'sealed in', however; over time, an item being baked will become dry. This is often an advantage, especially in situations where drying is the desired outcome, for example in drying herbs or in roasting certain types of vegetables. The most common baked item is bread. Variations in the ovens, ingredients and recipes used in the baking of bread result in the wide variety of breads produced around the world.

Some foods are surrounded with moisture during baking by placing a small amount of liquid (such as water or broth) in the bottom of a closed pan, and letting it steam up around the food, a method commonly known as braising or slow baking.

With the passage of time breads harden; they become stale. This is not primarily due to moisture being lost from the baked products, but more a reorganisation of the way in which the water and starch are associated over time. This process is similar to recrystallisation, and is promoted by storage at cool temperatures, such as in a domestic refrigerator.

Ingredients often used in baking are: flour, butter, margarine or other shortening, sugar, egg, salt, leavening agents, baking powder, baking soda and yeast.

The production of baker's yeast is the largest domestic use of a micro-organism for food purposes. Baker's yeast is a strain of *Saccharomyces cerevisiae*. The strain of the yeast is carefully selected for its capacity to produce abundant gas quickly, its viability during ordinary storage, and its ability to produce desirable flavour.

The organisms are mixed with bread dough to bring about vigorous sugar fermentation. The carbon dioxide produced during the fermentation is responsible for leavening or rising of the dough.

A pure culture of the selected strain of yeast is first grown in the laboratory and gradually built up to larger and larger volume by transfer from the test tube to the fermenter tank. Great care is taken to prevent contamination at any stage of development of the culture.

During manufacturing, the strain is inoculated into a medium which frequently contains molasses and corn steep liquor as sources of carbon, nitrogen and mineral salts. The reaction of the medium is adjusted to pH 4.4 to 4.6.

The inoculated medium is incubated at a temperature of 25° to 26°C, and is aerated during the incubation period. Yeasts oxidise sugars under aerobic conditions with the liberation of energy. A large part of this energy is utilised for the synthesis of cell protoplasm. The yeast cells multiply rapidly and exhaust the sugar supply within 10 hours.

At the end of incubation the yeast cells are removed from the fermented medium by centrifugation, washed and mixed with starch or corn meal, and then being pressed into cake form.

Yeast cakes must be kept cool to preserve the cells and to prevent spoilage by other micro-organisms. They may also be dried. Dried yeast remains viable for several months. Yeasts are rich in vitamins and in most of the essential amino acids required by man and animals.

YEAST STRAINS

Although genetic analyses and transformation can be performed with a number of taxonomically distinct varieties of yeast, extensive studies have been limited primarily to the many freely interbreeding species of the budding yeast *Saccharomyces* and to the fission yeast *Schizosaccharomyces pombe*. Although '*Saccharomyces cerevisiae*' is commonly used to designate many of the laboratory stocks of *Saccharomyces* used throughout the world, it should be pointed out that most of these strains originated from the interbred stocks of Winge, Lindegren and others who employed fermentation markers not only from *S. cerevisiae* but also from *S. bayanus*, *S. carlsbergensis*, *S. chevalieri*, *S. chodati*, *S. diastaticus* etc. Nevertheless, it is still recommended that the interbreeding laboratory stocks of *Saccharomyces* be denoted as *S. cerevisiae*, in order to conveniently distinguish them from the more distantly related species of *Saccharomyces*.

Care should be taken in choosing strains for genetic and biochemical studies. Unfortunately there are no truly wild-type *Saccharomyces* strains that are commonly employed in genetic studies. Also, most domesticated strains of brewers' yeast and probably many strains of bakers' yeast and true wild-type strains of *S. cerevisiae* are not genetically compatible with laboratory stocks. It is often not appreciated that many 'normal' laboratory strains contain mutant characters. This condition arose because these laboratory strains were derived from pedigrees involving mutagenised strains, or strains that carry genetic markers. Many current genetic studies are carried out with one or another of the following strains or their derivatives, and these strains have different properties that can greatly influence experimental outcomes: S288C; W303; D273–10B; X2180; A364A; Σ1278B; AB972; SK1; and FL100. The haploid strain S288C (*MATα SUC2 mal mel gal2 CUP1 flo1 flo8-1 hap1*) is often used as a normal standard because the sequence of its genome has been determined, because many isogenic mutant derivatives are available, and because it gives rise to well-dispersed cells.

However, S288C contains a defective HAP1 gene, making it incompatible with studies of mitochondrial and related systems. Also, in contrast to Σ1278B, S288C does not form pseudohyae. While true wild-type and domesticated bakers' yeast give rise to less than 2 per cent *p*-colonies, many laboratory strains produce high frequencies of *p*-mutants. Another strain, D273-10B, has been extensively used as a typical normal yeast, especially for mitochondrial studies. One should examine the specific characters of interest before initiating a study with any strain. Also, there can be a high degree of inviability of the meiotic progeny from crosses among these 'normal' strains.

Many strains containing characterised auxotrophic, temperature-sensitive, and other markers can be obtained from the yeast genetics stock culture centre of the American type culture collection, including an almost complete set of deletion strains. Currently this set consists of 20,382 strains representing deletants of nearly all nonessential ORFs in different genetic backgrounds. Deletion strains are also available from EUROSCARF and research genetics.

RAW MATERIALS

Ever since the 1920s, molasses has been the principal raw material in the production of baker's yeast. Both beet and cane molasses are used, separately or as a mixture, to supply fermentable supra as the major source of carbon and energy, together with minerals, trace elements, vitamins, and some organic nitrogen (amino acids). Additional nitrogen, in the form of ammonia, ammonium salts or urea and phosphorus (as phosphoric acid or phosphates) must always be supplied. Often some extra magnesium and/or zinc has to be added. When a mixture of beet molasses, with at least 20 per cent of cane molasses, is applied, no extra biotin supplement is needed; when pure cane molasses is used, pantothenate addition may be necessary. Although most molasses contain enough thiamine for optimum yeast growth, this vitamin is frequently added, since it stimulates the dough-leavening activity of the yeast.

One might conclude that molasses is not far from the ideal substrate for baker's yeast production. Certainly there is some truth in this conclusion. However, molasses may also contain harmful compounds deleterious to the growth yield and/or the quality of the yeast. These compounds include colloids and suspended solids, colouring substances, sulphurous acid, nitrates and nitrites, such substances as fungicides and sanitising agents (used at the sugar factory), short-chain fatty acids (especially butyric acid, which is highly toxic for yeast), hydroxymethylfurfural, and a vast number of compounds at the ppm-ppb level.

Carbon and Energy Sources

The main carbon and energy source present in molasses is sucrose. This disaccharide is hydrolysed to glucose and fructose by the enzyme invertase. Baker's yeast may express periplasmic as well as cytoplasmic invertase; these two enzymes are encoded by a single gene but are synthesised from different mRNAs.

Synthesis of invertase, as well as such other enzymes as maltase, galactokinase, cytochromes and gluconeogenic and glyoxylate bypass enzymes, is prevented by the presence of glucose in the medium. This phenomenon is termed glucose repression. Analogous to the situation in *Escherichia coli*, the term 'catabolite repression' has been used, but in yeast no evidence has been obtained for a role of a metabolite (e.g. cAMP) as an important effector in this respect. It has been suggested that regulation of invertase synthesis by glucose takes place at the levels of transcription, translation and maturation of the enzyme prior to excretion.

Evidence has been obtained indicating an important role for hexokinase PII in glucose repression. Hexokinase PII, one of two hexokinase isoenzymes, is 76 per cent homologous with hexokinase PI. Therefore, the difference between these two proteins must be involved in glucose repression. A part of hexokinase PII is likely to serve as a glucose detector, giving the triggering signal for glucose repression.

After exhaustion of glucose from the medium, specific genes responsible for release of glucose repression are activated. Until recently, explanation of the global regulatory system of glucose (de)repression at the molecular level remained confined to a nonspecified function of certain genes resulting in synthesis or prevention of synthesis, of enzymes such as invertase. Now it has become clear that the SNF1 gene (which stands for sucrose nonfermenting = CCR1), which is essential for release of invertase synthesis from glucose repression, encodes in fact a serine/threonine-specific protein kinase. This observation implies that protein phosphorylation serves as a signal in the process of glucose (de)repression. Unravelling the function of other genes required for release of glucose repression will indicate whether protein phosphorylation plays an essential role in glucose (de)repression.

The first step in the metabolism of glucose is its transport across the plasma membrane. The molecular mechanisms involved in transport of glucose by *Saccharomyces cerevisiae* have been the subject of discussion for years. There is general agreement, that glucose is transported via a facilitated mechanism. Controversy exists, however, about whether phosphorylation of glucose is a requirement for its transport. According to this hypothesis, polyphosphate localised at the periplasmic face serves as a P_i-source. Other models imply a close linkage of hexokinase with the glucose carrier, suggesting that glucose is phosphorylated in the cytoplasm in an ATP-consuming reaction catalysed by hexokinase. An association of hexokinase with the glucose carrier has not been observed, however.

As a compromise between these two models, a third hypothesis was formulated according to which the glucose carrier is phosphorylated at the expense of periplasmic polyphosphate. The phosphorylated carrier is recognised subsequently by cytoplasmic hexokinase, which phosphorylates the sugar. This model is in accordance with all experimental data, but more evidence is required in order to obtain general support.

S. cerevisiae exhibits two different types of transport system for glucose and fructose. For glucose, a high-affinity ($K_m \sim 2$ mM) and a low affinity ($K_m \sim 15$ mM) system have been described. The high-affinity component is subject to glucose repression. Fructose, on other hand, was shown to be transported by a high-affinity, low-capacity proton symport mechanism, in a strain of *S. cerevisiae*.

Nitrogen Sources

Since molasses does not contain sufficient amounts of assimilable nitrogen compounds to allow commercial yeast production, ammonia or urea is added during fermentation. Based on experiments with ^{14}C methylamine as an analogue for NH_4^+, evidence was obtained for the presence of two specific transport systems for NH_4^+, in baker's yeast, distinguished by a difference in affinity and V_{max}. The high-affinity uptake system ($K_m = 0.25$ mM) shows a relatively low V_{max}, whereas the high K_m carrier ($K_m = 2$ mM) exhibits a relatively high V_{max}. In addition, *S. cerevisiae* contains a nonspecific uptake system for monovalent cations, including NH_4^+. The mechanism for NH_4^+ transport is described as a secondary facilitated system associated with antiport of protons.

The extrusion of protons in media with NH_4^+ as a nitrogen source is the main reason for acidification of the medium.

The incorporation of ammonia in glutamic acid is catalysed by an NADPH-dependent glutamate dehydrogenase in *S. cerevisiae*. The yeast GDH1 gene encoding this enzyme has been cloned and sequenced. The alternative pathway for NH_4^+ assimilation, which is functional in various micro-organisms during nitrogen limitation proceeds via a coupled pathway involving glutamate synthetase and glutamine synthetase. Since *S. cerevisiae* expresses low activities of glutamate synthetase which do not increase during nitrogen limitation, it is generally considered unlikely that this pathway plays a significant role.

Glutamate serves as a source of nitrogen in the biosynthesis of other metabolites such as amino acids. Various L-amino acids may serve as sole nitrogen sources for *S. cerevisiae*. In addition to specific uptake systems for several amino acids, a general amino acid permease may be expressed which also shows affinity for D-amino acids. Not only is this general amino acid carrier inhibited by NH_4^+ ions, its synthesis is also prevented by the presence of ammonia. It has been shown that the latter type of regulation by NH_4^+ or a metabolite of NH_4^+, is effected at the level of transcription. This phenomenon, known as N-metabolite repression, has been discussed in detail.

Mammalian cells carry amino acids membranes via the glutathione cycle. Since it was found that baker's yeast expresses all enzymes involved, it was postulated that this cycle would play a significant role in the transport of amino acids. Subsequently it was argued, however, that the *in vivo* turnover rate of glutathione was too low to be of importance in this respect. Recently at least one of the glutathione cycle enzymes, γ-glutamyl transpeptidase, has been localised in the yeast vacuole. This finding leaves the intriguing possibility that in yeast, transport of amino acids across the vacuolar membrane would involve a glutathione cycle.

Oligopeptides may be transported as such across the plasma membrane by a transport system that is not inhibited by amino acids. The carrier functions independently of intracellular hydrolysis of the peptides.

Glutamate is an excellent nitrogen source for many yeasts. Its catabolism is catalysed by an NAD-dependent glutamate dehydrogenase in *S. cerevisiae*, yielding NH_4^+ and α-ketoglutarate. Since the biosynthesis of glutamine and carbamoyl phosphate requires ammonium ions, such catabolism of glutamate will occur when it is applied as the sole nitrogen source.

NAD-dependent glutamate dehydrogenase may be inactivated rapidly by the addition of NH_4^+ to cells growing on glutamate. It was shown that this is effected by a reversible phosphorylation of the enzyme, leading to a decrease in affinity for glutamate. This regulation system in combination with N-metabolite repression, is required to prevent excessive formation of intracellular ammonia. During severe nitrogen starvation intracellular proteins are hydrolysed by various proteases and peptidases in *S. cerevisiae*. Characterisation of enzymes involved intracellular proteolysis has progressed rapidly.

In Japan, in Latin America and elsewhere, urea instead of ammonia is applied as a nitrogen source for the industrial production of baker's yeast. *S. cerevisiae* expresses a constitutive low affinity, secondary facilitated transport system (K_m = 2.5 mM) far urea. When urea and ammonia concentrations are low, a high-affinity, secondary facilitated transport system for urea is derepressed (K_m = 14 µM). Assimilation of urea-N consumes more energy than with NH_4^+, since before glutamate synthesis urea is carboxylated in an ATP- and biotin-requiring reaction to allophanate which is subsequently hydrolysed to ammonia and carbon dioxide.

Vitamins

Baker's yeast requires biotin for growth, and compressed yeast contains about 0.75 to 2.5 ppm of this vitamin (dry weight basis). Cane molasses supplies ample amounts of biotin (0.5 to 0.8 ppm); beet molasses does not (0.01 to 0.02 ppm). Therefore, at least 20 per cent of cane molasses has to be blended with beet molasses in the preparation of the feed wort, or the fed has to be supplemented with synthetic biotin. For optimum growth it is also advisable to supplement the thiamin content of molasses with this vitamin. Thiamin is almost quantitatively taken up by baker's yeast during growth. Sufficient thiamin is usually added to the medium to obtain a content of 50 to 10 µg per g of final yeast solids because it improves the activity of compressed yeast in dough systems.

Minerals

For growth and good performance in fermentations, baker's yeast requires the addition of phosphates. The amounts added should give a final composition of the yeast of 2.5 to 3.5 per cent P_2O_5 for yeasts containing 7 to 9.5 per cent nitrogen (all based on dry weights). Phosphates are almost quantitatively taken up by the yeast during growth. The common sources of phosphorus are phosphoric acid, alkali phosphate salts, or ammonium phosphate. The latter can also serve as a source of nitrogen.

Molasses contains sufficient potassium to supply the requirements of yeast for this element. The same is generally true of calcium, but molasses has to be supplemented with a magnesium salt, generally magnesium sulphate. Molasses contains sufficient sources of sodium and sulphur to supply the elements. Yeast ash contains 0.4 to 0.5 per cent sodium as NaO_2 and 0.2 to 0.25 per cent sulphate as SO_3. If sodium chloride is added to yeast cream to aid in its filtration, the sodium concentrations may be somewhat higher.

Baker's yeast also requires the presence of some elements in trace amounts. These are Fe, Zn, Cu, Mn and Mo although the information in the scientific literature leaves some doubt as to whether these are the only trace elements required. As with vitamins, requirements are generally expressed in terms of nutrient concentration in the medium without reference to the amount of yeast grown. Therefore, quantitative interpretation is difficult. In general such trace elements are supplied in sufficient quantity by molasses with the possible exception of zinc. This metal may be added in the form of zinc sulphate.

Fermentation Activators and Inhibitors

Many products have been reported to be activators of yeast growth, such as flour milling waste, sludge from aerobic digesters, etc.

SO_2 inhibits yeast growth but concentrations up to 800 ppm in molasses can be well tolerated. *S. cerevisiae* adapts well to the presence of even higher concentrations of SO_2 as is known from the use of this species in the wine industry where fermentations are often carried out in the presence of 80 to 100 ppm of SO_2.

Molasses contains variable amounts of nitrate which can be reduced to nitrite by bacterial action during the production of yeast.

Leavening Agent

A leavening agent (also leavening or leaven) is any one of a number of substances used in doughs and batters that cause a foaming action which lightens and softens the finished product. The leavening agent—biological, chemical or even mechanical—reacts with moisture, heat, acidity, or other triggers to produce gas (usually carbon dioxide and sometimes ethanol) that becomes trapped as bubbles within the dough. When a dough or batter is mixed, the starch in the flour mixes with the water in the dough to form a matrix (often supported further by proteins like gluten or other polysaccharides like pentosans or xanthan gum), then gelatinises and 'sets', the holes left by the gas bubbles remain.

Biological leaveners

Micro-organisms that release carbon dioxide as part of their life cycle can be used to leaven products. Varieties of yeast are most often used, particularly *Saccharomyces* species (i.e. baker's yeast (*Saccharomyces cerevisiae*), though some recipes also rely on certain bacteria. Yeast leaves behind waste by-products (particularly ethanol and some autolysis products) that contribute to the distinctive flavour of yeast breads. In sourdough breads, the flavour is further enhanced by various lactic acid bacteria (lactobacilli) or acetic acid bacteria (acetobacilli).

Leavening with yeast is a process based on fermentation, biologically changing the chemistry of the dough or batter as the yeast works. Unlike chemical leavening, which usually activates as soon as the water combines the acid and base chemicals, yeast leavening requires proofing, which allows the yeast time to reproduce and consume carbohydrates in the flour.

Yeast can also be used to make alcoholic beverages like beer or wine. The resulting cast-off yeast, known as barm, can be used as a leavener and was probably ancestral to the use of modern pure-cultured yeast. While not as widely known, bacterial fermentation is sometimes used, occasionally providing a drastically changed flavour profile from a yeast fermentation; salt rising bread, which uses a culture of the *Clostridium perfringens* bacterium, is a well-known example.

Some typical biological leaveners are: (i) beer (unpasteurised—live yeast), (ii) buttermilk, (iii) ginger beer, (iv) kefir, (v) sourdough starter, (vi) yeast and (vii) yogurt.

Chemical leaveners

Chemical leaveners are chemical mixtures or compounds that typically release carbon dioxide or other gases when they react with moisture and heat; they are almost always based on a combination of acid (usually a low molecular weight organic acid) and an alkali. They usually leave behind a chemical salt. Chemical leaveners are used in quick breads and cakes, as well as cookies and numerous other applications where a long biological fermentation is impractical or undesirable.

Since chemical expertise is required to create a functional chemical leaven without leaving behind off-flavours from the chemical precursors involved, such substances are often mixed into premeasured combinations for maximum results. These are generally referred to as baking powders.

Chemical leavening agents include:

1. Baking powder.
2. Baking soda (sodium bicarbonate).
3. Monocalcium phosphate.
4. Sodium aluminium phosphate (SALP).
5. Sodium acid pyrophosphate (SAPP).
6. Other phosphates:
   (a) Ammonium bicarbonate (hartshorn, horn salt, bakers ammonia).
   (b) Potassium bicarbonate (potash).
   (c) Potassium bitartrate (cream of tartar).
   (d) Potassium carbonate (pearlash).
   (e) Hydrogen peroxide.

Mechanical leavening

Creaming is the process of beating sugar crystals and solid fat (typically butter) together in a mixer. This integrates tiny air bubbles into the mixture, since the sugar crystals physically cut through the structure of the fat. Creamed mixtures are usually further leavened by a chemical leavener. This is often used in cookies.

Using a whisk on certain liquids, notably cream or egg whites, can also create foams through mechanical action. This is the method employed in the making of sponge cakes, where an egg protein matrix produced by vigorous whipping provides almost all the structure of the finished product.

The Chorleywood bread process uses a mix of biological and mechanical leavening to produce bread; while it is considered by food processors to be an effective way to deal with the soft wheat flours characteristic of British Isles agriculture, it is controversial due to a perceived lack of quality in the final product. The process has nevertheless been adapted by industrial bakers in other parts of the world.

Other leaveners

Steam and air are used as leavening agents when they expand upon heating. To take advantage of this style of leavening, the baking must be done at high enough temperatures to flash the water to steam, with a batter that is capable of holding the steam in until set. This effect is typically used in popovers, Yorkshire puddings and to a lesser extent in Tempura.

Nitrous oxide is used as a propellant in aerosol whip cream cans. Large densities of N_2O are dissolved in cream at high pressure. When expelled from the can, the nitrous oxide escapes emulsion instantly, creating a temporary foam in the butterfat matrix of the cream.

Other Carbon and Energy Sources

Any sugar-containing raw material or any starchy material that can be hydrolysed to fermentable sugars may serve as a carbon and energy source for the production of baker's yeast. These sugars are sucrose, maltose, glucose, fructose, and mannose. Lactose is not fermented by bakers' yeast, and galactose is fermented only very slowly. Such sugar-containing raw materials may be sugar cane juice or molasses, grape juice concentrates, date juice, wood hydrolysates, starch hydrolysates, or waste sulphite liquor. Up to the present time economics have dictated the use of molasses. Waste sulphite liquor is used to some extent in Finland. This liquor from paper pulp mills contains a mixture of hexoses and pentoses at very low concentrations. *S. cerevisiae* assimilates only the hexoses, and consequently very large volumes of liquor have to be passed through the fermentors.

PRINCIPLE OF AEROBIC GROWTH

Extracellular concentrations of glucose affect to a great extent the metabolism of baker's yeast. A high concentration of glucose not only leads to glucose repression, it also affects the amount of biomass formed from substrate utilised due to the formation of ethanol. At glucose concentrations above about 50 mg/l, baker's yeast ferments part of the sugars, even under fully aerobic conditions, resulting in a substantial decrease in yield. To prevent this, manufacturers grow baker's yeast under sugar-limiting conditions in fed-batch cultures. The application of chemostats for the production of baker's yeast has not been successful for a variety of reasons.

Above a critical growth rate, which may be dependent on (pre)-growth conditions and on the strain used, glucose accumulates and ethanol formation starts. After addition of a glucose pulse to sugar-limited chemostats of *S. cerevisiae* grown at low dilution rates, identical effects are observed. This phenomenon, known as the 'Crabtree-effect', is explained in physiological terms by the limited capacity for the oxidation of the final product of the glycolytic pathway (i.e. pyruvate). When the flux from sugars to pyruvate exceeds the capacity to oxidise this metabolite, remaining pyruvate is converted to ethanol. Now that there is consensus about the conditions under which the Crabtree effect occurs, it is of scientific and economic interest to find out the cause of this limited oxidative capacity. It is well known that other yeasts (e.g. *Candida utilis*) are able to grow completely oxidatively at growth rates above the critical growth rate of *S. cerevisiae*. Isolated mitochondria from both species show similar oxidative capacities for NADH and pyruvate, however.

Consequently, a detailed explanation for the differences in response to an increase in glycolytic flux remains to be given. It is questionable whether it will be possible to pinpoint one step as the rate-limiting one based on enzyme activities measured *in vitro*. Another appealing approach to a problem like this would be to carry out flux control studies. Determination of flux control coefficients of the pathway described above may indicate which enzyme or enzymes determine the flux to an important extent.

When ethanol is synthesised it diffuses through the plasma membrane to the surrounding medium. Reports about intracellular accumulation of ethanol were based on erroneous results as explained by Dombek and Ingram.

COMMERCIAL FERMENTATION PROCESS

The objective in the final stage of commercial baker's yeast fermentation may be described as 'optimum quality of yeast at minimum cost'. The latter criterion often implies a compromise between maximum yield on raw materials and maximum productivity. Raw-materials include molasses, which forms a substantial part of the cost price of baker's yeast.

Here 'productivity' is defined as the amount of yeast produced per unit of time required for fermentation, unloading, cleaning, sterilisation and filling. This section deals with practical problems caused by areas of mutual incompatibility between: (i) maximum yield versus maximum productivity, and (ii) quality versus minimum costs. In addition, we discuss the current state of the art of modelling and control.

Quality versus Productivity

The feed pattern in Fig. 19.1 resembles some of the patterns presented by Reed. A consequence of this scheme is a decrease in growth rate during the second phase of the fermentation, which results in a decrease of the percentage of budding cells. Such a feeding pattern is known to be essential if yeast with a good keeping quality is to be obtained.

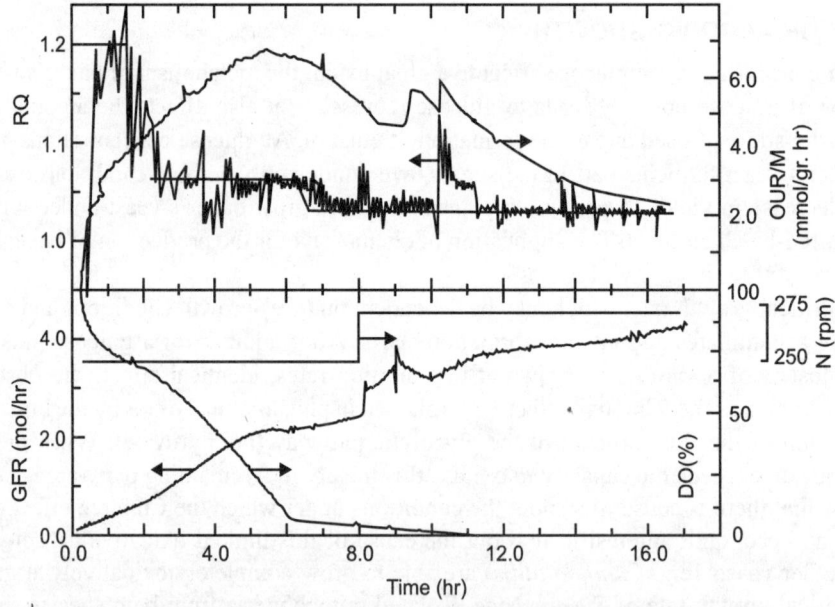

Fig. 19.1. Glucose feed rate (GFR), oxygen uptake rate (OUR), stirrer speed (N) and RQ as a function of fermentation time in an RQ-controlled, oxygen-limited baker's yeast fermentation on laboratory scale. RQ is the ratio of CPR to OUR, where CPR is the carbon dioxide production rate.

Another way to attain all cells in the G-1 phase—the phase (just) before budding—would be to induce synchronous growth. It has been stated, however, that it is unlikely that synchronisation can be induced in a manner that would allow industrial application. Ripening of cells may also be favoured by slight aeration for 1–2 hours at the end of the fermentation when the feed supply has been turned off. This may be explained in physiological terms; since storage compounds such as trehalose accumulate at low growth rates under carbon and nitrogen limitation when dissolved oxygen concentrations are rather high. It is evident that such a ripening period leads to a decrease in productivity. To obtain a product of good quality, which includes good gassing power and keeping quality; must be subjected to various profiles of growth rate, temperature and so on during propagation. This makes it difficult to grow yeast commercially in continuous culture. Other problems encountered include changes in morphology that may result in flocculation and an increase in frequency of infection. Until now, no lasting commercial plant operations of continuous cultures for baker's yeast are known.

Maximum Yield versus Maximum Productivity

In general only a limited amount of seed yeast is available for commercial fermentation, which follows from the necessity to make optimum use of the fermentors, including those used for the production of seed.

Control

Demands for consistently high yeast quality and yield require an accurate control of commercial fermentations. Thus critical process variables such as temperature, aeration and pH are under closed-loop control; feed rates for molasses and ammonia frequently are controlled according to preset schedules (open-loop control). This may not be sufficient, however, since no corrections can be made when problems caused by, for example, the following conditions are encountered.

1. Changes in the composition of raw materials (especially molasses, a waste product of the sugar industry, is notorious in this respect).
2. Changes in the physiological state of seed yeast.

To overcome such problems, control strategies have been developed, the application of which leads to prevention of excessive alcohol formation. This may be effected by on-line measurements of the respiratory quotient. The RQ value indicates whether alcohol is produced or consumed. In case cells neither produce nor consume alcohol, the RQ value equals $RQ_{critical}$. The numerical value of $RQ_{critical}$ follows from the overall mass balance. This may result in a value of $RQ_{critical}$ that differs from 1.00; a value of 1.02 has been reported.

Based on the difference between the set point and the measured RQ value, a closed-loop control has been described that regulates the sugar supply. Underaeration may be prevented in a similar way. It should be noted that this closed-loop control functions only when there is a net production or consumption of alcohol. When the supply of molasses or sugar to the fermentor increases exponentially, the closed-loop control system described may be too slow to allow adequate operation.

The following strategy, which leads to a more rapid control has been suggested (Fig. 19.2). Here, the supply rate of sugar is controlled not only by the difference of measured RQ value with the RQ set point (RQ_S) but also by the oxygen consumption rate, which is proportional to the biomass formation rate. This is true during growth on sugar as well as during conditions when alcohol consumption occurs.

A disadvantage of any RQ control loop is its dependence on the accuracy of oxygen and carbon dioxide analyses.

DRYING

Like commercial fermentation, the industrial practice of drying is based on technological as well as physiological knowledge. Dryers of four types—rotolouver, belt, fluidised-bed and spray dryers—have been reviewed. Application of spray drying for yeast cells is limited because the cell viability of the dried product obtained is very low even when a relatively low outlet air temperature (60°C) is used.

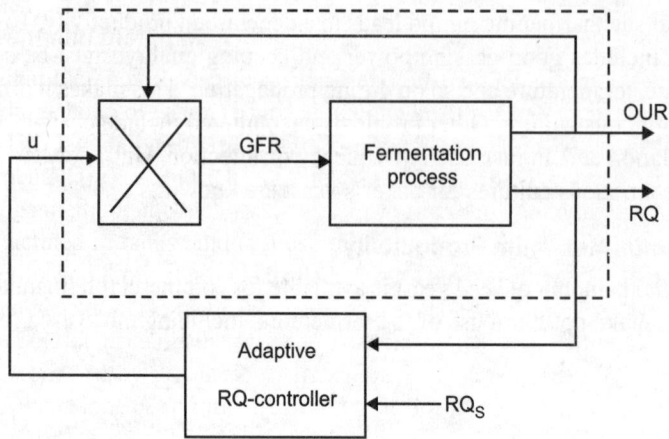

Fig. 19.2. Inner-loop feedback structure for RQ control.

The heat of evaporation is a function of the actual dry matter content of the yeast. Up to 90 per cent dry matter, the heat of evaporation is constant and equals 10 kcal/mol, whereas above 90 per cent dry matter, the value increases linearly with dry matter content, reaching a value of 20 kcal/mol at 95 per cent dry matter. This is understandable, since when the yeast contains up to 90 per cent dry matter, free water is evaporated. To obtain a higher dry matter content, physically bound water must be removed. However, dry matter contents of commercial samples of dried yeast never exceed 96 per cent, since a higher dry matter content leads to irreversible damage of metabolic functions, probably due to removal of chemically bound water.

During rehydration of dried yeast, the cells may lose up to 31 per cent of their dry matter, which includes proteins, peptides, amino acids, phosphate and vitamins. The leakage takes place only above 80 per cent dry matter content. This phenomenon may be explained by changes in membrane structures duo to liquid crystalline-gel transitions during the drying process. It is known that model membrane systems lose their barrier function when a gel phase is induced.

IMPROVING INDUSTRIAL FULL-SCALE PRODUCTION OF BAKER'S YEAST BY OPTIMISING AERATION CONTROL

Scientists have analysed the control of optimum dissolved oxygen of an industrial fed-batch procedure in which baker's yeast (*Saccharomyces cerevisiae*) is grown under aerobic conditions. Sugar oxidative metabolism was controlled by monitoring aeration, molasses flows, and yeast concentration in the propagator.

It has been found that proteins in yeast high yield, easy-to-use *K. lactis* expression at the later stage of the propagation, and keeping pH and temperature under controlled conditions. A large number of fed-batch growth experiments were performed in the tank for a period of 16 hours, for each of the three manufactured commercial products. For optimisation and control of cultivations, the growth and metabolite formation were quantified through measurement of specific growth and ethanol concentration. Data were adjusted to a model of multiple lineal regression, and correlations representing dissolved oxygen as a function of aeration, molasses, yeast concentration in the broth, temperature and pH were obtained. The actual influence of each variable was consistent with the mathematical model, further justified by significant levels of each variable, and optimum aeration profile during the yeast propagation was found. Baker's yeast is used extensively because of its ability to raise dough by fermenting mainly maltose and sucrose present in the dough to ethanol and carbon dioxide. It is also used in the leavening process because of its contribution to the aroma and flavour of bread. The conditions in dough differ from those in industrial baker's yeast production, since in the latter process, the environment is aerobic and the sugar concentration is low.

In a modern propagation plant, the question to be answered is how to control the process by ensuring optimal air supply and at the same time optimise the appropriate metabolic pathway that the yeast may encounter during its growth in the propagator. In particular, optimising processes under pre - and post-stationary phase conditions may produce a substantial economic. The production of baker's yeast involves the multistage propagation of the selected yeast strain using sugar as a carbon source. Baker's yeast is usually produced starting from a small quantity of yeast added to a liquid solution of essential nutrients (molasses, ammonia or ammonium salts, phosphate and vitamins) at a suitable temperature and pH. Once the cell population has grown enough, it is trans ferred into a larger bioreactor for a new growth stage; 4 or 5 stages are usually necessary to reach a satisfactory production quantity. The smaller bioreactors used for the initial stages operate under batch and anaerobic conditions, whereas in the larger bioreactors used for the later stages, aeration is provided and the fed-batch cultivation mode is adopted, i.e. the nutrients are fed to the culture medium at a variable rate.

The plant configuration and operative choices are the consequence of the effects that *Saccharomyces cerevisiae* metabolism produces on biomass yield and growth rate. During the aerobic growth of *S. cerevisiae*, both sugars and ethanol can be used as carbon and energy sources. Sugars can be metabolised via 2 different energy-producing pathways, oxidation or fermentation, depending on the sugar concentration in the medium.

Oxidative metabolism of glucose: Theoretically, glucose is entirely oxidised and provides a high level of energy for adenosine triphosphate (ATP) synthesis.

When the yeast production yield is maximised, 0.5 g of dry matter (biomass) is produced per gram of consumed glucose.

Fermentative metabolism of glucose: When the glucose concentration is sufficiently high, yeasts ferment glucose and ethanol is produced.

The low level of energy produced is related to low yeast growth. This work analyses the control of optimum dissolved oxygen of an industrial fed-batch procedure in which baker's yeast (*Saccharomyces cerevisiae*) is grown under aerobic conditions. Sugar oxidative metabolism was controlled by monitoring aeration, molasses flows and yeast concentration in the propagator.

Indeed, at a high sugar concentration, oxidation is suppressed and fermentation takes place [the phenomenon often referred to as the Crabtree effect]; oxidation predominates when sugar concentration is below 50–100 mg. On the other hand, under oxygen-limited growth conditions, the fermentative pathway leading to ethanol production predominates, even at a low sugar concentration.

Furthermore, an oxidative metabolism of ethanol may be produced. Without sugars, the ethanol produced during the initial fermentative metabolic pathway is reconsumed in the presence of molecular oxygen. Biomass yields on sugars are strongly related to the prevailing metabolic pathway, being maximal only when sugar is oxidised. At high growth rates, the biomass yield of baker's yeast (*S. cerevisiae*) decreases due to the production of ethanol. For this reason, it is standard industrial practice to use a fed-batch process whereby the growth rate is fixed at a level very close to the point of ethanol production. Optimally, growth should be maintained at this critical level, but in practice this is difficult because the critical growth rate is dependent upon strain and culture conditions.

The critical growth rate may vary from batch to batch and even during the experiment. In order to avoid the risk of decreasing the yield, an alternative approach is to use the overflow metabolite as an indicator of how close or far the actual growth rate is from the critical growth rate. Thus, if ethanol production is maintained constant, it is possible to fix the growth rate at a value slightly above the critical growth rate.

The effect of variables such as pH and temperature is well-known and their optimal set-points can easily be defined. On the contrary, yield and productiveness can largely be affected by the concentration of biomass, sugar, oxygen and ethanol formation, if any. The optimal conditions giving maximum yield and productiveness change along with time together with the biomass growth. Therefore, the feeding rate of the molasses is the most critical variable and the problem is to individuate the best feeding rate sequence. Furthermore, bioprocess control runs into a number of difficulties resulting from the nonlinear, nonsteady kinetic properties of the process dynamics as the micro-organisms multiply, adapt, and change their behaviour with time and with the environment, a lack of sensors providing direct measurements of the system state variables, such as biomass, substrates and metabolites. More often than not, sensors are not industrially available or used.

The optimal process control must maximise both cell yield and productivity. The way to overcome this productivity and yield conflict is by accurately regulating the molasses feeding to ensure that the sugar concentration is tightly maintained in such a way that only oxidation occurs and the respiratory capacity of the cells is utilised to the maximum.

The carbohydrate feedstock is an important cost factor in baker's yeast production and, consequently, biomass yield on sugar is an important optimisation criterion. In order to maintain competitiveness, the fermentations must be highly consistent, with minimum variation in product quality, maximum yield on raw materials and minimum production of undesirable side products.

Many parameters impact the metabolic activities of micro-organisms and need to be controlled. Hence, many researchers have focused their attention on optimising fed-batch processes for the production of baker's yeast with different aims (productivity, quality of the yeast, or energy saving). The majority of them commonly developed their research work under laboratory conditions, seldom under pilot plant conditions, but never on a large industrial scale.

Materials and Methods

In general, industrial fed-batch production of baker's yeast is carried out in open loop conditions, and the empirically established molasses feed profiles are kept as manufacturing secrets. Other than feed control, optimisation of the entire bioprocess through the choice of optimal bioreactor size, process duration, and initial concentration of inoculum is the goal of industrial production.

Fermentation was controlled in the last phase of commercial yeast production following a fed-batch procedure. Three commercial products were manufactured, with their 'recipe' characteristics (formulation used in the process for feeding the yeast) treated as confidential.

The traditional, fast, and acidic modes correspond to different needs and to different types of dough: traditional produces yeast used in slow-development dough (traditional dough), fast produces yeast used in quick-development dough (industrial dough), and acidic produces yeast used in acid-sugary dough (products which need long preservation, such as sliced bread).

With the addition of molasses to any original formulation, the medium used in this study contained glucose in the range of 5–100 g/l. During the fed-batch phase, ammonium salts and ammonia were used to provide a source of nitrogen; other minor nutrient requirements were satisfied by inorganic salts. Vitamins of the B group (factors of yeast growth) were added. Each fermentation was controlled for 16 hours, 1/2 hours of maturation to guarantee yeast stability.

Culture Conditions

An industrial strain (baker's yeast) of *S. cerevisiae* (property of the company) was used throughout the fermentative process. Full-scale tests were conducted in an industrial plant with a cylindrical propagator previously sterilised with water steam under the following conditions: 121°C, 103 kPa, 15–30 minutes.

The propagator tank incorporates an aeration grill through which air is introduced. The air flow, which is filtered at its entrance in order to block polluting elements, exercises three important functions: incorporation of oxygen for cellular metabolism, elimination of carbon dioxide accumulated in the broth, and shaking the substratum to avoid the decantation of the yeast. The air flow rate ranged from 7000 to 15000 hours.

An oxygen probe 'Inpro 6800 series O_2 sensors', placed inside the tank and coupled to a microprocessor Model 4100E, was used to monitor the oxygen dissolved. The probe was calibrated before each fermentation and after replacing the electrolyte or the membrane in the probe. Saturation percentages were measured for calibration: 100 per cent was measured before yeast spread and after vigorously airing the tank approximately 10 minutes with 3000 per hours of air; 0 per cent saturation value remained stable.

The pH was maintained in the range of 4–7. It was started at around 4 in order to control the microbial contamination and was slowly raised, never exceeding pH 7. The temperature process was maintained close to 33°C. Foam was controlled by addition of an antifoam agent at regular intervals throughout the process.

Analytical Methods

In the control room, online measurements of dissolved oxygen (percentage), aeration, molasses (kg/h), temperature (°C), and pH were recorded. Simultaneously, ethanol (ml/l), yeast concentration in the fermentation broth (g/kg), and specific growth were determined offline. Specific growths were calculated from yeast concentration data.

Yeast concentration in the fermentation broth was determined by filtering 10 ml of fermentation broth through preweighed glass fibre filters, washed and dried in a microwave oven for 7 hours at 100°C, and kept in a desiccator for 1 hour before reweighing. The molasses feed profile was controlled with a feedback loop based on previously collected data. Samples of the fermentation broth were distilled to determine ethanol concentration. The distilled product was collected in a flask containing potassium dichromate and sulphuric acid and neutralised against Mohr salt.

A large number of experiments were performed and the information acquired was stored in the system database in order to achieve a full optimisation. Statistica 5.0 was the program chosen to illustrate the model dependence of the dissolved oxygen on the operating variables.

Results and Discussion

Aeration, sugar and yeast concentration in the broth have been considered as fundamental variables influencing the concentration of dissolved oxygen. Air incorporates oxygen, and yeast and sucrose influence its consumption. However, the influence of temperature and pH on dissolved oxygen must also be kept in mind. Thus, air flow rate (A), concentration of molasses (M), yeast concentration (Y), pH, temperature (T) and time (t) were considered independent variables which had an effect on fed-batch aerobic yeast production, and dissolved oxygen (O) was selected as the dependent variable.

In order to optimise conditions for biomass growth in the fed-batch feeding of the industrial reactor, a large number of experiments for each type of fermentation were performed. In particular, a series of 26 fed-batch fermentations (16 hours from inoculation) were performed under controlled aerated conditions for traditional recipes.

In all the different fermentations, an upward trend in aeration is observed early in the process while a downward trend occurs in the later stages, associated with the feeding of molasses according to each of the recipes. In general, an excess of dissolved oxygen was observed in all the types of fermentations, in both the early and later stages of the process, as a negative factor in the overall cost of the full process.

These results are in agreement with previous results, whereby, at the initial stages of the process, the maximum feasible growth rate is dictated by the threshold-specific growth rate at which respirofermentative metabolism sets in. In later stages, the specific growth rate is decreased to avoid problems with the limited oxygen transfer.

The aeration is always a positive factor, since air flowing through the broth contributes to an increased amount of dissolved oxygen. The addition of sugar is a negative factor, because when substratum is fed, it is metabolised through the corresponding consumption of oxygen, thereby diminishing the oxygen concentration in the tank. Yeast concentration in fermentation broth is also a negative factor, since the yeast needs oxygen for its in-tank metabolising processes. It is necessary to point out an inconsistent positive factor in the case of the acidic fermentations, which is explained in the statistics, since the associated P-value of 0.6877 eliminates any effect of this variable and therefore can be neglected.

Temperature ought to remain constant, with no significant fluctuations, since growth should remain at its optimum level; for our strain, this corresponds to temperatures close to 33°C. The oxygen solubility in aqueous phase should decrease as temperature increases. However, the high P-values obtained correspond to a nonsignificant level of temperature. These high P-values can be explained by considering factors such as aeration and concentration levels of yeast or of molasses, which highly influence the percentage of dissolved oxygen affecting yeast growth, favouring a nonsteady equilibrium throughout each operation.

This work analyses the control of optimum dissolved oxygen of an industrial fed-batch procedure in which baker's yeast (*Saccharomyces cerevisiae*) is grown under aerobic conditions. Sugar oxidative metabolism was controlled by monitoring aeration, molasses flows and yeast concentration in the propagator.

PROPERTIES

Taste and Flavour

The properties of taste and flavour, to which yeast contributes, are part of the definition to the term 'bread aroma'. Flavour is the total of the sensations the consumer experiences: taste, aroma, structure, colour, temperature and mechanical chewing qualities. Research into bread aroma started some 50 years ago when the baking industry was in its infancy, and up to 1980 methods of analysis were based on analytical chemistry or comparative organoleptic tests. Most of the data have been obtained by these methods, which were not always reliable, and the conclusions drawn must sometimes be treated with caution. It is only in recent years that bread aroma research has involved sensorial analysis. This method requires the five sense organs to be trained in such a way that they can be used as an (objective) measuring instrument. At this moment, it seems to be the only reliable method of analysis, given the complexity of the bread aroma. To gain insight into the contribution of yeast to bread aroma, we need answers to the following questions:

1. Can bread aroma be measured?
2. What is the contribution of each of the dough components to bread aroma?
3. What is the influence of leavening and dough processing on bread aroma?

Gas chromatography analysis of volatile bread elements has thus far identified more than 200 compounds, belonging to 11 classes: alcohols, aldehydes, esters, acids, ketones, lactones, phenols, ethers, heterocyclic hydrocarbons, sulphur compounds and amines. It is, however, disappointing that these investigations have not lead to the identification of the causal agents of bread aroma.

Among dough components, the flour definitely contributes to bread aroma. Amino acids are precursors for many volatile compounds. They are also, together with such reducing sugars as glucose, fructose, and maltose, involved in nonenzymatic browning reactions and are essential for aroma. Flour lipids are highly unsaturated and quite unstable. They decompose to carbonyl compounds, possessing a specific aroma. Phenolic acids also occur in flour, but their organoleptic properties make them undesirable. Yeast cells serve as a source of amino acids and will thus stimulate the formation of browning products during baking. Use in dough of high yeast concentrations (5 per cent) will create a 'yeast-characteristic' aroma generally experienced as negative. Also, bacteria, normally present in baker's yeast, do contribute through their fermentation products.

The role of other constituents of dough — fat, sugar and enzymes should be mentioned. Fat, added for improved crumb and structure, may decompose into aroma-rich carbonyl compounds. Sugars, already mentioned in connection with flour, will also determine the fermentation speed of yeast and the quantity and type of browning products in the crust. Enzymes, added to the dough, do not contribute directly to bread aroma, but their action (i.e. proteolysis of wheat proteins) may lead, through an increased free amino acid concentration, to better flavour. Not only the dough components, but also their changes during the rising process, influence the final aroma.

Fermentation starts as soon as mixing begins. Not much is known about this phase, but it seems that the mixing speed influences the concentration of isobutyric and valeric acids in the dough. High-speed mixing, compared with the conventional process, increased the level of isoacids (having unpleasant flavours) up to fourfold. The importance of the first proof has been questioned by several authors. Conford reported that there was no difference in aromas of breads obtained from doughs that underwent a 3- and 8-hour first proof and doughs obtained by the Chorleywood process. Also Collyer and, Kilborn and Tipples found no significant difference in aroma between mechanically developed bread and the traditional leavened bread. It is emphasised again that these results were based on organoleptic tests. In any event, the introduction of the mechanical dough process in the United States was not successful. The main reason was that the public disapproved of the bread because it had less flavour and taste than a conventional bread. Moreover, in the past decade, a number of authors readjusted their opinion on the influence of the first proof on bread aroma. In any case, because of a lack of flavour in present-day bread, yeast bread flavour formulations have appeared in the past few years.

The influence of first-proof fermentation may be disputed but the contribution of final-proof fermentation is beyond doubt. As long ago as 1937, Cathcart showed that the duration of the final proof time influenced the bread aroma. Cole and coworkers showed that as a consequence of fermentation in the final proof, the concentrations of organic acids and carbonyl compounds in a baked bread increased by 30 and 65 per cent, respectively. Roiter and Borovokova showed a fourfold increase in oxyben-zaldehyde concentration during the final proof.

It was suggested by Fornet that not only yeast, but also the bacteria present in the compressed yeast, may contribute to bread aroma. Robinson and coworkers postulated that bacteria, through production of short-chain organic acids, influence bread aroma.

In addition to fermentation, bread aroma is determined by the duration, temperature and type of baking. Baking itself is a rather complex physical and chemical process. To the yeast, it means an initially increased fermentation rate with subsequent decreases until the dough reaches a temperature of around 55°C and the cells die. The trapped carbon dioxide expands, creating the well-known 'oven spring'. There is also transport of water and alcohol to the surface. The surface undergoes browning by Maillard-type reactions, whereby carbonyl groups of reducing sugars and amino groups of amino acids and proteins condense. Subsequent Amadori rearrangements and Strecker degradations create the final brown pigments or melanoidines in the crust. Precursors of these reactions are provided and influenced by yeast fermentation. To fermenting yeast in the dough, there are no such things as first, intermediate, and final proofs; only the duration of the fermentation period is important, and it has been clearly shown that in this process, yeast generates acids and carbonyl compounds and alters the free amino acid composition of the dough, thus suggesting a fermentative involvement in the production of bread aroma.

Yeast-based Applications in Bread Making

The application of baker's yeast remains of prime importance in bread making, There is no 'standard bread' by which to estimate the performance of a yeast. Recipes for bread vary worldwide, and so do the ingredients: in addition to wheat, milled corn, rye, sorghum and durum are used.

Physiological studies of baker's yeast during dough rise in typical conventional processes give an insight into possible shortcomings and determine new areas of research into strain improvement. There are a few basic methods for preparing a wheat dough: the traditional sponge and dough, and its variant the liquid ferment, and the straight dough process. Restricting ourselves to straight doughs, we can summarise that they are basically made by mixing flour, water and salt. The amount of ingredients is usually expressed as a percentage of the flour weight. In practice this means that a dough containing the regular 50 per cent of water and 2 per cent of salt will have a dissolved NaCl concentration of 3.1 per cent, slightly higher than seawater. The osmotic stress induces a 'secondary fermentation' whereby glucose yields glycerol, ethanol and carbon dioxide. We have established that as much as 10 per cent of the sugar now can go to such fermentation, leading to a final concentration of 0.4 per cent of glycerol in the water phase in doughs containing 6 per cent of yeast. Further increase in osmotic pressure by making the dough sugar-rich (5–20 per cent) certainly increases glycerol production, explaining at least partly the decreased gassing power.

Fermentation starts as soon as the ingredients have been mixed, and trehalase will be activated upon uptake to the preexisting hexoses from the dough. The physiological significance of trehalose degradation in the presence of glucose is still unknown; its degradation may be a condition of starting the cell cycle. We did not observe bud formation in less than 40 minutes at 28°C, coinciding with the lowest trehalose level in the cell. In the first half-hour of dough rise, the yeast is cofermenting the preexisting hexoses together with maltose, provided by the amylases of wheat. Initial levels of glucose and fructose are repressive. This discriminates between yeast strains with low and high maltose fermenting ability, which also indicated that this effect is hardly visible with low yeast input. From the K_m value of the high-affinity maltose uptake system, it can be calculated that the dough water phase must constantly contain some 4.5 g/l to sustain a maximum uptake rate and fermentation speed. This may be the case with low (< 2 per cent) yeast input. The introduction of short straight dough methods with a total process time of around 100 minutes created a need for additional sugar due to increase yeast input. This problem was solved by the use of fungal amylases, generating additional maltose, at the level of 100–200 ppm. A further increase in gassing rate was obtained by either increasing dough temperature (up to 35°C, end final proof) as practiced in England or by the increase in yeast input to 6 per cent as practiced in Portugal. Because of the presence of carbon and nitrogen sources, yeast is indeed able to grow during dough rise.

Chapter 20

Enzymes in the Food Industry

INTRODUCTION

From a futuristic viewpoint, added enzymes in the food industry will fall into two distinct categories: those added as proteins themselves or those added to the plant (and animal) sources of edible material in the form of genes (DNA). Further categories probable will include enzymes mimics: these are synzymes, enzyme analogues, catalytic antibodies (abzymes) and ribozymes (catalytic RNA). Food-processing operations may be still undeclared in details as today, whereas food additives will require even stricter labelling requirements, perhaps with both popular and chemical-naming on the package.

The food industries will continue to use added enzymes, to bioconvert natural biochemicals in foodstuffs into new food products with desirable colour, flavour, taste or texture. Many other food processes exploit hydrolytic enzymes, such as proteases, amylases and cellulases to lower the viscosity of foods by partial breakdown of proteins, starches and celluloses, respectively. This procedure saves on energy costs during pumping of viscous materials around the processing plant and so contributes to cheap processes. In addition, in assisting processing, most enzymes work rapidly even at moderate temperatures and near-neutral pH. Their action can be terminated by boiling, for example, as in the brewing industries. This allows fine control of such food-processing operations, including the sophisticated product improvements associated with changing consumer demands. Enzymes are natural extracts and are 'generally recognised as safe' (GRAS) where they have been extracted and purified from harmless sources, usually fungal (such as yeast) rather than bacterial. In addition, enzymes produce chiral chemical products by relatively clean processes that produce less harmful effluents. Enzymes are sold on a price per unit activity basis (not weight), and their catalytic power can be obtained very cheaply, provided that crude preparations are allowed for use in a particular food industry. Purification necessitated by food safety regulations may make some enzymes too expensive to use in cheap food products, in processing or product improvement, unless the profit is achieved by increased sales.

The presence of naturally-occurring toxicants in foodstuffs may have to be detailed on labels in the future: moreover, many of the enzymic processes in use will then be for purposes or detoxification rather than processing-convenience or cosmetic appeal. A variety of enzymic events occur naturally in the growth and ripening of fruits and vegetables, but only a few of these can be encompassed in this chapter. Added enzymes will achieve stereospecific and regioselective bioconversions by attacking their appropriate chemical substrates in the foodstuffs. Such biological conversion of utilisable chemical components of animals, plants and insects is essential in the digestion mainly of macromolecules of food derived from living organisms by other species: any non-digestible molecules are usually classified as micronutrients as distinct from macronutrients. Paradoxically, although we obtain most of our energy (ATP) from the oxidation of acetate to carbon dioxide and water through the Krebs tricarboxylic acid cycle in all aerated (oxygenated) body tissues, we do not find vinegar (acetic acid) to be a useful main component of our diet. Starch, fats and proteins predominate as macronutrients, so that added (and digestive) enzymes are often forms of amylase, lipase and protease. Much is now known about the chemistry of these, especially in terms of their specificity, efficacy, pH optimum and temperature optimum: the last is a result of enhanced reaction rate with increasing temperature, which is obliterated at higher temperatures by enzyme destruction (denaturation). Because enzymes must be bought and employed on the basis of their activity, the cost of particular enzyme preparations is thus mainly based on the necessity to incur labour costs in purification (and immobilisation) to acceptable (or legislative) composition, activity and absence of toxicity (sometimes noted as GRAS). Genetically engineered sources of enzymes may require additional classification based on overall recombinant DNA source and final composition.

With regard to bioconversions in the food industry, interest increased greatly in the 1980s, mainly because of the realisation that enzyme families will transform a wide range of unnatural compounds as well as their natural substrates, and also because the availability of a wide variety of enzymes was increased. Bioconversion (or biotransformation) is the term used to describe the use of enzyme-catalysed reactions in organic synthesis. It appears likely that enzyme-catalysed reactions and whole-cell-mediated bioconversions will contribute even more in the future to synthetic organic chemistry and its many applications, in addition to the food industry.

The transformations achieved are usually very energy efficient when compared with the relevant chemical process. Enzyme-mediated bioconversions include oxidoreductase, transferase, hydrolase, lyase, isomerase and ligase reactions. Both selectivity and energy economy are equally of value to the food industry, which not only converts foodstuffs themselves but is also concerned with the manufacture of additives such as colours and antioxidants. Bioconversions can be carried out either using pure or partially purified enzymes, or whole cells can be used. The disadvantages of using isolated enzymes include the expense involved in isolating highly purified enzymes and the possible requirements for the addition of enzyme cofactors (or enzyme cofactor recycling). The advantages include the fact that a particular enzyme may be specific for a selected reaction, cosolvents are better tolerated, and only simple apparatus and work-ups are required.

The use of whole cells, as an alternative approach, is inexpensive and the required enzyme cofactors are present in the cells. However, this approach requires 'the use of large-scale glassware, and side reactions can interfere with or dominate the substrate and/or the product. Growth *in situ* of whole-cell preparations may provide a renewable biocatalyst in some cases. It is of related interest that green algae of the *Chlorella* sp. have been used in the bioconversion of progesterone: hydroxylation and side-chain degradation reactions were observed.

Much of the chemical interest in enzyme utilisation has in food production involved the selection of an appropriate enzyme to bioconvert the targeted substrate present in a precise programme of biodegradation, as in the case of the commonly-occurring macromolecules. These are polysaccharides such as starches from a variety of plant sources, celluloses and lignocelluloses, hemicelluloses, glycans and glucans, xylans and pectins: other macromolecules are mainly proteins and fats (Fig. 20.1). Macromolecules are hydrolysed by appropriate naturally-occurring enzymes by the rapid addition of the elements of the water molecule to each bond cleaved. This process can be from one end of the polymer chain (e.g. exonucleases in nucleic acid hydrolysis) or at many locations within the polymer chain (e.g. endonucleases). The particular location of fastest attack is usually modulated by the backbone conformation or local configuration of monomer units and in addition gross structural features such as the crystallinity of cellulose or the particular regions of keratins play a role. Unfolding of the globular conformation (or dissociation of the subunits of quaternary structure) associated with the thermal denaturation of proteins may increase their susceptibility to hydrolysis by proteases: boiled egg protein (ovalbumen) is indeed more rapidly digestible in the human stomach and upper intestine (by pepsin and trypsin/chymotrypsin respectively) than is uncooked egg white ovalbumen. Here there is an excellent example of pH optimum: the pepsin required to operate in the acidity (due to hydrochloric acid) of the stomach has a main pH optimum of about 2.5, whereas the further digestion of proteins (and peptides) by trypsin and chymotrypsin operates most rapidly at the mildly alkaline pH (about 7.5) of the upper small intestine.

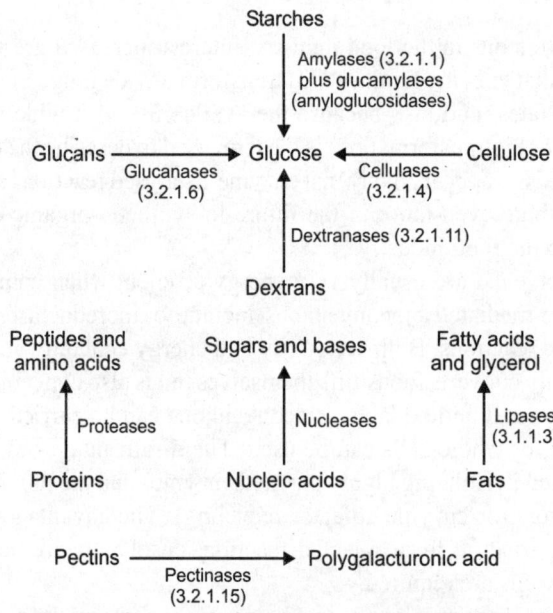

Fig. 20.1. Food macromolecules hydrolysed by added enzymes.

ADDED ENZYMES IN THE FOOD INDUSTRY

Simple hydrolytic enzymes (hydrolases) can be isolated from the appropriate animal tissues and used in their natural role, in food-processing industries (Table 20.1). Proteins in the diet are partially hydrolysed by pepsin in stomach secretions under acidic conditions. Further hydrolysis of some peptide bonds in dietary proteins occurs in the intestine, catalysed there by trypsin and chymotrypsin at slightly alkaline pH values. The structure and mechanism of these enzymes are well established, and improvements in the chosen enzyme can be made by genetic engineering recombinant DNA technology approaches (using protein engineering) or by direct chemical alteration in structure (protein tailoring) to achieve the modification of the chosen food substrate.

Table 20.1. Added enzyme utilisation in the food and beverage industries.

Enzyme	Industry/food	Enzymic action
α-Amylase	Baking	Starches to form glucose
α-Amylase	Brewing	Starch liquefaction and partial hydrolysis to glucose and limit dextrins
Amyloglucosidase	Brewing	Limit dextrins to glucose
Amyloglucosidase	Sugar	Corn starch to glucose
Glucose isomerase (immobilised)	High-fructose syrup	Glucose: half conversion to fructose-glucose equilibrium mixture
Invertase	Sugar beet	Sucrose to glucose and fructose
Dextranase	Sugar refining	Dextran hydrolysis to glucose
Rennins	Cheese and related foods	Milk kappa-casein to paracasein: curds with calcium ions to solid precipitate
Lactase (immobilised)	Ice cream/milk	Lactose to glucose and galactose
Lipases	Chocolate, oils, and fats	Fats to fatty acids and glycerol
Papain	Meat	Degradation of actinomyosin (muscle protein): meat tenderisation or dissolution
Proteases	Brewing	Proteins to amino acids
Lignocellulases, hemicellulases and cellulases	Fruit and vegetables	Hemicellulose and cellulose hydrolysis: softening
Pectinases	Fruit juice	Clarification or cloud-addition
Glucose oxidase plus catalase	Sauces	For removal of glucose or oxygen
Lipid peroxidation-removing enzymes	Fatty foods	Reduction of fatty-food toxicity
Polyphenol oxidase	Fruit and vegetables	Colour, taste, antioxidant and composition modification
Isolation and utilisation of appropriate genes (DNA), e.g. restriction enzymes plus ligases	Tomato	Tomato ripening control
Digestive enzymes	Baby food and health foods	Digestive aids
Reactive oxygen species (ROS)-removing enzymes	All foods	Reduction of food toxicity

Improvements in enzyme thermostability to excessive heating may also be useful. Enzymatic treatment of a non-viscous suspension such as milk is accomplished using reusable immobilised enzymes. Improvement in enzyme thermostability is often evident in practice, especially if the immobilised enzyme has been attached chemically to the solid support (plus some chemical cross-linking constraint that holds the enzyme conformation in native form). Improvements in enzyme thermostability have been achieved with a few extra hydrogen bonds (or electrostatic interactions).

Protein engineering has been achieved with the enzyme, glucose isomerase, which is used in large amounts world-wide to convert glucose into fructose (about 50 per cent conversion at equilibrium):

$$\text{Glucose} \rightleftarrows \text{Fructose}$$

The widely used mixture is known as high fructose syrup, and it has a consumer-desirable high sweetness relative to glucose. The glucose is made by the enzymic hydrolysis of corn starch using immobilised amyloglucosidase:

$$\text{Corn starch} \rightarrow \text{Glucose}$$

Thermostability of the glucose isomerase can be improved by specifically replacing the lysine at position 253 by an arginine residue in the same position. It is uncertain how the enzyme conformation is made more difficult to unfold at higher temperatures (unfolding is assumed to be the universal mechanism of protein thermodenaturation). Modified enzymes, such as glucose isomerase (Arg 253), constitute the first generation of redesigned biocatalysts for use in food industries. Better understanding will emerge of the basic design of enzymes (including abzymes: catalytic antibodies) and their mechanisms in relation to substrate specificity (including enantiospecificity), high efficacy, and pH and temperature stability (selected enzymes to operate in partially non-aqueous media). Immobilised enzyme systems such as those used in milk and other food-processing applications unfortunately have diffusion limitations of substrate access, and consequently often display a lower affinity for substrate [a higher Michaelis constant (K_m)] and a lower maximal velocity. Deleterious side effects of enzyme immobilisation are compensated for in processes by using greater quantities of the enzyme, around the surface of a solid support particle. Immobilised enzymes can be recovered and reused or used in continuous flow-through reactors with a liquid substrate such as milk (or water or alcoholic beverages). Nonetheless, immobilised enzyme applications fit in well with biochemical engineering unit operations associated with batch or continuous processes in the food industry.

Examples of the many bioconversions important in the food industry, some of which use immobilised enzymes, are given in Table 20.1. Protein engineering (genetic engineering) can be attempted, as noted for glucose isomerase, using site-directed mutagenesis of a few identified bases in the nucleotide-residue genomic DNA sequence of that particular enzyme made by the production micro-organism. Thus, a modified enzyme can be produced by redesign considerations to effect a carefully predicted and monitored change in enzyme conformation via an altered amino acid residue sequence and used after design. Cytochromes P-450 are especially interesting in this context. Studies on cytochromes P-450 (Fig. 20.2) are associated with identification of novel uses for this ubiquitous enzyme, with computer modelling playing an increasing role in this area. Genetic engineering of plants themselves has significance also in the food industry. For example, antisense RNA technology has been used to decrease pectin degradation during tomato fruit processing. The extent of pectin degradation during processing affects the quality of processed tomato products such as tomato ketchup or purée. Such degradation is caused by the combined action of two endogenous enzymes, polygalacturonase (EC 3.2.1.15) and pectinesterase (EC 3.1.1.11), which can be inactivated by so-called 'hot break' processes. These involve flash-heating the pulp to at least 85°C within minutes of its preparation to destroy the natural pectolytic enzymes in the fruit and thus preserve cloud stability. However, these operations are expensive and may adversely influence the flavour and aroma of the final paste. Tomato lines have been generated that contain antisense genes for polygalacturonase and the expression of antisense RNA reduced endogenous polygalacturonase levels to less than 1 per cent of normal. The pectin isolated from these genetically engineered tomatoes was much less degraded than normal.

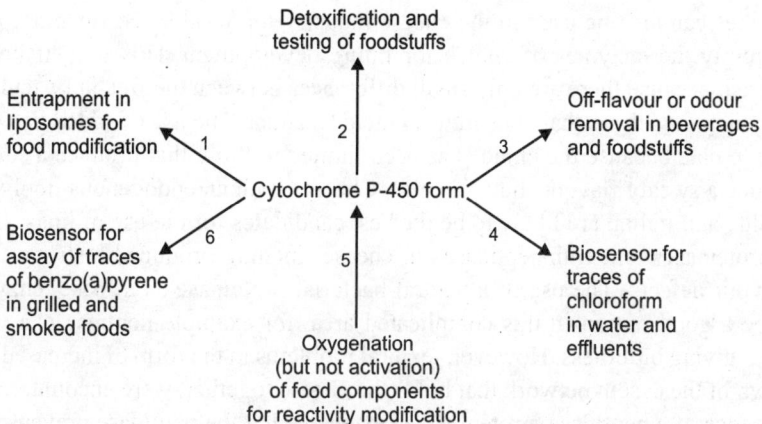

Fig. 20.2. The possible utilisation of cytochromes P-450, produced in recombinant yeasts, in the food processing industries is shown [form 1A1 is genotoxic: it activates benzo(a)pyrene to the ultimate carcinogen, DNA-binding form]. Applications 1–5 use different forms of cytochromes P-450, and form 1A1 in No. 6 (a harmful activation of a carcinogen if it were to occur in the body-activation products such as epoxides react with DNA to cause mutagenesis and cancer in some cases).

Milk and Cheese Industries

Cheese-making

The enzyme chymosin (EC 3.4.23.4 rennin) is used in cheese manufacture to coagulate the milk casein. Replacement of the natural enzyme rennin (in its unpurified form known as rennet) in the cheese-making process is essential because natural rennin is obtained from the fourth stomach of the unweaned calf. This not only limits enzyme availability, but also renders the resultant cheese unattractive to some vegetarians who do not consume animal tissue extracts. The specific attack by rennin on a single peptide bond in milk casein is difficult with other enzymes. Rennin attacks this single peptide bond in κ-casein, and converts it to paracasein (with release of a peptide fragment). The paracasein is then precipitated by calcium ions present to form the casein curd (clot) required for cheese manufacture.

A rennin substitute must be readily water-soluble, it must be non-toxic, and free from antibiotic activity, which might destroy essential micro-organisms required for the cheese-ripening process. An enzyme substitute must also be free of unwanted micro-organisms that can be process-spoilers, or even human pathogens. Unwanted extra protease ability must be avoided, as the k-casein to paracasein conversion should be the only proteolytic step.

The curd formed must display normal body and texture with no off-flavours, unwanted colours or malodours in the cheese. In early studies, pepsins seemed to meet some of those requirements but some loss of fat into the whey occurred and non-specific hydrolysis of other peptide bonds resulted in the formation of bitter-tasting peptide contaminants. Useful thermostable enzymes with lower pH-sensitivity than rennin have been obtained from *Mucor pusillus* and *Endothecium parasitica*. However, now that calf rennin itself can be made in yeast by recombinant DNA technology, it (chymosin) may be the enzyme of choice in cheese-making. Attempts to improve rennin by enzyme designer techniques includes the partial removal of its sensitivity to the pH of milk. Lowering of milk pH is caused by production of lactic acid by lactobacilli associated with milk souring.

Added enzymes can also be used in the cheese industry for accelerated ripening: proteinases and lipases are currently the enzymes of choice for future development. However, if lipases are added caution is required, because there are only small differences between the free fatty acid levels required for a normal Cheddar and those that constitute a rancid Cheddar. The use of added lipases has not been very successful to date because the choice has been limited to those that produce a soapy flavour and those that produce a sweaty flavour (butyric acid). Cheeses with an endogenous lipolytic flavour note such as Feta, Blue and Italian are likely to be the best candidates for the use of lipases. Indiscriminate use of added proteinases and endopeptidases in cheese ripening produced a strong flavour but also texture and flavour defects. The use of a neutral bacterial proteinase as a 'base' enzyme for flavour building may be a good option in this complicated area, for example neutrase can increase flavour intensity without giving bitterness. However, textural problems in the form of increased brittleness, due to the breakdown of the casein network that holds the cheese together, were encountered. If neutrase is used in the presence of a peptidase, proteolysis is extensive but the peptidase prevents the build up of bitter peptides. Neutral proteinases are thus a good choice because they produce flavour without bitterness. They provide peptidase substrates early in ripening (they are relatively short-lived at the pH of the cheese) but do not persist to cause problems later in the process.

Enzyme encapsulation in liposomes may be a good future option for incorporating enzymes into cheese: phospholipid liposomes are food-compatible and do not alter the overall cheese composition. Liposomes can be added to cheese in the vat such that they stay intact through curd formation and only begin to lyse, releasing enzymes into the curd, when the curd has been hooped after it has been pressed. When free enzymes are added to milk only 3–4 per cent of the added enzyme is retained in the curd. With the use of liposomes this could be increased to 90–95 per cent: the enzymes are held in the curd in close proximity to the casein substrate. This liposomal delivery system has been used to ripen Feta cheese enzymically (by trapping lipases and proteolytic systems from the milk): flavour and texture were improved by this procedure.

Added enzymes may also be useful in cheese preservation. In particular, lysozyme (EC 3.2.1.17) may be of value because of its ability to hydrolyse the carbohydrate polymers of alternating N-acetylglucosamine and N-acetylmuramic acid that together with peptide chains forms the cell wall of Gram-positive bacteria. Lysozyme is stable in cheese and can inhibit *Clostridia* without inhibiting the starter lactic acid bacteria. Cheeses containing this enzyme initially had a fall in *Listeria* numbers but this was later followed by an increase in growth after 31 days. The usefulness of this enzyme as an antimicrobial agent may be improved in the future by genetic engineering.

Milk quality

The added enzymes xanthine oxidase (EC 1.1.3.22) and glucose oxidase (EC 1.1.3.4) are useful in milk preservation because they generate the hydrogen peroxide required by the endogenous raw milk enzyme lactoperoxidase (EC 1.11.1.7) to kill bacteria; hydrogen peroxide cannot be added to food in most developed countries for legal reasons. The use of these added enzymes has been shown to prevent the multiplication of a lipase-producing strain of *Pseudomonas fluorescens* that in untreated milk caused the development of fatty acid rancidity in Cheddar cheese.

The hydrolysis of lactose in milk to glucose and galactose by the added enzyme acid β-galactosidase during food processing, prevents lactose crystallisation in frozen, condensed milk products. Furthermore, hydrolysis of the lactose in milk can decrease the sucrose requirement by 20–40 per cent and reduce the calories of flavoured milk drinks by 10 per cent. Lactose is also a major component of whey, comprising

70–75 per cent of whey solids which are produced in large quantities as a by-product in the cheese manufacturing industry.

The sweet syrup formed from hydrolysed whey has many potential uses including the production of lactose-free products for the 70 per cent lactose-intolerant population worldwide and as a nutritional sweet syrup for use in the confectionery, baking, soft drinks and dairy industries. Possible sources of β-galactosidase include plants such as almond, peach and apricot fruit, fungi such as *Aspergillus niger*, yeasts such as *Saccharomyces lactis*, bacteria such as *Escherichia coli* and animal organs such as intestine and skin tissue.

Enzyme assays for determining milk quality have been developed that make use of either endogenous milk enzymes (direct assays) or added microbial enzymes (indirect assays). Direct assays using enzymes include the phosphatase test: the thermal destruction characteristic of alkaline phosphatase (EC 3.1.3.1) enables it to be used as a quick, cheap and largely successful assay to ascertain whether the suitable temperature/time treatment for achieving pasteurisation has been applied. However, apparent reactivation of enzyme activity can occur probably due to phosphatase production by micro-organisms. Enzyme markers for mastitis, which affects milk quality, may include catalase (EC 1.11.1.6) and *N*-acetyl-β-D-glucuronidase. Bacterial contamination (in raw or pasteurised milk) may be detected by assays of bacterial cytochrome *c* oxidase (EC 1.9.3.1) or catalase.

Application of the enzyme tests that have been developed for heat-stable microbial lipases and proteases, which influence dairy product quality, would also be worthwhile. Indirect assays of milk quality using added enzymes include the assay of microbial ATP to give a result equivalent to total bacterial count using firefly luciferase (EC 1.13.12.17) to produce light, which is measured by photometry.

Meat Industry

Added enzymes in the meat industry (in addition to control of endogenous enzymes) contribute to the development of tenderness, which is judged to be the most important textural consideration. There are three main causes of toughness in meats. First, an excessive amount of heat-resistant connective tissue: here proteolytic activity should be directed preferentially to breakage of collagen fibres; second, cold-shortening due to too rapid chilling; and third, inadequate time for conditioning. In the last two cases tenderising may be achieved by proteinases that disrupt muscle myofibrillar proteins. Early meat tenderising processes included the practice by Mexican Indians (500 years ago) of using leaves of the papaya tree (*Carica papaya*) to wrap their meat in, such that during cooking vegetable juices would be absorbed. A family of thermostable cysteine proteinases (papain is the best characterised one) is responsible for the tenderising effect of the plant extracts. However, papain is not as effective against collagen as ficin from fig (*Ficus* spp.) and bromelain from pineapple (*Ananas comosus*), but all three are effective at degrading myofibrillar proteins. Nevertheless, crude papain (derived from the dried latex and applied in powder form) because of its safety, low cost and ready availability compared with ficin and bromelain, is the most widely used added enzyme in meat tenderisation. Crude papain preparations in fact contain papain, chymopapain (most abundant enzyme in the preparation) proteinase Ω (III) and proteinase IV.

Papain is most active in the temperature range used for normal cooking of meat (40°–70°C) and is not very active in chilled meat. It is of interest that a thermostable cysteine protease from ginger rhizome has been shown to preferentially degrade the thin filaments of the muscle in the band I region and thus achieve tenderisation of beef, without causing the mushiness induced by papain at similar high levels. Problems with the use of added enzymes to achieve meat tenderisation include poor enzyme distribution resulting in mushy spots upon cooking due to the presence of high concentrations of enzymes. A commercial process for achieving an even distribution by injecting the papain into the living animal before slaughter has been developed. Emulsions in oil of the added tenderising enzymes may be distributed through the meat more effectively than when used as an aqueous solution.

Collagenases may be of particular use in upgrading muscles from older animals or coarser muscles, where collagen is more resistant to gelatinisation during cooking. Some bacterial collagenases appear to be able to deal with connective tissue toughness as they are able to cleave collagen and degrade native collagen with much greater activity than mammalian ones. However, these bacterial enzymes may not be produced by suitably safe organisms (e.g. *Clostridium histolyticum* is a known pathogen). On the other hand, collagenase from *Vibrio* (*Achromobacter*) was found to be more effective than *Clostridium* collagenase, and a collagenase from *Flavobacterium* spp. may be of use as an added tenderising enzyme because of its demonstrated weakening effect on intramuscular collagen.

Confectionery Industry (Sugars and Oils)

Lipases (EC 3.1.1.3) carry out a number of reactions including the simple hydrolysis of triglycerides (in the presence of water) to mono- and diglycerides and free fatty acids and also interesterification and randomisation (a variation on interesterification) reactions. The manufacture of chocolate utilises cocoa butter (a high-value fat): its particular mixture of distearyl oleyl glycerol and palmityl oleyl stearyl glycerol confers its characteristic melting point and crystal structure, which are vital to its use. Enzymic interesterfication of cheaper oils may be able to produce a cocoa butter substitute. It is possible to enrich palm oil in distearyl oleyl glycerol and palmityl oleyl stearyl glycerol using a 1–3-specific lipase from *Aspergillus* and, following fractionation, a product close to cocoa butter in composition results, which is usable as a confectionery fat. Monoglycerides are often used as emulsifiers in the food industry and these are made by partial hydrolysis of triglycerides by lipases followed by fractionation. There is also the potential to use lipases of very narrow specificity to selectively release fatty acids of value: the Δ9-specific enzyme from *Geotrichum* could be used to selectively release oleic acid from suitable sources.

A number of added enzymes are used in the food industry to hydrolyse starch slurries to form useful glucose syrups and maltose syrups (extensive starch hydrolysis) and also maltodextrins (partial starch hydrolysis). These include bacterial and fungal α-amylases (EC 3.2.1.1, α-1,4-glucan glucanohydrolase), β-amylases, glucoamylase (EC 3.2.1.3 amyloglucosidase), also the debranching enzymes pullulanase (EC 3.2.1.41) and isoamylase (EC 3.2.1.68). Maltodextrins with appropriate properties for a particular food application such as viscosity, fermentability and sweetness can be produced by controlled hydrolysis of the starch slurries with α-amylases. A new group of maltodextrins called 'starch hydrolysis products', which have a similar mouthfeel to fats can be produced by the milder enzymic hydrolysis of starch by α-amylase. These products can successfully entirely or partially replace oils and fats in a number of oil/fat-containing formulations. Fatty diets have been implicated in obesity and the aetiology of heart disease; therefore, a number of fat-mimetics have been devised by food manufacturers. However, fat mimetics (such as sucrose polyesters) can, it is claimed, reduce the absorption of fat-soluble vitamins and can have undesirable laxative side-effects. A reduction in the contribution of fats and oils to the caloric content of the diet and an increase in complex carbohydrates suggests that there are promising opportunities for the production and use of digestible and safe fat-mimetics from 'starch hydrolysis products'. Invertase (EC 3.2.1.26) is derived from *Saccharomyces cerevisiae* and is used in the hydrolysis of sucrose to glucose and fructose. In the confectionery industry invertase is used in the production of soft-centred chocolates. Glucose isomerase is used to convert glucose syrups into high-fructose corn syrups (known to be sweeter than glucose syrups), which have many applications in the food industry. Glucose oxidase (EC 1.1.3.4) can be derived from *Aspergillus niger* and used to oxidise glucose to gluconic acid: this prevents the Maillard (browning) reaction occurring between glucose and amino groups, which can for example adversely affect the taste and appearance of powdered egg products.

Baking Industry

Malt (malted barley) is an important source of the added enzymes used in the baking industry: it contains a wide range of enzymes including proteases, pentosanases and diastase. Diastase can be used to compensate for overly low levels of endogenous α-amylase. The main enzymes used in the baking industry are starch-degrading enzymes, proteases, pentosanases, lipases and oxidoreductases. If the requirements for starch-degrading enzymes are examined then it appears that wheat flour needs to contain a minimum amount of amylase activity, and in those with low-activity added amylases from a range of sources including malt, *Aspergillus niger* and *Bacillus subtilis* can be used.

Amylases are used on a wide scale in the breadmaking process and this is their main application in the baking industry: amylases may improve or control dough-handling properties and enhance product qualities such as colour, volume and shelf-life. The availability of amylases with intermediate thermostability has enabled their use in desired anti-firming action.

Added proteases in the baking industry are used in the destruction of gluten protein cohesiveness; papain or the neutral protease from *B. subtilis* is thus used in the manufacture of crackers, cakes and wafers. However, in the case of biscuits some cohesiveness is required and thus care must be taken with the use of proteases. Breadmaking requires a very selective and controlled modification and so problems can arise in choosing the correct protease.

Pentosanases (enzymes that hydrolyse pentose polymers) influence the distribution of water in a dough and thus its rheological properties.

However, even closely related microbial xylanases can possess differences in activity, resulting in marked differences in dough stickiness; thus, specific examples of these enzymes appear good candidates for production by genetically modified micro-organisms.

Redox enzymes such as lipoxygenase, glucose oxidase and sulphydryl oxidase appear set to play an increasingly important role in baking. Glucose oxidase is likely to be used as a flour-improving agent as it increases the gas-retaining ability of dough, and in combination with sulphydryl oxidase is a dough-strengthening agent (due to disulphide bond formation).

Lipoxygenase (EC 1.13.11.12) has a useful bleaching action (oxidation of carotenoid pigments) and acts as a dough conditioner, giving the dough a better tolerance to mixing and an improved loaf volume. However, normally lipoxygenases are considered undesirable in food processes because they attack polyunsaturated fatty acids of nutritional value, resulting in the oxidation products that contribute to rancidity. Indeed, antioxidants such as vitamin E or butylated hydroxy toluene are often added to prevent rancidity development on storage.

Lipids have an important role in breadmaking: dough can be considered to be a lipid-stabilised foam and lipase activity converting triglycerides to a di- or monoglyceride can beneficially influence the foam-stabilising properties of lipids. Soya flour has a definite improving effect on bread and is an important source of the lipase used in baking. It may act by generating the substrate (linoleic acid) for lipoxygenase (another soya flour enzyme). It should be noted that care should be taken with lipases as they could cause an adverse effect on the sensory (taste and smell) characteristics of bread, i.e. by causing rancidity.

Brewing and Winemaking Industry

Modern brewing makes great use of added enzymes. For example, at the malting stage fungal amyloglucosidase (EC 3.2.1.3) can be added to increase the amount of fermentable sugar by further breakdown of the so-called limit dextrins, which are α-1,6-linked glucose oligomers. Many American beers are made from maize (corn), which requires the addition of added amylases to produce sufficient starch breakdown, as the natural diastases are insufficient to achieve this. Bacterial amylases appear to offer better temperature stability (required by modern technological requirements) than fungal ones. Although the use of added enzymes in wine making has traditionally been rare, in recent years there has been a greater use of added pectolytic enzymes, which are added before fermentation of white wine 'musts' (made from pressed juice without any grapeskin contact) to achieve the faster clarification of the wines after fermentation. Added pectolytic enzymes during wine making is also associated with the mass production of red wines by the process known as thermovinification; this achieves well-coloured wines with acceptable astringency levels rapidly and thus economically. The grape mash is heated to solubilise pigmented anthocyanins from the skin and this is achieved without excessive leaching of the astringic procyanidin polyphenols. However, heating releases pectin, which needs to be removed by the added pectolytic enzymes to reduce juice viscosity.

Fruit Juice Industry

The added enzymes pectin methyl esterase (EC 3.1.1.11) and polygalacturonase (pectinase: EC 3.2.1.15) are used in the removal of cloudiness in apple juice. Pectin methyl esterase demethoxylates the free soluble pectin in the juice, allowing it to be depolymerised by the polygalacturonase. This results in a decreased viscosity of the juice but is still insufficient to ensure its clarification. The pectin methyl esterase/polygalacturonase complex then acts on some of the pectin coat of the particles responsible for the cloudiness, exposing a positively charged protein core (at juice pH of around 3.5). This enables electrostatic aggregation with the outer negatively charged cloud particles nearby: aggregates grow until they sediment under gravity. The enzymes added are usually a mixture of fungal enzymes containing pectin methyl esterase, polygalacturonase and pectin lyase (another depolymerising enzyme) activities.

Added enzymes are also useful in the removal of bitterness from citrus fruits. In particular, considerable work has been done on the application of fungal naringinase preparations to remove the bitter component of grapefruit (the glycosylated flavanone, naringin; Fig. 20.3). The fungal extracts contain both α-rhamnosidase (EC 3.2.1.40) and β-glucosidase (EC 3.2.1.21) activities and thus will break down naringin to a less bitter mixture of naringinin and prunin.

POLYPHENOL OXIDASE AND BROWNING OF FRUITS AND VEGETABLES

Polyphenol oxidase is a plastid-associated ubiquitous copper-containing plant enzyme (associated in particular with the thylakoid membrane and photosystem. This enzyme catalyses the hydroxylation of monophenols to o-diphenols (monophenol monooxygenase or tyrosinase activity, EC 1.14.18.1). Also the oxidation of o-diphenols to o-quinones utilising molecular oxygen is catalysed (catechol oxidase or diphenol oxidase, or diphenol oxygen oxidoreductase activity, EC 1.10.3.2.). The laccases, found in fungi and higher plants (EC 1.10.3.1) oxidise p-diphenols (in addition to o-diphenols) to their corresponding quinones. The organisation of the polyphenol oxidase gene family has been described in tomato. Similar oxidation reactions are important in the degradation of aromatic xenobiotic compounds.

Enzymic browning in a number of plant tissues including potato tubers, bananas, grapes, pears, green olives, kiwis, strawberries, plums and apples is thought to involve polyphenol oxidase. In apples, enzymic browning is undesirable because of the unpleasant appearance and development of an off-flavour; it is thus important from both the consumer and food industry viewpoint. Such browning occurs when plant tissues are damaged, thereby exposing them to oxygen. Polyphenol oxidase then catalyses the oxidation of phenolic compounds to quinones that condense to form darkened pigments. This is clearly an important economic problem and considerable effort has been devoted to inhibiting this reaction by a number of strategies.

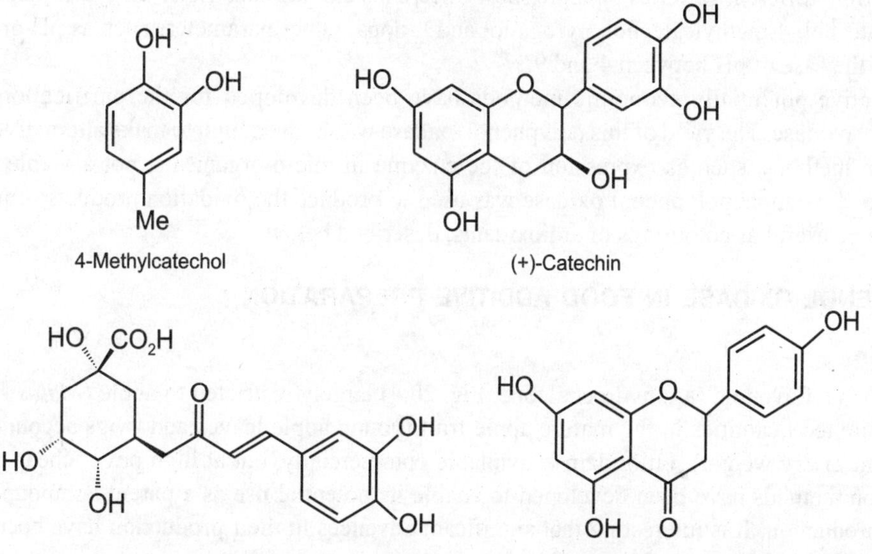

4-Methylcatechol

(+)-Catechin

Chlorogenic acid

Narininging; R = glucosyl-rhamnosyl
Prunin; R = glucosyl

Fig. 20.3. The glycosylated flavanone, naringin.

The most widespread method used in the food industry to control browning is the addition of reducing agents such as sulphites. However, health concerns over sulphites have led to the search for alternatives to chemical methods. EDTA (a chelating agent) may be used as an inhibitor of polyphenol oxidase: this either binds to the active-site copper or reduces the level of copper available for incorporation into the holoenzyme. A copper-binding metallothionein from *Aspergillus niger* has also been reported to inhibit polyphenol oxidase (mushroom tyrosinase) activity.

Prevention of browning is best approached by the use of antisense inhibition of polyphenol oxidase gene expression using constitutive promoters (e.g. CaMV 35S) to express antisense polyphenol oxidase RNA; melanin formation is then specifically inhibited in the potato tuber because polyphenol oxidase is not expressed. Lack of bruising sensitivity achieved in this way in transgenic potatoes and the absence of any apparent detrimental side effects suggests that this is a novel possibility for the prevention of enzymic browning in a wide variety of fruit and vegetable crops. In contrast, the useful action or added polyphenol oxidase ill the food industry in the production or antioxidant and colourant products is imminent and is discussed below.

Ironically, polyphenol oxidase is considered to be an enzyme that is difficult to purify because of the presence of the phenolics with which it reacts, resulting in the modification and inactivation of the protein molecule. Solubilisation of particulate polyphenol oxidase is difficult, although a number of methods for its extraction and purification from apple (and other sources) have now been reported. A partial purification of polyphenol oxidase has been achieved (by ammonium sulphate precipitation and hydrophobic chromatography on phenyl Sepharose CL4B) from the fruit of 12 apple cultivars grown in France, analysed for polyphenol oxidase activity in both the cortex and peel. The red delicious apple cultivar showed the highest polyphenol oxidase activity and the Elstar cultivar the lowest. Polyphenol oxidase has been purified 120-fold from the cortex of red delicious with a yield of around 40 per cent. Enzymes from different varieties of apple show different substrate specificity for typical plant phenols such as catechol, 4-methylcatechol, pyrogallol and L-dopa. Other parameters such as pH optima vary widely, in the case of pH between 4 and 9.

Alternative potentially economic methods have been developed for the purification of apple polyphenol oxidase. The yield of this polyphenol oxidase was high enough to make alternative potential production methods, such as expression of the enzyme in micro-organisms, not a viable economic alternative. This apple polyphenol oxidase was used to produce the oxidation products of phloridzin, which can be useful as colourings or antioxidants, described below.

POLYPHENOL OXIDASE IN FOOD ADDITIVE PREPARATION

Phloridzin

Phloridzin is a flavonoid (a dihydrochalcone, Fig. 20.4) largely restricted to apple (*Malus* sp.), and is found in limited quantities in the mature apple fruit (young apple leaves and twigs account for up to 10 per cent of dry weight). Phloridzin is available commercially, but at high price; cheap alternative purification methods have been developed to enable its potential use as a parent compound for food additive production. It is interesting that significant advances in their production have been achieved using polyphenol oxidase in a biotransformation.

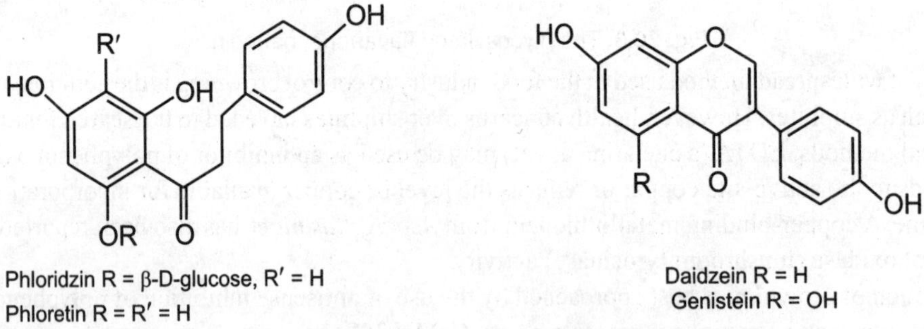

Phloridzin R = β-D-glucose, R′ = H
Phloretin R = R′ = H

Daidzein R = H
Genistein R = OH

Fig. 20.4. A dihydrochalcone.

If reliance is placed upon natural sources for the supply of phloridzin, the most important determinant in a particular tissue of its phloridzin content is its period of development; cultivar, including rootstock type was found to have a much less pronounced effect. Nevertheless, the effect of cultivar can be dramatic in relation to total tissue growth. This gives wide variation in total phloridzin production by particular cultivars; as illustrated by the results obtained for different rootstocks. Production of phloridzin is best achieved by the coppicing of fast-growing rootstocks, such as M25 or MM106. This is comparable with the production of willow or poplar for biomass, and for which mechanical harvesting equipment has been developed.

Production of Phloridzin Derivatives Using Polyphenol Oxidase

The 3-hydroxylation of phloridzin has now been achieved using L-ascorbic acid to block partially a polyphenol oxidase reaction: apple-derived polyphenol oxidase is particularly effective at catalysing this hydroxylation step. Many forms of polyphenol oxidase such as commercial fungal tyrosinase, do not carry out this reaction effectively. The L-ascorbic acid acts by inhibiting the accumulation of quinones by continually reducing them to the *o*-diphenol as they are formed. Recovery of the 3-hydroxyphloridzin was achieved by partition against ethyl acetate, and precipitation with chloroform, followed by water recrystallisation. If the reaction is allowed to proceed in the absence of L-ascorbic acid, quinones are produced, which after shifting the pH to pH 8 (from the enzyme optimum of pH 5), form two isomeric dimers. However, the structure of these two dimers has not been fully characterised while significant biotechnological problems also remain to be solved in this process.

The apple polyphenol oxidase employed shows optimal activity at approximately 30 per cent oxygen saturation of water, and this was taken into account for the reaction vessel design used to produce the phloridzin oxidation products (in addition to its function in replenishing the oxygen consumed in the reaction). The desirability for relatively slow reaction rates led to the optimum design as a 'balanced oxygen type' that essentially consisted of a stirred tank in which oxygen uptake by stirring was balanced at 30 per cent saturation for the oxygen used as part of this reaction process. In practice, because the reaction rate is determined by oxygen uptake, excess enzyme may be added and the tank stirred at a defined rate. Polyphenol oxidase is inactivated as a result of its own activity. Fixing it to a support material would therefore be uneconomic for this procedure, especially considering the loss of activity then incurred: it is clear that the development of a suitably protective antioxidant support might be useful here. The specific example of hydroxylating and dimerising phloridzin has been discussed: moreover, many other flavonoids could give useful products if subject to similar bioconversions. For example, Taylor and Clysdale investigated the potential for generating useful coloured products by the oxidation of phenolics. 3-Hydroxyphloridzin could also be manufactured *in situ* in apple juice by the addition of L-ascorbic acid followed by stirring with the pressed apple pulp that contains endogenous polyphenol oxidase.

Other Biotransformations Using Polyphenol Oxidase

Monophenolic flavonoids and soya isoflavonoids such as daidzein and genistein, which have a relatively poor antioxidant activity (Fig. 20.4), could have their antioxidant activity enhanced by hydroxylation to form *o*-diphenolics. Currently there is some concern about the presence of phyto-oestrogens in some foodstuffs given to infants. During processing it is possible that added polyphenol oxidases may achieve their removal or indeed modify them such that they become beneficial. This is because flavonoids and isoflavonoids (many of which demonstrate oestrogenic activity), for example phloretin and daidzein may have their oestrogenic functionality decreased or even obliterated by *o*-diphenol formation in the particular molecule. Concomitantly this would provide enhanced antioxidant ability, as shown for 3-hydroxyphloretin. This would evidently be possible only if high levels of reducing agents (such as L-ascorbic acid) were present. In the absence of reducing agents, the *o*-diphenols formed would be likely to undergo tannin-type cross-linking reactions (making them biologically non-functional).

Tea Fermentation by Polyphenol Oxidase

The well-appreciated and popular beverage, tea has been made from selected leaves of *Camellia sinensis* for thousands of years. Black tea, by virtue of its more complex colour and flavour, is largely consumed in preference to green tea. The conversion of green into black tea is incorrectly referred to as fermentation (no micro-organisms are involved). Enzymic conversions occur because the leaves of the tea bush contain large amounts of catechins (up to 30 per cent dry weight; Fig. 20.3) that are prone to the action of both polyphenol oxidase and peroxidase (EC 1.11.1.7). In the intact leaf the catechins are segregated from the enzymes. Upon leaf disruption however, rapid enzymic oxidation of catechins occurs to form two major groups of pigments, the theaflavins and thearubigins (Fig. 20.5). Polyphenol oxidase acts on catechins to produce mostly theaflavins, whereas peroxidase produces mostly thearubigins (perhaps by further oxidation of theaflavins). The activity of peroxidase is dependent upon hydrogen peroxide (generated by polyphenol oxidase) and therefore on the activity of catalase (EC 1.11.1.16), which can remove the hydrogen peroxide as quickly as it is produced. Lipoxygenase activity produces the leaf aldehyde, hexenal, responsible for the characteristic refreshing aroma of 'brewed' tea beverages. It is the combined activity of all of these endogenous enzymes that controls the final characteristics of the tea as consumed.

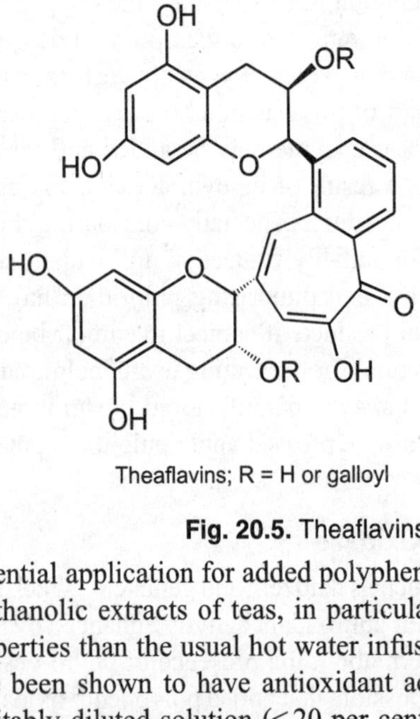

Theaflavins; R = H or galloyl 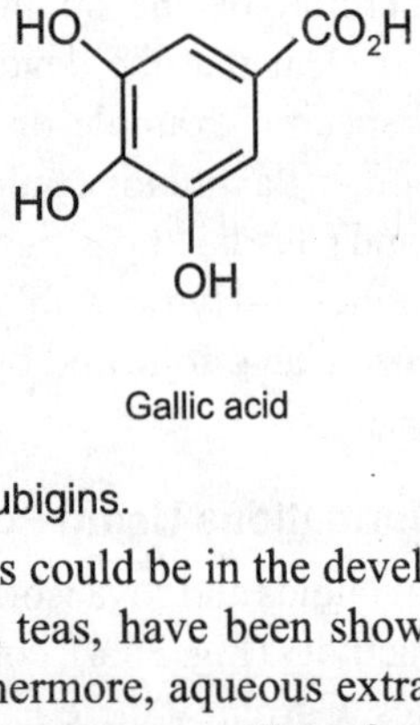   Gallic acid

Fig. 20.5. Theaflavins and thearubigins.

Another potential application for added polyphenol oxidases could be in the development of novel tea products. Ethanolic extracts of teas, in particular of green teas, have been shown to have better antioxidant properties than the usual hot water infusions. Furthermore, aqueous extracts of green and black teas have been shown to have antioxidant activity *in vivo* in man. Use of added polyphenol oxidase to a suitably diluted solution (< 20 per cent ethanol) may then lead to the production of the desired black tea taste. According to the quantity of polyphenol oxidase added this could range from a light 'Oolong' type flavour to a strong 'Assam' type flavour. There could also be advantages in the development of more water-soluble derivatives by this approach, limiting the potential for tanning-type reactions.

Endogenous polyphenol oxidase is used in producing clarified ciders and wines: here, a high degree of phenolic oxidation causes tanning reactions and this leads to a clearing of the beverages. This 'hyperoxidative' effect leads to a light (relatively astringent-free) taste.

Interest has been expressed by commercial sources in using added polyphenol oxidases for this purpose: apple polyphenol oxidase, especially considering its acceptable source, would seem particularly suited for this purpose.

USE OF ENZYMES TO REMOVE OXYGEN FROM FOODSTUFFS

Lipid rancidity due to the products of free radical reactions in the presence of oxygen and redox metal ions must be avoided. Especially harmful in the onset of one-electron recycling due to reducible natural [and xenobiotic (X)-foreign chemicals] present. Many redox metals, especially Fe^{III} can be reduced to the Fe^{II} form coupled with oxidation of X(reduced) to X(oxidised). Fe^{II} can then be involved in reactions that convert atmospheric oxygen to the reactive superoxide free radical (O_2^-):

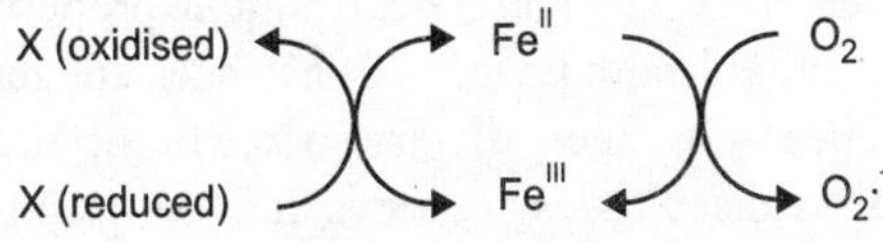

Fe^{II} is often responsible for Fenton chemistry that can produce a range of oxygen radicals including the highly reactive hydroxyl radical that can also be produced in aqueous media by ionising radiation. The hydroxyl radical is particularly destructive if formed within the human body. The superoxide radical however can be removed by the enzyme superoxide dismutase and this can be added to foodstuffs if necessary. Other reactive oxygen species can be removed with other appropriate enzymes: thus hydrogen peroxide is removed by catalase:

$$2H_2O_2 \rightleftharpoons 2H_2O + O_2$$

Catalase contains iron, while superoxide dismutase contains copper (a redox metal, as Cu^{II} and Cu^{I}) plus zinc a nonredox metal Zn^{II} whose role is mainly structural and mechanistic.

Glucose is often removed from foodstuffs by the addition of glucose oxidase, isolated from the fungus *Aspergillus niger*. This yellow enzyme contains flavins as bound cofactor (prosthetic group) and is able to convert glucose rapidly to gluconic acid by oxidation at the hydroxyl group at carbon 6 of the glucose molecule, plus hydrogen peroxide (Fig. 20.6). The hydrogen peroxide formed is simultaneously degraded to water and oxygen by added catalase, and the oxygen formed is used up along with glucose by glucose oxidase.

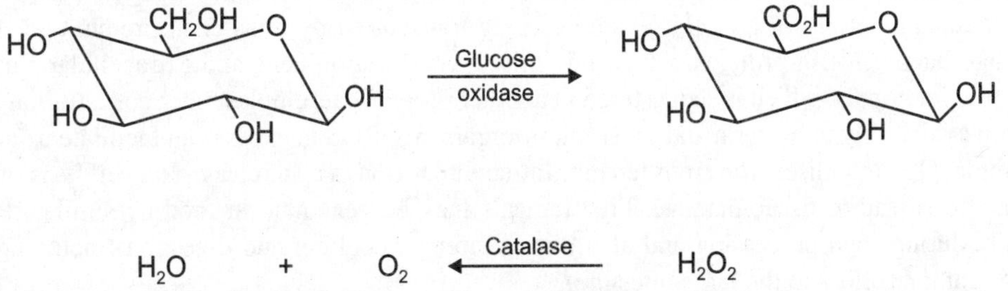

Fig. 20.6. Conversion of glucose to gluconic acid by oxidation.

Overall, therefore, glucose is fully removed in the presence of excess oxygen, while oxygen is fully removed in the presence of excess glucose. The easily tasted rancid flavour due to oxidation of fats by free radicals in, for example, salad cream can be prevented by incorporating some immobilised glucose oxidase/catalase on to an inside disc in the lid so that air-space oxygen is removed down to fine limits. Alternatively, glucose can be removed from many foodstuffs where brown pigmentation will occur in the presence of glucose due to its reaction with particular amino acids (such as with lysine in the Maillard reaction) (see Table 20.1).

FOOD ENZYMOLOGY IN THE PREVENTION OF FOOD TOXICITY

There is much effort currently being devoted to food enzymology in relation to food toxicology. Thus, added enzymes could be used as antioxidants to prevent oxidative damage to food (or to repair it), or to convert endogenous or added food molecules/substrates into potent antioxidants, which would then themselves protect both the food and the consumer against oxidative damage. One novel example of this would be the use of the enzyme polyphenol oxidase from an apple source to produce new apple-derived flavonoids with improved antioxidant and other desirable properties (e.g. colourant properties) for use as food additives with potential health benefits. It has been suggested that oxidative damage to DNA in foods (e.g. meats) could be a subsequent dietary source of the altered DNA bases implicated in cancer. Furthermore, ingestion of oxidised lipids could result in the seeding of the lipid hydroperoxides into low-density lipoproteins (LDL: one of the carriers of cholesterol in the blood) that are degraded, for example, by transition metal ions; this results in oxidative damage to LDL implicated in the development of atherosclerosis. Prevention of free radical damage to DNA, membrane lipids and proteins in food components will become a priority in the food industry, and much more use will be made of dietary antioxidants, including antioxidant enzymes.

Free Radicals in the Food Industries

The collective term reactive oxygen species (ROS), refers to not only oxygen-centred radicals such as superoxide ($O_2 \cdot^-$) and the hydroxyl radical ($OH \cdot$) but also to hydrogen peroxide (H_2O_2), singlet oxygen ($^1O_2$), hypochlorous acid (HOCl) and ozone (O_3). Free radicals are produced as the by-products of normal cellular metabolism: thus, $O_2 \cdot^-$, $OH \cdot$ and $NO \cdot$ (nitric oxide: a reactive nitrogen species or RNS) and ROS such as H_2O_2 are all formed *in vivo*. The production of superoxide as a by-product of metabolism can be considered to be a chemical accident resulting from autooxidation reactions and the leakage of electrons from the electron transport chains of mitochondrial respiration in cells that convert oxygen to water and produce ATP in bioenergetic uses of oxygen. The dangerous hydroxyl radical is produced in living organisms first by splitting of covalent bonds in water by background ionising radiation; and second by reaction of transition metal ions with H_2O_2, Cu^I and Fe^{II} to reduce H_2O_2 to $OH \cdot$. However, iron is handled carefully *in vivo*, for example being transported by transferrin protein and stored in ferritin and haemosiderin proteins, which minimises 'free' iron in cells and extracellular fluids. The same is true for copper, which is sequestered in another protein, caeruloplasmin. Sequestration restricts 'free' iron availability to bacteria and other micro-organisms. ROS in excess can facilitate iron release, for example, $O_2 \cdot^-$ mobilises iron from ferritin. Intracellular iron is also released on cell lysis (after cell death) and can lead to tissue damage. Free radicals may be generated in food by similar reactions, especially during food processing and also during storage, cooking and digestion (including by the action of gut microflora in the large intestine).

DNA Damage in Food Processing and its Repair using Added Enzymes

The endogenous reactions that are likely to contribute to ongoing DNA damage are oxidation, methylation, depurination and deamination. Methylation of cytosines in DNA is important for the regulation of gene expression and normal methylation patterns can be altered during carcinogenesis. Conversion of guanine to 8-hydroxyguanine, a frequent result of ROS attack (Fig. 20.7), has been found to alter the enzyme-catalysed methylation of adjacent cytosines, thus providing a link between oxidative DNA damage and altered methylation patterns. The chemistry of DNA damage by several ROS has been well-characterised *in vitro*, although more information is needed about the changes produced by $RO_2 \cdot$, RO^- and O_3.

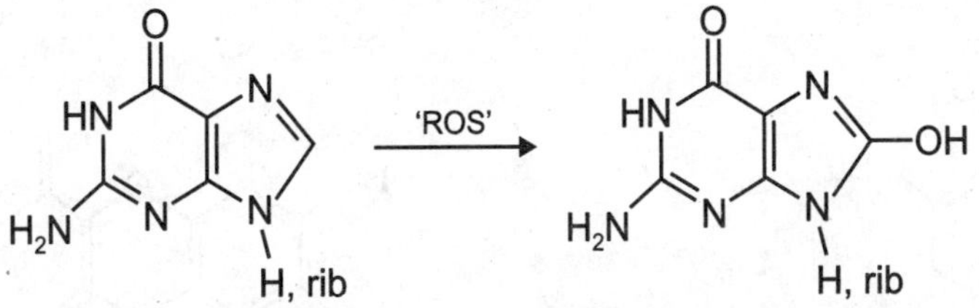

Fig. 20.7. Conversion of guanine to 8-hydroxyguanine, a frequent result of ROS attack.

In DNA, the phosphate group linking the sugars (the acids of nucleic acids) presents a powerful chelating agent for transition metal ions in all foods, and oxidative processing may cause the release of intracellular iron and/or copper ions into forms that could then bind to DNA. Thus, $O_2\cdot^-$ releases some iron ferritin and H_2O_2 can release iron from heme proteins. DNA-associated copper ions in tissues might also react with phenolic compounds to produce ROS and electrophilic phenolic intermediates. This could cause DNA lesions including base modifications, strand breaks and phenol adducts to the DNA bases, some or all of which might contribute to any possible carcinogenicity of particular phenolic compounds in foods. Phenolic compounds that cause DNA damage in the presence of copper ions include 2-hydroxyoestradiol, 2-methoxyoestradiol, diethylstilboestrol, butylated hydroxy toluene (BHT), butylated hydroxyanisole (BHA), L-DOPA, dopamine, ferulic acid and caffeic acid. It is of interest that BHT and BHA are used as antioxidants in foods. Phenols thus have pro- and antioxidant effects, depending on the assay system used: many synthetic and dietary polyphenols [including quercetin, catechin, gallic acid ester and caffeic acid ester (Figs 20.3 and 20.8)] can protect mammalian and bacterial cells from the cytotoxicity induced by peroxides such as H_2O_2. Thus, food processing, which will ensure their retention and enzymic modification will be developed by food scientists.

Lipid-free radicals formed during lipid peroxidation can also attack DNA and these may damage cell organelle (mitochondrial) DNA, which is in close proximity to the inner mitochondrial membrane. New antioxidant enzymes will be developed for use in the food industry to protect DNA from attack by particular ROS. Some of these will be enzyme analogues (synzymes) and enzyme mimics, if any problems of toxicity of these proposed additives can be definitely eliminated.

DNA damage can be repaired by the action of a series of enzymes. However, DNA from human cells and tissues contains low levels of DNA base-damage products, suggesting that these enzymes do not achieve complete removal of modified bases (present in the diet or formed *in situ* by mutagenic agents), perhaps because they operate at close to maximum capacity *in vivo*. A rise in DNA base-damage products could be due to either increased oxidative damage and/or decreased repair activity. DNA glycosylases exist for the repair of several DNA base lesions, including oxidised, methylated and deaminated bases. A repair system for the abasic (apurinic, apyrimidinic: AP) sites produced by spontaneous depurination also exists. Areas of current interest include the role of poly(ADP-ribose)polymerase (PARP) in the rejoining of DNA strand breaks, including those caused by ROS. Studies using gas chromatography/mass spectrometry (GC-MS) have investigated the ability of enzymes to repair DNA containing a wide range of lesions, and have shown that they can sometimes have a broader specificity than expected. The dietary ingestion of damaged DNA may be undesirable if modified bases produced by DNA hydrolysis (digestion) are later incorporated into the body DNA. Appropriate repair enzyme treatment of damaged foodstuffs may be deemed necessary in the future, perhaps even being regulated by international agencies. Some relaxation however, of the requirement for the complete absence of known human carcinogens in foodstuffs is evident, in view of new analytical techniques that can detect even 'a few molecules of these'.

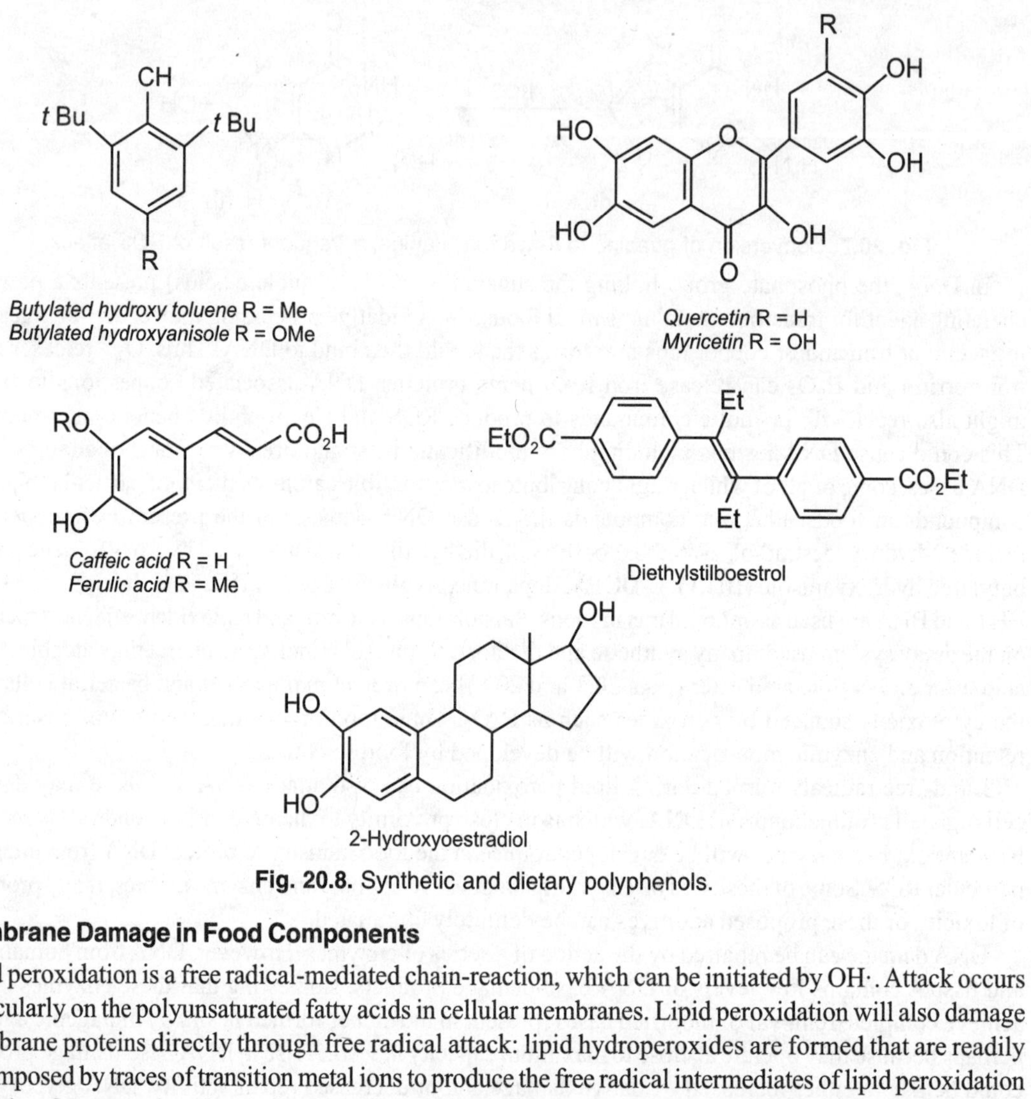
CH
t Bu
t Bu
R
Butylated hydroxy toluene R = Me
Butylated hydroxyanisole R = OMe
R
OH
HO
O
OH
HO
OH
O
Quercetin R = H
Myricetin R = OH
RO
CO2H
HO
Caffeic acid R = H
Ferulic acid R = Me
Et
EtO2C
CO2Et
Et
Diethylstilboestrol
OH
HO
HO
2-Hydroxyoestradiol

Fig. 20.8. Synthetic and dietary polyphenols.

Membrane Damage in Food Components

Lipid peroxidation is a free radical-mediated chain-reaction, which can be initiated by OH·. Attack occurs particularly on the polyunsaturated fatty acids in cellular membranes. Lipid peroxidation will also damage membrane proteins directly through free radical attack: lipid hydroperoxides are formed that are readily decomposed by traces of transition metal ions to produce the free radical intermediates of lipid peroxidation capable of propagating the chain reaction. Protein modification includes oxidation of thiol groups to disulphide bridges. Lipid peroxidation of the membrane components of food contributes to rancidity and thus food spoilage.

FOOD ANTIOXIDANTS INCLUDING ADDED ENZYMES AND PROTEINS

From the discussion in the previous section, it is clear that the prevention of oxidation of foodstuffs is of major importance. An antioxidant is 'any substance that, when present at low concentrations compared to those of an oxidisable substrate, significantly delays or prevents oxidation of that substrate'. Oxidisable substrates include, as noted above, DNA, lipids, proteins (including membranes and lipoproteins) and carbohydrates. Other antioxidants include proteins and enzymes such as superoxide dismutase, glutathione peroxidase, catalase and caeruloplasmin. Antioxidants useful in foods include vitamin E (including α-tocopherol), vitamin C (ascorbic acid or ascorbate), glutathione, selenium, β-carotene and albumin (Fig. 20.9). Flavonoids, isoflavonoid type phytoestrogens and coenzyme Q (ubiquinone) are also antioxidants that may be important. Cells have multiple antioxidant defences to protect themselves against ROS: however, if these were entirely effective oxidative damage would not occur and repair mechanisms would not be required. Instead, oxidative damage occurs continuously in cells and tissues, including those eaten as foods. Various enzymic reactions occur in the ripening of fruit and vegetables and added enzymes can be employed to accelerate these reactions in favourable cases.

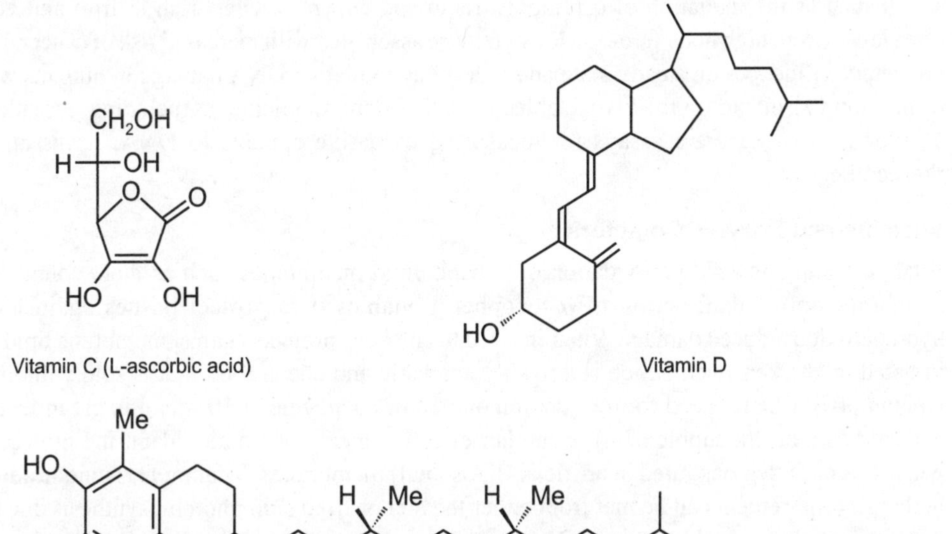

Fig. 20.9. Antioxidants useful in foods include vitamin E (including α-tocopherol), vitamin C (ascorbic acid or ascorbate), glutathione, selenium, β-carotene and albumin.

Many antioxidants are present in the diet: fruit: grains and vegetables are the main sources of these antioxidants. So-called 'functional foods' protect the eater against oxidative damage, and resulting disease.

Dietary intake of fresh fruit and vegetables appears to be inversely correlated with cancer of the stomach, pancreas, oral cavity and oesophagus and to a lesser extent of the breast, cervix, rectum and lung. Emphasis has been placed on the protective role of ascorbate and there is evidence that ascorbate can react with and/or inhibit the formation of carcinogenic *N*-nitroso compounds such as *N*-nitrosamines. There is much interest in the development of antitoxicity enzymes for use in the food industry, where toxicity may be inherent in the foodstuff or accidentally developed by inappropriate food processing.

The protective effects of fruits and vegetables can also be due to other mechanisms than antioxidant action such as the induction of carcinogen-removing enzymes. Diets rich in fruit and vegetables are often low in iron; high body free-iron levels may be associated with increased risk of cancer. Investigations on dietary influences on steady-state and total-body oxidative DNA damage in humans will be related to the optimal intake of fruit, vegetables or antioxidant supplements including enzymes. The rapid development of accurate assays for measuring oxidative damage to DNA, lipids and proteins is proceeding.

Vitamins and Enzyme Cofactors

Vitamin E inhibits lipid peroxidation of phospholipid membranes such as those found in foods. The membrane antioxidant action of α-tocopherol enables it to protect tissues against linoleic acid hydroperoxide induced damage. Vitamin E fed to chickens protects against membrane lipid peroxidation initiated in chicken liver, which is a readily available and cheap food that is sold without processing. Ubiquinol-10 (the reduced form of ubiquinone-10 or coenzyme Q-10 found in green leafy vegetables and sold as a health supplement) is another effective membrane antioxidant, the protective action of which has been demonstrated in artificial (liposomal) membranes. Vitamin D is unique among vitamins in that its requirement can be met from either the diet or from skin photobiosynthesis due to ultraviolet light in sunlight (or both). Vitamin D is a membrane antioxidant in that it inhibits lipid peroxidation in artificial (liposomal) membrane systems and may also function as an antioxidant in the animal or plant that is eventually eaten. The similar antioxidant efficacy of its precursor in the skin (7-dehydrocholesterol) is worth noting. Vitamin C (a dietary necessity in humans) is another important dietary antioxidant: it protects against oxidative damage to membranes and proteins and is widely used in the food industry.

Flavonoids and Isoflavonoids

As mentioned above, diet is a major influence on health and consequently not only vitamins but also other endogenous compounds such as antioxidants are important. Interestingly, there are relationships between diet and some of the disease states discussed. Flavonoids such as quercetin and myricetin (Fig. 20.8; found in red wine, tea, apples and onions) have been widely reported to inhibit membrane lipid peroxidation. Isoflavonoid phytoestrogens (found in soya products) such as genistein and daidzein (Fig. 20.4) also protected microsomal membranes against lipid peroxidation and liposomal membranes against lipid peroxidation. This action is observed also for endogenous oestrogens such as 17 β-oestradiol, catechol oestrogens and tamoxifen.

Pulse radiolysis (of aqueous solutions) has been used to study the spectral, acid-base and redox properties of the phenoxyl radical derived from 3,4-dihydroxybenzene derivatives and selected flavonoids. The favourable reduction potentials of the phenoxyl radicals suggests that flavonoids may act as efficient antioxidants of alkylperoxyl and superoxide/hydroperoxyl radicals. In addition, the relative antioxidant activities of a number of flavonoids have been measured, including the catechins found in tea, as they scavenger radicals in the aqueous phase and also lipid peroxyl radicals. The order of potency, measured as chemiluminescence intensity, of flavonoids such as the benzoic and cinnamic acids (in the presence of hydrogen peroxide or hydroxyl radicals) has been shown to correlate well with their radical-scavenging abilities. Flavonoids may also be potent scavengers of nitric oxide, the anthocyanidins being more effective than the hydroxyethylrutosides. Some flavonoids and tannins have been reported to have xanthine oxidase inhibitory action. In addition, the total antioxidant capacity of fruits and fruit juices (rich in flavonoids and antioxidant vitamins) has been measured. The antioxidant properties of flavonoids on LDL may contribute to the reduced risk of coronary heart disease in wine drinkers, the so-called French paradox. Another phenolic compound found in wine (resveratrol) also protects LDL against oxidative damage. Dietary phenolic acids from each of the three groups present in the human diet such as caffeic and chlorogenic acids (hydroxycinnamic acid derivatives), ellagic acid (a tannic compound) and protocatechuic acid (a hydroxybenzoic acid derivative) each protects isolated LDL against oxidative damage. Therefore, the 3-hydroxylation and o-diphenol bioconversions of phenolics, particularly the improvement of the antioxidant properties of flavonoids, may have an important impact on processes employed in the food industry and ultimately on human health.

The bioconversion of phloridzin to 3-hydroxyphloridzin by the added enzyme polyphenol oxidase, greatly enhanced its ability to inhibit lipid peroxidation. Furthermore, 3-hydroxylation of phloretin to form the highly potent 3-hydroxyphloretin provides greatly enhanced inhibition of lipid peroxidation which is of comparable efficacy to that of quercetin. Moreover, the efficacy of the aglycone dimer in inhibiting lipid peroxidation was greater than that of phloretin. The overall order of potency of the phloridzin derivatives in this system was 3-hydroxyphloretin > aglycone dimer > 3-hydroxy-phloridzin > phloretin > phloridzin = glycone dimer. It is clear, therefore, that while phloridzin is not a good inhibitor of lipid peroxidation in the liposomal model membrane system, its derivatives are much more effective. Phloridzin has antioxidant properties in an aqueous-based system used for measurement of antioxidant capacity. Its lack of ability in the ox brain phospholipid liposomal system is presumably because of the influence of its glucose group: this results in a decreased lipophilicity, which influences its uptake and orientation within the liposomal membrane. This hypothesis is supported by the much improved ability to inhibit lipid peroxidation shown by the aglycone forms.

The antioxidant action of oestrogens, for example 17-β-oestradiol, may contribute to their cardioprotective action. Phloretin, the aglycone form of phloridzin, has been shown to be oestrogenic and its 3-hydroxy derivative may have a much decreased oestrogenic activity. This, together with its enhanced antioxidant properties, could enable it to act in a manner similar to the antioxidant antioestrogen/ weak oestrogen drug tamoxifen. Alternatively, combinations of phloretin and 3-hydroxyphloretin may offer the best combination of weak oestrogenic and antioxidant properties. Functional foods (sometimes known as nutraceuticals) are being sought, and promoted, worldwide and phloridzin derivatives may be candidates for such use. A sophisticated approach to food modification in relation to beneficial effects of functional foods will be based on improved public knowledge of food additives, including acceptability of antioxidant 'chemicals' and proteins.

Further Studies on Antioxidants and Colourants: Phloridzin Derivatives

The investigation of colourants has centred on the extraction and processing of existing types or the synthetic production of 'nature-identical' compounds. All of these developments are likely to have little difficulty in gaining permission for use (i.e. an 'E' listing in the EU), and require no additional toxicity testing. Substances including novel anthocyanins may also experience little difficulty due to their similarity to existing products. Entirely new dyes or antioxidants would, however, have to pass toxicity tests and achieve food manufacturer acceptance. An intermediate position may apply to one group of potential new compounds, the dimerised oxidation products of phenolics, that can be produced as a result of traditional food processing and to which the phenol oxidation enzyme technology described earlier is relevant. Many phenolic oxidation productions investigated by Taylor and Clysdale were potentially useful colours. Lea and Goodenough have shown that most of the colour of apple juice is due to the oxidation product of phloridzin, which has a hue similar to that of the synthetic colourant tartrazine (E102) (over which there has been much consumer concern because of reports of hyperactivity in children). In addition, yellow dimers have been produced from the grape polyphenol oxidase-mediated coupling or (+)-catechin. The yellow/orange properties of the phloridzin oxidation product indicates potential use as a food colourant. Hunter Lab colourimetric profiles have demonstrated similarity with tartrazine at soft-drink pH values (2.7–4.0): specific absorbance at peak wavelength (420 nm) has been shown to be greater than that of tartrazine, and stability trials in foods have shown the oxidation product to be more stable than tartrazine, particularly in light. The phloridzin dimerisation product also has greater light stability than tartrazine in some actual products (lemonade and cider) and thus shows greater technical performance in addition to greater potential marketability as a 'nature-identical' substance. The phloridzin dimer oxidation product has been shown to comprise a large proportion of the colour of apple juices and ciders and hence represents a potential natural or 'nature-identical' product with performance superior to that of synthetic tartrazine.

The antioxidant properties of 3-hydroxyphloretin suggest its potential use as a technological food antioxidant. Studies of antioxidant applicability in lard (i.e. prevention of rancidity) showed that an o-diphenolic structure as part of the A-ring of a dihydrochalcone (e.g. 3-hydroxyphloretin; Fig. 20.4) produces a compound that is more effective as an antioxidant than when the o-diphenolic is attached to either a pyran ring (e.g. as in flavanones, flavones or flavanols) or to an unsaturated α-β bond (e.g. as in chalcones). Butein (Fig. 20.10), which is a tetrahydroxychalcone and hence a less potent antioxidant than 3-hydroxyphloretin (a pentahydroxydihydrochalcone), was found to be six-fold more effective in preventing fat rancidity than the commercial food antioxidant BHT. 3-Hydroxyphloretin would be expected to be at least six times more potent than BHT. 3-Hydroxyphloridzin has greater water solubility than 3-hydroxyphloretin and could find application therefore in aqueous systems: a particular application could be in the protection of the colourant properties of flavopoids. Depending on the concentration used, 3-hydroxyphloridzin itself is able to show coloured properties upon the formation of dimerised oxidation products: combinations of 3-hydroxyphloridzin and the dimerised oxidation product of phloridzin could then provide a highly stable mixture. Loss of colour of the oxidation product could be compensated for by colour formation that occurs upon oxidation of the 3-hydroxyphloridzin.

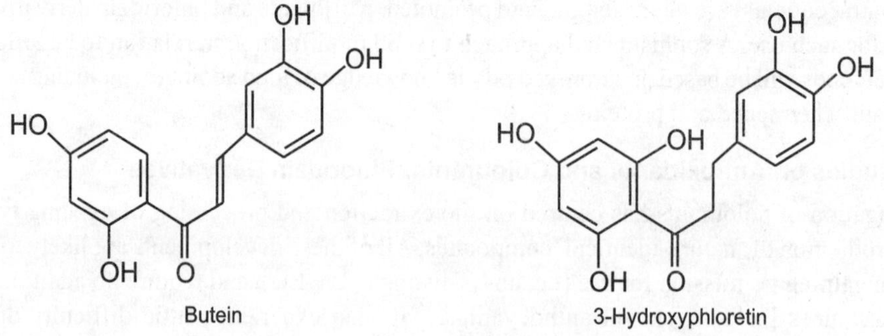

Fig. 20.10. Butein and 3-hydroxyphloretin.

ADDED ENZYMES IN THE FOOD INDUSTRY: FUTURE PROSPECTS

The future holds many exciting possibilities for the use of soluble enzymes and for the use of immobilised enzymes that are covalently attached to solid supports. Greater apparent stability is achieved (especially if cross-linking of the protein conformation is achieved with glutaraldehyde) and flow-through of liquid substrates (such as milk) fit in better with biochemical engineering features (unit operations). Added enzyme applications in food processing are becoming widespread for traditional purposes such as lowered cost of pumping after viscosity decreases using hydrolase enzymes.

Nevertheless, it is becoming clear that a combination of public awareness and consequent legislation will switch urgent interest to food detoxification. A knowledge of the subtle changes associated with food quality deterioration—often due to problems with ROS—will necessitate the urgent development of enzymic and other ways (use of novel antioxidants) of overcoming the perceived health risks of both naturally occurring and additive (or contaminant) toxicants. Attention will focus on even very low levels of hitherto undetected materials because of the development of extremely sensitive analytical techniques, often using antibodies to the analyte. Public opinion in some developed countries may demand legislation that food manufacturers (and governments) may consider to be inappropriately stringent on the content of naturally occurring or accidentally introduced 'toxins' in foodstuffs. Labelling of the exact content of such undesirable compounds may clarify some of these situations, especially with regard to foreign-gene content (DNA) in genetically engineered foods.

Chapter 21

Citric Acid

INTRODUCTION

Citric acid is a weak organic acid, and it is a natural preservative and is also used to add an acidic, or sour taste to foods and soft drinks. In biochemistry, it is important as an intermediate in the citric acid cycle and therefore occurs in the metabolism of virtually all living things. It can also be used as an environmentally benign cleaning agent and acts as an antioxidant and a lubricant.

Citric acid exists in greater than trace amounts in a variety of fruits and vegetables, most notably citrus fruits. Lemons and limes have particularly high concentrations of the acid; it can constitute as much as 8 per cent of the dry weight of these fruits (1.44 and 1.38 grams per ounce of the juices, respectively). The concentrations of citric acid in citrus fruits range from 0.005 mol/l for oranges and grapefruits to 0.030 mol/l in lemons and limes. These values vary depending on the circumstances in which the fruit was grown.

CITRIC ACID FROM LEMONS

Citric acid derives its name from the Latin citrus, the citron tree, the fruit of which resembles a lemon. Citric acid was produced commercially from Italian lemons from about 1826 in England by John and Edmund Sturge, but with the increasing importance of citric acid as an item of commerce, production was started in Italy by the lemon growers, who established a virtual monopoly during the rest of the nineteenth century. Lemon juice remained the commercial source of citric acid until 1919 when the first industrial process using *Aspergillus niger* began in Belgium.

Synthetic Citric Acid

Citric acid had been synthesised from glycerol by Grimoux and Adams and later from symmetrical dichloroacetone: (i) by treating with hydrogen cyanide and hydrochloric acid to give dichloroacetonic acid, (ii) converting this into dicyano-acetonic acid, (iii) with potassium cyanide, which on hydrolysis yields citric acid, as shown in Fig. 21.1.

Several other routes using different starting materials have since been published. All chemical methods have so far proved uncompetitive or unsuitable, mainly on economic grounds, with the starting material worth more than the end product, although poor yields due to the number of reaction steps in the synthesis and precautions necessary when handling hazardous compounds involved have contributed to the problem.

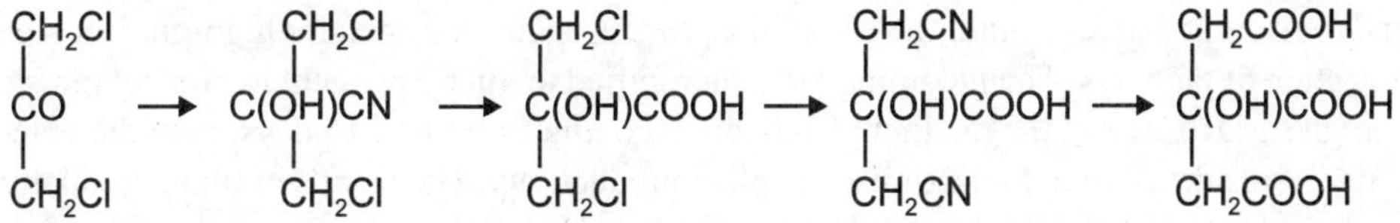

CH₂Cl ... CH₂Cl ... CH₂Cl ... CH₂CN ... CH₂COOH

CO → C(OH)CN → C(OH)COOH → C(OH)COOH → C(OH)COOH

CH₂Cl ... CH₂Cl ... CH₂Cl ... CH₂CN ... CH₂COOH

(i) ... (ii) ... (iii) ... (iv)

Fig. 21.1. Synthesis of citric acid.

Microbial Citric Acid

The concept of microbiological action yielding useful products followed from Pasteur's pioneering studies on fermentation and resulted in systematic investigations of fungi and bacteria. Amongst them Wehmer, in 1893, showed that a '*Citromyces*' (now *Penicillium*) accumulated citric acid in a culture medium containing sugars and inorganic salts. This work did not lead directly to a commercial process but the subsequent search for other organisms capable of this synthesis did. Many other organisms were found to accumulate citric acid including strains of *Aspergillus niger, A. awamori, A. fonsecaeus, A. luchensis, A. phoenicus, A. wentii, A. saitoi, A. lanosius, A. flavus, Absidia* sp., *Acremonium* sp., *Aschochyta* sp., *Botrytis* sp., *Eupenicillium* sp., *Mucor piriformis, Penicillium janthinellum, P. restrictum, Talaromyces* sp., *Trichoderma viride* and *Ustulina vulgaris*.

Currie found strains of *A. niger* that produced citric acid when cultured in media with low pH values, high sugar levels and mineral salts. Prior to this *A. niger* was known to produce oxalic acid; the key difference was the low pH which, as we now know, suppressed both the production of oxalic acid, which would be toxic, and gluconic acid, which has a significantly higher production rate from sugar than citric acid. In biotechnological terms, citric acid is known as a bulk, or low value, product. The market is, and always has been, very competitive, so the profit margins are small. Improvements in productivity depend on the detail of the various processes, many of which are not easily protected by patents, so that secrecy is important and understandable.

Citric Acid by the Surface Method

The general details of the original process are straightforward. The fungal mycelium is grown as a surface mat on a liquid medium in a large number of shallow trays with a capacity of 50 to 100 litres. Each tray has a surface area of about 5 m² and a depth of between 5 and 20 cm. The trays are manufactured from high purity aluminium or stainless steel and usually can be lifted by just two men. The trays are stacked in racks in a chamber to allow operation under relatively aseptic conditions. Various sucrose sources were used initially but cane molasses and then beet molasses soon became the norm as the sugar source. The molasses are diluted to the required concentration, usually 15 per cent and the pH adjusted to 5–7. After sterilisation, the medium is pumped into the trays and inoculation carried out directly from spores, either by adding a liquid suspension or by blowing the spores in with the air stream. Aerating the chambers is important for two purposes, oxygenation and heat removal. The air requirement depends on the stage of growth. Initially sterile air at low rates is used to prevent contamination during the germination stage, which takes about 12 hours. Later, when growth is maximal, rates of up to 10 m³ per cubic metre medium per minute are needed to ensure heat dispersal. The heat generation is considerable, around 1 kJ hr⁻¹ m⁻³ medium and the surface and medium temperatures are ideally around 28° to 30°C. This high volume air is not necessarily sterile, as contamination is normally not a problem once the pH has fallen, after about 24 hours growth. The pH falls to about 2, or slightly lower, and remains at that level until the end of the process, hence the need for high-grade materials for the construction of the trays. The incoming air is humidified to 40–60 per cent to prevent moisture loss from the high surface area of the medium. Cultivation continues for 8 to 15 days, with the objective of minimising the residence time to maximise the plant productivity. The details of time, productivity and yield are closely guarded secrets, but productivity of the order of 1 kg per square metre per day can be obtained and yield is up to 75 per cent of the initial sugar level. At the end of the process, which can be monitored by total acid production or judged by experience, the mycelial mat is removed by filtration and washed, as it contains up to 15 per cent of the total citric acid. The washings and spent medium are treated with lime (calcium hydroxide) at about 90°C to precipitate the insoluble tricalcium tetrahydrate salt of citric acid. It is not possible to crystallise the acid directly from the crude molasses medium although this can be done if pure sucrose is used as the carbon source. The precipitate of calcium citrate is washed and suspended in enough sulphuric acid to precipitate the calcium as calcium sulphate. This releases the citric acid into solution from where it can be treated further as required.

The surface process, though commercially profitable for many years, is labour intensive and inefficient in its use of space; there is a limit as to how high a large tray can be lifted. The production of citric acid by surface culture was challenged at the beginning of the 1940s by the development of submerged fermentation processes. When Shu and Johnson published their work on the effect of medium ingredients and their concentrations on citric acid production in submerged culture, the fundamental technology for submerged production was ready to be exploited on an industrial scale.

Submerged Process for Production of Citric Acid

The submerged process has become the method of choice in the industrialised countries because it is less labour intensive, gives a higher production rate, and uses less space. Several designs of reactor have been used, particularly in pilot scale systems; the stirred tank reactor is the most common design although air-lift reactors, with a higher aspect ratio than the stirred tank reactor are also used. The reactors are constructed of high-grade stainless steel, an important requirement in view of the low pH levels developed, the ability of citric acid to solubilise metal ions and the presence of manganese in stainless steels. Inferior grades of steel have caused problems in the past, both of leaching and pitting or general corrosion. Industrial rumours suggest it may still happen though not by design. The empirical process of 'conditioning' a reactor, whereby a few batches are processed before optimal production levels are achieved, may be related to this problem.

The other general requirement for reactors for citric acid production is the provision of aeration systems that can maintain a high dissolved oxygen level. With both tank and tower reactors sterile air is sparged from the base, although extra inputs are often used with tower reactors. The reactor may be held above atmospheric pressure to increase the rate of oxygen transfer into the fermentation broth. The influence of dissolved oxygen on citric acid formation has been examined and the dissolved oxygen levels are routinely monitored. The oxygen levels are also affected by the rheology of the broth.

A typical plant will consist of four areas: medium preparation, reactor section, broth separation and product recovery. The medium preparation will involve dilution of the molasses, or other raw material, addition of nutrients and other pretreatment such as ferrocyanide, and sterilisation, either in line or in the reactor. Where in line sterilisation is used the reactors are steam sterilised separately. It is usual to prepare an inoculum for the production reactor in a smaller reactor, in which the conditions may be modified to give rapid growth rather than product formation. Primary inoculation is by spores and the initial phase of the growth is critical.

When a separate inoculum stage is used, the correct stage for transfer, characteristically between 18 and 30 hours, is judged by pH level. Production temperature, like the inoculum temperature, is about 30°C. The process is allowed to continue until the rate of citric acid production falls below a predetermined value, which is reached many hours before the production ceases altogether.

Many reports suggest that the morphology of the mycelium is crucial to the ultimate yield; not only with respect to the shape of hyphae, but also their aggregation. Several studies suggest that hyphae should be abnormally short, bulbous and heavily branched. It is recognised that this condition is brought about by manganese deficiency or related to the addition of ferrocyanide, which is probably the same thing. The mycelium should also form small (less than 0.5 mm) pellets with a smooth, hard surface. Such pellets are produced when a number of factors are controlled, such as ferrocyanide levels, manganese levels, low iron (less than 1 ppm), low pH, control of aeration and agitation or the amount of spore inoculum.

It is clear that this morphological appearance is not in itself necessary for a successful yield, but is a result of the correct process parameters. Pellet formation is not necessary, but does give a broth with a lower energy requirement for mixing. When a change to a filamentous growth type occurs, the dissolved oxygen level may fall by 50 per cent for a fixed input. That filamentous growth can give satisfactory yields has been demonstrated and consideration of the diffusion characteristics of pellets versus filamentous mycelium would suggest that while yields may be similar, productivity should be greater without the additional diffusional constraint of pellets.

Aeration is a significant factor in the cost of the process, and although a constant aeration rate is used in many laboratory scale studies, the industrial practice is to use relatively low aeration rates initially (0.1 vvm) rising to 0.5–1 vvm as growth proceeds. Such aeration rates will lead to foaming and various devices and agents are available to minimise the problem. Although very high yields are possible, the productivity is a more important consideration on an industrial basis, and it is rare that the process is allowed to continue to the maximum yield.

The processes run today owes much to the pioneering work carried out by Clark and his co-workers at the Northern regional research laboratories in Canada during the 1950s and early 1960s. Here, the technology for large-scale production of citric acid with *A. niger* using molasses was established. After the fermentation characteristics were worked out, attention was given to the controlling mechanisms of the fermentation. Numerous reports have been published on the role of metal ions on the citric acid cycle, in particular. After decades of academic discussion, there is general agreement about the factors that regulate the fermentation and give rise to the high yields obtained in industry.

Continuous and Immobilised Processes

A process for continuous production of citric acid has been described, but no commercial application of this has been made in spite of the high productivity values obtained. The process does not use the carbon source as the limiting substrate so that excess sugar will pass out of the reactor. As the carbohydrate substrate is one of the major cost factors, the continuous process will be less efficient than the batch process. This might be overcome by using several reactors in series, but this offsets any advantage from the continuous process.

Fed-batch processes have been used industrially so that the conversion of sugar concentrations greater than 15 per cent can be achieved, but the gain does not seem to be sufficient to allow the fed-batch method to become standard. The possibility of using the mycelium in an immobilised system has occurred to several workers and attempts on a small scale have been reported. Immobilisation of mycelium in alginate beads or collagen proved possible, but with very low production rates. The difficulties of avoiding oxygen limitation when preparing beads, and preventing further growth, which reduces oxygen transfer rates, have led to the immobilisation of conidia which are then grown under nitrogen limitation to the desired compact pellet. While giving a manageable system, the productivity was still too low to be of industrial interest.

Other constructs for immobilisation that have been more successful are the use of exchange filtration, and a rotating disc with an adhering mycelial film, reminiscent of sewage treatment techniques. These radical methods are unlikely to gain acceptance, even were they to give economic productivity gains, unless the engineering problems of scale-up can be overcome without making the capital costs too large.

Yeast-based Processes

From about 1965 methods using yeasts were developed, first from carbohydrate sources, then from n-alkanes. At this time hydrocarbons were relatively cheap and plants were built to use the method. The economics have altered since then and plants that have been built to utilise both yeast technologies have apparently switched back to carbohydrate feedstocks.

The potential advantages of using yeasts rather than filamentous fungi are the higher initial sugar concentrations that can be tolerated and the faster conversion rates possible. Further, the insensitivity to metal ions means that crude (and hence cheaper) grade molasses can be used without costly pretreatment. Since 1968, when the patent for citric acid production from molasses by eight genera of yeasts was allowed, there have been many process modifications reported. *Candida, Hansenula, Pichia, Debaromyces, Torulopsis, Kloekera, Trichosporon, Torula, Rhodotorula, Sporobolomyces, Endomyces, Nocardia, Nematospora, Saccharomyces* and *Zygosaccharomyces* species are known to produce citric acid from various carbon sources. Out of these genera the *Candida* species, including *C. lipolytica, C. tropicalis, C. guillermondii, C. oleophila* and *C. intermedia* have been used.

The original process incorporated calcium carbonate into the medium to maintain a neutral pH, and generally a pH above 5.5 was used. Various additions have been proposed to reduce the isocitric acid contamination that afflicts yeasts even on carbohydrate media. Halogen substituted alkanoic mono- or di-substituted acids, n-hexadecyl citric acid or *trans*-aconitic acid, and even lead acetate have been patented, despite the possibility of toxic residues in the resulting citric acid. Many mutants have been selected for reduced isocitrate production. An osmophilic strain, which would convert sugar concentrations as high as 28 per cent without pretreatment of the molasses substrate, has been patented.

Tower reactors of fairly standard design are used, but with improved cooling systems as the rate of heat production is high. A continuous process has been described where the pH is maintained at 3.5 with ammonium hydroxide.

The industrial production of citric acid from n-alkanes is not now economic, although a plant was built, and operated, around 1970 at Saline, Reggio Calabria, Italy (Liquichimica). This process was based on a low aconitase mutant of *C. lipolytica* in a batch process with stirred, aerated tank reactors of 400 m^3, operating on a 72 hours cycle. The conversion from alkanes was reported to exceed 130 per cent (by weight). The theoretical yield is 250 per cent, but part of the alkanes was converted to biomass and carbon dioxide. The yeast was removed by centrifugation and the purification was traditional.

The medium used was based on the process developed for the yeast strain that had a substrate concentration of 10 per cent n-decane, although n-alkanes from 9 to 20 carbons could be used. The availability and cost of Libyan n-alkanes, which lead to the development of this and other plants, including the dual substrate plants, has changed over the last three decades. One unique feature of the *n*-alkane process is the insolubility of the substrate. To ensure a rapid conversion the *n*-alkane has to be thoroughly dispersed, so additives such as polyoxypropylene glycol ether, at concentrations from 20 to 200 ppm, are used to enhance this.

Koji Process

A third method for the production of citric acid is the koji process, using *Aspergillus* species. This is the solid state equivalent of the surface process described previously. It was originally developed in Japan where it uses the readily available rice bran and fruit wastes. It is confined to southeast Asia and is a relatively small-scale process. The carbohydrate source, which is principally starch and cellulose, is sterilised by steaming and the resulting semisolid paste (about 70 per cent water), at a pH of about 5.5, is inoculated by spraying on spores of *A. niger*. Additions of ferrocyanide or copper may be made. The incubation temperature is 30°C and the process takes about four to five days. Yields are low because of the difficulty of controlling trace metals and the process parameters. The fungus produces sufficient cellulases and amylases to break down the substrate, though the low yields may reflect the rate limitations of this step.

Uses of Citric Acid

Citric acid is used in food, confectionery and beverages, in pharmaceuticals and in industrial fields. Its uses depend on three properties: acidity, flavour and salt formation. Chemically citric acid is 2-hydroxy-1,2,3-propane tricarboxylic acid (77-92-9). It has three pK_a values at pH 3.1, 4.7 and 6.4. As these three values are relatively close together the second H^+ is appreciably dissociated before the first is completed, and similarly with the third. Because of this overlapping the solution is well buffered throughout the titration curve and there are no breaks from about pH 2 (the approximate pH of a 0.2 M solution) to pH 7.

Citric acid forms a wide range of metallic salts including complexes with copper, iron, manganese, magnesium and calcium. These salts are the reason for its use as a sequestering agent in industrial processes and as an anticoagulant blood preservative. It is also the basis of its antioxidant properties in fats and oils where it reduces metal-catalysed oxidation by chelating traces of metals such as iron. There are two components to its use as a flavouring: the first is due to its acidity, which has little aftertaste; the second to its ability to enhance other flavours.

A process to remove sulphur dioxide from flue gases has been developed where citric acid is used as a scrubber, forming a complex ion which then reacts with H_2S to give elemental sulphur, regenerating citrate. This may become more important with increased environmental pressures.

Citric acid esters of a range of alcohols are known; the triethyl, butyl and acetyltributyl esters are used as plasticisers in plastic films and monostyryl citrate is used instead of citric acid as an antioxidant in oils and fats. A summary of the uses of citric acid is given in Table 21.1.

Effluent Disposal

Regardless of the method of production the disposal of waste is an increasing problem for manufacturers both from a cost and a regulatory viewpoint. Gypsum (calcium sulphate) is not valuable enough to purify and use in, for example, plaster. It may be disposed of to landfill sites, at a cost, and in some cases may be pumped out to sea, where tidal conditions permit. A more serious problem is the disposal of the filtrate from the precipitation where molasses has been used as a raw material; the waste is non-toxic, but has a high biological oxygen demand, so that it cannot be disposed of to rivers untreated. Anaerobic digestion, with fuel gas as a useful by-product, is probably the future method of choice, although animal feedstuff formulation in the form of condensed molasses solubles is another possibility. It can also be used as a medium for the growth of yeasts for animal feeds.

Table 21.1. Applications of citric acid.

Industry	Property	Use	Market share
Food			About 75%
Beverages	Acidulant	Flavouring	
Jellies, jams, etc.	Flavouring	Acidulant	
Fats and oils	Antioxidant	Metal complexing	
Frozen foods	Antioxidant		
Pharmaceutical			About 10%
Effervescent	Acid	Flavour	
Vitamins	Antioxidant		
Anticoagulants	Sequestering	Buffering	
Iron preparations	Salt formation		
Cosmetics	Buffering	Antioxidant	
Industrial			About 15%
Cleaning (metals)	Sequestering		
Detergents	Buffering	Sequestering	
Photographic	Buffering		
Primer binding	Sequestering		
Polymerisations	Sequestering		

BIOCHEMISTRY OF CITRIC ACID ACCUMULATION BY *ASPERGILLUS NIGER*

The biochemical mechanism by which *Aspergillus niger* accumulates citric acid has attracted the interest of researchers since the late 1930s when the optimisation of this accumulation to give a commercial process began. In this sense, the various theories which have been proposed to explain the accumulation of citric acid in such high yields also reflect the general biochemical knowledge at the time the respective research was done. In view of the high input into this research through more than 50 years it is, therefore, rather disappointing that there is still no explanation of the biochemical basis of this process which would consistently explain all the observed factors influencing this fermentation. Reasons for this are manifold.

First, citric acid is only accumulated when several nutrient factors are present, either in excess (i.e. sugar concentration, H^+, dissolved oxygen), or at suboptimal levels (trace metals, nitrogen and phosphate), and thus is subject to multifactorial influence. Hence it is unlikely that single biochemical events are solely responsible for citric acid overflow.

Secondly, an appreciable part of the literature consists of work which has been performed using low or only moderately producing strains or by applying nutrient conditions not optimal for citric acid production, and while this may be justified for special reasons in individual cases, the respective results are not comparable to those obtained by others. Moreover, their significance for the understanding of the commercial citric acid fermentation is questionable. Thirdly, the biochemical knowledge of filamentous fungi is still significantly inferior to that of, for example, *Saccharomyces cerevisiae* or higher eukaryotes and, moreover, results from these sources cannot be uncritically transformed to filamentous fungi, which impedes a biochemically correct interpretation of results in several areas. Hence, although a considerable amount of basic biochemical research has been carried out with *A. niger*, the present state of understanding of the events relevant for citric acid accumulation (not to say production) is still a poorly resolved puzzle.

This section attempts to draw the currently recognisable picture and to aid in the further fitting together of the other scattered bits and pieces.

Glucose Catabolism in *A. niger* and its Regulation

Citric acid biosynthetic pathway

It is well known, since the famous tracer studies by Cleland and Johnson, and Martin and Wilson, that citric acid is mainly formed via the reactions of the glycolytic pathway. Like most other fungi *Aspergillus* spp. utilise glucose and other carbohydrates for energy and cell synthesis by channelling glucose into the reactions of the glycolytic and the pentose phosphate pathway, respectively. The pentose phosphate pathway accounts for only a minor fraction of metabolised carbon during citric acid fermentation, and this decreases throughout prolonged cultivation. Legisa and Mattey speculated that this may be due to inhibition of 6-phosphogluconate dehydrogenase by citrate, but evidence for this is lacking. It should be noted that both arabitol and erythritol are accumulated as by-products until late stages of the fermentation; hence a complete blockage of the pentose phosphate pathway is obviously not taking place.

A. niger possesses a further pathway of glucose catabolism which is catalysed by glucose oxidase. This enzyme is induced by high concentrations of glucose and strong aeration in the presence of low concentrations of other nutrients, conditions which are also typical for citric acid fermentation; glucose oxidase will hence inevitably be formed during the starting phase of citric acid fermentation and convert a significant amount of glucose into gluconic acid. However, due to the extracellular location of the enzyme, it is directly influenced by the external pH and will be inactivated at pH < 3.5. Because of the pK_a values for citric acid, its accumulation decreases the pH of the culture filtrate to pH 1.8 thereby inactivating glucose oxidase. It is not known if, and by which mechanism gluconic acid can be catabolised to citric acid during further fermentation.

The catabolism of glucose via glycolytic catabolism leads to 2 moles of pyruvate, and their subsequent conversion to the precursors of citrate (i.e. oxaloacetate and pyruvate). Cleland and Johnson were the first to show that *A. niger* uses 1 mole of the carbon dioxide which is released during the formation of acetyl-CoA and 1 mole of pyruvate to form 1 mole of oxaloacetate (Fig. 21.2a). This reaction is of utmost importance to high citric acid yields, because oxaloacetate could otherwise only be formed by one turn of the tricarboxylic acid cycle, which would be accompanied by the loss of two moles of CO_2 and only two thirds of the carbon of glucose could therefore accumulate as citric acid (Fig. 21.2b). The enzyme catalysing this reaction was shown to be pyruvate carboxylase, which was characterised by Feir and Suzuki and Wongchai and Jefferson.

Unlike the enzyme from several other eukaryotes, the pyruvate carboxylase of *A. niger* is localised in the cytosol. Glycolytic pyruvate will therefore be converted to oxaloacetate, and further to malate by the cytosolic malate dehydrogenase isoenzyme, thereby also regenerating 50 per cent of the glycolytically produced NADH (Fig. 21.3). It has been postulated that, analogous to higher eukaryotes, the cytosolic malate may serve as the cosubstrate of the mitochondrial tricarboxylic acid carrier, and that such an enhanced malate concentration may stimulate export of citrate from the mitochondrion.

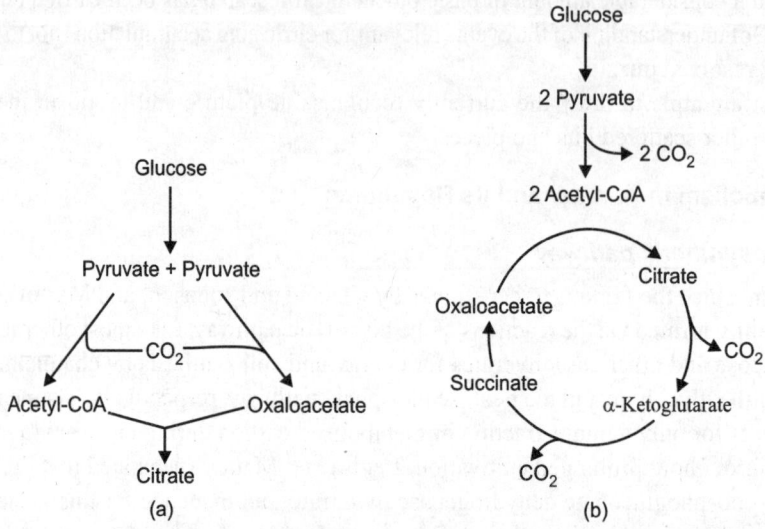

Fig. 21.2. Metabolic pathways from glucose to citric acid by (a) involvement of an anaplerotic carbon dioxide fixation, and (b) sole involvement of the citric acid cycle. Only relevant intermediates are given, and arrows may indicate more than a single enzymatic step. Note that in (b), each of the two acetyl-CoA molecules is subject to one turn of the tricarboxylic acid cycle.

It should be noted that the fixation of carbon dioxide, while convincing and experimentally verified, does not seem to occur during the early phases of fermentation: Kubicek, by continuously quantifying carbon dioxide and oxygen in the exit air of a pilot plant citric acid fermentation, observed that during the first 70 hours of fermentation the respiratory coefficient (i.e. CO_2 released/O_2 taken up) is close to 1; it starts to decrease thereafter and reaches the level predicted from the operation of the pyruvate carboxylase reaction (0.66) only at stages where citrate accumulation is already taking place at a constant rate (e.g. < 120 hours). The Cleland and Johnson reaction may therefore only be important at later stages of fermentation, whereas the initial phase of citric acid accumulation takes place without anaplerotic carbon dioxide supply.

It should be noted that *A. niger* is also capable of accumulating another organic acid – oxalic acid – as a (toxic) by-product of citric acid fermentation. The biosynthesis of this compound is controversial, and appears to depend on whether glucose or citric acid is used as the carbon source.

In the latter case, the glyoxalate cycle has been implicated in its biosynthesis. Its biosynthesis on glucose as a carbon source occurs by the hydrolysis of oxaloacetate catalysed by oxaloacetate hydrolase, which is cytosolically located and appears to act as a valve by which the carbon overflow can be channelled into an energetically neutral pathway (Fig. 21.4) and so compete with citrate overproduction. Although production of oxalate is, because of its toxicity, of considerable interest to citric acid fermentation, the regulation of its biosynthesis is controversial.

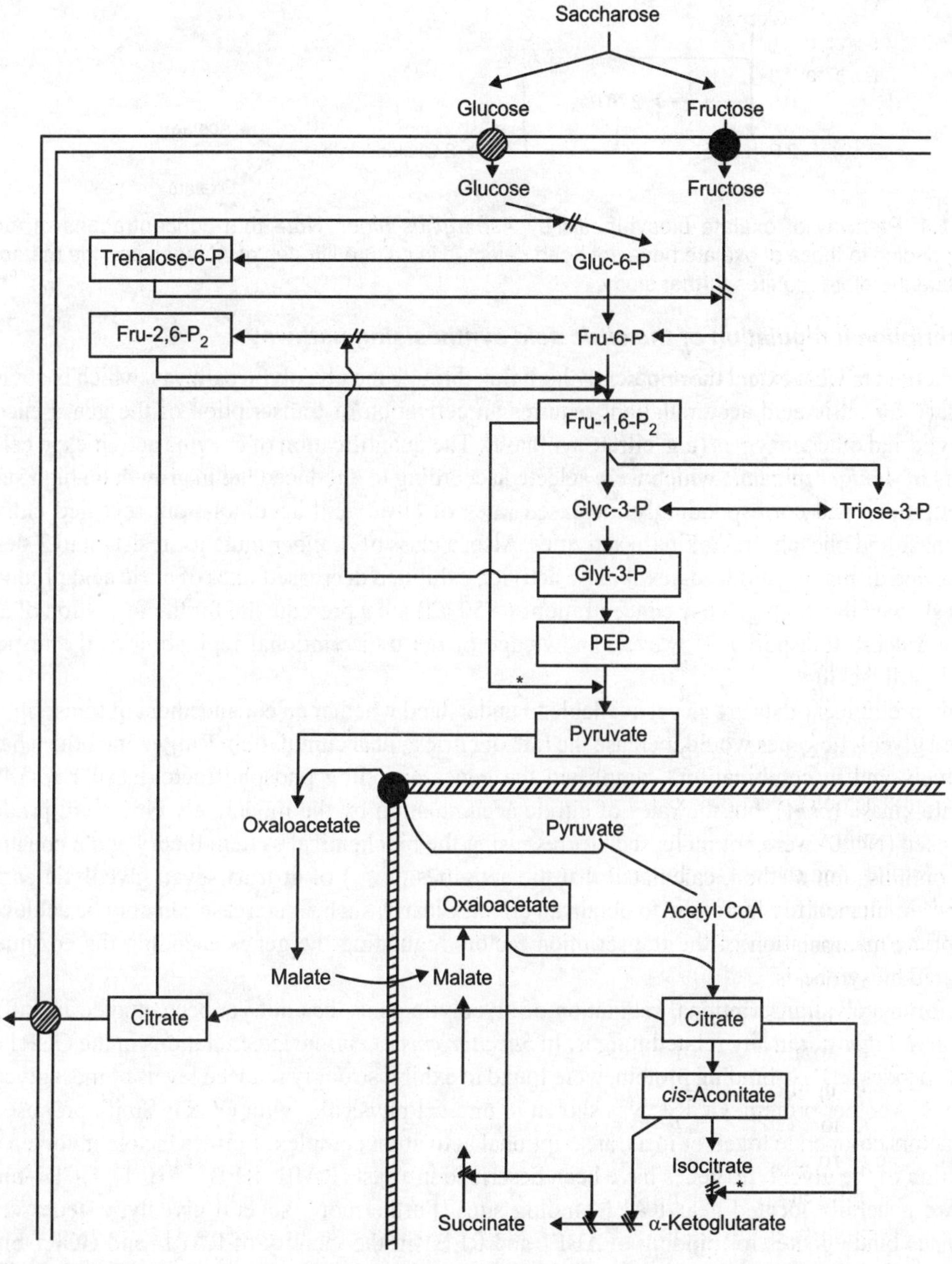

Fig. 21.3. Metabolic and regulatory network of citric acid biosynthesis from sucrose in *A. niger*. For convenience, sucrose is assumed to be split into glucose and fructose by invertase extracellularly and only the monosaccharides are taken up. The double line indicates the plasma membrane, the hatched double line the mitochondrial membrane. Circles inserted into the membranes indicate known or assumed transport steps (hatched: characterised in *A. niger*; full: assumed, but not yet characterised; empty: countertransport, to be verified). Thick lines and arrows indicate metabolic reactions; thin lines and arrows indicate regulatory interactions (*activation: // inhibition). Intermediates of regulatory importance are boxed.

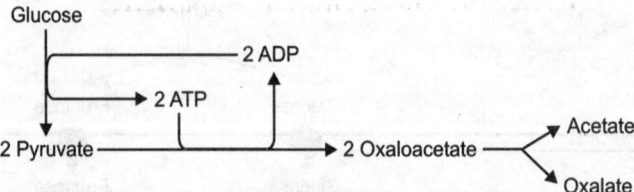

Fig. 21.4. Pathway of oxalate biosynthesis by *Aspergillus niger*. Note that concentrations of acetate corresponding to those of oxalate have not been detected in culture filtrates of *A. niger*, and the metabolism of acetate therefore requires further study.

Transcriptional regulation of the citric acid synthesising pathway

It is uncertain to what extent the apparently high flux through the glycolytic pathway, which is obviously necessary for citric acid accumulation, requires an activation of transcription of the genes encoding glycolytic and other enzymes (e.g. citrate synthase). The quantification of enzyme activities in cell-free extracts of *A. niger* mutants, which were selected according to a reduced lag in growth on high sucrose concentrations and correspondingly increased rates of citric acid accumulation, revealed enhanced hexokinase and phosphofructokinase activities. Also, a class of *A. niger* mutants, resistant to 2-desoxy-glucose and displaying reduced hexokinase activity, exhibited decreased rates of citric acid production. Torres showed that high glucose concentrations (> 50 g/l) are a prerequisite for the formation of a low-affinity glucose transporter. However, knowledge of the transcriptional regulation of the respective genes is still lacking.

Only preliminary data are as yet available to understand whether an enhancement of transcription of selected glycolytic genes would increase the rate of citric acid accumulation. Ruijter and others have — selectively and in combination—amplified the genes encoding phosphofructokinase 1 (*pfkA*) and pyruvate kinase (*pkiA*), but the rates of citrate accumulation by the moderately citric acid producing strain used (N400) were not increased. Torres, using the biochemical system theory and a constrained linear optimisation method, calculated that the activities (V_{max}) of at least seven glycolytic enzymes must be simultaneously increased to obtain an effect. Clearly, such an increase can only be achieved by appropriate manipulation of the transcription factors regulating the genes encoding the enzymes for citric acid biosynthesis.

Unfortunately, transcriptional regulation of glycolytic genes has not yet been studied in sufficient detail in *A. niger* nor in any related fungus. In *Saccharomyces cerevisiae*, mutations in the GCR1 gene, which encodes a DNA-binding protein, were found to exhibit strongly reduced levels of most glycolytic enzymes. Another protein, GCR2, was shown to interact physically with GCR1. Smith proposed that both factors co-operate together in a transcriptional activation complex. Further factors involved in the regulation of the glycolytic genes have been described in yeast (RAP1, REB1, ABF1). GCR1-binding sites are generally located near RAP1-binding sites. Furthermore, several glycolytic genes contain consensus binding sites for binding of ABF1 and REB1 in the vicinity of RAP1- and GCR1-binding sites. It is intriguing that the above named binding sites have so far not been detected in the 5′-noncoding sequences of the few glycolytic genes studied in *A. niger* or the close relative *Aspergillus nidulans* (Table 21.2, Fig. 21.5). Transcriptional regulation of glyceraldehyde-3-phosphate dehydrogenase and of 3-phosphoglycerate kinase has been studied in some detail in the closely related fungus *A. nidulans*. Its transcription depends on positive control by several co-operating DNA-binding proteins since a truncated core promoter of the *pgkA* gene only containing the CAAT, TATA and CT-rich elements could not trigger transcription. Punt identified a 'glycolytic box' as responsible for transcription. No differences in expression of *gpdA* were observed on 1 per cent glucose or 0.1 per cent fructose.

Table 21.2. Genes encoding enzymes involved in the biosynthesis of citric acid by *A niger*, which have already been cloned from *A. niger* or other *Aspergillus* spp.

Organism	Gene
A. niger	*suc1* (invertase)
A. niger	*glkA* (glucokinase)
A. niger	*tpsA* and *tpsB* (trehalose-6-phosphate synthases A and B)
A. niger	*pfkA* (phosphofructokinase)
A. niger	*gsdA* (glucose-6-phosphate dehydrogenase)
A. nidulans	*tpiA* (triosephosphate isomerase)
A. nidulans	*gpdA* (glyceraldehyde-3-phosphate dehydrogenase
A. nidulans	*pgkA* (3-phosphoglycerate kinase)
A. oryzae	*enoA* (enolase)
A. nidulans	*pkiA* (pyruvate kinase)
A. niger	*pkiA* (pyruvate kinase)
A. niger	*cisA* (citrate synthase)

A 24-bp region, which shares 60 per cent similarity with the 'glycolytic box', is also present at −638 and −488 of the *pgkA* promoter (Fig. 21.5). However, another sequence, located between −161 and −120, in the *pgkA* promoter was shown to be essential for expression of the respective gene. It consists of two non-overlapping octameric sequences that match in seven out of eight nucleotides to the higher eukaryotic consensus ATGCAAAT.

A 17-base pair sequence was found in the 5′-regions of the *A. nidulans* and *A. niger pkiA* genes that may act as an upstream regulating sequence.

This sequence was shown to be distinct from the proposed *cis*-acting element mediating increased transcription of pyruvate kinase on glycolytic carbon sources.

Glucose metabolism and its regulation

The disappointing result that amplification of selected genes did not lead to an increase in the rate of citric acid accumulation by *A. niger* indicates the operation of very tight fine control of at least some of the enzymes involved. In fact, this fine control was already a major target of investigation throughout the early 1980s, and as a consequence several of the enzymes involved in it have been comparably well characterised (Table 21.3).

Most recently, the method to study the concentration of intracellular metabolites in *A. niger* has also been critically reassessed. Based on these data, Fig. 21.3 shows those regulatory interactions between metabolites and enzymes which are believed to be of major importance to the regulation of citric acid biosynthesis in *A. niger*.

Similar to the situation in yeast and higher eukaryotes, citrate and phosphoenolpyruvate (PEP) seem to be the major factors negatively affecting the glycolytic flux, whereas fructose-2,6-diphosphate (Fru-$2,6$-P_2) and Fru-$1,6$-P_2 appear to be the major activators.

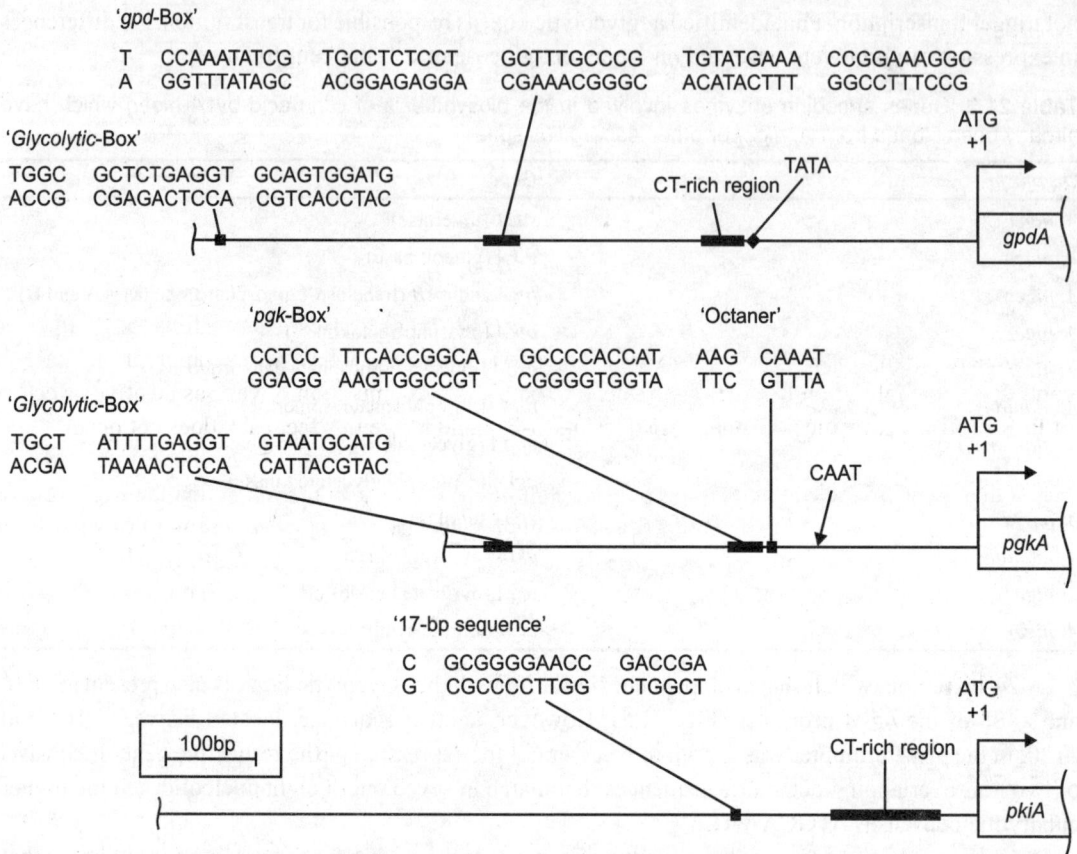

'gpd-Box'

| T | CCAAATATCG | TGCCTCTCCT | GCTTTGCCCG | TGTATGAAA | CCGGAAAGGC |
| A | GGTTTATAGC | ACGGAGAGGA | CGAAACGGGC | ACATACTTT | GGCCTTTCCG |

'Glycolytic-Box'

| TGGC | GCTCTGAGGT | GCAGTGGATG |
| ACCG | CGAGACTCCA | CGTCACCTAC |

ATG +1

CT-rich region TATA

gpdA

'pgk-Box' 'Octaner'

| CCTCC | TTCACCGGCA | GCCCCACCAT | AAG | CAAAT |
| GGAGG | AAGTGGCCGT | CGGGGTGGTA | TTC | GTTTA |

'Glycolytic-Box'

| TGCT | ATTTTGAGGT | GTAATGCATG |
| ACGA | TAAAACTCCA | CATTACGTAC |

ATG +1

CAAT

pgkA

'17-bp sequence'

| C | GCGGGGAACC | GACCGA |
| G | CGCCCCTTGG | CTGGCT |

ATG +1

100bp

CT-rich region

pkiA

Fig. 21.5. Regulatory nucleotide motifs present in the 5′-nontranscribed sequences of three glycolytic genes of *A. nidulans* (*gpdA*, *pgkA*) and *A. niger* (*pkiA*). Only characterised nucleotide sequences are given. The boxed bar marker indicates 100 bp, and all genes are not drawn to scale.

Table 21.3. Enzymes of *A. niger*, involved in citric acid biosynthesis and catabolism, with noteworthy regulatory properties.

Enzyme	Activators	Inhibitors	Comments
Low-affinity glucose transporter			Only formed in the presence of high glucose concentrations
Hexo/glucokinase		Tre-6-P*	
Phosphofructokinase 1	Fru-2,6-P_2, AMP, NH_4^+	Citrate PEP	
Phosphofructokinase 2			No significant regulation
Pyruvate kinase	Fru-1,6-P_2 NH_4^+		
Pyruvate carboxylase			Higher activities found in the presence of high glucose concentrations
Citrate synthase			No significant regulation

(Contd ...)

Enzyme	Activators	Inhibitors	Comments
NADP-specific isocitrate dehydrogenase	ATP*, citrate*	–	–
α-Ketoglutarate dehydrogenase	cis-Aconitate, oxaloacetate	–	–

*Effectors which show only a weak effect, whose significance in vivo is doubtful.

Regulation of citric acid biosynthesis

Citrate is one of the best known inhibitors of glycolysis, and the ability of A. niger to overproduce citrate by an active glycolytic pathway has therefore attracted biochemical interest for a long time; it is considered to be of major consequence for the fermentation rate. However, under appropriate nutrient conditions, this inhibition is more than counteracted by the accumulation of various positive effectors of PFK1 (NH_4^+, inorganic phosphate, AMP, Fru-2,6-P_2), and hence this feedback does not occur.

A series of investigations by Kubicek and co-workers favour the assumption that Fru-2,6-P_2 may play a major role in the counteraction of citrate inhibition: Kubicek-Pranz found that the triggering of citric acid accumulation by replacing A. niger in high concentrations (14 per cent w/v) of sucrose or glucose is paralleled by a rise in the intracellular concentration of Fru-2,6-P2. Also, mycelia cultivated on carbon sources which allow higher yields of citric acid (i.e. those which are taken up rapidly) showed higher concentrations of Fru-2,6-P_2. The concentration of Fru-2,6-P_2 correlates, therefore, positively with the rate of citrate production, and this fact may be responsible for the lack of citrate inhibition of PFK1. The reason for the increased F-2,6-P_2 level is not completely clear, but it appears to be due to an increased Fru-6-P supply for PFK2, since this enzyme is only poorly regulated in A. niger.

The biosynthesis and regulation of Fru-2,6-P_2 links regulation of PFK1 to that of earlier steps in glycolysis. Torres has recently concluded from theoretical calculations that a major part of the actual control of citric acid production must occur at hexose uptake and/or phosphorylation, which is in accordance with such an assumption. The biochemistry of these early steps in A. niger glycolysis is not completely clear, however Steinböck found a single hexo/glucokinase only in the citric acid producing strain ATCC 11414, which was inhibited by citrate and weakly sensitive to trehalose-6-phosphate. The inhibition by citric acid was due to chelation of Mg^{2+} which is required to chelate the co-substrate ATP, and is most probably irrelevant under physiological conditions where Mg^{2+} is present in excess. However, the inhibition by trehalose-6-phosphate appears to be relevant to the flux towards citric acid, since a recombinant strain of A. niger, which carries a disrupted copy of the constitutively expressed trehalose-6-phosphate synthase gene tpsA, produces citric acid at increased rates. Similarly, a strain bearing multiple copies of tpsA and hence overproducing trehalose-6-phosphate synthase exhibited a reduced rate of citrate production. These data indicate that the cellular level of trehalose-6-phosphate regulates the flux from glucose to citric acid and are thus in accordance with the conclusions of Torres that hexokinase most likely accounts for the major part of regulation at the early steps of glycolysis, thereby supplying an increased concentration of substrate for PFK2.

However, most recently Panneman reported on the isolation and characterisation of a glucokinase from A. niger N400, a strain producing only low levels of citric acid, which has properties different from the hexo/glucokinase purified by Steinböck. They also concluded that by analogy with A. nidulans there may be also at least one separate hexokinase as well. The difference between the results of Steinböck and Panneman are currently unresolved. Hybridisation of an A. niger ATCC 11414 DNA with a Kluyveromyces lactis hexokinase-encoding gene as a probe showed hybridisation to a single fragment only. The gene from strain ATCC 11414 has recently been cloned in laboratory, and its characterisation has to be awaited for clarification of this situation. Whatever the results of this investigation, the results by Arisan-Atac clearly show that a relief from trehalose-6-phosphate inhibition positively influences the glycolytic flux at high sugar concentrations, and the hexose-phosphorylating step is therefore a major regulatory point in this fermentation.

Glucose uptake by *A. niger* was investigated by Torres. *A. niger* ATCC 11414 contains two transporters with different K_m, and V_{max}. However, the high-affinity permease can only be detected during growth on low glucose concentration (1 per cent w/v), whereas the low-affinity permease is detectable in the presence of high glucose concentrations. The latter may therefore contribute to the increased glycolytic flux during growth on high glucose concentrations.

Several lines of evidence suggest that the regulation of PFK1 by Fru-2,6-P_2 may not be the only parameter regulating citrate accumulation. Citrate inhibition of PFK1 also seems *in vivo* to be antagonised by ammonium ions. This antagonism is functionally linked to the well known effect of trace metal ions (particularly manganese ions) on citric acid accumulation, as one of the effects caused by manganese deficiency is an impairment of macromolecular synthesis in *A. niger*, which causes increased protein degradation. As a consequence, mycelia accumulate elevated concentrations of NH_4^+. Proof for the role of manganese ions in this process has been obtained by the isolation of mutants of *A. niger* whose PFK1 was partially citrate-insensitive and whose citric acid accumulation was simultaneously more tolerant to the presence of Mn^{2+}. Furthermore, several authors have reported that the exogenous addition of NH_4^+ during citric acid fermentation even stimulates the rate of citrate production, which is consistent with this effect of NH_4^+ on PFK1. The latter authors documented that both the time of addition as well as the concentration of NH_4^+ were important, and its addition during inappropriate fermentation phases even decreased acid accumulation.

The reason for the impairment of macromolecular synthesis under manganese deficient cultivation conditions had originally been assumed to be at the translational level. However, Hockertz and other have demonstrated that the absence of manganese ions from the nutrient medium of *A. niger* causes a reversible inhibition of DNA, but not RNA biosynthesis. This is supported by the findings that the effect of manganese deficiency can be mimicked by addition of hydroxyurea, an inhibitor of ribonucleotide reductase. They proposed that manganese deficiency may primarily impair DNA synthesis by causing a shortage of desoxyribonucleotides required for DNA replication.

A further mechanism of regulation of PFK1 was proposed by Legisa and co-workers, who postulated that PFK1 is regulated by phosphorylation by cyclic-AMP dependent protein kinase A. They speculate that a high concentration of sucrose causes an increase in mycelial cyclic-AMP levels which trigger the phosphorylation of PFK1, thereby converting an inactive (non-phosphorylated) form into an active (phosphorylated) form. The support for their model is their observation that PFK1 was inactivated by treatment with alkaline phosphatase. However, this model, while intriguing, has to be treated cautiously until solid evidence for it has been obtained, as the molecular weight of the PFK1 purified by Legisa and Bencina and used for their studies was 48 kDa which is not that of native PFK1 (84 kDa). Moreover, the method section does not indicate whether (and how) the alkaline phosphatase had been removed or inactivated prior to the PFK1 assay. If this was not done, the 'inactivation of PFK1' may have been due to a removal of Fru-6-P from the assay and thus be an artefact. Proof for a regulation of PFK1 by phosphorylation is therefore still needed.

A stimulation of citric acid accumulation by increased cyclic-AMP levels had also been postulated earlier. Smith showed that the stimulatory effect was dependent on the zinc concentration of the medium.

Adenylate cyclase from *A. niger* has been described as Zn^{2+} dependent by Wold and Suzuki. A bottleneck of their investigations, however, is that they were using 1 per cent (w/v) sucrose throughout, and hence the relevance of their findings to the effect of zinc under citric acid fermentation conditions is unclear. Smith and studied the intracellular concentration of cyclic-AMP in *A. niger* during citric acid biosynthesis on media with and without Mn^{2+} ions added, and with high (14 per cent) and low (1 per cent) sucrose concentrations. They reported that the cyclic-AMP levels were growth rate dependent, and comparable if phases of similar growth rates were compared. Whether or not cyclic-AMP is in fact involved in the regulation of citrate overproduction remains to be assessed.

Role of Citrate Breakdown in Citrate Accumulation

Role of the citric acid cycle

The reason why *A. niger* accumulates such massive amounts of citric acid has, since the early studies by Ramakrishnan, attracted numerous investigations. Although citrate has been considered an 'overflow' product, which implies that it accumulates as a result of an excessive substrate supply rather than a limited catabolism, an excessive amount of work has been concerned with the attempt to identify a bottleneck in the tricarboxylic acid cycle as the reason for its accumulation. Numerous workers claimed that inactivation of an enzyme degrading citrate (e.g. aconitase or the isocitrate dehydrogenases) would be essential for the accumulation of citric acid. While this view has an extraordinary long half-life in the review literature, solid evidence for the presence of an intact citric acid cycle during citric acid fermentation was presented 25 years ago, and explanations based on this view are therefore simply incorrect.

The requirement of citric acid accumulation of a deficiency in some metal ions (e.g. Mn^{2+}, Fe^{3+}) has frequently been used to explain an inhibition of some enzymes of the TCA cycle. Thus, iron deficiency has been claimed to inhibit aconitase. However, the activity of this enzyme during citric acid accumulation has been demonstrated clearly by others both *in vitro* as well as *in vivo*. It should be kept in mind that the enzymes of the respiratory chain, which also require iron, are highly active during citric acid accumulation. By a similar rationale, the necessity for Mn^{2+} deficiency has been used to claim an inhibition of either of the two isocitrate dehydrogenases which require divalent metal ions for activity. However, this requirement is for chelation of the substrate (i.e. isocitrate). In view of the fact that Mg^{2+} (which is present in excess) can take over the chelating role of Mn^{2+} efficiently, this interpretation is unlikely to explain the effect of Mn^{2+}.

Several other explanations for citric acid accumulation are based on the postulation of a metabolic inhibition of the NADP-specific isocitrate dehydrogenase by citrate or glycerol, which would create a bottleneck in the tricarboxylic acid cycle and—because of the K_{eq} of aconitase—lead to a spilling over of citrate. Unfortunately, none of the explanations which are based on an inhibition of NAD- or NADP-specific isocitrate dehydrogenases have ever been supported by evidence from *in vivo* experiments. The 'glycerol theory', has recently been reassessed by studying the effect of increased mycelial glycerol concentrations on the oxidation of 1,5-^{14}C-citrate by mycelia and isolated mitochondria of *A. niger*. The appearance of ^{14}C-labelled CO_2—which because of the labelling position applied can only be released during the metabolic conversion of citrate to α-ketoglutarate—was virtually unaffected by the glycerol concentration, thereby clearly disproving an effect of glycerol on the activity of isocitrate dehydrogenases and consequently this theory. Also, in contrast to the enzyme from crude cell-free extracts, the purified NADP-specific isocitrate dehydrogenase was not inhibited by citrate.

It is surprising that the question of whether the isocitrate dehydrogenase step of the TCA cycle is active during citric acid fermentation or not has never been viewed from a theoretical point of view: using the cellular concentration of free and protein-bound glutamic acid as an indicator of metabolic flux from glucose to α-ketoglutarate, there is no indication for a significant change in this flux unless at late stages of fermentation where the fungal growth (and also the need for glutamic acid) has stopped, and this flux is only 17 per cent lower than that occurring in a culture accumulating 78 per cent less citric acid, and hence may not be of high relevance to the mechanism of citric acid accumulation.

With regard to the mechanisms which trigger the initial accumulation of citrate from the mitochondria, a fact completely overlooked so far is the activity of the tricarboxylate transporter. This carrier competes directly with aconitase for citrate, and if its affinity for citrate were much higher than that of aconitase, would pump citrate out of the mitochondria without any necessity for inhibition of one of the TCA cycle enzymes. As the tricarboxylate carrier of mammalian tissues and yeast occurs by countertransport with malate, such a situation is conceivable when its counter-ion malate accumulates in the cytosol. Malate accumulation has in fact been shown to precede citrate accumulation. However, the mitochondrial citrate carrier of *A. niger* has not yet been investigated, and this hypothesis clearly needs thorough investigation before it can be used to explain citrate accumulation. It is also not known to what extent changes in the flux through the NAD-dependent, NADP-dependent isocitrate dehydrogenases, α-ketoglutarate dehydrogenase and succinate dehydrogenase, contribute to a rise in the intramitochondrial citrate concentration. As these enzymes are known to be regulated by the mitochondrial NADH/NAD and NADPH/NADP ratios, as well as by AMP, *cis*-aconitate and oxaloacetate, fluctuations in the level of mitochondrial TCA metabolites are likely.

Respiratory activity and the role of NAD regeneration

Formation of citric acid is dependent on strong aeration, and dissolved oxygen tensions higher than those required for vegetative growth of *A. niger* stimulate citric acid fermentation. On the other hand, sudden interruptions in the air supply cause an irreversible impairment of citric acid production without any harmful effect on mycelial growth. The biochemical basis of this observation appears to be related to the presence of an alternative respiratory pathway, which is obviously required for reoxidation of the glycolytically produced NADH, by a continuously maintained, high oxygen tension, whose activity is impaired by short interruptions in the air supply. Weiss and colleagues studied the role of the standard and alternative respiratory pathways in citric acid accumulation in detail. They detected that the assembly of the proton pumping NADH:ubiquinone oxidoreductase is impaired during citric acid accumulation, which could be the reason for the importance of the activity of the alternative pathway. Interestingly, disruption of the gene encoding the NADH-binding subunit of complex I in a low producing strain of *A. niger* increased its catabolic overflow, yet this strain excreted much less citrate than its parent. These findings stress the fact that citric acid accumulation is not a mono-causal process, and citrate accumulation in high amounts depends on a delicate balance of several factors, whose interrelationship is not yet fully understood.

The requirement of a high oxygen supply is also related to another effect of Mn^{2+} ions on *A. niger*, i.e. on the morphology of the fungus: whereas *A. niger* grows in long and smooth filaments when supplied with optimal concentrations of Mn^{2+} ions, Mn^{2+} deficient grown mycelia are strongly vacuolated, highly branched, contain strongly enthickened cell walls and exhibit a bulbous appearance. This type of morphology has been shown to provide a much better rheology and enables a higher oxygen transfer; it may thus be required for optimal citric acid yields.

NAD regeneration may also be related to the effect of pH on citric acid fermentation: the almost quantitative conversion of glucose to citric acid, as occurs during the idiophase of fermentation, yields 1 ATP and 3 NADH. While part of the NADH pool can be reoxidised by the alternative, salicylhydroxamic acid (SHAM) sensitive respiratory pathway described above, this yield of ATP probably still exceeds that of the cell's maintenance demands. Roehr speculated that the ATP will be consumed by the plasma membrane bound ATPase during maintenance of the pH gradient between the cytosol and the extracellular medium. The involvement of this enzyme in the maintenance of the pH gradient in citric acid producing *A. niger* has been shown by Mattey. Hence the requirement of a low pH for citric acid accumulation may be, at least in part, related to a high turnover of the ATP formed, which otherwise would lead to a metabolic imbalance and so stop acidogenesis. However, this explanation still requires experimental verification. Most recently, single-point mutagenesis of a plant ATPase and its expression in yeast resulted in increased H^+-pumping and increased growth rates at low pH.

Export of citric acid from A. niger

Torres proposed that the two citric acid transport steps, i.e. that from the mitochondria to the cytosol, and that from mycelia into the culture filtrate, are among the most important regulatory points for the obtention of high yields.

The mechanism of transport of mitochondrial citrate into the cytosol is still completely unknown, except for the hypothesis that it occurs by countertransport with the glycolytically overproduced malate. ATP-citrate lyase, an enzyme which in other cells uses the cytosolic citrate for lipid biosynthesis, appears to be unable to manage this high efflux but its precise regulation under citric acid producing conditions is not understood. The latter authors have also purified a cytosolic and a mitochondrial carnitine acetyltransferase from *A. niger*, which exhibited similar kinetic and physicochemical properties. As the activity of this enzyme was in considerable excess of that of ATP-citrate lyase, they concluded that transfer as a carnitine ester may be the major physiological source of acetyl-CoA for lipid biosynthesis. If this is indeed the case it would explain why the cytosolic citrate pool is rather stable. Because of their findings of a cytosolic isoenzyme of carnitine acetyltransferase, Jernejc and Legisa also speculated that this enzyme transfers acetyl-CoA to the mitochondria and thus for citrate biosynthesis. This is an intriguing speculation, but requires the identification of a cytosolic pathway from pyruvate to acetyl-CoA which is not yet known.

Mattey and co-workers explained the export of citrate through the plasma membrane in terms of the large pH gradient between the cytosol and the extracellular medium, and postulated that citrate efflux from the cells may occur by diffusion of the 2(−) citrate anion, driven by a gradient. If this assumption is correct, the low pH would be responsible for the citrate gradient necessary for transport and consequently less citrate would be secreted at higher pH values. However, recent studies in our laboratory clearly showed that citrate export requires ATP, and its V_{max} is not strongly affected by the external pH; this renders the diffusion hypothesis rather unlikely.

Netik also reported that citrate export is strongly increased in mycelia grown under manganese deficiency, which is consistent with previous observations that the intracellular concentration of citrate in manganese sufficient and deficient grown mycelia is not greatly different, despite the five- to seven-fold higher extracellular levels under the latter conditions. The reason for the requirement of manganese deficiency for citrate export is not clearly understood, but may be related to an absolute requirement of citrate uptake for manganese ions, probably because of a requirement for chelated citrate as a substrate for the permease.

The reason for the reciprocal effect of Mn^{2+} ions on export and import of citric acid may also be related to yet another effect of manganese deficiency, i.e. inhibition of triglyceride and phospholipid synthesis as well as a shift in the ratio of saturated to unsaturated fatty acids of whole mycelial lipids and of isolated plasma membranes. The different behaviour of the citrate export and import system of *A. niger* may also be seen in the light of earlier studies on the antagonism of several membrane affecting compounds on the detrimental action of manganese ions, e.g. lower alcohols, lipids or tertiary amines. Also the technically important ability of Cu^{2+} ions to antagonise the deleterious effect of Mn^{2+} may be related to citrate excretion, as Cu^{2+} strongly inhibited the uptake of citric acid from the medium. However, the effect of Cu^{2+} may also reside in its inhibition of the uptake of Mn^{2+} by *A. niger*, which occurs by a specific, high affinity transport system. The properties of the uptake and the export system are otherwise similar (ΔpH driven proton symport) and it may be speculated that they are catalysed by the same enzyme system.

BIOCHEMISTRY OF CITRIC ACID PRODUCTION BY YEASTS

In terms of bulk production citric acid is widely regarded as one of the most important of the organic acids produced by microbiological methods, although reliable estimates of world production are not easily obtained. A widespread perception has been that most of the production is achieved with *Aspergillus niger*, in what has come to be regarded as the 'traditional' fermentation process, although the first indications of a microbiological process for the production of citric acid were from Wehmer, who noted that 'Citromyces' (now *Penicillium*) could accumulate citric acid.

Indeed until around 1970 *A. niger* was almost exclusively the organism used for the production of citric acid; the ability of other filamentous fungi to excrete citric acid was known and has been reviewed, but they are of limited importance. A more important class of production organisms found within the *Candida* yeasts, and an increasing proportion of the total production of citric acid is now manufactured using strains of *Yarrowia lipolytica* (the asexual form is *Candida lipolytica*, syn. *Saccaromycopsis*).

The *Candida* genus (family Cryptococcaceae, subfamily Cryptococcoideae) contains 30 species, and six varieties, many of which are pathogenic to animals, including humans. With increasing numbers of immunodeficient people, either through retroviral disease or the anti-rejection drugs used in organ transplantation, the pathogenic species such as *C. albicans* have assumed a new importance. Many *Candida* species have been isolated from fruit, seeds, soil, and similar sources.

Vegetative growth consists of budding cells and pseudomycelium, or true mycelium with blastospores. *C. lipolytica* was isolated from margarine (hence its name, Gr. *Lipos*, fat; *lysis*, breaking). The cells are variable, long oval to almost cylindrical and short oval. A well developed pseudomycelium is frequently formed with some true mycelium. The organism, as well as hydrolysing fats, will liquify gelatine, but does not ferment sugars.

As well as the industrial importance of the organism, it is being developed as a cloning vehicle for the expression of heterologous proteins. Some understanding of the pathways involved in citric acid production has resulted from the cloning of particular genes as a result of this development; in particular our knowledge of the peroxisomal pathways has been advanced through developments in the understanding of protein targeting. It is rarely known whether the perfect or imperfect form is being used in a particular process. Indeed, *C. lipolytica* is a dimorphic yeast and the morphology may vary, particularly during the course of a batch process.

The impetus for the study of citric acid production from *Candida* yeasts appears to have had two aspects: first the availability in the 1960s of relatively cheap hydrocarbons as feedstock; and secondly the use of hydrocarbons for the production of glutamic acid by *Corynebacterium*. Particularly in Japan the further use of this feedstock in a number of fermentation processes was explored. This phase came to a halt in 1973 when the price of crude oil was increased dramatically. This process is reflected in the number of patents granted: from one in 1967 and two in 1968 up to 15 in 1972, then dropping to three by 1975.

Possibly as a result of the extent of industrial commitment to yeast-based processes, alternative carbon sources were explored; the finding that alkane-utilising yeasts can also use sugars to produce citric acid formed the basis of the present expansion of the industrial importance of *C. lipolytica*. The potential advantages of using yeasts rather than *A. niger* are the higher initial sugar concentrations that can be tolerated and the faster conversion rates possible. The sensitivity of *A. niger* to metal ions, particularly manganese, is well-known, and a source of increased costs associated with the pretreatment of molasses. This is avoided with *Candida* yeast that is far less sensitive to metal ions.

The fermentation with *Candida* yeasts appears to be biphasic with citric acid accumulating after the growth phase, when nitrogen is exhausted. Although nitrogen limitation, with nitrogen usually supplied in the form of ammonium salts, is the trigger for acid accumulation, other parameters influence the yield and productivity of the process. The pH is maintained above pH 5.0, unlike the situation in *A. niger* where a medium pH below 2 is required for a good yield. Lowering the pH with the *C. lipolytica* fermentation results in the production of polyols, mainly erythritol and arabitol.

The addition of iron salts to the medium lowers the yield of citric acid, although some iron is required for normal growth. The addition of iron increases the activity of aconitate hydratase, and this is thought to result in the conversion of citric to isocitric acid. The influence of iron on the growth and synthesis of citric and isocitric acid in ethanol-containing media showed similar effects. Changes in the concentration of iron caused abrupt switching between the predominant formation of either citric or isocitric acids.

One noteworthy feature of the process is the requirement for thiamine. Unless this is added, oxoacids, mainly oxoglutarate, accumulate and the yield of citric acid is reduced. The reason for this requirement is not known but is likely to be related to the level of oxidative decarboxylation required, where thiamine pyrophosphate (TPP) is a cofactor. When β-oxidation is the main assimilatory pathway the requirement for pyruvate dehydrogenase would not be significant, but the flux through oxoglutarate dehydrogenase might be elevated. The other obvious requirement for TPP is for the transketolase reaction; although the role of the pentose phosphate cycle in the metabolism of *C. lipolytica* during citric acid accumulation is not known, the production of erythritol and arabitol under conditions of low pH might be indicative of its activity. The activities of enzymes of the TCA cycle have been measured after thiamine-limited growth with ethanol as a substrate. This will use essentially the same pathway as growth on alkanes, and thiamine limitation is similarly accompanied by oxoglutarate production. The activity of the oxoglutarate dehydrogenase complex is greatly reduced and oxidative decarboxylation of oxoglutarate becomes the limiting reaction in the TCA cycle. This leads to oxoglutarate accumulation within the cells and secretion into the culture medium. The glyoxylate cycle is used as an alternative pathway when the TCA cycle is impaired in this way.

Although growth is usually limited by nitrogen exhaustion, limitation of growth by sulphur, magnesium or phosphorus gives a similar effect. Citric acid levels between 50 and 220 mM were measured after 168 hours, with nitrogen and sulphur limitation giving the highest specific production rates. Potassium limitation was ineffective (6 mM), and the glucose uptake rate was only 50 per cent of that achieved when nitrogen or sulphur was limiting.

Synthesis of Citric Acid from *n*-Alkanes

Growth on alkanes

An important feature of the growth of yeast on alkanes is that the flow of carbon from the substrate to the cellular materials is significantly different to that found during conventional growth on a carbohydrate, in that during growth on carbohydrates fatty acids are synthesised while carbohydrates are degraded, whilst the opposite is true for growth on alkanes. The metabolic sequence when growth on alkanes occurs is therefore:

1. Uptake of alkanes into the cell.
2. Oxidation of alkanes into the corresponding fatty acids.
3. Conversion of the fatty acids to acyl CoA esters.
4. Metabolism of fatty acyl CoA esters to acetyl CoA, or incorporation into cellular lipid.
5. Synthesis of TCA cycle intermediates.
6. Gluconeogenesis, synthesis of amino acids, nucleic acids, etc.

Since the utilisation of alkanes overlaps considerably with the metabolism of fatty acids the oleaginous yeasts such as *C. lipotytica* were obvious targets for fermentation processes with this type of feedstock.

Uptake of alkanes

Alkanes are of limited solubility in water so that the uptake of alkanes by cells could be of three types: by direct contact between the alkane droplets and the microbial cells; through the soluble phase; or by 'solubilisation' by micelle formation in an emulsion with subsequent uptake. All three mechanisms are believed to occur. Once contact between a hydrophobic alkane droplet and the hydrophobic cell membrane has been made the alkane will dissolve in the lipid phase and be transported across the membrane. Despite this, particular areas of the membrane may become specialised for the rapid uptake of alkanes. Meissel have observed distinctive channels in the cell wall of yeast grown on alkanes when studied by electron microscopy.

Similar channels have been observed by Osumi, together with protrusions on the cell surface which reach the cell membrane through electron-dense channels. The hypothesis has been put forward that alkanes attach to these channels and migrate through them to the membrane and into the endoplasmic reticulum which appears to be particularly associated with the cytoplasmic end of these channels. The endoplasmic reticulum is the site of the initial oxidation of the alkanes.

Alkane emulsions adhere to the cell wall of *Candida* yeast by a non-enzymatic mechanism. The binding is due to a lipopolysaccharide in the cell wall that is induced by alkanes. The lipopolysaccharide, which is mannan with about 4 per cent covalently linked fatty acid, has been isolated and characterised.

Initial oxidation of n-alkanes

Three oxidation mechanisms are known but the one most likely to be operating in *Candida* yeast is the mixed function oxidase (mono-oxygenase). A cytochrome P-450 hydroxylase system, dependent on $NADPH^+$ and H^+, has been described in several species of *Candida*, (Fig. 21.6). The formation of P-450 has been shown to be inducible by long-chain alkanes, alkenes, secondary alcohols and ketones with hexadecane increasing the specific activity by 150-fold relative to cells grown on glucose. As well as the P-450, a microsomal NADPH-cytochrome c-reductase was increased. The influence of carbon and nitrogen sources on a number of NAD^+- and $NADP^+$-linked dehydrogenases was examined; no significant effects other than on the $NADP^+$-cytochrome c-reductase were seen.

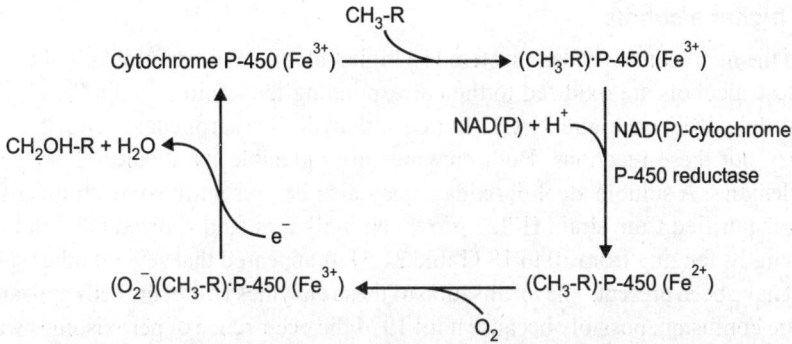

Fig. 21.6. Hydroxylation of an alkane by cytochrome P-450 dependent mono-oxygenase.

The cytochrome P-450 concentration was linearly related to hexadecane uptake rates when cells were cultivated under conditions of oxygen limitation in a chemostat, leading to the suggestion that cytochrome P-450 is the rate-limiting step in alkane uptake and oxidation. It is unlikely however that flux control is in fact dependent on a single step in a steady state system such as this.

Alkane molecules are susceptible to such oxidations at one or both of the terminal methyl groups. A monoterminal oxidation pathway appears to be operating in *C. lipolytica*. The fatty acids in cell lipids of active, alkane degrading cells of *C. lipolytica* grown on various alkanes showed a pattern corresponding to the *n*-alkane chain length.

The alkanes are oxidised to the corresponding fatty acids that are incorporated into lipids, either directly, after chain elongation or by β-oxidation.

Table 21.4 shows the relationship for *C. lipolytica* grown on a variety of substrates. The correlation between odd chain length alkane substrate and odd chain length fatty acids in the cells is clear. The high activity of a mono-oxygenase system, with its oxygen radical mechanism, suggests that protection against damage by free radicals might be important when yeast grows on alkanes. Indeed a considerable increase in copper and zinc superoxide dismutase (SOD) is seen during growth on *n*-alkanes as compared to glucose. A correlation between SOD and catalase was noted and resistance to oxygen free radicals observed as a result of the high levels of copper/zinc SOD, which also protected against deleterious effects of Cu^{2+} and Zn^{2+} in the medium.

Table 21.4. Ratio of odd chain fatty acids and C17 acids to total cellular fatty acids in *Candida lipolytica* cells grown on *n*-alkanes and glucose.

Substrate	Odd chain acids (%)	C17 acids (%)
Glucose	2.9	1.6
n-Undecane	9.6	5.7
n-Dodecane	0.9	0.9
n-Tridecane	60.0	33.1
n-Tetradecane	1.0	1.0
n-Pentadecane	80.9	58.0
n-Hexadecane	1.6	1.0
n-Heptadecane	97.8	94.9
n-Octadecane	3.4	3.4

Oxidation of higher alcohols

The product of the microsomal oxidase system is a higher alcohol corresponding to the chain length of the alkane. These alcohols are oxidised to the corresponding fatty acid through the aldehyde. NAD^+-linked alcohol dehydrogenase and NAD^+-linked aldehyde dehydrogenase, specific to long-chain substrates, carry out these reactions. Both enzymes are inducible by alkanes as well as long-chain alcohols or aldehydes. A soluble alcohol oxidase may also be present in some strains of *Y. lipolytica*. The enzyme was purified from strain H-222 grown on *n*-alkanes, and showed maximum activity with carbon chain lengths ranging from 10 to 18 (Table 21.5). It appeared that several other specific alcohol oxidases might have been present. The localisation of these enzymes within the cells appears generalised. Early reports are confusing, possibly because until 1974 the occurrence of peroxisomes was not known. Osumi have detected both dehydrogenases in peroxisomes, mitochondria and microsomes.

Table 21.5. Substrate specificity of soluble alcohol dehydrogenase from *C. tropicalis*.

Substrate chain	Relative activity	Substrate chain	Relative activity
2	0	9	75
3	0	10	100
4	3	11	85
6	25	12	120

Peroxisomes in yeast metabolising n-alkanes

When grown on alkanes, specific organelles, less than 1 µm in diameter, infrequently seen in cells grown on carbohydrate substrates, become numerous. These organelles have been identified as peroxisomes by cytochemical staining for catalase. Indeed their appearance is directly related to the increased catalase activity seen during the metabolism of alkanes. These organelles contain several of the enzyme systems involved in the initial oxidation of alkanes and similar substrates, and transport between the various compartments of substrates and intermediates is a complex area. Two peroxisomal targeting signals are known (PTS1 and PTS2) and it is suggested that PTS receptors, which have been found in several subcellular locations, shuttle between the cytosol and the peroxisomal membrane. The PTS1 protein is highly conserved and the human homologue (PTS1R) has been cloned as a result. Interestingly this is mutated in a group of patients afflicted with a fatal peroxisomal disorder. Protein unfolding is not required for the import of peroxisomal matrix proteins, which is markedly different from other mechanisms for the translocation of proteins. The gene *pay5* encodes a peroxisomal integral membrane protein in *Y. lipolytica*, pay5p, of 380 amino acids (41.7 kDa) homologous to the mammalian PAF-1 protein which is essential for peroxisome assembly. Pay5p is targeted to mammalian peroxisomes in an interesting example of the evolutionary conservation of targeting mechanisms. In humans, mutation of PAF-1 results in the Zellweger syndrome. Mutants of *Y. lipolytica* (pay5-1) also show defective peroxisome synthesis.

Activation of fatty acids to CoA esters

Two acyl CoA synthetases have been isolated from *C. lipolytica* with different locations, specificity functions and regulation. Their properties are summarised in Table 21.6. Synthetase I is constitutive while synthetase II is inducible by fatty acids. The enzymes could be distinguished immunochemically. The synthetase I is widely distributed including mitochondria where glycerophosphate acyltransferase is also located, while synthetase II is located in the peroxisomal compartment where β-oxidation occurs. Evidence for β-oxidation has been obtained from the study of peroxisomes from *C. tropicalis*. The stoichiometry of the process demonstrated that the β-oxidation system was similar to that described for castor bean and liver.

Table 21.6. Comparison of the properties of acyl CoA synthetases for *C. lipolytica*.

Properties	Acyl-CoA synthetase I	Acyl-CoA synthetase II
Induction by fatty acid	No	Yes
Phosphatidylcholine	No	Yes
Stability	High	Low
Substrate specificity	Narrow	Wide
Chain length specificity	Below C16	All
Solubilisation (Triton X)	Easy	Hard
Subcellular location	General	Peroxisomes
Function	Lipid synthesis	Fatty acid degradation

Acyl CoA esters are oxidised by acyl CoA oxidase, a FAD-containing enzyme, to enoyl CoA, forming hydrogen peroxide from molecular oxygen. The catalase present in the peroxisome breaks down the hydrogen peroxide. The enoyl CoA is then metabolised to give acetyl CoA with CoA and NAD^+ as hydrogen acceptor. Acyl CoA oxidase has been purified from *C. lipolytica* and *C. tropicalis* from which organism it has been crystallised. Its substrate specificity is summarised in Table 21.7.

Table 21.7. Substrate specificity of acyl CoA oxidase from *C. tropicalis*.

CoA ester	Relative activity	CoA ester	Relative activity
Butyryl	5	Myristoyl	50
Hexanoyl	2	Palmitoyl	37
Octanoyl	16	Stearoyl	17
Decanoyl	97	Oleoyl	64
Lauroyl	100	Arachidoyl	7

The peroxisome contains an NAD^+-dependent glycerol-3-phosphate dehydrogenase which is thought to act as a shuttle hydrogen carrier with the FAD-dependent glycerol-3-phosphate dehydrogenase present in the mitochondria, regenerating NAD^+ and generating energy.

Synthesis of intermediates of the tricarboxylic acid cycle

While growing on alkanes it is clear that the substrate is degraded to the level of acetyl CoA, or propionyl CoA in the case of odd chain length acids, and while lipids may be incorporated from the fatty acids all other intermediates must be synthesised from the two-carbon precursor. In general, yeast growing under gluconeogenic conditions utilises the glyoxylate cycle as an anaplerotic mechanism. The role of this cycle has been demonstrated in *Candida* yeast grown on alkanes. The two characteristic enzymes of the glyoxylate cycle, isocitrate lyase and malate synthase, are induced by growth on *n*-alkanes. However, while the level of isocitrate lyase is considerably elevated compared to the levels in glucose grown cells, the level of NAD-dependent isocitrate dehydrogenase is lower. The distribution of the flux of intermediates between the TCA cycle and the glyoxylate cycle is determined by the relative activities of these two enzymes which therefore suggests that a high level of glyoxylate cycle activity occurs during growth on *n*-alkanes. Much of the isocitrate lyase is present in the particulate fraction of the cells, and the enzymes of the glyoxylate cycle have been localised to the peroxisomal compartment. However, citrate synthase, aconitase and malate dehydrogenase, the characteristic enzymes of the TCA cycle, are present in the mitochondrial compartment as might be anticipated. Fatty acid β-oxidation is not present in the mitochondria of *C. lipolytica* or *C. tropicalis* but appears confined to the peroxisome. This implies that acetyl CoA required for citrate synthesis must be transported to the mitochondria from the peroxisome, probably by the carnitine acyltransferase system (Fig. 21.7).

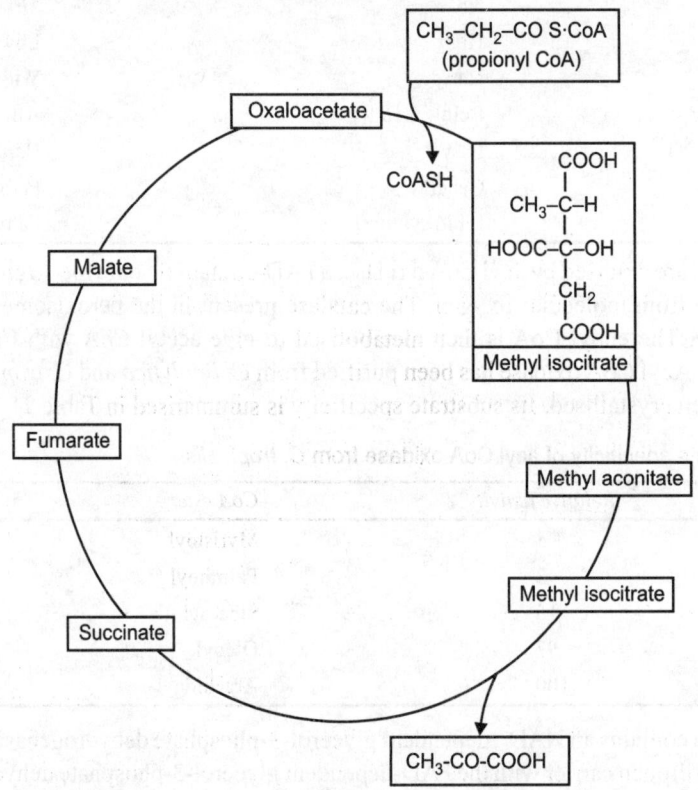

Fig. 21.7. Methyl isocitrate cycle in *C. lipolytica*

Methyl isocitrate cycle

The propionyl CoA, derived from odd chain length *n*-alkanes, is metabolised by a cyclic pathway analogous to the first steps in the TCA cycle. This pathway is based on the accumulation of pyruvate and seven carbon tricarboxylic acids in *C. lipolytica* grown on odd chain length alkanes. Methyl citrate, methylaconitate and methylisocitrate were detected as were the key enzymes described in the methyl citrate cycle. In this pathway propionyl CoA from the odd chain fatty acid β-oxidation sequence reacts with oxaloacetate via a methyl citrate-condensing enzyme, analogous to citrate synthase. The resulting methylcitrate is isomerised to methylisocitric acid, possibly by aconitase and the methylisocitrate is cleaved in a manner analogous to citrate lyase to give succinate and pyruvate.

The two key enzymes, methylcitrate synthase and methylisocitrate lyase, clearly differ from citrate synthase and isocitrate lyase. Both the methyl tricarboxylic acid converting enzymes seem to be constitutive, like the TCA cycle enzymes, while the key enzymes of the glyoxylate cycle are inducible. The overall effect of this path is to convert propionate to pyruvate. The main factor in the level of citric acid production from alkanes is the amount of isocitrate lyase.

The role and control of isocitrate lyase has been examined in *C. lipolytica* and *C. tropicalis*, and it has been suggested to be a rate limiting enzyme for the process. The characteristics of the enzyme were determined in crude extracts by Marchal; the main features were a K_m value of 0.6 mM (at pH 7.0) with inhibition by phosphoenolpyruvate and succinate.

Significantly, citrate at 5 mM was not inhibitory. When grown on glucose the level of isocitrate lyase was only 2 per cent of that found when grown on alkanes, where the level was four times that found when grown on acetate, the classic two-carbon substrate. Induction of this enzyme is clearly greater in the presence of alkanes (Table 21.8).

Table 21.8. Adenine nucleotide levels (mM) during a batch fermentation.

Time (hr)	ATP	ADP	AMP	Total
20	0.35	0.28	0.17	0.81
25	0.3	0.22	0.20	0.72
30	0.6	0.03	0.01	0.64
50	0.72	0.02	0.005	0.745
70	0.8	0.02	0.004	0.824

The role of isocitrate lyase in the production of citrate from carbohydrate substrates is unlikely to be significant and it might well be that the critical factor in the overproduction is not the details of the regulation but that maximal fluxes are obtained, that is, the absence of effective regulation. A similar situation may occur in *A. niger*. The control of flux through the TCA cycle versus the glyoxylate cycle is usually thought of in terms of competition between NAD^+-dependent isocitrate dehydrogenase and isocitrate lyase, with adenine nucleotide regulation of isocitrate dehydrogenase and repression/derepression of isocitrate lyase but with no metabolite level control of isocitrate lyase, which is the situation in *E. coli*. This situation cannot occur in *Y. lipolytica* as isocitrate lyase is apparently in the peroxisome and the NAD^+-dependent isocitrate dehydrogenase is mitochondrial, with no common pool of isocitrate (Table 21.9).

Table 21.9. Relationship of adenine nucleotide ratios, cell mass and citric acid production.

Time (hr)	Cell mass (g)	Citric acid (g/l)	ATP:ADP	ATP:AMP	Energy charge
20	11	0	1.25	1.95	0.6
25	14	0	1.36	1.5	0.57
30	16	6	20	60	0.96
50	15	24	36	144	0.98
70	14	40	40	200	0.98

The isocitrate lyase from *Yarrowia lipolytica* has been purified and characterised. The active form was obtained as a single peak from an ion exchange column, with a specific activity of 7.4 U/mg. The molecular mass was estimated to be between 200 and 210 kDa, and appears to have four subunits of about 50 kDa. The pH optimum was pH 6.0 and a K_m of 0.3 mM was estimated. The enzyme was noncompetitively inhibited by succinate and oxalacetate. The gene for isocitrate lyase has been cloned by complementation of a mutation (*acuA3*) in the structural gene of isocitrate lyase of *E. coli*. The open reading frame was 1668 bp long and had no introns in contrast to the genes sequenced from other filamentous fungi. The deduced protein was 555 amino acids with a molecular mass of 62 kDa, which is similar to that observed for the purified monomer. The enzyme has a putative glyoxosomal targeting sequence S–L–K at the carboxy-terminus and contained a partial repeat which is typical for eukaryotic isocitrate lyases, but is absent from the *E. coli* sequence. Deletion mutants, as expected, were unable to utilise acetate, ethanol, fatty acids or alkanes, but surprisingly the growth on glucose was also reduced. Citrate synthase from several strains of *Y. lipolytica* which are citrate producers have been isolated and purified to homogeneity. The enzyme was a dimer with a subunit molecular mass of 40 kDa, and exhibited a K_m value of 10 and 5 µM with acetyl CoA and oxalacetate respectively. The enzyme activity observed in extracts is greater than that of isocitrate lyase, aconitase or isocitrate dehydrogenase. *Candida lipolytica* has both an NAD^+ and an $NADP^+$-dependent isocitrate dehydrogenase. The $NADP^+$-dependent enzyme had Michaelis-Menten type kinetics with respect to isocitrate, and a K_m of 80 µM for isocitrate at pH 7.0. There was inhibition by oxalacetate at 5 mM of about 40 per cent. The energy metabolism of *C. lipolytica* has been examined during growth on *n*-alkanes; in particular, the concentration of adenine nucleotides during a batch fermentation was measured.

After 25 hours there was a sharp drop in the concentration of ADP and AMP while the ATP level rose. The total adenine nucleotide levels fell slightly, then recovered. These changes coincided with the exhaustion of nitrogen in the medium and the effective cessation of growth. At this point citric acid excretion began, together with isocitric acid. The proportion of isocitric to citric acid was high, about 40 per cent, although the intracellular citric to isocitric ratio was close to that expected from the aconitase equilibrium at about 90 per cent citric: 10 per cent isocitric acid. The adenylate energy charge reflected the changes in adenine nucleotides, rising to approach 1. However, the dramatic changes are seen in the ATP:AMP ratio, and the most common allosteric effectors amongst the adenine nucleotides are AMP and ATP, so that the ATP:AMP ratio is a better indicator of regulatory changes. The enzyme that is regarded as a significant target for allosteric regulation during growth on alkanes is mitochondrial NAD^+-specific isocitrate dehydrogenase. The activity of this enzyme with respect to isocitrate and AMP is sigmoidal, consistent with its structure which has four co-operative binding sites. The enzyme is totally dependent on AMP for activity, with maximal activity shown at 0.1 mM AMP and 50 per cent activity at 0.05 mM. At values below 0.01 mM the enzyme is virtually inactive (Fig. 21.8).

Magnesium also behaved as an allosteric activator of the enzyme, apparently with two co-operative sites. Since the substrate for the enzyme is magnesium isocitrate this is perhaps surprising. There was no correlation between the rate of *n*-alkane uptake and nitrogen exhaustion or changes in adenine nucleotide levels. This is unexpected since the cessation of growth should greatly reduce the energy demand and hence the substrate uptake. The implication is that the coupling between electron transport and ATP synthesis becomes 'loose', or that energy is used in, for example, a transport process.

The mitochondrial ATP synthase genes have been studied in *Y. lipolytica* and a 6.6 kilobase region sequenced. This closely resembled the human mitochondrial genome with ATP synthase subunits 8 and 6 being followed by the genes for cytochrome *c* oxidase subunit 3, NADH-ubiquinone oxidoreductase subunit 4 and ATP synthase subunit 9. All the genes were transcribed from the same strand of DNA into multigenic RNAs starting from a nonanucleotide sequence, 5'-ATA-TAAATA-3', similar to other yeast mitochondrial promoters. In addition to these apparently normal mitochondrial genes there is a cyanide-resistant oxidase located in the inner membrane. Its activity is typically blocked by benzohydroxamic acid. This resembles the situation found in *A. niger* and the circumstances of uncoupled electron transport are also similar.

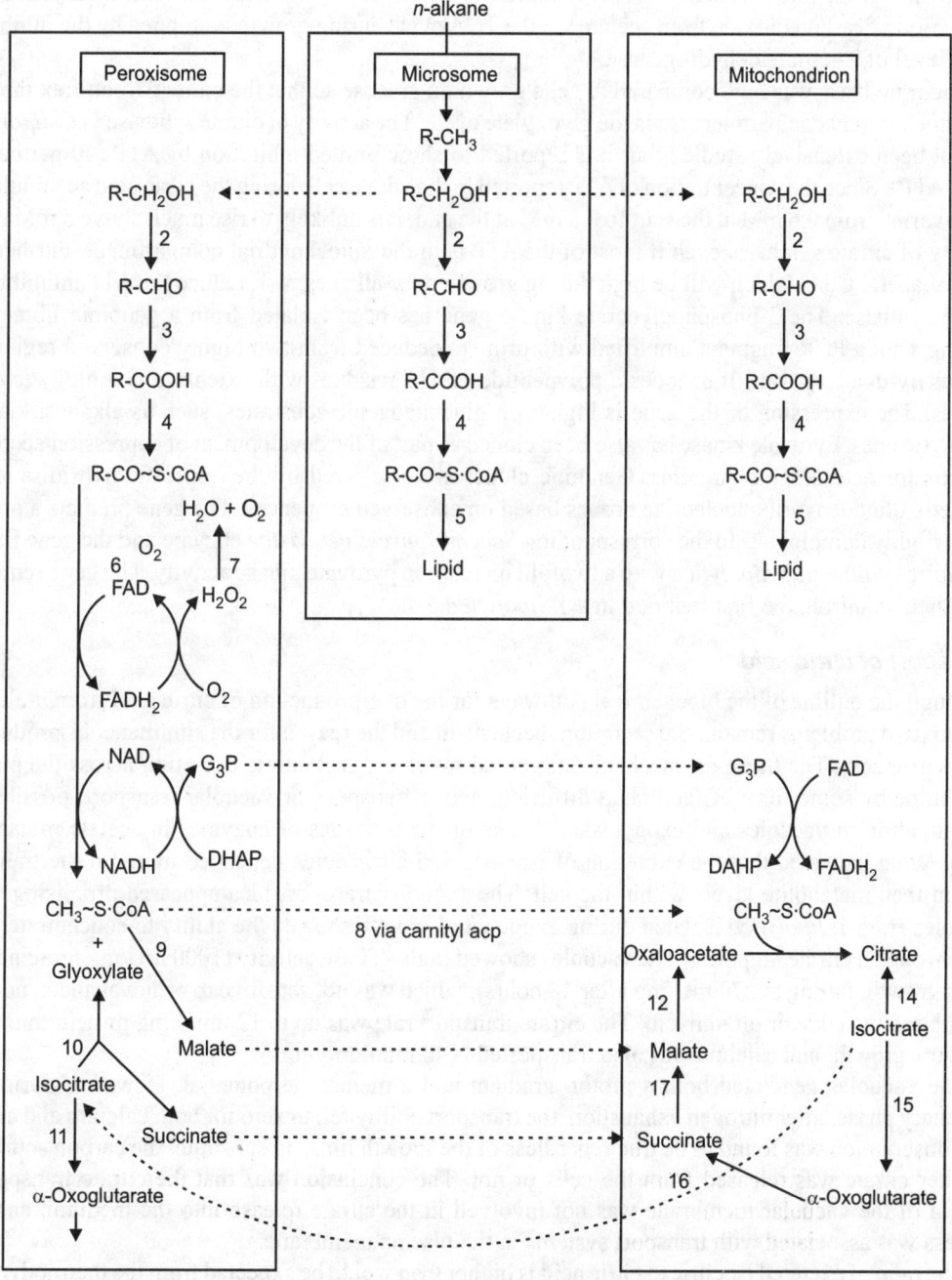

Fig. 21.8. Compartmentation in *C. lipolytica* during growth on *n*-alkanes.

The activity of the NAD⁺ isocitrate dehydrogenase, which is already low compared to the level found in cells grown on glucose, is almost totally inhibited by the drop in AMP, and the evolution of carbon dioxide mirrors this, being sharply reduced to very low levels when growth ceases. The metabolic production of carbon dioxide from acetate via the TCA cycle during growth is stopped by the inhibition at the level of isocitrate dehydrogenase.

Isocitrate lyase was high compared to cells grown on glucose so that the entire carbon flux through the mitochondrial compartment is via the glyoxylate cycle. The activity of citrate synthase in *C. lipolytica* has not been extensively studied, but it is reported to show limited inhibition by ATP (40 per cent at 5 mM ATP). Since the concentration of ATP reported in the whole cell during the citric acid accumulation phase varied from 0.6 mM at the start to 0.8 mM at the end, it is unlikely to rise much above 5 mM in the vicinity of citrate synthase, even if most of the ATP is in the mitochondrial compartment. Further, the level of acetyl CoA, which will be high during growth on *n*-alkanes, will reduce the ATP inhibition of citrate synthase. The 3-phosphoglycerate kinase gene has been isolated from a genomic library, by probing with a PCR fragment amplified with primers deduced from two highly conserved regions of various pyruvate kinases. It encodes a polypeptide of 417 residues with extensive homology to other kinases. The expression of the gene is higher on gluconeogenic substrates, such as alkanes, than on glycolytic ones. Pyruvate kinase has also been cloned as part of the development of expression/secretion systems for heterologous proteins. Genomic clones were selected by their specific hybridisation to synthetic oligodeoxyribonucleotide probes based on conserved sequences. The gene predicts a protein that is highly homologous to the corresponding *Saccharomyces cerevisiae* enzyme and the gene further transforms wild type *Y. lipolytica* with a twofold increase in pyruvate kinase activity. The gene sequence contained an intron, the first reported in a *Y. lipolytica* gene.

Transport of citric acid

Although the outline of the biochemical pathways for the overproduction of citric acid from *n*-alkanes is clear, two problems remain: the secretion mechanism and the reason for the simultaneous production of isocitric acid. The transport mechanism(s) could involve direct citrate excretion across the plasma membrane by some form of facilitated diffusion, active transport, or vacuolar transport, possibly by accumulation in vacuoles and exocytosis. Studies of the activities of enzymes in acetate mutants of *Y. lipolytica* indicated that the excretion of isocitric and citric acids depended more on the transport system than metabolite levels within the cell. The vacuolar transport idea appeared promising when vacuoles from *Y. lipolytica* isolated during exponential growth showed the ability to concentrate citric acid through a citrate uniporter. The vacuoles showed high ATPase activity (1000 mU/mg protein at six hours growth, falling to 270 mU/mg after 48 hours), which was not sensitive to orthovanadate, nor was it inhibited by azide or oligomycin. The citrate transport rate was up to 12 nmol/mg protein/min. after 12 hours growth, and calcium was also transported (140 nmol/mg/min.).

The vacuoles generated both a proton gradient and a membrane potential. However, during the stationary phase, after nitrogen exhaustion, the transport ability fell to zero for both calcium and citrate. This observation was found to be true regardless of the growth limiting substrate, the carbon source, or whether citrate was released from the cells or not. The conclusion was that the citrate transporting system of the vacuolar membrane was not involved in the citrate release into the medium, and that process was associated with transport systems in the plasma membrane.

The ratio of excreted isocitric to citric acid is higher than would be expected from the thermodynamic equilibrium of aconitase, being as high as 40 per cent in wild-type yeasts, rather than the 7 per cent expected on an equilibrium basis. Nonetheless it is apparent that the strategies used to mitigate this unwanted production of isocitric acid all have a common theme in that they inhibit or delete aconitase. By limiting the formation of isocitrate in the first place the problem is resolved. The strategies reported include: the use of iron-free medium, which resulted in impairment of aconitase activity; the addition of sodium tetraborate, which may complex with iron to give a similar outcome; and the selection of mutants with low aconitase activities.

These have been selected by their ability to grow on n-alkanes but not citric acid and the low aconitase results in improved citrate to isocitrate ratios and decreased biomass, but the complete absence of aconitase would presumably be lethal. Other strategies are the use of inhibitors such as monofluoroacetate which is metabolised to monofluorocitrate and acts as a competitive inhibitor of aconitase, and 2,4-dinitrophenol, an uncoupler of oxidative phosphorylation; and the addition of alcohols, up to oleyl alcohol. The first two strategies are of use in selecting mutants but would be undesirable in a commercial fermentation. The relative levels of isocitrate lyase and aconitase in determining the ratio of isocitrate to citrate was underlined by Finogenova with a study of a series of *C. lipolytica* mutants. Mutants with a high isocitrate lyase activity and a low aconitase level synthesised citric acid almost exclusively regardless of whether the carbon source was glucose, alkane, ethanol, acetate or glycerol. The mutant low in isocitrate lyase but with a high level of aconitase produced primarily isocitric acid on alkanes, where the ratio of citrate to isocitrate was 1:3.6, while on glucose the ratio was 1.8:1. Wild-type strains with high levels of both enzymes gave intermediate results. In the wild-type strains the ratio could be shifted towards isocitrate synthesis by inhibiting isocitrate lyase with aconitate, the reverse of the industrial strategy. The explanation advanced by Marchal is still valid. Marchal suggested that the high isocitrate ratio was a result of compartmentation within the cell. Whereas citrate is mainly mitochondrial, isocitrate is in the mitochondrial, the cytoplasmic and the peroxisomal compartments. Isocitrate will be exported from the mitochondrial compartment to the cytosol and then to the peroxisome where it will be converted to glyoxylate and succinate. The absence of aconitase from the cytoplasmic compartment will result in higher isocitrate levels with lower citrate levels, and it is presumably from the cytoplasm that the acids are exported. It is further possible that citrate and isocitrate have differential transport, but no mutants have been reported to suggest that there is a separate export mechanism for each acid.

Synthesis of citric acid from glucose

The production of citric acid from glucose by *C. lipolytica* was established before the industrial production from alkanes was initiated, although an inhibitor of aconitase was required to minimise isocitric acid production. The productivity on glucose was found to be similar to that on n-alkanes, so that the industrial process, which in some cases had started out to make citric acid from alkanes, was adapted to synthesis from glucose without major problems. Such industrial plants were designed for yeasts, but the feedstock could be altered. To overproduce citrate from glucose, the same obstacles must be overcome as with synthesis from n-alkanes: an undiminished supply of precursors for citrate synthesis in the form of oxaloacetate and acetyl CoA, a reduction in the catabolism of the citrate, an unregulated citrate synthase and a transport mechanism.

Pathway for citrate synthesis from glucose

The pathways involved in the synthesis of citrate in *Candida* yeasts are similar to those of other organisms in basic properties; the over-accumulation is a result of differences in regulation rather than differences in mechanisms. The outline of the biochemical pathways is shown in Fig. 21.9. The basic difference between the pathways on n-alkanes and glucose lies in the source of acetyl CoA: in the case of n-alkanes, β-oxidation from fatty acids; in the case of glucose, by glycolysis. In both cases oxalacetate is synthesised by an anaplerotic route, either the glyoxylate cycle or in the case of glucose, pyruvate carboxylase; the immediate reaction leading to citrate is citrate synthase with both substrates. The differences lie in the direction of the pathways: with n-alkanes as a substrate, gluconeogenesis is required for the synthesis of metabolites derived from the glycolytic sequence; when glucose is the substrate, fatty acids must be synthesised from acetyl CoA. Pyruvate carboxylase was shown to be the source of oxalacetate by Aiba and Matsuoka. Its relative activity in glucose-grown cells is almost ten times that in cells grown on n-alkanes, but it was only 10 per cent of the activity of citrate synthase.

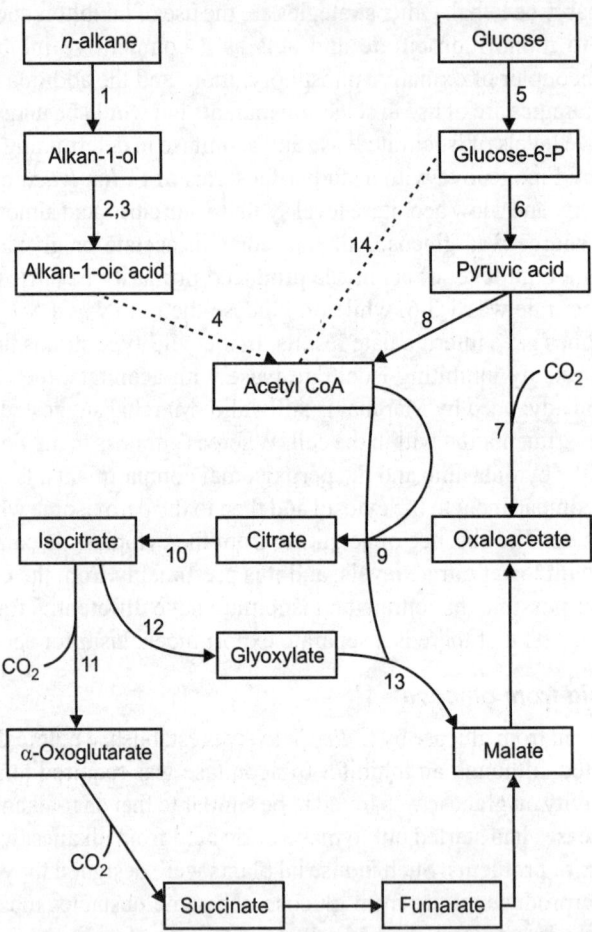

Fig. 21.9. The metabolic relationships of citrate metabolism in yeasts with n-alkanes or glucose as substrate. (1) Alkane monooxygenase; alkane, reduced rubridoxin:oxygen 1-oxidoreductase, 1.14.15.3. (2) Alcohol dehydrogenase; alcohol:NAD⁺ oxidoreductase, 1.1.1.1. (3) Aldehyde dehydrogenase; aldehyde:NAD⁺ oxidoreductase, 1.2.1.3. (4) β-oxidation. (5) Hexokinase; ATP:D-hexose 6-phosphotransferase, 2.7.1.1. (6) Glycolysis. (7) Pyruvate carboxylase; pyruvate:carbon dioxide ligase (ADP), 6.4.1.1. (8) Pyruvate dehydrogenase; pyruvate:lipoate oxidoreductase (acceptor acylating), 1.2.4.1. (9) Citrate synthase; citrate:oxaloacetate lyase (CoA acylating), 4.1.3.7. (10) Aconitase; citrate (isocitrate) hydrolyase, 4.2.1.3. (11) Isocitrate dehydrogenase; threo-DS-isocitrate:NAD oxidoreductase (decarboxylating), 1.1.1.41(42). (12) Isocitrate lyase; threo-DS-isocitrate:glyoxylate-lyase, 4.1.3.1. (13) Malate synthase; 1-malate glyoxylate-lyase (CoA-acetylating), 4.1.3.2, and (14) Gluconeogenesis.

The incorporation of carbon dioxide into pyruvate and thence into citrate appears to involve both carbon dioxide from metabolism within the cell and from the medium. In theory, however, the amount of carbon dioxide released in the pyruvate dehydrogenase reaction to yield acetyl CoA should be enough to form the oxaloacetate needed for citrate synthesis. When grown at a medium pH of 4.5, *C. lipolytica* showed 20 per cent incorporation of exogenous carbon dioxide into one of the carboxyl groups of citrate, but this fell to 8 per cent at pH 6.0 (Table 21.10).

Table 21.10. Activities of enzymes of a *Candida lipolytica* strain grown on glucose.

Organism	Citrate synthase	Aconitase	NAD+-ICDH	Pyruvate carboxylase	Ratio citric: isocitric
Wild	0.6	0.28	0.17	0.06	5.3:1
Low aconitase	0.66	0.22	0.21	0.08	32:1
High aconitase	0.47	0.38	0.11	0.02	1.8:1

Enzyme activities in U/mg cell protein. The aconitase mutants were selected for their differences on hexadecane, where the relative activities were 0.61:0.22:0.73 (wild:low:high).

The subcellular location of the various enzymes has been determined. Pyruvate carboxylase was found in the cytoplasmic compartment in *C. lipolytica*, and many other yeasts. The NADP+-dependent isocitrate dehydrogenase was found to be distributed in both cytoplasmic and mitochondrial compartments, while ATP-citrate lyase was found in the cytoplasmic compartment. The presence of this latter enzyme would be required for lipid synthesis, but is presumably regulated so that it does not degrade a significant amount of the cytoplasmic citrate. The number of peroxisomes in yeasts grown on glucose is very small.

The properties of the NAD+-dependent isocitrate dehydrogenase are thought to be central to citrate accumulation when glucose is used as a substrate as well as *n*-alkanes. The AMP requirement for activity means that the very low AMP levels found during the stationary phase induced by nitrogen depletion will result in very low activity of the isocitrate dehydrogenase. The enzyme was shown to be allosterically regulated by AMP although with excess isocitrate the rate became AMP independent. It is also inhibited by ATP which is high during citric acid accumulation.

The export of isocitrate from the mitochondrial compartment is presumably reduced when glucose is a substrate, as the glyoxylate cycle is non-functional because of the low level of isocitrate lyase and the absence of malate synthase. This may be the reason for the improved ratio of citrate to isocitrate produced when glucose is a substrate. The presence of the NADP+-dependent isocitrate dehydrogenase in both cytoplasm and mitochondria has been noted but its role, if any, is not known.

An important factor in the over-production of citric acid is the maintenance of the flux through glycolysis when metabolite levels rise. In particular the inhibition of phosphofructokinase by citrate might be expected to regulate the precursors for citrate production when citrate levels are high. In citrate producing strains of *Y. lipolytica* the citrate inhibition of phosphofructokinase appears to be weak, while AMP has no effect. Ammonium suppressed the inhibitory effect of citrate and activated the enzyme, a similar mechanism to that suggested for *A. niger*. However, in *Y. lipolytica* under conditions of nitrogen exhaustion, when growth has ceased it is less likely that there is a significant pool of intracellular ammonium.

The entry of glucose into the cell is normally regulated, and under conditions of citrate accumulation there is indeed a reduction in the glucose uptake rate, suggesting that the regulation is present to some extent. The regulation of hexokinase has been shown to be sensitive to trehalose-6-phosphate, which occurs in yeasts at about 0.2 mM. This is well above the apparent K_i for *Y. lipolytica* hexokinase and it was concluded that this compound was physiologically significant. There was, however, no activity against glucokinase up to 5 mM so that high levels of glucose might avoid the regulatory step at hexokinase.

A related substrate, glycerol, has attracted some attention, and the activities of glycerol kinase and the NAD^+ and FAD-dependent glycerol-3-phosphate dehydrogenases, involved in the glycerol phosphate shuttle between cytoplasm and mitochondria, were determined. Glycerol kinase was localised in the cytoplasm but both glycerol phosphate dehydrogenases were associated with the membrane fraction of the cells. The glycerol kinase was purified and found to be inhibited by AMP, but insensitive to fructose-1,6-bisphosphate.

Nitrogen metabolism during growth on glucose

Yeasts and fungi contain both NAD^+ and $NADP^+$-dependent forms of glutamate dehydrogenase as well as glutamine synthetase. Glutamate dehydrogenase functions both as an anabolic and catabolic enzyme:

$$\alpha\text{-oxoglutarate} + NH_3 + NAD(P)H + 2H^+ \leftrightarrow \text{Glutamate} + H_2O + NADP^+$$

The NADPH form acts primarily in the direction of glutamate synthesis although it is reversible; the NADH form acts as a catabolic enzyme providing α-oxoglutarate for the citric acid cycle. The activity of the NADPH enzyme is increased under the nitrogen depletion which precedes citric acid excretion in *Y. lipolytica*, while that of glutamine synthetase is decreased as might be expected. Both the NADPH and the NADH glutamate dehydrogenases were located in the cytosolic compartment in *Y. lipolytica* which is consistent with a role in synthesis of glutamate rather than energy metabolism. Glutamine synthetase was also cytoplasmic. Interestingly the enzymes in the closely related *C. maltosa* are mitochondrial, and the organism does not produce citric acid. Aspartate aminotransferase was located in the mitochondria in *Y. lipolytica*. Glutamate dehydrogenases are normally allosterically regulated by inhibition by ATP or GTP and activation by ADP or GDP. It is not known whether this situation occurs in *Y. lipolytica*, but it would be consistent with the high level of ATP and low ADP seen during the period of nitrogen starvation.

The importance of nitrogen levels to citric acid production was demonstrated by Moresi who determined kinetic constants for a *Y. lipolytica* strain at different initial glucose concentrations in the medium. Although increasing the glucose concentration from 40 to 108 g/l gave a negative effect on the growth rate, the yield coefficients for glucose and nitrogen were approximately constant. By using a production medium without nitrogen, a citrate lag phase was observed during which the intracellular nitrogen fraction decreased from about 8 per cent to a new low equilibrium value of less than 3 per cent. The idiophase was found to be a non-growth associated process, and the citric acid formation rate was dependent only on the cellular nitrogen concentration. The strain used in this study was capable of equalling the productivity of the best *A. niger* mutants (about 1.05 g/l/hr), but not the selectivity as citric acid was only 85.5 per cent of the acid excreted; the majority of the rest was isocitric acid.

Transport of citric acid during growth on glucose

The effect of various inhibitors on the excretion of citric acid has indicated that the export of citric acid is energy requiring. The addition of protein synthesis inhibitors to cultures of *C. lipolytica* at the time of nitrogen exhaustion inhibited the production of citric acid. At the same time, dinitrophenol (an uncoupler of oxidative phosphorylation), reumycin (respiratory chain shunting agent), or arsenate (which forms

ADP-arsenyl instead of ATP) all decreased the yield of citric acid in proportion to the concentration of the agent. There was no significant effect on biomass yield. Since the overproduction of citric acid appears to involve some 'uncoupling' of the electron transport chain from ATP synthesis, with maximal levels of ATP resulting, the requirement for ATP shown here may be connected with export rather than synthesis, as may be the requirement for protein synthesis.

On the other hand, Kulakovskaya and others showed that the activity of the plasma membrane ATPase of *Y. lipolytica* decreased by a factor of ten during the course of nitrogen limited growth with glucose as a carbon source. Citric acid excretion was independent of glucose concentration and resistant to diethylstilboestrol, an inhibitor of the plasma membrane ATPase, for the first 30 minutes of the excretion process. They concluded that the process is independent of energy provision.

Thus, the overproduction of citric acid by yeasts from both alkane and carbohydrate sources is now well established, both commercially and scientifically. The basic pathways and some of the enzymology are understood, although many details remain to be resolved. With both substrates the overproduction appears to represent a mechanism for recycling reducing equivalents and energy produced by unbalanced growth conditions in the form of the absence of, and subsequent intracellular restriction on, a primary substrate from the growth medium. Further developments in enzymology may arise coincidentally from the use of the organism as a cloning vehicle, but one of the main unresolved problems is the mechanism of excretion, which is central to the problem of high productivity.

STRAIN IMPROVEMENT

Many factors need to be considered by citric acid producers to obtain the economically most favourable process. Strain breeding is one of these factors. In this section we will summarise ways to improve citric acid production genetically. Commercial production of citric acid is performed mainly with *Aspergillus niger* and to some extent with *Candida* (or *Yarrowia*) *lipolytica*. As the existing fermentation processes usually give high yields, the main objective of strain breeding nowadays is shortening of fermentation time. However, other factors may also be relevant for strain improvement. For example, accumulation of a high concentration of citric acid by *A. niger* results from quite extreme culture conditions and strain breeding may decrease the sensitivity of the process to these conditions.

The number of reports considering strain improvement that have appeared in literature is limited. Rohr, Kubicek and Rohr and Mattey have reviewed much of the older work. However, some research and screening activities are 'hidden', i.e. performed by industry and not published for obvious reasons. This section is structured more or less on the basis of the methodology used for strain improvement of *A. niger*:

1. Mutagenesis and selection.
2. The use of the parasexual cycle.
3. Genetic engineering.

As strain breeding involves fungal genetics, some aspects of the genetic methodology used have been included.

General Aspects of Strain Improvement

The initial *A. niger* production strains were isolated from their natural habitat, soil. Better strains have been derived from these isolates by various procedures. Basically, two methods can be distinguished for strain selection. In the first method, acid production is tested for individual colonies obtained from single spores (single spore method). Such a method requires automated screening procedures that enable testing of thousands of colonies and is therefore usually done by plate tests. A pH indicator is commonly included in the medium to estimate acid production, but since a pH indicator does not distinguish between citric acid and other acids, improved methods have been developed, e.g. using p-di-methylamino-benzaldehyde, which specifically measures citric acid. Yields are evaluated by determining the ratio between acid zone and colony diameter. Obviously, statistical analysis of screening results is quite important to evaluate the significance of a difference in acid production between the parental strain and strains derived from it. Liquid cultures, such as shake flasks, are not suitable in the initial stage of screening, but can be used in later steps for a limited number of selected strains. An alternative to screening by plates would be the use of 'high throughput' screening procedures, making use of microtitre plate technology. This has an even higher capacity than plates as it can be automated to a large extent. Nowadays, microtitre plate technology is commonly used by industry in all kinds of screening processes, but it is not clear whether citric acid producers also employ it.

The second method comprises selection of mutants with a specific trait from a large population using a suitable discriminative growth condition (passage method). Selection may be on the basis of resistance against an antimetabolite or failure to grow on a particular carbon source. Mutants can arise spontaneously or be produced by mutagenic treatment. A variety of methods are used for mutagenesis including exposure to chemicals, UV light, γ- and X-ray radiation. A serious drawback of mutagenic treatment is that high doses increase the chances of obtaining more than one mutation per genome at a time. Thus, in addition to a mutation that results in improved citric acid production, an isolate may have other mutations that might, for example, result in (slightly) reduced viability. To minimise the chances to introduce such unwanted mutations, mutagenic treatment should be performed in such a way that a high percentage of survival is obtained. When a better producing mutant is isolated it should be maintained in a proper way to prevent decay, i.e. lose its particular characteristics favourable for citric acid production. Decay is most pronounced during the vegetative stage and therefore storage of spores is the best way to preserve a strain. The optimal storage method depends on the organism. *A. niger* conidiospores are usually stored on silica beads at 4°C or suspended in a 20 to 30 per cent glycerol solution and frozen. Apart from natural variation certain mutations may be particularly unstable, i.e. losing such mutation may be advantageous for the fungus. For example a certain mutation may result in improved citric acid production, but concomitantly cause reduced vitality. This necessitates careful preservation of original strains and possibly frequent reisolation.

The biochemistry of citric acid biosynthesis has been reviewed before and will not be treated at length here. Some aspects will however be discussed in order to understand the rationale behind some strategies. Biosynthesis of citric acid from hexoses is depicted in Fig. 21.10. Following uptake, hexoses are degraded mainly via glycolysis yielding pyruvate. Part of the pyruvate is converted to acetyl CoA, part to oxaloacetate. Finally, these two compounds are condensed to citric acid, which is secreted and accumulated in the medium. Only in a few cases is the genetic basis or biochemical mechanism of the improved performance by a mutant known. Schreferl-Kunar isolated several mutants that grew better than the parent on 14 per cent sucrose. The rationale of this selection procedure is the notion that a high rate of citric acid production requires the ability for fast sugar metabolism. Four mutants consumed sucrose faster and gave higher citric acid yields than the parental strain. Unfortunately, it is not clear whether the productivity or just the final yield is improved in these mutants, although faster sucrose consumption suggests increased productivity. Interestingly, all four mutants had about twofold higher activity of the glycolytic enzymes hexokinase and phosphofructokinase, suggesting that the activity of these two enzymes is important in controlling the rate of sugar consumption. In the following sections a few specific objectives for strain improvement will be discussed.

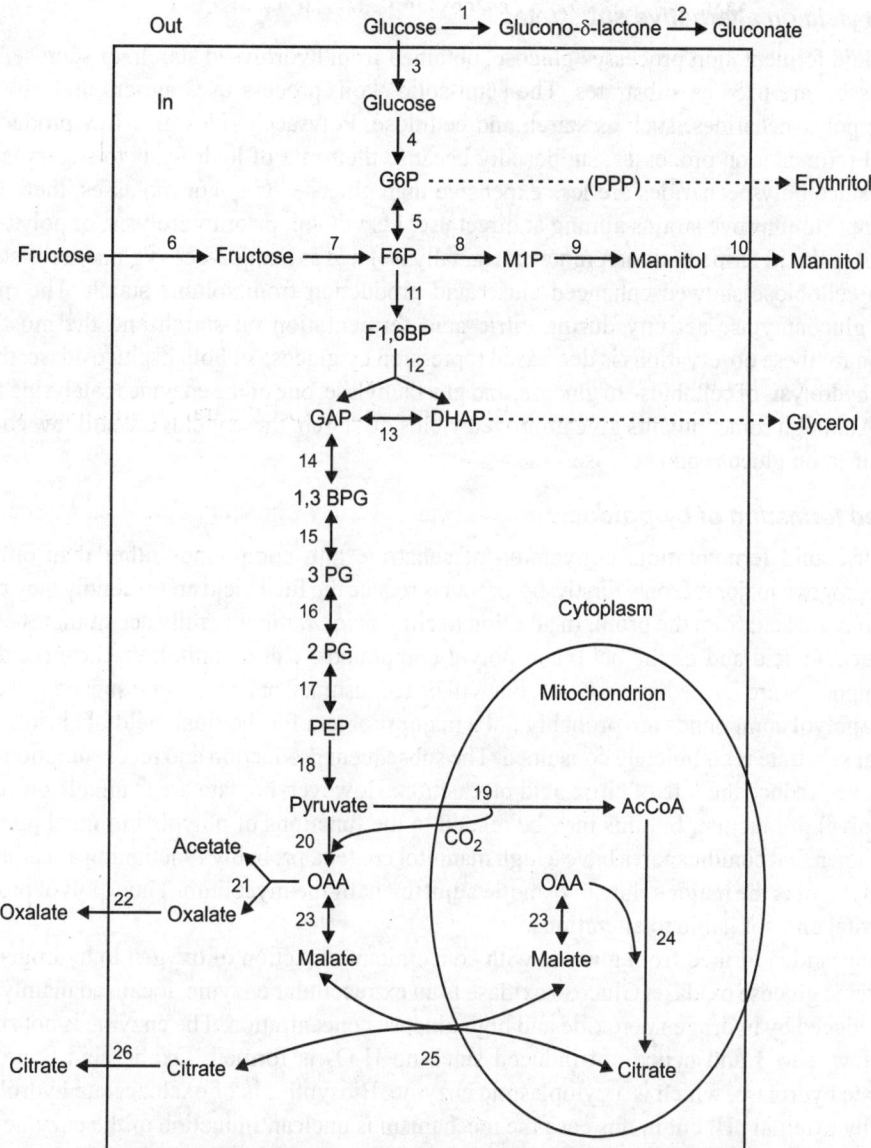

Fig. 21.10. Schematic representation of biosynthesis of organic acids and polyols with *A. niger*. The following steps are depicted: 1, glucose oxidase; 2, lactonase; 3, glucose transport; 4, hexokinase or glucokinase; 5, phosphoglucose isomerase; 6, fructose transport; 7, hexokinase; 8, mannitol-1-phosphate dehydrogenase; 9, mannitol-1-phosphate phosphatase; 10, mannitol transport; 11, phosphofructokinase; 12, aldolase; 13, triosephosphate isomerase; 14, glyceraldehyde-3-phosphate dehydrogenase; 15, phosphoglycerate kinase; 16, phosphoglycerate mutase; 17, enolase; 18, pyruvate kinase; 19, pyruvate dehydrogenase; 20, pyruvate carboxylase; 21, oxaloacetate hydrolase; 22, oxalate transport; 23, malate dehydrogenase; 24, citrate synthase; 25, tricarboxylate carrier; 26, citrate transport. Dashed arrows are used for multiple steps in biosynthesis of erythritol and glycerol. PPP, pentose phosphate pathway.

Improved yield on alternative substrates

In most liquid fermentation processes glucose, obtained from hydrolysed starch, or sucrose, in beet or cane molasses, are used as substrates. The semi-solid 'koji' process uses agricultural raw materials containing polysaccharides, such as starch and cellulose. Polysaccharides give low productivities in submerged fermentation processes, supposedly because their rate of hydrolysis to sugars is too slow. However, since polysaccharides are less expensive than glucose syrups or molasses, there have been some attempts to improve strains aiming at direct use, i.e. without prior hydrolysis, of polysaccharides (e.g. starch) in liquid fermentation. A mutant originally isolated as being 2-deoxyglucose resistant during growth on cellobiose showed enhanced citric acid production from soluble starch. The mutant had increased glucoamylase activity during citric acid fermentation on starch and the most probable explanation for these observations is decreased repression by glucose of both β-glucosidase, the enzyme catalysing hydrolysis of cellobiose to glucose, and glucoamylase, one of the enzymes catalysing hydrolysis of starch. Although some mutants give improved yields on starch, these yields are still low compared to those obtained on glucose and sucrose.

Decreased formation of by-products

During citric acid fermentation, conversion of substrate into compounds other than citric acid is undesirable for two major reasons. Firstly, by-products reduce the final yield and secondly they complicate recovery of citric acid from the broth. In addition to citric acid, *A. niger* readily accumulates other acids, mainly gluconic acid and oxalic acid, and polyol compounds, e.g. mannitol, erythritol and glycerol. Polyol compounds are formed from sugars, but will be reconsumed once the sugar substrate is exhausted. Therefore, polyol compounds are probably not a major problem for the final yield of citric acid as long as the sugar substrate is completely consumed. The subsequent production and reconsumption of polyols may, however, reduce the rate of citric acid production. However, no data are available on strains with reduced polyol production, but this may be related to the functions of polyols in fungal physiology. It has been shown that conidiospores have a high mannitol content, probably functioning as carbon storage, whereas glycerol is the major solute in osmotic adjustment of the mycelium. Thus, polyol production is probably vital and not liable to alterations.

Gluconic acid is formed from glucose with concomitant reduction of oxygen to hydrogen peroxide by the enzyme glucose oxidase. Glucose oxidase is an extracellular enzyme, localised mainly in the cell wall and induced by hydrogen peroxide and high glucose concentration. The enzyme is not stable at pH values below 2 to 3 and hence not induced since no H_2O_2 is formed. Oxalic acid is produced by oxaloacetate hydrolase, which is a cytoplasmic enzyme. Biosynthesis of oxaloacetate hydrolase is also regulated by external pH, but in this case the mechanism is unclear. Induction of the enzyme is optimal at pH 5 to 6, whereas a very low oxaloacetate hydrolase activity is observed at pH 2. In pure sugar fermentations, production of gluconic and oxalic acid can thus be kept to a minimum by starting the fermentation at a relatively low pH.

In fermentations using molasses as a substrate, an initial pH of 5 to 6 is commonly employed, because conidiospores will not germinate at lower pH values. Therefore, in processes using molasses, production of gluconic and oxalic acid may be a problem favouring production strains lacking glucose oxidase and oxaloacetate hydrolase. In one laboratory a number of *gox* mutants have been isolated. One of the mutations, *goxC*, results in the absence of glucose oxidase activity and strains carrying *goxC* do not produce gluconic acid from glucose. Interestingly, a *goxC* mutant produces more oxalic acid from glucose than wild-type *A. niger*.

The major problem with production of citric acid by *C. lipolytica* is the simultaneous production of considerable amounts of isocitric acid. Wild-type *C. lipolytica* strains produce approximately equimolar amounts of citric acid and isocitric acid from *n*-alkanes, whereas less isocitric acid is produced from sugar substrates. Akiyama and other reasoned that a low activity of aconitase, the enzyme catalysing the conversion of citric acid to isocitric acid, was essential to reduce production of isocitric acid. They selected a mutant that was more sensitive to fluoroacetate than the wild-type strain. This mutant had approximately 1 per cent of the wild-type aconitase activity and produced virtually no isocitric acid.

A. niger mutants with a decreased sensitivity towards manganese

It is commonly known that the manganese concentration should be extremely low during citric acid fermentation with *A. niger*. Any addition of manganese results in a lower yield. Manganese deficiency has multiple effects on physiology, e.g. increased protein turnover and altered cell wall composition, which probably means that the manganese effect is not clearly related to a particular cellular function. In pure sugar fermentations, manganese is usually removed by cation exchangers, whereas in molasses, manganese is precipitated with ferrocyanide. Obviously, mutants with a higher manganese tolerance would be advantageous, as this would make removal of manganese less critical. Smith and others reported an *A. niger* mutant which was more tolerant to manganese; it seems however that their parental strain is already quite tolerant as addition of 0.5 ppm manganese does not decrease the yield, while usually a level below 1 ppb is recommended. Nevertheless, in the presence of 1.5 ppm manganese, citric acid production by the mutant was threefold higher than obtained with the parental strain and similar to production in the absence of manganese.

One of the effects of manganese deficiency is a relatively high intracellular NH level, which presumably is due to increased protein turnover. This high NH concentration partially counteracts inhibition of the glycolytic enzyme, phosphofructokinase, by citrate. A mutant isolated by Schreferl contained a phosphofructokinase that was less sensitive to citrate than the one in the parental strain; this mutant accumulated approximately threefold more citric acid compared to the parent on a medium containing 20 mM manganese.

However, the citric acid yield of the mutant in the presence of manganese was only half that obtained with the parental strain on manganese deficient medium, indicating that the effects of manganese cannot be attributed to phosphofructokinase alone.

Morphology of A. niger

Characteristic for citric acid fermentation with *A. niger* is a rather abnormal morphology, which has been attributed to manganese deficiency, although other process conditions, such as pH, impeller speed and seeding level also affect morphology. Hyphae are abnormally short and stubby and the mycelium shows excessive branching. The aggregation of mycelium into compact pellets is also reported to be important, but this may vary between strains and with process conditions. An important benefit of such compact pellets is better rheology of the broth. A lower viscosity of the broth makes it easier to mix, requiring a lower power input for mixing and resulting in a higher dissolved oxygen tension. Efficient aeration is quite important as productivity decreases at lower dissolved oxygen tension and interruption of the oxygen supply even results in cessation of citric acid formation. For processes operating with a filamentous mycelium, mutants with altered morphology, i.e. more branching, resulting in more compact aggregates, might be beneficial. Such mutants were easily obtained in the case of *Fusarium graminearum*.

Isolation of Recombinant Strains Using the Parasexual Cycle in *A. niger*

Crossing these strains might combine beneficial characteristics of different strains. *A. niger* does not have a sexual cycle and crossings therefore involve the so-called 'parasexual cycle', which is not a life cycle, but a series of independent steps, i.e. fusion of hyphae resulting in heterokaryon formation, fusion of the nuclei of the different parents to form a diploid, mitotic recombination and finally haploidisation of the diploid strain to yield haploid strains again. If crossing of strains is impossible due to heterokaryon incompatibility, fusion of protoplasts can be used to obtain heterokaryons. Protoplasts can be prepared by treatment of mycelium with cell wall lysing enzymes in an osmotically stabilised medium.

Usami and coworkers have investigated the application of *A. niger* diploids and haploid recombinants in citric acid fermentation. They have fused protoplasts of a strain optimised for submerged fermentation and a strain optimal for semisolid fermentation. Some of the resulting diploid strains and haploid recombinants were better producers than both parents, but most were without significant improvement. The reason for higher production by diploids or haploid recombinants may be combination of beneficial mutations or complementation of adverse mutations introduced in the parents during previous mutagenic treatment. In the case of diploids the presence of two copies of the genome might result in overproduction of certain enzymes.

Genetic Engineering

Strain improvement by the techniques described in the previous sections is largely a trial and error process involving laborious screening procedures. Moreover, in many cases the improved performance is 'magic', as the underlying mechanism is not identified. Genetic engineering, on the contrary, is a rational approach as particular metabolic steps are manipulated. The use of recombinant DNA technology to improve citric acid production has been employed only recently, although transformation of *A. niger* was reported in 1985. *C. lipolytica* transformation is also possible, but we are not aware of any reports of genetic engineering of *C. lipolytica* to improve citric acid production. Different protocols for transformation of *A. niger* exist, but the most commonly used method involves polyethyleneglycol mediated uptake of DNA by protoplasts, followed by regeneration on a suitable selective medium. Introduction of DNA fragments (either circular or linearised) into *A. niger* results in integration of the DNA into the genome of the recipient strain. Integration can occur either at the homologous locus or at other loci. Multiple copies (tandemly integrated or scattered over the genome) of the gene introduced can be obtained. Expression of the gene introduced depends on the copy number and on the site of integration. To date there are three cases of genetic engineering concerning citric acid production by *A. niger*, which will be addressed in later sections, but first we will discuss some aspects of metabolic modelling.

Quantitative analysis of metabolism

For genetic engineering it is necessary to have at least some idea of which enzymatic step should be altered to increase the metabolic flux through the pathway of citric acid biosynthesis. However, to find the optimal strategy for metabolic engineering, it is necessary to analyse the metabolism involved quantitatively. For example, the simple finding that an enzyme has a low activity *in vitro* does not mean that it is 'rate-limiting' *in vivo*, since the activity of an enzyme in the cell also depends on the concentrations of its substrates, products and possible effectors. To understand the control properties of a metabolic pathway, two major theoretical frameworks have been developed. Metabolic control analysis (MCA) was established independently by Kacser and Burns and Heinrich and Rapoport, whereas biochemical systems theory (BST) was developed by Savageau. The majority of the literature concerns MCA and the formalism of MCA and its applicability in biotechnology have been reviewed extensively. Only a few of the basic concepts of MCA and BST will be discussed here. Both theories use the characteristics of the metabolic pathway under study, i.e. the kinetic properties of the enzymes, to describe it quantitatively. With this description it is possible to perform a sensitivity analysis. The effect of a small variation in, for example, the activity of an enzyme on the steady-state flux through the pathway (which is the rate of conversion of the primary substrate to the final product) can be calculated. In MCA the 'flux control coefficient' (C) was introduced, which is defined as the fractional change in flux (J) divided by the fractional variation in enzyme activity (e): $(dJ/J)/(de/e)$. In most cases flux control coefficients have values between 0 (the flux does not change upon an increase in enzyme activity, i.e. no flux control) and 1 (the change in flux is proportional to the change in enzyme activity, i.e. the enzyme is completely rate-limiting).

An important feature of MCA is the summation theorem, which states that the sum of the flux control coefficients of the enzymes in a pathway is equal to 1. As a consequence, the flux control coefficient of any enzyme in a very long pathway is probably very small as there are many enzymes contributing to control. Moreover, when an enzyme with some flux control is overproduced, control readily shifts to another step in the pathway. In practice this means that genetic engineering is not easy in complex pathways.

The benefit of control analysis in designing strategies to optimise biotechnological processes depends heavily on the availability of enzyme kinetic data and on the reliability of these data. In the case of citric acid biosynthesis by *A. niger* quite a few enzymes have been studied now but a few, such as the transport steps, are less well or not at all investigated, hampering a precise analysis.

Recently, a few attempts have been performed to analyse flux control in citric acid biosynthesis by *A. niger*. Torres performed modelling of the first part of the pathway, i.e. up to pyruvate (Fig. 21.10) using BST formalism and suggested that sugar transport and phosphorylation, which are lumped into one step in the model, form the most important step in controlling the flux through the pathway. Thus, according to this model, the cellular amount of sugar transporter and/or hexokinase should be increased to obtain a higher metabolic flux. To a certain extent these findings correlate with experimental data. As discussed already, certain mutants with improved citric acid production had increased activity of hexokinase and phosphofructokinase and Steinböck found that some 2-deoxyglucose resistant mutants had lower hexokinase activity and produced less citric acid than the parent. From an investigation of glucose transport in *A. niger*, Torres concluded that hexokinase contributed more to flux control in glycolysis than glucose transport.

In a subsequent study it was concluded from flux optimisation calculations that simultaneous overproduction of seven enzymes was required for a significant increase in flux. For practical reasons this is not achievable at the moment. Firstly, most of the *A. niger* genes required for this approach are not available and secondly, simultaneous overexpression of seven enzymes in a controlled way is experimentally difficult to accomplish.

Notably, this model has not incorporated the metabolism from pyruvate to extracellular citric acid and hexokinase might have flux control in the conversion of glucose to pyruvate, but the control in the complete pathway (hexose to citric acid) might be in later steps, i.e. between pyruvate and citric acid. Nevertheless, a modelling approach is worthwhile. It may not produce an exact solution to improve the process, but it provides a guideline for genetic engineering of *A. niger*.

Manipulation of the respiratory chain in A. niger

In addition to the normal respiratory chain, *A. niger* possesses alternative respiratory enzymes, including an NADH oxidase and an ubiquinol oxidase (Fig. 21.11). In the course of a citric acid fermentation the activities of the normal respiratory enzymes decrease whereas the activities of the alternative oxidases increase. The alternative oxidases do not pump protons concomitantly with electron transport and their physiological function is thought to be removal of excess reducing equivalents. Such a function is in agreement with the presence of the alternative oxidases during citric acid production. Conversion of hexoses to citric acid results in net production of ATP and NADH. Since there is no growth in the stage of citric acid accumulation, the cells probably do not require much ATP, and a switch from normal respiration to alternative oxidases would enable the fungus to reoxidise its NADH without concomitant ATP production.

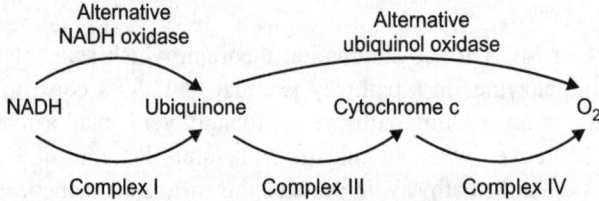

Fig. 21.11. Schematic representation of the normal and alternative respiratory chains. The normal respiratory chain (lower part) contains three complexes: NADH:ubiquinone oxidoreductase (complex I), ubiquinol:cytochrome c oxidoreductase (complex III) and cytochrome c oxidase (complex IV). In the alternative respiratory chain (top part) electrons are transferred directly from ubiquinol to oxygen.

A very attractive hypothesis has been put forward by the group of Weiss and others. They found that the proton-pumping NADH:ubiquinone oxidoreductase (complex I) is very fragile in *A. niger* B-60, which is a good citric acid producer, compared to a wild-type *A. niger* strain. The selective loss of complex I might result in an increased NADH/NAD$^+$ ratio in the cell, because the affinity of the alternative NADH oxidase for NADH is approximately one order of magnitude lower than that of complex I. Excretion of citric acid is a possibility in order to get rid of the excess, reducing equivalents. As such, the switch to alternative oxidases is not a reaction of the fungus to citric acid production, but the loss of complex I results in initiation of citric acid accumulation. To test this hypothesis one of the subunits of complex I was inactivated in a 'wild-type' (bad producing) *A. niger* strain by disruption of the corresponding, gene, *nuo*51, by molecular genetic techniques. The mutant was unable to form a functional complex I and should accordingly accumulate citric acid as B-60 does. Unexpectedly, the mutant excreted virtually no citric acid, whereas the wild-type *A. niger* strain produced approximately 30 per cent of the yield obtained with B-60. However, the mutant accumulated high intracellular levels of TCA cycle intermediates, including citrate. Apparently, the mutant is indeed unable to reoxidise NADH under these conditions, resulting in accumulation of TCA cycle intermediates. Prömper and others propose that, in contrast to wild-type *A. niger* and strain B-60, the mutant is unable to excrete citric acid (or other TCA cycle intermediates). This postulate, i.e. the presence of a citrate carrier, may explain the differences in citric acid production between wild-type *A. niger* and B-60, but does not resolve the discrepancy between wild-type *A. niger* and the mutant lacking complex I. It would be interesting to test the effect of disruption of *nuo*51 in strain B-60. In addition to the effect it might have on initiation of citric acid accumulation, it might also bring about an increase in the rate of acid production. Assuming an excess of ATP during citric acid production, inactivation of complex I would be a way to decrease such an excess, since less ATP is produced per NADH.

Engineering of glycolysis in A. niger

Obviously a high metabolic flux is necessary for fast citric acid accumulation. To date, two reports have been published in which attempts to increase metabolic flux and hence productivity are described. Arisan-Atac describes an increase in the rate of citric acid accumulation by a mutant of *A. niger* strain B-60 in which the gene encoding a subunit of trehalose-6-phosphate synthase, *ggsA*, was disrupted. This mutant lacks trehalose-6-phosphate synthase activity and the rationale for construction of this strain was the following. Trehalose-6-phosphate and the enzyme catalysing its biosynthesis have recently been shown to play a role in regulation of glycolytic flux in the yeast *Saccharomyces cerevisiae*. Trehalose-6-phosphate inhibits hexokinase activity in *S. cerevisiae in vitro* and this was found to be also the case in *A. niger*. Inactivation of trehalose-6-phosphate synthase would result in the inability to synthesise trehalose-6-phosphate and if, under citric acid producing conditions, trehalose-6-phosphate inhibits glycolysis in *A. niger*, the absence of trehalose-6-phosphate synthase might result in an increased glycolytic flux and increased citric acid production. This was indeed found to be the case. The *ggsA* disruption strain produced the same final yield of citric acid as the wild-type strain, but reached this yield in a shorter fermentation time. This is the only case where genetic engineering of *A. niger* results in improved citric acid production.

Recently a study was conducted in laboratory, the effects of overproduction of two glycolytic enzymes, phosphofructokinase and pyruvate kinase (Fig. 21.10) on citric acid production by *A. niger*. A few experimental studies have suggested that phosphofructokinase might be an important step in control of the glycolytic flux. Firstly, cultivation on a high concentration of sucrose, glucose or fructose stimulated citric acid accumulation by *A. niger* and these conditions also led to increased intracellular levels of fructose-2,6-bisphosphate, a potent activator of phosphofructokinase. Secondly, as already discussed, mutants selected for the ability to grow fast on high concentrations of sucrose exhibited increased citric acid production and in these strains the activities of hexokinase and phosphofructokinase were twofold higher than in the parental strain. We have overexpressed phosphofructokinase and pyruvate kinase, both individually and simultaneously, in *A. niger* N400. Unfortunately, moderate overexpression of these enzymes (three to five times the wild-type level) did not enhance citric acid production by the fungus significantly (Fig. 21.12). Overexpression of pyruvate kinase even appeared to have a negative effect on citric acid production. Thus, phosphofructokinase and pyruvate kinase do not seem to contribute in a major way to flux control of the metabolism involved in the conversion of glucose to citric acid. However, it must be noted that in cells overproducing phosphofructokinase, the concentration of fructose-2,6-bisphosphate was decreased approximately twofold compared to the wild-type. Hence, the fungus appears to adapt to overexpression of phosphofructokinase by decreasing the specific activity of the enzyme through a reduction in the level of fructose-2,6-bisphosphate. From his modelling studies Torres also concluded that phosphofructokinase and pyruvate kinase did not have flux control. In the model of Torres, however, regulation of phosphofructokinase by fructose-2,6-bisphosphate was not included. However, overproduction of phosphofructokinase, while maintaining or increasing fructose-2,6-bis-phosphate levels, may still increase glycolytic flux in *A. niger*.

Although the strains utilised for commercial production of citric acid are undoubtedly high-yielding, further strain improvement will most certainly be attempted. At the moment the primary strategy for strain breeding is probably still mutagenesis and selection. Quantitative analysis of metabolism and metabolic pathway engineering are only just being implemented, but this is a promising approach, not so much as an alternative to the traditional strain breeding methods, but complementary to it.

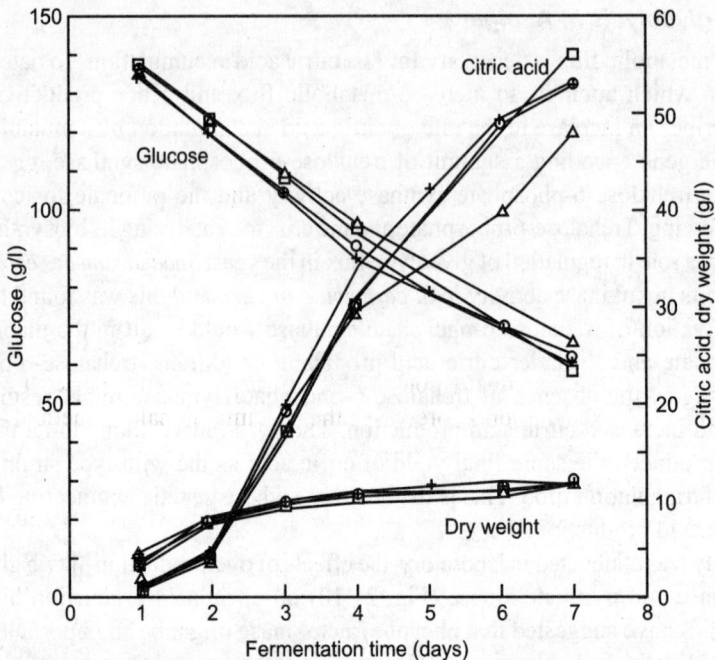

Fig. 21.12. Citric acid fermentation from glucose by an *A. niger* N400 wild-type strain(+) and transformants overproducing phosphofructokinase (O), pyruvate kinase (Δ) or phosphofructokinase and pyruvate kinase (□). Citric acid, glucose and dry weight are indicated.

FUNGAL MORPHOLOGY

In submerged culture the morphology of filamentous micro-organisms varies between pellets and free filaments depending on culture conditions and the genotype of the strain. All the growth forms have their own characteristics concerning growth kinetics, nutrient consumption and broth rheology. Of the two extremes, pellet suspensions exhibit Newtonian rheological behaviour, while the filamentous form produces more viscous media with consequent effects of poor mixing and mass transfer. This is unfortunate, as it is very often the case that the disperse filamentous form is the productive form. Another drawback with the pelleted suspension is that cell growth occurs only at the surface of the pellets where contact with oxygen and other nutrients is adequate, and the cells growing within a pellet respond to a very different environment. Further into the pellet, mass transfer limitation will gradually occur and cells could autolyse.

This section deals with the factors that affect *Aspergillus niger* morphology in submerged culture and the influence of morphology on productivity in citric acid fermentation.

Factors Affecting *Aspergillus niger* Morphology in Submerged Culture

According to many reports, the morphology of the mycelium is crucial to the process of fermentation, not only in relation to the shape of the hyphae themselves and the aggregation into microscopic clumps (micro-morphology), but also in the pelleted form of growth (macro-morphology). In all cases reported, the mycelium of acidogenic *Aspergillus niger* was found to conform to the morphological type described by Snell and Schweiger: short, swollen branches which may have swollen tips. The mycelial pellets should be small with a hard, smooth surface. It is known that this is brought about by adjustment of aeration and agitation, adjustment of pH, concentration of manganese and other trace metals, and inoculum level. However, it is not known whether the pelleted or filamentous form is more desirable for citric acid production.

Since the morphological form can strongly influence the overall process productivity, research on various aspects of morphological development has attracted the interest of academia and industry and attempts have been made to induce a particular form of growth and to relate morphology to product synthesis.

Initial investigations of mycelial morphology relied on manual measurements from photographs and little quantitative work was presented until the 1970s. Detailed morphological characterisation of the tree filamentous form was first presented by Metz. Their method, which made use of an electronic digitiser to make measurements from microphotographs, was time consuming, inaccurate and also difficult to automate. In 1988, Adams and Thomas presented the first image analysis method for morphological measurements of a filamentous fungus, using images taken directly from the microscope to an image analyser. Since then, highly automated methods have been developed which have many applications and allow detailed characterisation of growth and simple differentiation of filamentous micro-organisms. With the large variety of products produced by filamentous organisms and their complex physiology, a method that provides accurate and reproducible quantitative morphological characterisation is invaluable in studies of process optimisation and modelling.

In this section, the effects of agitation, nutritional factors (type and concentration of carbon source, nitrogen and phosphate limitation, pH, dissolved oxygen tension, trace metals levels) and inoculum size will be discussed with respect to the micro-morphology of *A. niger*.

Effect of Agitation

In submerged fermentation, agitation is important for adequate mixing, mass transfer and heat transfer. For aerobic fermentation, mixing is required to ensure sufficient oxygen transfer throughout the reactor vessel and aeration has been shown to have a critical effect on the submerged process of citric acid fermentation. Agitation creates shear forces that affect micro-organisms in several ways, causing morphological changes, variation in their growth and product formation and also damage in the cell structure.

For the dispersed form, in filamentous fermentation the effects of agitation superimposed on the fermentation process are difficult to quantify. Changes in morphology of filamentous fungi as a result of intensive agitation conditions have been observed in many cases. Under these conditions hyphae were thick, short and densely branched and this morphological type is usually associated with increased product yields. However, high impeller speeds were found to promote mycelial growth and possibly to stimulate the occurrence of metabolic pathways which resulted in low productivity of citric acid. The effect of stirrer speed on growth and productivity of three *Aspergillus niger* strains was reported by Ujcova. Higher speeds resulted in thicker and highly branched filaments. There was a drop in productivity at higher speeds although growth remained rapid. A similar effect for penicillin fermentation was reported by König. At higher speeds only a short period of penicillin production was maintained and a large fraction of the substrate was converted into carbon dioxide.

It has been reported that increased agitation can lead to breakage of hyphae for a number of micro-organisms. Although *A. niger* cultures are normally resistant to shear damage, mycelial fragmentation due to mechanical forces has been reported. The damage of hyphae and the consecutive release of intracellular material may account for the decreased productivities reported in many cases under intensive agitation conditions.

This has been proven for *Penicillium chrysogenum*. Smith and Makagiansar observed that the lower rates of penicillin synthesis at high agitation speeds were due to increased damage of hyphae, since it involved a greater frequency of circulation of mycelia through the high energy dissipation zone around the impeller.

In Figs 21.13 and 21.14 the effect of agitation on citric acid production and the relation between production and morphology is shown. In both reactors low dissolved oxygen levels were observed under conditions of low agitation intensities.

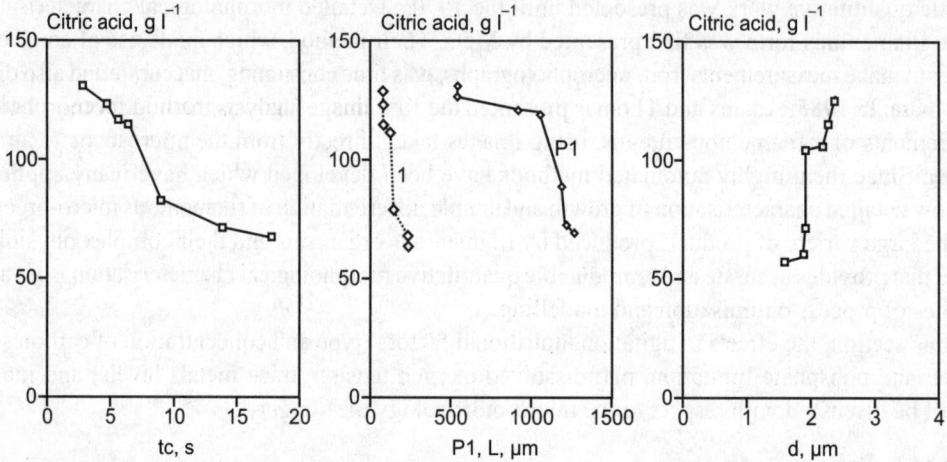

Fig. 21.13. Effect of agitation on citric acid production and the relation between production and morphology parameters in the tubular loop reactor.

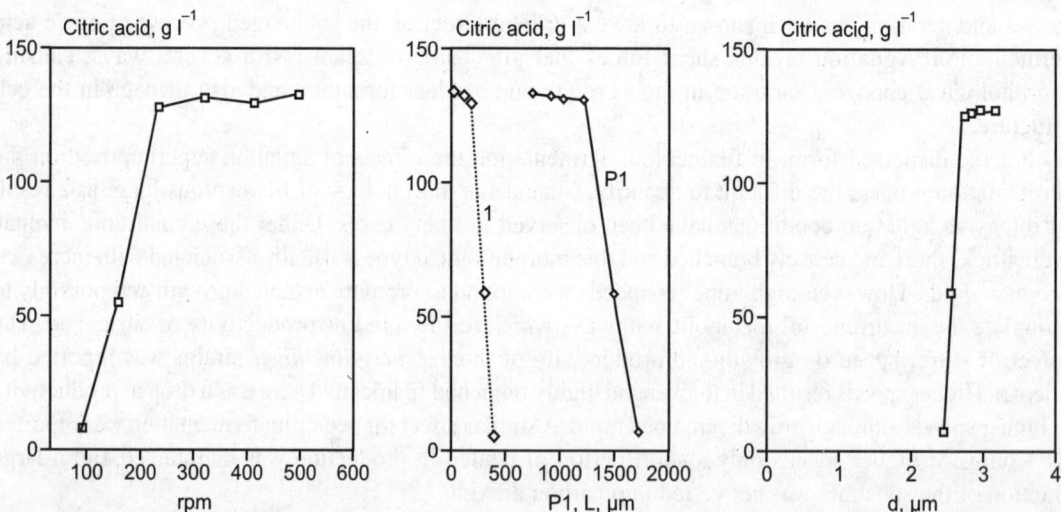

Fig. 21.14. Effect of agitation on citric acid production and the relation between production and morphology in the stirred tank reactor.

Effect of Nutritional Factors

Citric acid accumulation is strongly influenced by the composition of the nutrient medium. The medium constituents which have been found to exert an effect on citric acid fermentation are: type and concentration of the carbon source, supply of nitrogen and phosphate, pH, dissolved oxygen levels and concentration of certain trace metals. The influence on morphology of *A. niger* or other filamentous micro-organisms in submerged culture for most of these factors has been studied.

Type and concentration of carbon source

The carbon source for citric acid fermentation has been the focus of much study, frequently with a view to the utilisation of polysaccharide sources. The nature of the source has been shown in many cases to affect citric acid production, since it exerts a strong effect on levels of enzyme activity within the TCA cycle. In general, only sugars, which are rapidly taken up by the fungus, allow a high final yield of citric acid. Polysaccharides, unless hydrolysed, are not included in this category. Information concerning the role of the nature of sugar source on *A. niger* morphology in citric acid fermentation is limited. However, it has been observed that factors favouring increased growth rates, such as media rich in easily assimilated nutrients, affect morphology by reducing pellet formation in filamentous organisms.

Not only the type, but also the concentration of the carbon source is critical to this fermentation, influencing the rate of production and the final yield, in addition to growth of the fungus.

Nitrogen and phosphate limitation

In order to accumulate citric acid, growth must be restricted, but it is not clear whether phosphate or nitrogen is the necessary limiting factor. According to Shu and Johnson, phosphate does not have to be limiting, but when trace metal levels are not limiting, additional phosphate results in side reactions and increased growth. Kubicek and Rohr showed that citric acid accumulated whenever phosphate was limited even when nitrogen was not. In contrast, Kristiansen and Sinclair, using continuous culture, concluded that nitrogen limitation was essential for citric acid production.

Pellet formation in filamentous fungi has been discussed in many cases and among the factors considered to induce it, is the limitation of particular nutrients, including nitrogen. On the other hand, factors favouring increased growth rates, including excess phosphate concentrations, have been shown to reduce pellet formation.

pH

Culture pH can have a profound effect on citric acid production by *A. niger*, since certain enzymes within the TCA cycle are pH sensitive. The maintenance of a low pH during fermentation is vital for a good yield and it is generally considered necessary for the pH to fall to around pH 2 within a few hours of the initiation of the process, otherwise the yields are reduced. Information concerning the effect of pH upon the morphology of citric acid producing *A. niger* is very limited. Reports on the effect of pH on morphology for other fungi are contradictory; either it influences morphology greatly or it has no effect at all.

Dissolved oxygen tension

It has been shown that oxygen acts as a direct regulator of citric acid accumulation as it is favoured by increasing the dissolved oxygen tension of the fermentation medium. As already mentioned in the agitation, lower dissolved oxygen levels occurred with morphologies not associated with high yields on citric acid. However, reports on the effect of dissolved oxygen tension on the macro-morphology of *A. niger* suggest that no direct relationship exists between the two. Gomez and others, in their work on citric acid production from *A. niger*, found that no difference in morphology for pellets and filaments could be ascribed to dissolved oxygen levels, although production on citric acid was enhanced, particularly from pellets, by increasing the dissolved oxygen at different fermentation stages. Similarly, Van Suijdam and Metz showed that oxygen tension in the range of 12 to 300 mg Hg had no influence on the morphology of *P. chrysogenum*. These reports contradict the limitation hypothesis made by Hemmersdorfer, which suggests that lack of any particular nutrient, including oxygen, induces pellet formation.

Trace metal levels

A number of divalent metals have been suggested as being required in limiting amounts for a successful citric acid process. These include Fe^{2+}, Cu^{2+}, Zn^{2+}, Mn^{2+} and Mg^{2+}. Only the effect of manganese concentration has been shown to influence *A. niger* morphology. Manganese ions are known to be specifically involved in many cellular processes, such as cell wall synthesis, sporulation and production of secondary metabolites. Cellular anabolism of *A. niger* is impaired under Mn deficiency and/or nitrogen and phosphate limitation. The protein breakdown under Mn deficiency results in a high intracellular NH_4^+ concentration. This causes inhibition of the enzyme phosphofructokinase (essential enzyme in the conversion of glucose and fructose to pyruvate), leading to a flux through glycolysis and the formation of citric acid.

Kisser studied morphology and cell wall composition of *A. niger* under conditions of Mn sufficient and deficient cultivation in an otherwise citric acid producing medium. Omission of Mn ions (less than 10^{-7}) from the nutrient medium resulted in abnormal morphological development that was characterised by increased spore swelling and squat, bulbous hyphae. The inhibition of glucoprotein turnover caused by the presence of Mn ions led to a possible loss of hyphal polarity and increased branching and chitin synthesis. Clark also discussed changes in *A. niger* morphology following the addition of Mn. The authors noticed an undesirable change in morphology from the pellet like form to filamentous form with the addition of 2 ppb Mn to ferrocyanide-treated molasses. Morphological changes, which included prevention of clumping, absence of swollen cells and reduced diameters of filaments, accompanied by a 20 per cent reduction in citric acid yield, following the addition of 30 mg l^{-1} Mn to a Mn-free medium, were also reported by Papagianni.

Effect of Inoculum

Among the factors that determine morphology and the general course of fungal fermentations, the amount and type of inoculum is of prime importance. Early attempts have been made to standardise inocula for citric acid production in submerged culture. Van Suijdam reported that *A. niger* pellets would only form at inoculum sizes below 10^{11} spores per m^3. However, the effect of inoculum on mycelial morphology in submerged culture has been assessed mainly by the presence or absence of pellets and their characteristics. The reason for this was the lack of an adequate method to monitor mycelial morphology during fermentations. Morphology was quantified by an image analysis method in the work of Tucker and Thomas; a sharp transition from pelleted to dispersed forms of growth for *Penicillium chrysogenum* was reported, as inoculum levels rose towards 5×10^5 spores per m^3. This suggests that research on the inoculum in citric acid fermentation could now be more systematic, making use of the technological advances in characterisation and monitoring of morphology in fungal fermentations.

Thus, discussion of the factors influencing *A. niger* morphology in submerged culture should distinguish between macro- and micro-morphology although a number of similarities exist in relation to citric acid production and responses to the environment. This section has concentrated on micro-morphology. The observations indicate that it might be possible to manipulate the morphology parameters in order to improve bioreactor performance and process yields. Image analysis provides the tools for monitoring these parameters; however, further research is required to reveal possible general trends in metabolite regulation in relation to morphology of the producer micro-organism.

REDOX POTENTIAL IN SUBMERGED CITRIC ACID FERMENTATION

In living organisms oxidation-reduction systems play such an intimate and essential a part, that life itself might be defined as a continuous oxidation-reduction reaction. It is not surprising, therefore, that theoretical speculations and experimental studies on oxidation and reduction processes in animals and plants have been actively pursued since the isolation of oxygen over 150 years ago.

Helmholtz was the first to describe the decolourisation of litmus in a medium containing decaying protein. This was a reductive process since on passing air into solution, the original colour could be obtained again. Ehrlich injected redox dyes into living animals, killed them and investigated the redox state of the dyes in the organs. He attributed the varying state of reduction to the oxygen uptake of the organs. These dyes could therefore be used as indicators for particular reducing conditions. (Potter carried out the first electrometric measurement of reducing conditions in bacterial cultures. He detected with a platinum electrode that the bacterial culture had a more negative potential than uninoculated nutrient medium.) Gillespie followed the development of bacterial cultures and showed that strongly negative potentials become more positive when air is passed into the culture. Gillespie was also the first who applied the physical-chemical term 'redox potential' although the terms redox potential, reduction-oxidation potential, electrode potential and reduction potential were and are still used synonymously by various authors.

Redox potential detectors are usually not added to standard bioreactor instrumentation for a number of reasons, most of them related to conventional thinking in bioreactor instrumentation practices. As pH measurement represents the sum of all pH influencing compounds, redox potential measurement represents the sum of all redox potential influencing compounds in fermentation broth.

Overview

Redox potential is, however, a parameter that can give valuable information about metabolism taking place in various aerobic and anaerobic microbial cultures. The significance of redox potential levels for high yielding citric acid biosynthesis has been demonstrated in submerged citric acid fermentation.

Although only limited attention has been paid to this phenomenon in the past, some interesting and informative research work has been presented. Some workers have advocated the use of redox potential measurements for monitoring and controlling dissolved oxygen. At constant pH the relation between redox potential and dissolved oxygen partial pressure can be simplified by logarithmic relation. During the last few years a great deal of the attention for redox potential measurement and it uses, has been given to anaerobic bioprocesses. The importance of redox potential measurements was referred in waste water bioprocessing, as in the case of propionate degrading *Methanospirillum* and *Methanocorpusculum* bacteria in a fluidised bed reactor, where degradation was inhibited at redox potential below -300 mV, and in anaerobic digestion in methanogenic fermentation where volatile fatty acids were used as the substrate.

Redox potential measurements have also been found to be important in extremely thermophilic *Thermotoga* sp. bioprocessing, where most thermodynamic problems were associated with the relatively high redox potential. In various aerobic processes the importance of the redox potential has been observed. In the case of the biochemical transformation of *l*-sorbose to 2-keto-1-gluconic acid by a mutant strain of *Pseudomonas*, it was found that the redox potential indicated the oxygen demand of the culture. The importance of redox potential was also very significant in fermentations with *Proteus vulgaris*, *Clostridium paraputrificium* and *Candida utilis*, *Lactobacillus sanfrancisco* and *Lactoccocus lactis*. In *Acetobacterium malicum* degradation of fatty acids, there were differences in redox potentials at which electrons were released during oxidative pyruvate formation. In acetone-butanol fermentation by *Clostridium acetobutylicum*, redox potential measurements were used in batch and continuous fermentation. A correlation between redox potential and switch from an acidogenic to solventogenic metabolism was reported. Although the redox condition in a fermentation broth is reflected in the redox potential values measured, its characteristics cannot be generalised and the role of redox potential should be studied for each microbial process.

Publications on regulation of redox potential levels are rare. In the experiments of Lengel and Nyiri and Kjaergaard, on various bioprocesses, the redox potential was regulated by addition of reductants, while in *Candida guilermondii* fermentation by Huang and Wu, the addition of *n*-paraffins was used.

THEORY

Oxidation is a process in which a substance, molecule or ion loses or gives up electrons. Reduction, on the other hand, is a process in which a substance, molecule or ion, is involved in the taking up of electrons. Whenever one substance in a system is oxidised, another substance must be reduced. The relation between reduction and oxidation may be expressed as:

$$\text{Reduced form} \rightleftharpoons \text{Oxidised form} + \text{electron(s)}$$

However, since free electrons never exist in any noteworthy concentration, reduction and oxidation reactions are always coupled together, so that one reaction releases just as many electrons as the other one consumes. Thus, a pair of reactions always takes part in such a process. These simultaneous and complementary reduction and oxidation processes are generally known as redox reactions. The oxidation (or reduction) capacity of a solution is characterised by the free electron activity in it. Despite the fact that the lifetime of a free electron is extremely short (10^{-1}–10^{-15} seconds) there is a statistical possibility of free electron existence at the moment of transformation from electron-donor systems to electron-acceptor systems.

The thermodynamic probability of electron emergence under activated reaction capable conditions is understood as electron activity in a solution:

$$a_e = (1/k)^{1/n} (a_{red}/a_{ox}) \qquad \qquad \text{... (21.1)}$$

The oxidation potential is a quantitative measure of redox capacity of a solution. It is an electrical unit of charge of free energy in a redox interaction of the given system with a standard system. The system:

$$2H^+ + 2e^- \longleftrightarrow H_2$$

is a standard one. The oxidation potential is related to the electron activity in solution:

$$E_h = -RT/F \ln a_e \qquad \qquad \text{... (21.2)}$$

$$E_h = -RT/F \ln[(1/k)^{1/n}(a_{red}/a_{ox})] \qquad \qquad \text{... (21.3)}$$

$$E_h = kRT/nF + RT/nF \ln(a_{red}/a_{ox}) \qquad \qquad \text{... (21.4)}$$

In the first part of Eq. 21.4, kRT is equal to E_o, the standard redox potential of a 50 per cent reduced substance, based on a standard hydrogen electrode.

$$E_h = E_o + RT/nF \ln(a_{red}/a_{ox}) \qquad \text{... (21.5)}$$

Equation 21.5 is the well-known Nernst equation.

The redox potential of the measured substance, or substrate, depending on pH, is expressed in the Kjarergaard equation:

$$E_h = E_{O_2/H_2O} + RT/4F \ln a_{O_2} - RT/4F \ln 2.303 \text{ pH} \qquad \text{... (21.6)}$$

The potential values measured are dependent on pH, so that in each case measurements of redox potential should be accompanied by a statement of the pH value at which they were taken. In general a pH variation of one unit causes a potential variation of 57.7 mV.

Measurement of Redox Potential

In principle there are two ways of measuring a redox potential: by redox dyes and by electrodes. Measurement of the redox potential by dyes is not exact and requires a number of different dyes to obtain semi-quantitative measurements; furthermore, many of these dyes may be toxic to the cells or may inhibit the enzyme activities in biological liquids. Therefore, this method is not used in biochemical engineering. In bioreactors, combined sterilisable platinum as indicator and calomel or silver/silver chloride electrode as reference electrodes are employed. As electrolyte 3M KCl solution or sometimes KCl-gel are used.

It has been suggested that a decrease in E_h for a tenfold decrease in concentration of dissolved oxygen amounts to 14.8 mV. Clark and Cohen introduced the concept of rH in order to eliminate pH dependence on the potential:

$$\text{rH} = -\log a_{H_2} \qquad \text{... (21.7)}$$

An rH of 0 corresponds to a pO_2 of 0 atm and pH = 0, and rH = 42 corresponds to a solution in which pO_2 = 1 atm and pH = 0 (Fig. 21.15).

Calibration of redox electrodes

For calibration of the redox electrodes various redox buffers are in use. In this case two saturated solutions of quinhydrone at two different pH values at 25°C are recommended:

$$E_{h \text{ qinhydrone}} = 699 - 59.1 \text{ pH} \qquad \text{... (21.8)}$$

A relatively easier method is to use ascorbic acid at various pHs:

$$E_{h \text{ ascorbic acid}} = 375 - 60 \text{ pH} \qquad \text{... (21.9)}$$

Significance of Redox Potential

Redox potential in microbial cultures is caused by the existence of reversible oxido-reduction couples, irreversible reductors, and the action of free oxygen and free hydrogen. It is dependent on pH value, dissolved oxygen concentration, equilibrium constant and oxido-reduction potentials in the liquid. Mass transfer of oxygen in aerobic cultures requires a potential difference between oxygen concentration in the cell and the surrounding medium. The concentration of oxygen decreases from the solution towards the cells, and it is highly probable that the intracellular redox potential of micro-organisms is always slightly more negative than the extracellular redox potential.

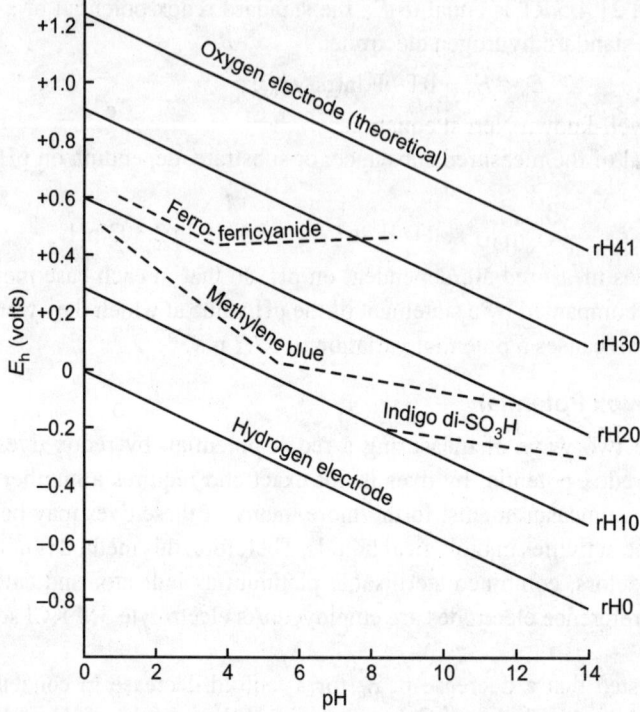

Fig. 21.15. Electrode potential versus pH. Continuous line, theoretical curves, broken line, actual system.

Several investigations have revealed that the redox potential yields more information about the oxidative status in aerobic or partially aerobic microbial cultures than concentration of dissolved oxygen. Most commercial dissolved oxygen probes, when used in industrial conditions, are often susceptible to failure or erratic signal behaviour during the fermentation cycle, especially when dissolved oxygen is a limiting factor. In L-leucine fermentation, the redox signal was useful in determining the oxygen transfer requirements when dissolved oxygen was practically zero.

At constant pH the relation between redox potential and dissolved oxygen partial pressure can be simplified by the following equation, demonstrated in Fig. 21.16:

$$\log pO_2 = aE_h + b \qquad \qquad ...(21.10)$$

A similar relationship between pO_2 and E_h has been observed in amino acid production by *Corynebacterium glutamicum*:

$$\log pO_2 = 0.0157\ E_h - 0.071 \qquad \qquad ...(21.11)$$

Shibai carried this further for inosine production by *Bacillus subtilis*; pO_{2crit} was determined by measuring the dissolved oxygen, the redox potential and cell respiration rate in pH and temperature controlled culture. When the dissolved oxygen partial pressure was above 1.10^{-2} atm, the redox potential had a linear relationship with the logarithm of the dissolved oxygen partial pressure. Therefore $pO_2 = 1.10^{-2}$ atm was estimated by determining the redox potential, on the assumption that there was a linear relationship even at the pO_2 level less than 1.10^{-2} atm. The redox potential was markedly lowered by the physiological change in the cells, when cell respiration was inhibited at $E_h = -180$ mV, which corresponded to $pO_2 = 2.10^{-4}$ atm.

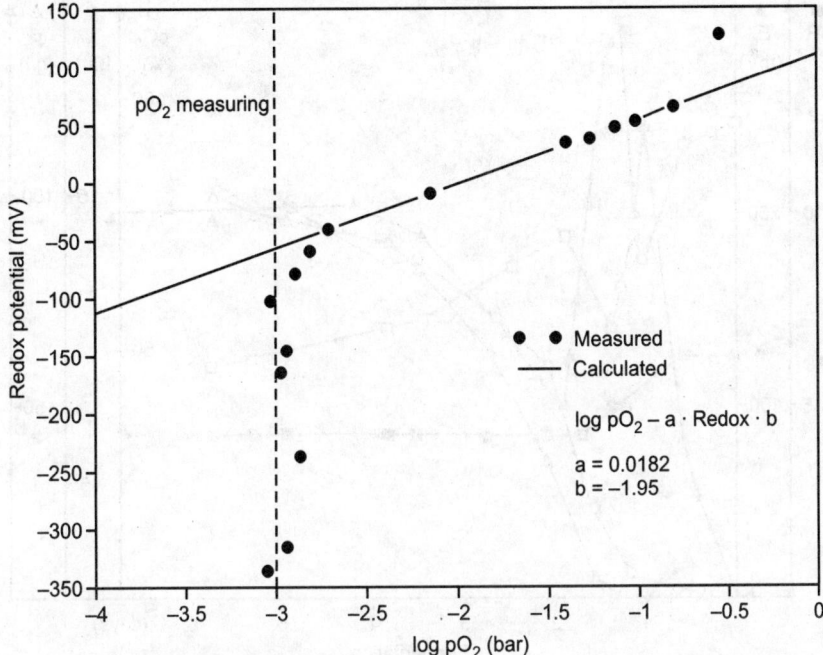

Fig. 21.16. Relationship between oxygen tension and redox potential.

pO_2 in this culture was recorded as nearly zero when the cell rapidly biosynthesised the product. It went up above 1.10^{-2} atm at the end of fermentation, when the substrate was almost completely assimilated. The data showed that maximum production was obtained under limited oxygen supply, where cell respiration was inhibited. When cell respiration was not inhibited, as the pO_2 level rose above 1.10^{-2} atm, the cell did not produce the maximum amount of L-leucine.

The lowest values of pO_2 that have been reported were 4.10^{-3} atm for *Saccharomyces cerevisiae*, 3×10^{-4} atm for inosine and 2×10^{-4} atm for the leucine producer.

Redox Potential in Citric Acid Fermentation

Although citric acid production is the oldest industrial process, in addition to our own work, there are only two other publications on redox potential measurements. In one research on submerged citric acid fermentation using beet molasses as a substrate, the relevance of redox potential levels for high product yielding biosynthesis has been demonstrated. For a high citric acid yielding fermentation there is an optimal course of the redox potential profile with two maxima of 260 and 280 mV and two minima of 180 and 80 mV of essential importance. This redox potential course has been evaluated by analysis of more than 200 fermentations. The time course for a typical batch fermentation is shown in Fig. 21.17.

Beet molasses contains different organic and inorganic redox couples, substances and several metal ions that could significantly influence redox potential of the whole fermentation broth. Addition of $K_4Fe(CN)_6$, a well-known redox substance, to the substrate causes the formation not only of metal ion complexes, but also the Fe^{3+}/Fe^{2+} redox couple, which regulates the ion balance of the substrate. The balance of various redox couples and especially metal ion in fermentation broth is of essential importance for citric acid biosynthesis. Related to this the influence of various influent factors and substances on redox potential levels of beet molasses substrate have been studied (Fig. 21.18).

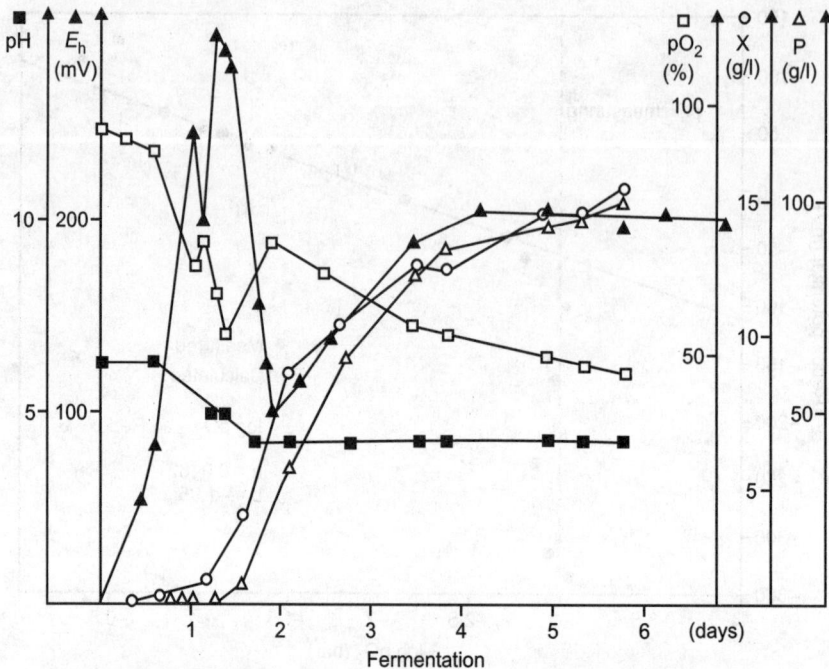

Fig. 21.17. Process parameters of high citric acid yielding fermentation.

A reference redox potential profile was obtained for sterile medium only, with no addition of $K_4Fe(CN)_6$ (curve 1). After 24 hours of aeration, the redox potential reached a stationary phase that was unchanged until the end of the experiment. In experiments where inoculated substrate was used in absence of any addition of $K_4Fe(CN)_6$ (curve 2), and with an initial addition of this compound (curve 3), the redox potential profile exhibited a typical single peak. Only in the case where inoculated substrate with primary and secondary addition of $K_4Fe(CN)_6$ was used (results shown in Fig. 21.17), was the twin peak redox potential course observed. The different metabolic activities in the fermentation process are summarised in all the redox reactions and detected in redox potential measurement. From these experiments it was concluded that only in the presence of *Aspergillus niger* were the relevant changes detected. Similar observations were made by Kwong and Rao in amino acid fermentation using *Corynebacterium glutamicum*. Redox potential measurements in citric acid fermentation might also give valuable indications of product biosynthesis in the fermentation. From evaluation of more than 200 batches, it was concluded that a high yielding fermentation is directly related to levels and time course of redox potential. The yield of citric acid is reflected in the time course of the redox potential. This is shown in Figs 21.19 and 21.20, where experiments with different histories are shown. Figure 21.19 presents the characteristics of an unsuccessful fermentation with respect to citric acid production. Growth was diffused and the low citric acid production was therefore expected. This is also reflected in the course of the redox potential. The second peak is low and almost negligible (190 mV).

The effect of temperature change is well reflected in the course of redox potential. Figure 21.20 presents the data from an experiment started at an initial temperature of 20°C. The temperature was changed after 20 hours to 30°C. The effect of this change can be clearly seen from the redox curve. In the same experiment foaming caused a loss of the substrate (89 hours), which was also indicated in a new peak of the redox potential.

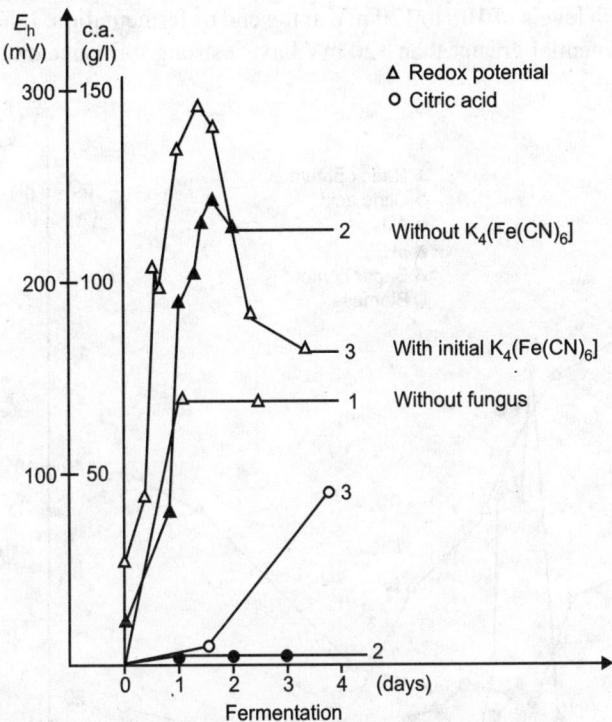

Fig. 21.18. Redox potential measurements and citric acid formation by *Aspergillus niger*. Curve 1: aerated sterile sugar beet molasses substrate including potassium ferrocyanide; curve 2: inoculated and aerated sterile sugar beet molasses substrate excluding potassium ferrocyanide; curve 3: inoculated and aerated sterile sugar beet molasses substrate including potassium ferrocyanide.

In a high yielding fermentation on beet molasses substrate, the redox potential course starts at a level of 0 to 20 mV, as shown in Fig. 21.17. After 12 hours, the culture reaches a level of oxygenation which significantly influences germination of conidia in the lag phase and the subsequent development of bulbous cells that appears at the first peak of the redox potential at 260 mV. After the first peak, a period of inhibition followed by the first redox minimum at 180 mV occurs. In this phase it seems that microbial activity stops. Oxygen partial pressure in fermentation broth increases and the carbon dioxide and redox potential decreases, indicating a reduced level of activity for the micro-organism. This phase is a progressive transition from glucose to fructose consumption. For this reorganisation, a low redox potential level is needed, resulting in the change in morphology.

After this phase, the microbial growth mode changes to spherical pellets. This was indicated by the second redox peak at 280 mV. After a decrease in redox potential to 80 mV, the second minimum, citric acid production starts. As reported by Tengerdy, at the lowest redox potential level, the peak oxygen demand and initiation of rapid excretion of citric acid can be observed. The low redox potential reveals the reducing state of the complex redox system of the fermentation broth, where the respiratory enzyme system signifies strong metabolic activity. It seems that citric acid biosynthesis, as well as some other microbiological reactions, proceeds favourably at the redox potential near the minimum of the redox curve for the particular culture involved. This was found to be true in riboflavin fermentation.

The redox potential time-course in a high citric acid yielding fermentation reaches a final level of 180 mV. Interestingly if significant amounts of oxalic acid, up to 20 mg/l, are produced, the redox potential will only reach levels of 100 to 120 mV at the end of fermentation. It has also been found that oscillations in redox potential greater than ±20 mV have a strong influence on further development of fermentation.

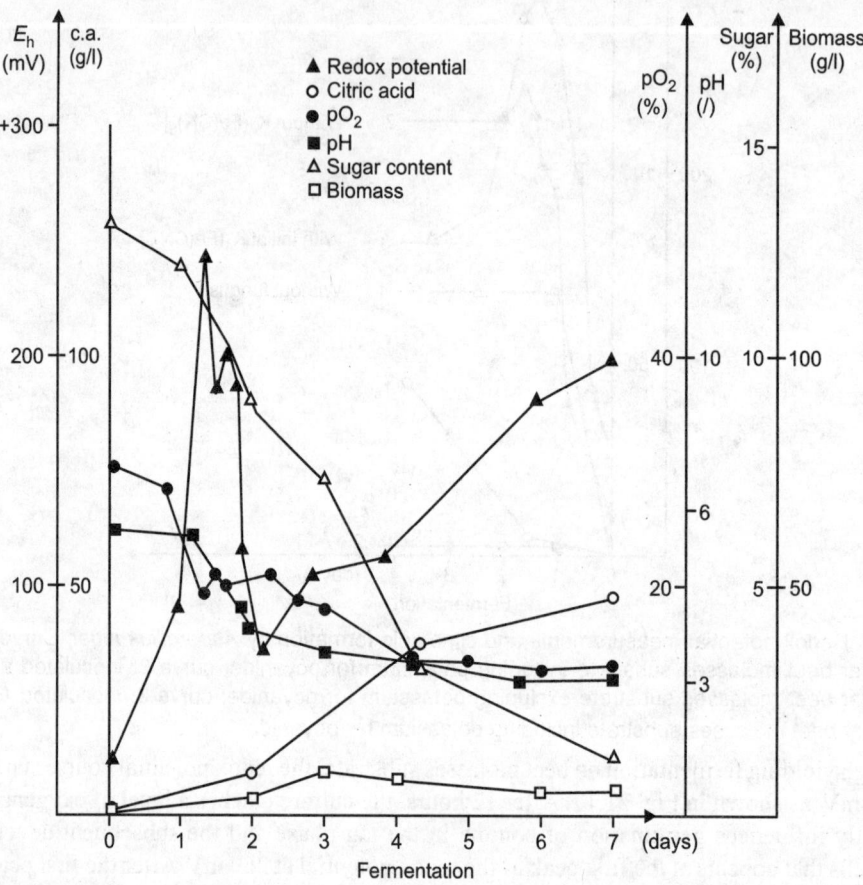

Fig. 21.19. Process variables in a low yielding, abnormal citric acid fermentation.

Regulation of the Redox Potential

Although measurements and observation of redox potential have been published in several articles, its regulation and process control have only rarely been discussed. In a few fermentation processes, as in *Bacillus lichenoformis* cultivation, a chemical method based on addition of glucose has been used. Huang and Wu added *n*-paraffins for regulation of redox potential in a *Candida guilermondii* fermentation. In a continuous process for production of xylanase by *Bacillus amiloliquefaciens*, a physical method based on regulation of dilution rate and agitation was used. Constant maintenance of redox potential in various bioprocesses were reported by Lengel and Nyiri. Radjai found that the redox potential minimum for amino acid fermentations with *Corynebacterium glutamicum* was directly influenced by the agitation rate. The minimum redox potential of the culture became less negative as the rate of agitation was increased. This is consistent with the increase obtained in the oxygen transfer rate and subsequently in dissolved oxygen partial pressure as agitation speed is increased.

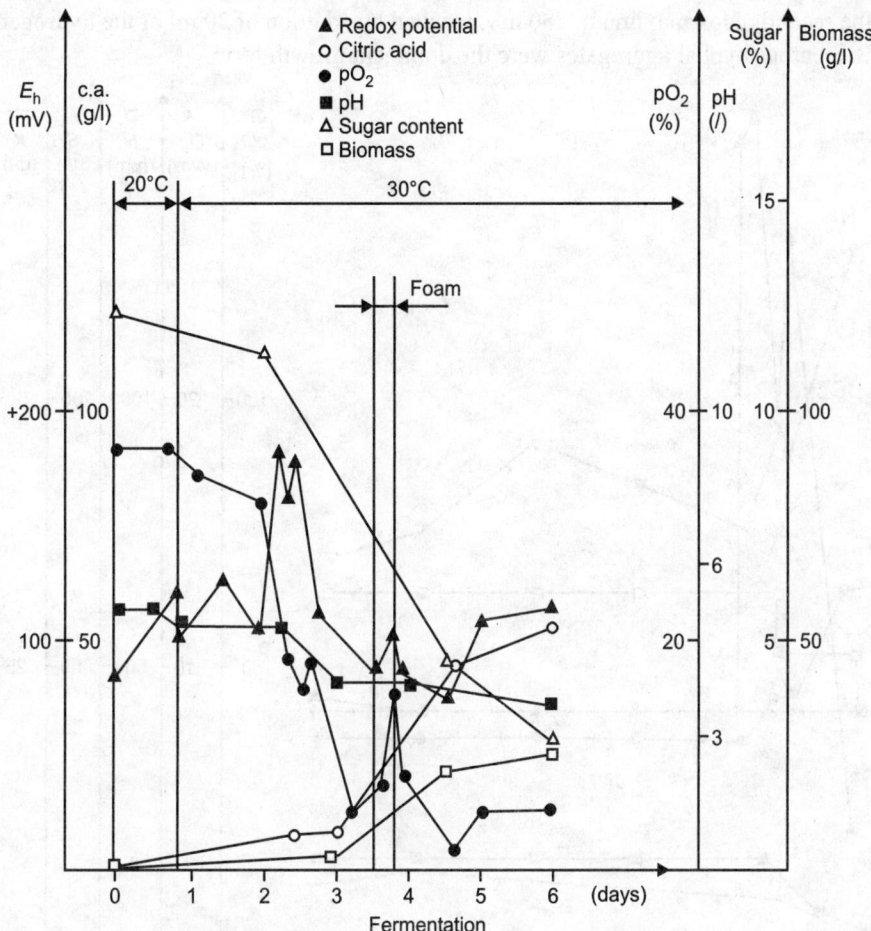

Fig. 21.20. Effect of temperature shift on citric acid fermentation with *Aspergillus niger* and sugar beet molasses medium.

Regulation of Redox Potential in Citric Acid Fermentation

The aim of using regulation of redox potential in citric acid fermentation was to establish a method for redox potential regulation that will conduct a fermentation process towards the essential redox levels needed for high citric acid production. According to this, two different methods, a chemical method, similar to those used for pH control by using oxidants and reductants, and a physical method, based on simultaneous agitation and aeration control were tested.

Chemical methods

In the first experiment, 0.1 per cent hydrogen peroxide was used as oxidant, and 0.1 per cent sodium sulphite as reductant. The results of the experiment are presented in Fig. 21.21. The first redox peak reached 260 mV. At this level no oxidant was added. The microbial growth form was bulbous cells. After the first redox maximum, the first minimum of 180 mV was obtained by addition of 80 ml of the sodium sulphite. After this addition microbial growth turned from bulbous to filamentous hyphae growth forms. At the second redox maximum, 280 mV, reached by addition of 20 ml of the hydrogen peroxide solution, filamentous hyphal aggregates were the dominant growth form.

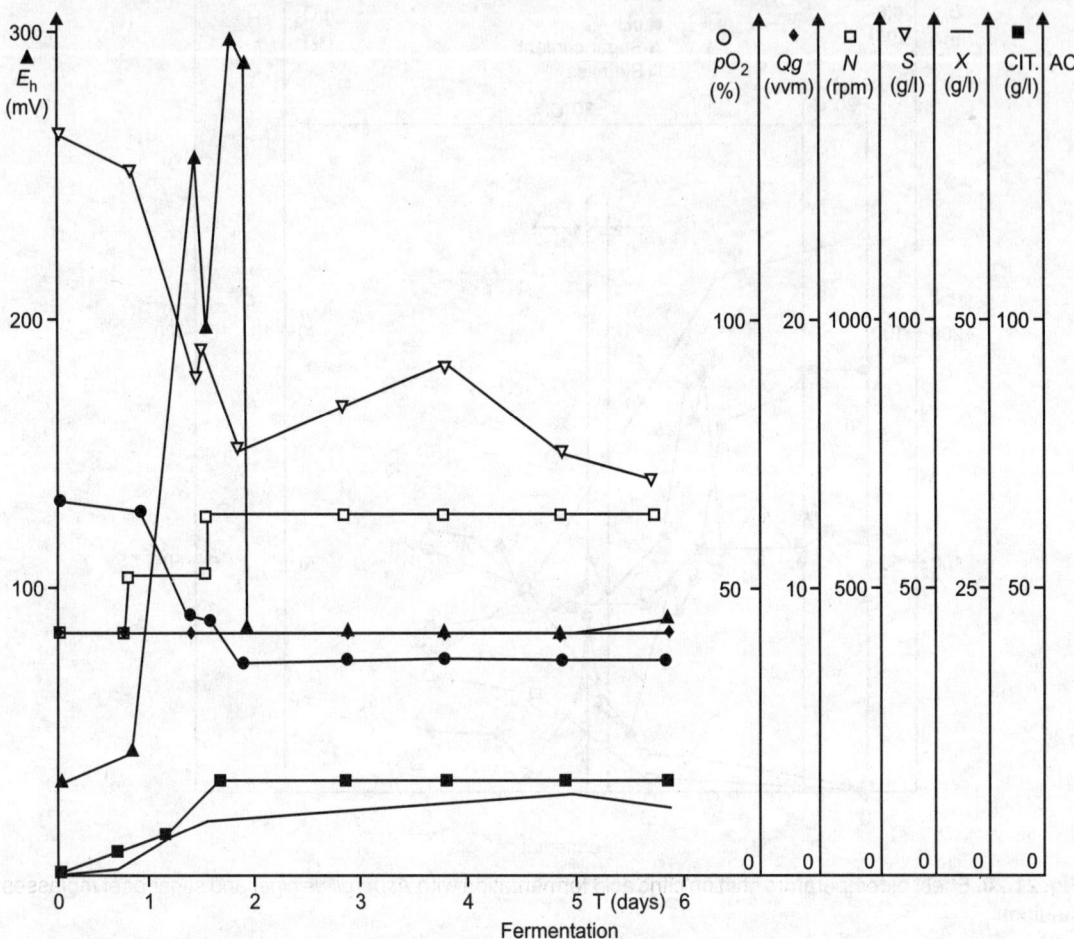

Fig. 21.21. Process parameters of citric acid fermentation at chemical regulation of redox potential using 0.1 per cent sodium sulphite as reductant and 0.1 per cent hydrogen peroxide as oxidant.

The second redox minimum was obtained by addition of 195 ml of sodium sulphite solution. After this the microbial form did not change. Shear in the bioreactor caused formation of hyphal fragments which were present until the end of fermentation. This period also exhibited an unchanged redox potential of 80 mV. Although this method gave a redox time-course which was similar to the time-course in high yielding fermentations, the microbial growth after addition of sodium sulphite turned completely to low citric acid producing filamentous growth forms. The addition of reductant did not stop microbial growth, but it produced an unproductive growth form. At the end of fermentation a biomass level of 5.5 g/l and 12.8 g/l citric acid were obtained.

In a further experiment, a water solution of 0.1 per cent hydrogen peroxide as oxidant and a 20 per cent solution of glucose as reductant were used. In Fig. 21.22 the results of such an experiment are presented. The first maximum of 260 mV was obtained at 25 hours. In this period, bulbous cell agglomerates appeared. Following this the regulation of redox potential levels started. The first redox minimum of 180 mV was obtained at 30 hours by addition of 275 ml of the glucose solution. The second maximum of 280 mV was reached soon after by addition of 26 ml of hydrogen peroxide.

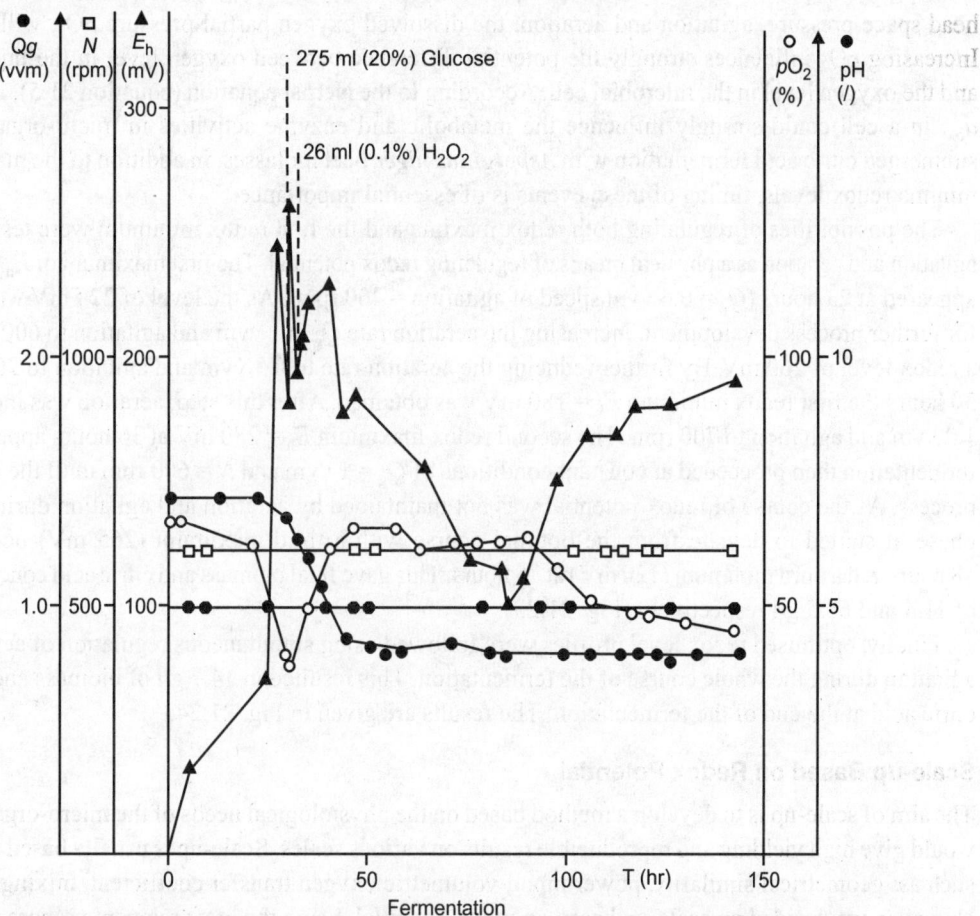

Fig. 21.22. Process parameters of citric acid fermentation at chemical regulation of redox potential using 20 per cent glucose as reductant and 0.1 per cent hydrogen peroxide as oxidant.

This phase was characterised by formation of small spherical pellets with short and thin peripherial hyphae. The second minimum of 200 mV appeared after the second peak soon after the regulation was stopped. This was followed by a slow, unaided drift up to a third peak of 240 mV. In this phase mycelium growth in the pellet form with thin and long peripherial hyphae appeared. The redox then fell slowly to a third minimum of 100 mV followed by a gentle increase to 180 mV at the end of fermentation.

Using these agents, regulation of redox potential of the fermentation broth was possible. The redox potential time-course was close to the optimal and addition of either compound did not inhibit the development of a productive growth mode, mycelial pellets with thick and long peripherial hyphae being the typical morphology feature. At the end of the fermentation, a biomass level of 11.1 g/l and 40 g/l of citric acid were obtained (Fig. 21.22).

Physical methods

Physical parameters such as temperature, head space pressure, agitation and aeration strongly influence the oxygen transport coefficient in the liquid phase. Therefore by lowering the temperature and increasing head space pressure, agitation and aeration, the dissolved oxygen partial pressure pO_2, will increase. Increasing pO_2 influences strongly the potential difference between oxygen level in the liquid phase and the oxygen level in the microbial cell. According to the Nernst equation (equation 21.5), increasing a_{ox}, in a cell could strongly influence the metabolic and enzyme activities in micro-organisms. In submerged citric acid fermentation with *Aspergillus niger* beet molasses, in addition to the maxima and minima redox levels, timing of these events is of essential importance.

The possibilities of regulating both redox maxima and the first redox minimum were tested, using agitation and aeration as a physical means of regulating redox potential. The first maximum of $E_h = 220$ mV appeared at 23 hours ($Q_g = 0.4$ vvm speed of agitation = 400 rpm). As the level of 220 mV was too low for further process development, increasing the aeration rate Q_g to 1 vvm and agitation to 600 rpm gave a redox level of 260 mV. By further reducing the aeration rate to 0.3 vvm and agitation to 200 rpm, at 30 hours the first redox minimum $E_h = 180$ mV was obtained. After this step, aeration was increased to 1.2 vvm and agitation to 700 rpm. The second redox maximum $E_h = 280$ mV at 36 hours appeared. The fermentation then proceeded at constant conditions of $Q_g = 1$ vvm and $N = 600$ rpm until the end of the process. As the course of redox potential was not maintained by aeration and agitation during the last phase, it started to deviate from the optimal course with a third maximum (265 mV) occurring at 48 hours and a third minimum (120 mV) at 75 hours. This gave final biomass and citric acid concentrations of 11.4 and 68.5 g/l respectively (Fig. 21.23).

Finally, optimised redox level profiles were followed using simultaneous regulation of aeration and agitation during the whole course of the fermentation. This resulted in 14.7 g/l of biomass and 95 g/l of citric acid at the end of the fermentation. The results are given in Fig. 21.24.

Scale-up Based on Redox Potential

The aim of scale-up is to develop a method based on the physiological needs of the micro-organism that would give high yielding and reproducible results on various scales. Scale-up is usually based on criteria such as: geometrical similarity, power input, volumetric oxygen transfer coefficient, mixing time, etc. However, we decided on scale-up based on redox potential, being the most relevant process parameter for our process. As redox potential indicates oxygen demand of the culture, the basic idea was to use a physiological criterion of our bioprocess for scale-up. If redox potential indicates a microbial demand for oxygen, it could also reflect information on the appropriate aeration and agitation conditions needed to meet this demand.

Bioreactor dimensions

The experiments were performed in 10 l Bioengineering AG, and 100 and 1000 l Chemap AG bioreactors. These were all equipped with Rusthon turbines, but were not geometrically similar. The reactor dimensions are given in Table 21.11.

Media composition

The fermentation substrate consisted of diluted beet molasses with 12.5 per cent of total reducing sugars. It was treated by addition of potassium hexacyanoferrate $K_4[Fe(CN)_6]$, which balanced the ratio of heavy metals ions by the formation of metal complexes. $K_4[Fe(CN)_6]$ was added in two stages, before sterilisation (primary addition) and after (secondary addition). The fermentations were carried out at $T = 30°C$.

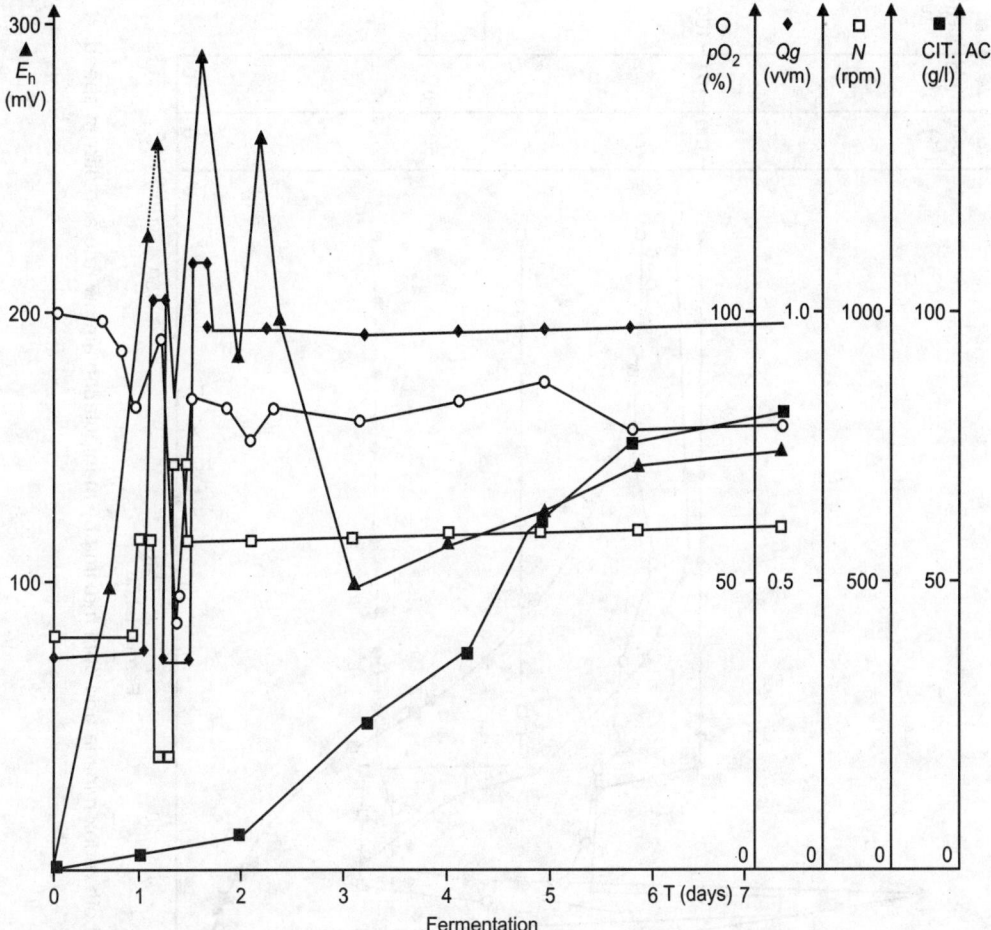

Fig. 21.23. Regulation of the first redox minimum and both maxima by manipulating airflow rate and stirred speed.

Table 21.11. Stirred tank reactor dimensions.

Parameter	Reactor volume (1)		
	10	*100*	*1000*
d – Impeller diameter (m)	0.072	0.220	0.400
D – Reactor diameter (m)	0.150	0.410	0.888
H – Liquid height (m)	0.310	0.860	2.700
H/D	2.060	2.100	3.145
Imp. tip speed (m/s)	1.1–2.2	3.4–5.7	6.9–11.1

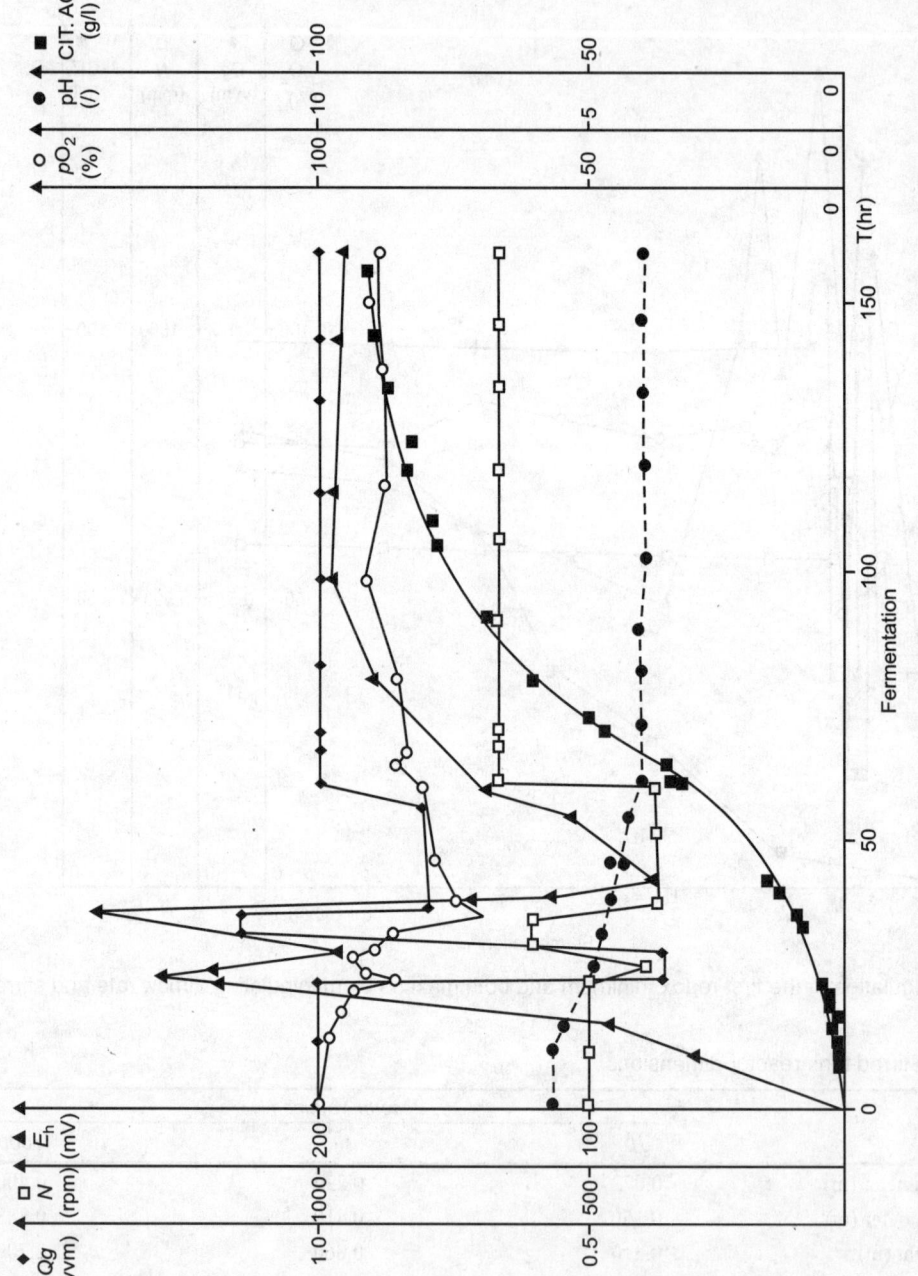

Fig. 21.24. Regulation of both redox minima and both maxima by manipulating airflow rate and stirred speed.

Laboratory scale experiments

Basic research for scale-up was performed in a 10 1 laboratory fermentor. The best redox profile was determined from some 200 fermentations. The objective of the scale-up was to obtain a similar redox profile in the larger reactors by regulating the agitation and aeration.

Pilot scale experiments

Fermentations were carried out in the 100 1 and 1000 1 reactors; aeration and agitation were increased and decreased stepwise as outlined above to obtain the two desired redox potential maxima and minima. This was achieved as indicated in Table 21.12. The results from the experiments are summarised in Table 21.13, with similar results obtained on all scales.

Table 21.12. Scaling up redox profiles.

Reactor volume	1 l	100 l	1000 l
First maximum	260 mV/27 hr	260 mV/31 hr	260 mV/28 hr
First minimum	180 mV/30 hr	191 mV/31 hr	190 mV/32 hr
Second maximum	280 mV/36 hr	280 mV/38 hr	280 mV/39 hr
Second minimum	120 mV/48 hr	100 mV/48 hr	110 mV/52 hr

Table 21.13. Results of scale-up experiments.

	Bioreactor		
	10 l	100 l	1000 l
T (hr)	160	160	160
S(g/l)	0.0	2.0	0.0
X(g/l)	14.5	13.8	15.2
P(g/l)	95.0	91.5	105.0
$Y_{P/S}(\%)$	78	74	84
$Y_{P/X}$	6.5	6.6	6.9
$Y_{X/P}(\%)$	15.2	15.0	14.4
$Y_{X/S}(\%)$	11.6	11.2	12.1

Thus, for high citric acid yielding submerged fermentation on beet molasses the optimal redox potential time course and its typical redox levels, with two maxima, 260 and 280 mV, and two minima, 180 and 80 mV, are essentially important. It is possible to influence the fermentation by changing the redox potential profile as well as the magnitude of the maxima and minima. Regulating the redox by using hydrogen peroxide as oxidant and sodium sulphite or glucose as reductant, resulted in a favourable redox profile for the whole process, but the fermentation was affected to such an extent that poor growth and reduced citric acid yields were obtained. A better method for regulating the redox potential during fermentation is through alteration in aeration and agitation. The desired redox profile is attained by respectively increasing, and decreasing the aeration and agitation to obtain the desired maximum and minimum values. It is a simple practical approach based on changing the gradient of oxygen transfer in the fermentation broth, which influences changes in intracellular oxygen concentration and therefore the microbial physiology of the cell.

This method of regulating the redox profile was used as a scale-up criterion with the process successfully scaled up from 10 to 1000 l. Considering the results obtained, it is evident that this new scale-up method leads to very reproducible results even in geometrically non-similar bioreactors.

DOWNSTREAM PROCESSING IN CITRIC ACID PRODUCTION

Pretreatment of Fermentation Broth

On completion of the citric acid fermentation the obtained solution contains, besides the desirable product, the mycelium and varying amounts of other impurities, e.g. mineral salts, other organic acids, proteins, etc. The method of citric acid recovery from the fermentation broth may vary depending on the technology and raw materials used for the production.

In the surface process the fermentation fluid is drained off the trays and hot water is introduced to wash out the remaining amount of citric acid from the mycelial mats. Thorough washing at this stage is necessary, because the mycelium retains about 15 per cent of the product formed in the fermentation. After 1–1.5 hours the wash water is drained off and then added to the fermentation liquor and mycelial mats are removed from trays, disintegrated and flushed into the washing vessel using limited amounts of water. In this vessel the mycelium is heated to about 100°C by steam. The hot pulp is subsequently dewatered by pressure filtration. The solution containing 2–4 per cent of citric acid is added to the fermentation fluid, whereas the filtration cake, containing not more than 0.2 per cent of citric acid, is dried to yield a protein-rich feed-stuff.

In the submerged fermentation the mycelium is far more difficult to separate from the fermentation broth. After the fermentation process is completed the mycelium containing broth is heated to a temperature of 70°C for about 15 minutes, to obtain partial coagulation of proteins, and then filtered, usually by means of the continuous filters (e.g. a rotating vacuum drum filter or a belt discharge filter). Because of the slimy consistency of mycelium forming in the submerged process, filter aids may be required. If the mycelium is to be used as a feedstuff, the filter aid must also be digestible, e.g. from cellulosic materials.

If during the fermentation process oxalic acid is formed as a side product due to suboptimal control of the fermentation process, it has to be removed from the broth. This is usually achieved by increasing the pH of the fermentation fluid with the calcium hydroxide to pH = 2.7–2.9 at a temperature of 70°–75°C. Calcium oxalate thus precipitated may be removed from the solution by filtration or centrifugation, and the citric acid remains in solution as the mono-calcium citrate. Oxalate removal increases the rate of filtration of the calcium citrate and gypsum in the subsequent steps of downstream processing and reduces the yellow hue of the citric acid solution.

Recovery of citric acid from pretreated fermentation broth may be accomplished by several procedures: classical method of precipitation, solvent extraction, adsorption/absorption on ion-exchange resins, and recently developed, more sophisticated methods such as electrodialysis, ultra- and nanofiltration or application of liquid membranes.

Precipitation

The standard method of citric acid recovery has involved precipitating the insoluble tricalcium citrate by the addition of an equivalent amount of lime to the citric acid solution. Successful operation of the precipitation depends on citric acid concentration, temperature, pH and rate of lime addition. To obtain large crystals of high purity, milk of lime containing calcium oxide (180–250 kg/m^3) is added gradually at a temperature of 90°C or above and pH below, but close to 7. The concentration of citric acid in the solution should be above 15 per cent. The process of neutralisation usually lasts about 120–150 minutes. The minimum loss of citric acid due to solubility of calcium citrate is 4–5 per cent.

If precipitation is properly done, most impurities remain in the solution and may be removed by washing the filtered calcium citrate. Washing is performed with the smallest amount possible of hot water (approx. 10 m^3 of water per ton of acid at the temperature 90°C until no saccharides, chlorides or coloured substances can be detected in the effluent. The calcium citrate is then filtered off and subsequently treated with concentrated sulphuric acid (60–70 per cent) to obtain citric acid and the precipitate of calcium sulphate (gypsum). After filtering off the gypsum a solution of 25–30 per cent of citric acid is obtained. The filtrate is treated with activated carbon to remove residual impurities or may be purified in ion-exchange columns. The purified solution is then concentrated in vacuum evaporators at temperature below 40°C (to avoid caramelisation), crystallised, centrifuged and dried to obtain citric acid crystals. If crystallisation is performed at temperatures below 36.5°C, the citric acid monohydrate is formed and above this transition temperature citric acid an-hydrate may be obtained. The schematic flowchart of the standard precipitation method is shown in Fig. 21.25.

The disadvantage of this technology is the large amount of lime required for citric acid neutralisation and of sulphuric acid for calcium citrate decomposition. Moreover, it results in the formation of large amounts of liquid and solid wastes (solution after calcium citrate filtration and gypsum). For one ton of citric acid, 579 kg of calcium hydroxide, 765 kg of sulphuric acid and 18 m^3 of water are consumed and approximately one ton of waste gypsum is produced.

With the aim of decreasing the amount of lime and sulphuric acid by about one third, Ayers has proposed recovery of citric acid by precipitation of di-calcium acid citrate. An additional advantage of this method is that di-calcium acid citrate has a definite crystalline structure and washes cleaner than the amorphous tri-calcium citrate. Moreover, fewer impurities are precipitated from a fermentation fluid with the di-calcium salt than with the normal salt, when the reaction mixture is completely neutralised.

Di-calcium acid citrate precipitates from a citric acid solution that has been partially neutralised by the addition of calcium hydroxide, calcium oxide or calcium carbonate at an elevated temperature. It is believed that an equilibrium exists between tri-calcium citrate and citric acid on the one side, and di-calcium acid citrate on the other. At room temperature the rate of calcium hydrogen citrate formation is negligible, but if the temperature is elevated above 40°C the complete conversion of tri-calcium citrate mixed with aqueous solution of citric acid occurs within a reasonable length of time (about 24 hours). According to this principle a new method of citric acid recovery has been developed.

The citric acid solution, obtained from the fermentation broth, is divided in two parts. The first part, about two-thirds of the total volume, is completely neutralised with milk of lime, and the tricalcium citrate is filtered off and added to the remaining part of the original citric acid solution. If the obtained mixture is heated above 40°C, a precipitate of dicalcium acid citrate will result. As an alternative method, an amount of calcium hydroxide no greater than two-thirds of that required for complete neutralisation may be added directly to a citric acid solution.

This mixture of tricalcium citrate and citric acid may then be converted to dicalcium acid citrate by heating above 40°C, preferably to 80°–95°C (depending on the boiling point of the solution). It has been found that the results of the process may be improved, both by shortening the time and by increasing the yield, if the mixture is seeded with dicalcium acid citrate crystals (practically about 10 to 25 per cent of the expected yield).

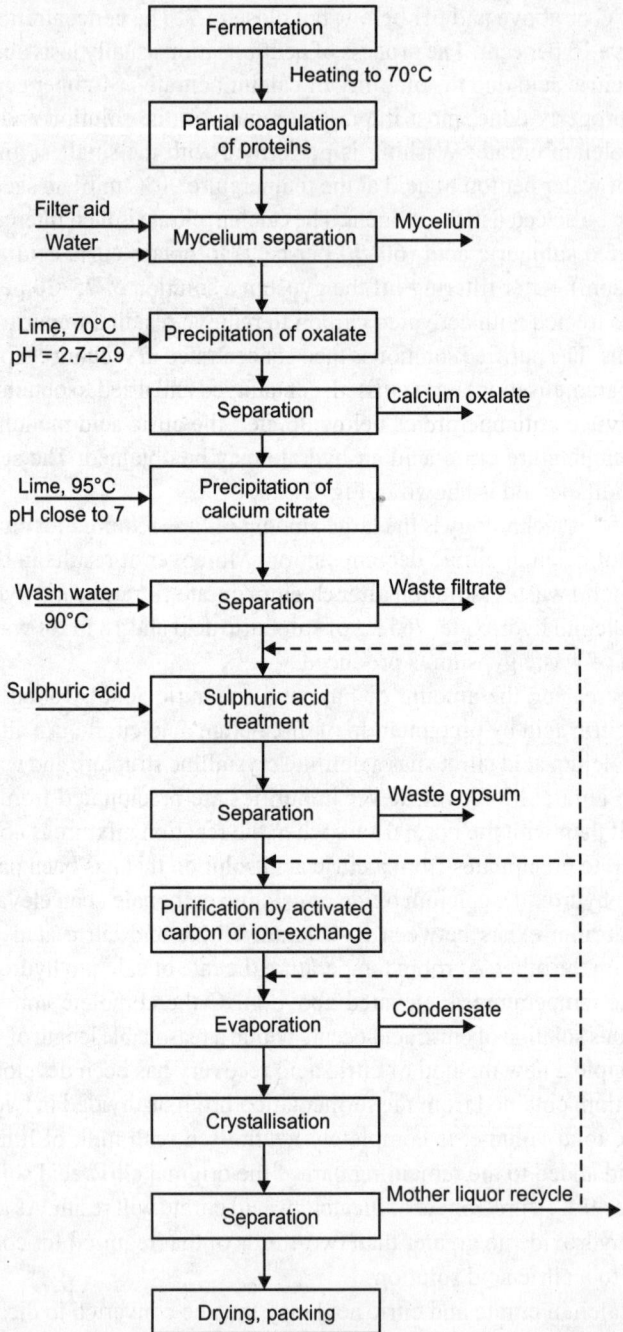

Fig. 21.25. Flowsheet of the standard precipitation method of citric acid recovery from fermentation broth.

As an alternative to the classical methods of precipitation, separation and purification of citric acid from fermentation solutions, Schultz has suggested isolating the citric acid from the fermentation solution in the form of its alkali metal salts and recovery of the acid from such salts directly in one single operation. This process is based on the fact that certain alkali metal salts of citric acid crystallise from a fermentation solution after neutralisation of the acid by the addition of alkaline alkali metal compounds (hydroxides, bicarbonates or carbonates) in such a manner that the mono-, di- or tri-alkali metal citrates are obtained.

The impurities contained in fermentation broth influence or even inhibit crystallisation of salts, so not all the theoretically possible alkali metal salts of citric acid can be produced in crystalline form according to the process. Of the sodium salts, however, all three possible salts can be recovered in the form of crystals.

Before neutralisation the fermentation solution may be concentrated by vacuum evaporation to a concentration of at least 40 per cent, calculated for free citric acid. After neutralising the alkali metal salts crystallise on standing or on slowly stirring the solution; seed crystals may be added to enhance the rate of the process. Crystallisation is ordinarily completed within 24 hours. Separation of the crystals from the solution is performed by the usual methods (filtration, centrifugation). After washing the crystals with a small amount of water, an almost white or slightly yellowish-brown precipitate is obtained, depending upon the type of alkali, metal citrate recovered. Subsequent purification of citric acid may be performed by ion exchange on cation exchange resins or by electrodialysis.

The yield of citric acid on recovering it in the form of its alkali metal salts is between 50 per cent and about 80 per cent depending on the salt used. Citric acid remaining in the fermentation broth may be recovered by the 'classical' method of precipitation in the form of a calcium citrate and following treatment with the sulphuric acid. According to this process considerable savings in chemicals are achieved and the amount of the spent gypsum produced is reduced. Moreover, the obtained gypsum filters more rapidly, due to the presence of alkali metal ions, than gypsum from the 'classical' technology, produced in the absence of the alkali metal ions. The use of purer raw materials than molasses (e.g. sucrose or glucose) in citric acid production leads to simplified methods for its recovery and purification. Crystalline or raw sugar are the best raw materials in view of the high acid yield and relatively short fermentation times attained. Crystalline sugar is also favoured by the reduced risk of infection with foreign micro-organisms due to the low initial pH value of the nutrient medium (2.5 to 3), and by the considerable reduction of the total amount of wastes and effluents.

Crystalline sugar based fermentation makes it possible to use a modified, citrate-free method of citric acid recovery, applied in industrial practice in several citric acid manufacturing plants in Poland and the Slovak Republic. This technology consists of direct removal of impurities from the post-fermentation liquor, i.e. colloids (proteins), mycelium derived substances, coloured substances formed on heating the fermentation solution, and mineral salts introduced with the nutrient medium, substrate and water. These impurities must be removed as they interfere with the subsequent crystallisation process. The first step of purification of the solution is achieved using suitably selected coagulating agents and activated carbon and then filtering off the precipitates. Further treatment involves the removal of the remaining impurities by ultrafiltration and retention of the mineral salts using ion-exchange resins. The purified citric acid solution is concentrated, crystallised, centrifuged and dried according to the classical production process flowsheet.

After the separation of citric acid crystals the supernatant liquid from the centrifuge is recycled back to the concentration section where the so-called second crop and then a third crop of crystals is obtained. The supernatant liquid obtained after removing the third crop crystals by centrifugation contains a large amount of impurities and must be purified by the classical method involving the precipitation of calcium citrate. Thus the citrate free method can be used for purifying only up to 80 per cent of the whole amount of citric acid. This necessitates the construction of a separate process line in order to avoid plants using the above technology to manufacture merely a 50 per cent solution of citric acid, making it necessary to purify a part of the citric acid by the calcium citrate method. It is also possible to produce half of the acid amount in crystalline form and the rest in liquid form. In this case, citric acid solution purified by the citrate free method is thickened, crystallised and centrifuged to obtain the first crop. The supernatant liquid from the centrifuge (citric acid concentration of about 50 per cent) is purified by the described method so as to meet the quality standard requirements in liquid form. The advantage of this technology lies in the fact that about half of the product is obtained in crystalline form and the use of lime and sulphuric acid is eliminated as well as the formation of large amounts of effluents and solid wastes. The flowsheet of the simplified, non-citrate method of citric acid recovery is shown in Fig. 21.26.

Solvent Extraction

An alternative method of citrate-free recovery of citric acid from a fermentation broth is extraction by means of a selective solvent which is insoluble or only sparingly soluble in the aqueous medium. The solvent should be chosen so as to extract the maximum amount of citric acid and the minimum amount of impurities. The citric acid can then be recovered from the extract either by distilling off the solvent or by washing the extract with the water. From the aqueous solution purified citric acid is subsequently crystallised by concentration.

In the first patent concerning citric acid solvent extraction it has been proposed to apply *n*-butanol and then to wash the solution of citric acid in *n*-butanol with water. Since the first report a number of solvent combinations have been suggested and a great amount of information and patents have been published. In general, extraction methods may be divided into three basic groups:

1. Extraction with organic solvents which are partly or wholly immiscible with water, such as certain aliphatic alcohols, ketones, ethers or esters.
2. Extraction with organophosphorus compounds, such as tri-*n*-butylphosphate (TBP) and alkylsulphoxides, e.g. trioctylphosphine oxide (TOPO).
3. Extraction with water-insoluble amines or a mixture of two or more of such amines, as a rule dissolved in a substantially water-immiscible organic solvent, and extraction with amine salts.

Each solvent used for extraction is characterised by its equilibrium distribution coefficient which is defined as the ratio of the acid concentration of the extract to the acid concentration of the aqueous phase. For low concentrations of citric acid in the raw fluid the distribution coefficient depends strongly on the type of solvent; at higher acid concentrations differences between solvents are much reduced.

Extraction with organic solvents (in practice ketones and alcohols are used) may be useful in cases where the acid has a relatively high concentration in the aqueous system from which it is to be extracted. These solvents have rather low distribution coefficients (0.02–0.36), thus the extract is always more diluted than the raw liquor and multistage extraction is necessary as a rule. Moreover, solvents with relatively higher distribution coefficients (such as butanols) are too water-miscible, so they require energy-consuming steps of subsequent solvent recovery. Thus, these extraction systems are relatively inefficient for acid recovery from the dilute aqueous solutions found in most fermentation streams.

Organophosphorus extractants have a significantly higher distribution ratio than carbonbonded solvents under comparable conditions, e.g. using undiluted TPB for citric acid extraction a distribution ratio of about 2 may be obtained at a 0.1 mol initial acid concentration at 25°C. Alkylosulphoxides have been shown to extract carboxylic acids with a distribution ratio even higher than that of TBP. The value of the distribution coefficient is influenced not only by acid concentration but also by temperature. In TBP the distribution ratio for citric acid decreases by a factor of 4 in the 0°–80°C range. This property allows perfect control of the process: extraction at low temperature (10°–30°C) and reextraction with water at higher temperature (70°–90°C).

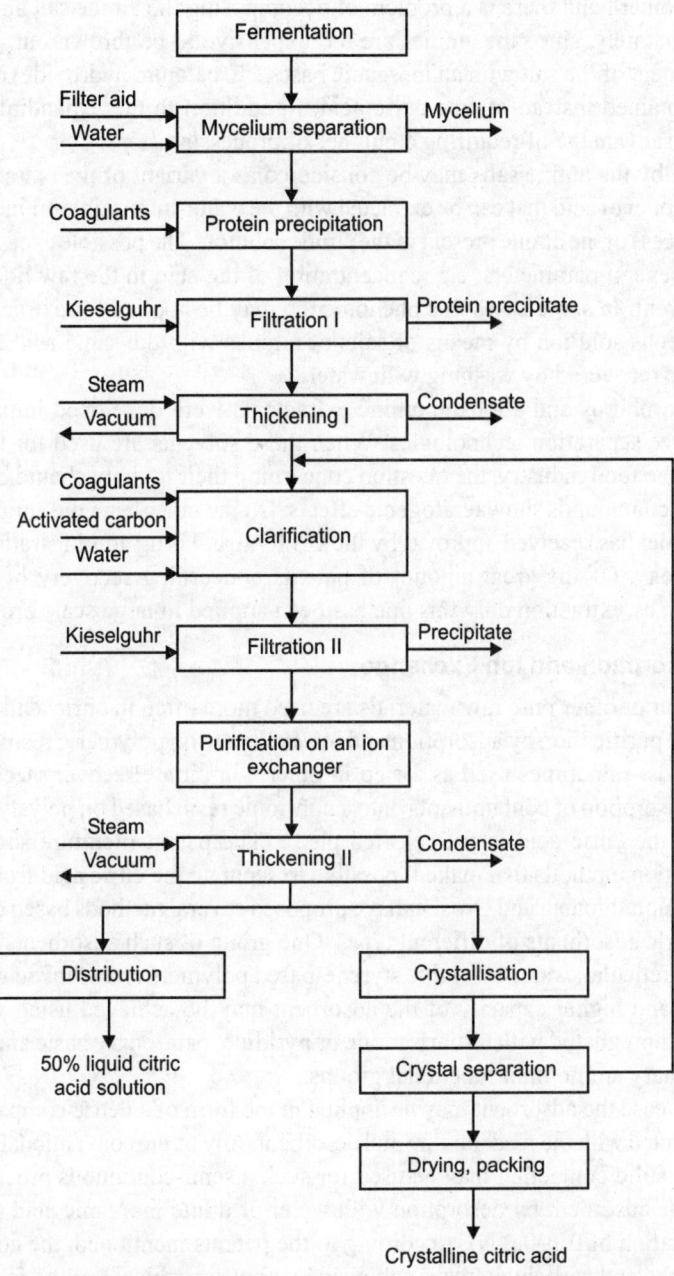

Fig. 21.26. Flowsheet of the simplified non-citrate method of citric acid separation and purification.

For the extraction by means of amines, aliphatic, araliphatic or aromatic amines, or their mixture, preferably with the average aggregate number of carbon atoms at least 20 for each amino group, may be used. These reagents have the advantage of providing a favourable coefficient of distribution of the citric acid between the aqueous and amine phases so the acid may be extracted even from highly dilute solutions. On the other hand there is a problem of decomposing the amine salt and recovering the acid and the amine separately, since the amines are too expensive to be thrown out. Usually the amine is liberated by treatment of the salt with an inorganic base (e.g. calcium hydroxide) or inorganic acid, and the salt is thus obtained instead of free citric acid. In addition to the expenditure of chemicals, this process has the disadvantage of requiring a number of processing steps.

The extraction by the amine salts may be considered as a variant of the extraction with amines. In some cases the amount of acid that can be extracted with the water-immiscible amine is stoichiometrically considerably in excess of the amine present in the amine solution. The possible excess amount of extracted acid depends on several parameters, e.g. concentration of the acid in the raw liquor, the nature of the amine and its solvent. In some cases this phenomenon may be applied for extracting the acid from its concentrated aqueous solution by means of salts of amines with the same acid. From the extract the excess acid can be recovered by washing with water.

The organophosphorus and aliphatic amine extractants were developed initially for the needs of inorganic extractive separation technologies. When these solvents are used for the recovery of citric acid intended for the food industry, the question concerning their toxicity should be settled. It is known that some of these compounds show teratogenic effects. On the other hand the amine extractant patented by Baniel and Baniel has received approval by the US food and drug administration for the use in food and drug technology. Of the great amount of patents concerning recovery of citric acid from the fermentation broth by extraction only this one has been applied in large scale production.

Adsorption, Absorption and Ion Exchange

As crystalline sugar or other pure raw materials are used more often in citric acid production, methods of its recovery and purification by adsorption and ion exchange on polymeric resins are gaining interest. One of the methods, sometimes used as a step in other non-citrate recovery technologies mentioned above, involves adsorption of contaminants onto a non-ionic resin based on polystyrene or polyacrylates and collection of the citric acid in the rejected phase. The patent literature suggests more efficient adsorption/absorption methods that make it possible to separate the citric acid from fermentation broth in a single step. Kulprathipanja and Oroskar have proposed several methods based on a similar principle, involving polymeric adsorbents of different types. One group of such adsorbents may be neutral, non-ionogenic, macro-reticular, water-insoluble styrene-based polymers cross-linked with di-vinylbenzene. Better selectivity and higher capacity of the adsorbent may be achieved using weakly basic anionic exchange resins, impregnated with tertiary amine or pyridine, or strongly basic anionic exchange resins containing quaternary ammonium functional groups.

In the simplest case the adsorbent may be applied in the form of a dense compact fixed bed which is alternatively contacted with the feed mixture and desorbent. Any of the conventional equipment employed in static bed fluid-solid contacting may be used for such a semi-continuous process. The citric acid is recovered from the adsorbent by desorption with water or dilute inorganic acid (preferably sulphuric acid of a concentration of 0.1–0.2 N). According to the patents mentioned, the complete separation of citric acid from salts and carbohydrates is achieved by adjusting the pH of the feed solution below the first ionisation constant of citric acid. The pH value required to maintain adequate selectivity is inversely proportional to the concentration of citric acid in the feed mixture. Polymeric resins proposed for use in citric acid recovery are manufactured by several chemical companies and sold under different trade names, so they are commercially available. They may differ slightly in physical properties such as porosity, skeletal density, specific surface area and dipole moment. The preferred adsorbents should have a surface area of 100–1000 m^2/g. The various types of polymeric adsorbents were originally designed for different chemical technologies, e.g. for decolourising dye wastes, decolourising pulp mill bleaching effluent or removing pesticides from waste effluent. Their effectiveness in the separation of citric acid from *A. niger* fermentation broth is rather unexpected.

The efficiency of the ion-exchange separation process may be greatly enhanced by applying a so-called simulated moving bed counter-current flow system. In this case the apparatus consists of at least two static beds, connected with appropriate valving so that the feed mixture is passed through one adsorbent bed while the desorbent material can be passed through the other. Progressive changes in the function of each ion-exchange bed simulate the counter-current movement of the adsorbent in relation to liquid flow. In such a system, the adsorption and desorption operations are continuously taking place, which allows both continuous production of an extract and a raffinate stream and the continual use of feed and desorbent streams. The simulated moving bed system applied for citric acid recovery in a pilot scale is proposed by Edlauer.

The disadvantage of the ion-exchange method may be seen in the fact that elution of citric acid from the adsorption bed may require a large amount of desorbent, due to the tailing effect known in chromatography, causing considerable dilution of the resulting citric acid solution. The periodical regeneration of the ion-exchange resins by inorganic bases may also be a source of unwanted effluent wastes.

Liquid Membranes

Recently more sophisticated methods of citric acid separation with the application of liquid membranes are being developed. Liquid membranes containing mobile carriers consist of an inert, micro-porous support impregnated with a water-immiscible, mobile ion-exchange agent. The mobile carrier, which is held in the pores of the support membrane by capillarity, acts as a shuttle, picking up ions from an aqueous solution on one side of the membrane, carrying them across the membrane and releasing them to the solution on the opposite side of the membrane. The flow of the complexed ion is coupled to the flow of the second ion (e.g. the hydrogen ion). This process is categorised as 'coupled transport', and the membranes in which it takes place are called coupled transport membranes. The coupling of the flows of the two ions permits one of the ions to be pumped 'up-hill' from a solution in which it is dilute to a solution in which it is more concentrated.

For citric acid separation by liquid membranes, the tertiary amines which give the best results in solvent extraction can also be used. In the extraction step, the basic amine reacts with hydrogen ions in the feed solution to form a tertiary alkylammonium cation. This cation then associates as an ion pair with the citrate anion to form an alkylammonium salt, which is transported across the membrane and stripped from the organic carrier solution into the aqueous product phase. This reaction regenerates the tertiary amine, which then diffuses back to the feed side of the membrane, where it recomplexes with hydrogen and citrate ions.

Supported liquid membranes have not been adopted for industrial scale, primarily due to a lack of long-term stability resulting from loss of membrane by solubility, osmotic flow of water across the membrane, progressive wetting of the support pores, and pressure differential across the membrane. To eliminate these problems microporous hollow fibres have been employed by Basu and Sirkar. In this case the permeator consists of two sets of identical hydrophobic microporous hollow fibres.

One set carries the feed solution of citric acid and the other the strip solution flowing in the lumen. The organic liquid membrane is contained in the shell side between these two sets of hollow fibres. This technique has been shown to be promising for citric acid separation even in the large scale, as the extent of citric acid recovery of up to 99 per cent was linear with the membrane area, suggesting easy scale-up. The use of liquid membranes for the recovery of citric acid from fermentation broths offers unique advantages over conventional techniques: lower energy consumption, higher separation factors in a single stage, the ability to concentrate citric acid during separation and smaller size of the complete separation apparatus. These advantages may result in a reduction in overall recovery costs and in amount of wastes.

Electrodialysis

Another environmentally friendly alternative to the conventional methods of citric acid recovery may be electrodialysis. This process enables separation of salts from a solution and their simultaneous conversion into the corresponding acids and bases using electrical potential and mono or bipolar membranes. Bipolar membranes are special ion-exchange membranes which, in an electrical field, enable the splitting of water into H^+ and OH^- ions. By integrating bipolar membranes with anionic and cationic exchange membranes a three- or-four compartment cell may be arranged, in which electrodialytic separation of salt ions and their conversion into base and acid takes place. According to Karklins, complete transformation of sodium tri-citrate into citric acid in a four-compartment cell may be achieved a little faster, but voltage on electrodes is higher than in a three-chamber cell. Specific electroenergy consumption of the four-compartment cell was about 40 per cent higher than that of a three-chamber apparatus.

When converting organic salts, high final acid concentrations may be achieved, as opposed to mineral salts. It makes the process especially advantageous for citric acid recovery, as the evaporation step normally required can be omitted. On the other hand organic salts such as sodium citrate have a relatively large molecular weight and the solution also shows relatively low conductivity. These properties make the separation more difficult and lead to higher energy consumption, as in the case of inorganic compounds. The energy consumption (excluding pumping) for the separation of 1 kg of citric acid using bipolar membranes is in the range of 6.1×10^3 to 7.2×10^3 kWs. Due to low mass transfer at low pH values it is advantageous to adjust the pH of the feed acid stream to 7.5.

Before the fermentation solution comes to the electrodialysis some pretreatment steps are normally necessary: filtration of the broth, removal of ionogenic substances (especially Ca^{++} and Mg^{++} ions) and neutralisation by means of sodium hydroxide. In the subsequent electrodialytic step the sodium citrate solution is converted into base and citric acid, which is simultaneously concentrated and for the most part purified. The produced NaOH may be reused for the neutralisation.

Although there have been several patents published concerning recovery and purification of organic acids by electrodialysis, this method is still applied only in laboratory scale and requires optimisation. The economics are mainly influenced by the relatively high energy consumption, the membrane costs and the membrane lifetime. However, due to the wider commercial availability of bipolar membranes in the past few years and various advantages of the electrodialysis technique it is expected that this technology will soon be competitive with other processes. Besides the elimination of environmental problems, the use of electrodialysis enables continuous separation of the citric acid from the broth during fermentation, leading to the decrease of an inhibiting influence of the product. It is also possible to apply this technique for recovery of the citric acid in continuous fermentation processes. The scheme of the proposed method for citric acid separation by means of electrodialysis with bipolar membranes is shown in Fig. 21.27.

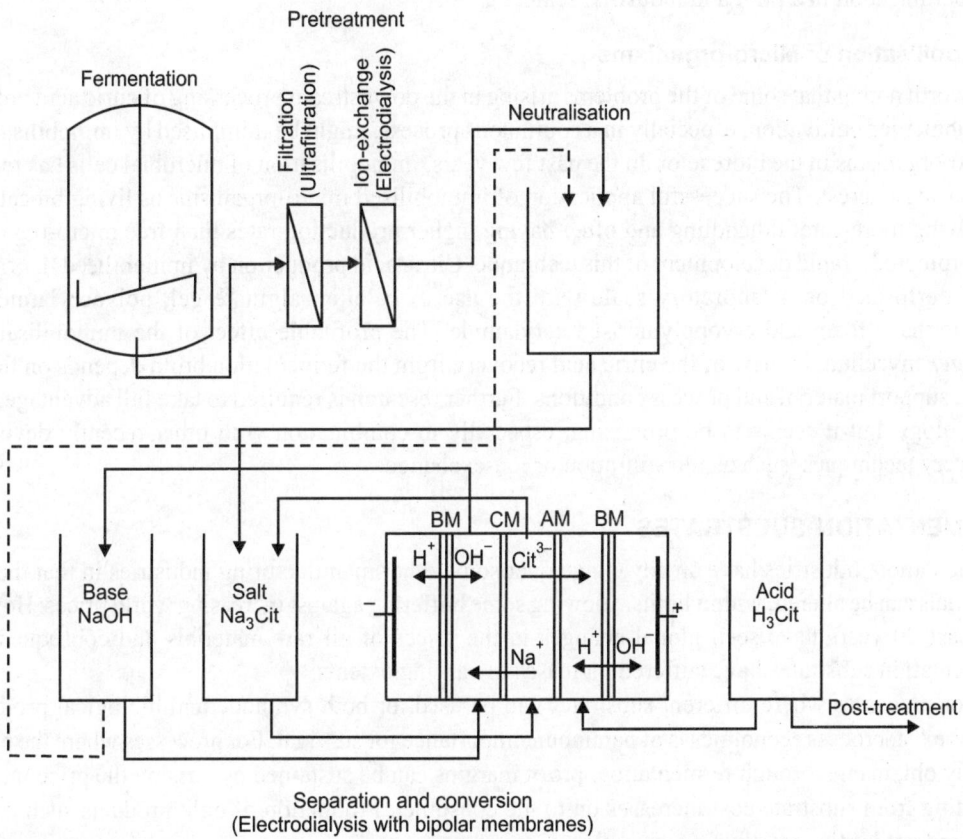

Fig. 21.27. Scheme of citric acid separation by means of electrodialysis with bipolar membranes.

Ultrafiltration

Continuous separation and concentration of citric acid may be also achieved by ultra and/or nanofiltration. Visacky verified in a laboratory scale a two-stage membrane process for citric acid recovery from the broth obtained in *A. niger* cultivation on sucrose. Polysulphone membrane with cut-off 10,000 used in the first stage allowed the product to pass through to the permeate stream, while the retentate stream contained most of peptides and proteins from the broth. The rejection coefficient for the product in this step was 3 per cent, for the reducing sugars 14 per cent and for the proteins 100 per cent. Tighter nanofiltration membrane with cut-off 200 in the second stage rejected approximately 90 per cent of citric acid and 60 per cent of reducing sugars (mono-saccharides). Concentration of the product in the retentate stream was increased three times in comparison to the feed. A similar two-stage membrane technique was adapted by Bohdziewicz and Bodzek for simultaneous separation and concentration of pectinolytic enzymes and citric acid from a fermentation broth. The dilute citric acid solution obtained as a permeate in the first step of the post-fermentation fluid ultrafiltration was then concentrated up to 20 per cent using reverse osmosis. Such membrane processes may give important benefits in industrial technologies of citric acid recovery: low energy consumption, no wastes in comparison to the conventional chemical methods, possibility of use in continuous processes. However, they require practical verification and optimisation in a pilot and industrial scale.

Immobilisation of Micro-organisms

It is worth noting that some of the problems arising in the downstream processing of citric acid produced by submerged cultivation, especially in a continuous process, might be minimised by immobilisation of micro-organisms in the bioreactor. In the past few years, immobilisation of microbial cells has received increasing interest. The successful application of immobilised micro-organisms as living biocatalysts, involving more careful handling and often having higher production rates than free micro-organisms, has prompted a rapid development of this technique. Citric acid production by immobilised *A. niger* has been performed on a laboratory scale with the use of calcium alginate gel, polyacrylamide gel, polyurethane foam and cryopolymerised acrylamide. The profitable effect of the immobilisation of *A. niger* mycelium in view of the citric acid recovery from the fermentation broth depends on the type of the support material and process conditions. Further research is required to take full advantage of this technology, but it seems to be promising, especially in combination with other recently developing recovery techniques, such as ultrafiltration or ion-exchange.

FERMENTATION SUBSTRATES

Fermentation industries have an advantage over some other manufacturing industries in that their raw materials can be altered, within limits, allowing some buffering against increasing world prices. However, the past 20 years have seen global changes in the prices of all raw materials and consequently all fermentation substrates have suffered increases to varying extents.

For processes where different substrates can be used, or both synthetic and biological production routes exist, process economics is of paramount importance for survival. For processes where the product is only obtainable through fermentation, profit margins can be sustained by passing the price increases resulting from substrate cost increases on to the consumer. Production of bulk products such as citric acid and antibiotics are obvious examples.

These products therefore may have had less pressure on them than the others to search for the cheapest possible substrate, but even here there is competition between rival companies and ways to lower costs and increase profits are thus continually being sought. The choice of substrate is therefore always under review.

There is always pressure to find a cheaper or better substrate, but the new substrate may present storage problems, may be difficult to sterilise or have an unwanted variability in composition. Increased productivity is not the only yardstick to be used. The substrate may have a residue which poses product recovery and purification problems. The cheapest substrate is therefore not often the best. In addition to these problems, any change in substrate or amendment to the formulation of the medium will influence the characteristic of the fermentation process, and has to be carefully evaluated.

A substrate must be readily available throughout most of the year. Seasonably produced crops from which process wastes are used as fermentation feedstock are not suitable if the harvest period is short and the material to be used is subject to contamination and spoilage.

    Thus the industry must have substrates that are relatively stable and can be stored reasonably easily for more than half a year.

    A process, for example, citric acid production, can be changed to accommodate a new substrate. The advent of cheap hydrocarbons in the 1960s led to many companies switching over to this substrate. *Aspergillus niger*, the traditional producer, cannot grow on alkanes, but a variety of yeast can and some will accumulate citric acid sufficiently enough for industrial processes to be established.

    The price of the substrate is crucial. However, it is important to take into consideration the amount of available carbon. This differs according to the type of substrate being used (Table 21.14). This suggests that if the choice of substrate is not limited, a carbohydrate could be replaced by alkanes with no loss in process productivity (an important optimisation parameter for the citric acid process). However, others factors have to be taken into consideration before this is accepted—increased aeration or agitation rates may be necessary with alkanes (being a more reduced substrate) and this factor must be met by the savings from the change of substrate.

Table 21.14. Relative carbon contents of fermentation substrates.

Substrate	Carbon content (g/mol carbon/mol substrate)	Carbon content relative to glucose (%)
Carbohydrates (glucose, sucrose, starch, etc.)	0.40	100
Acetic acid	0.40	100
Methanol	0.50	125
Ethanol	0.70	175
Methane	0.75	188
Triolein	0.80	200
n-Hexadecane	0.87	218

    Transport costs for substrates from the collection or production point to the fermentation plant have to be considered. These costs may become significant if too much water is present and will mitigate against the use of some waste materials at sites removed from their point of production. One substrate may be more attractive to use than another simply because it poses fewer problems in the processes both before and after the fermentation.

    Fermentation media for citric acid biosynthesis should consist of substrates necessary for growth of the producer micro-organism and its citric acid biosynthesis, primarily the carbon, nitrogen, phosphorus and microelements sources. Moreover, process water and air can be included as fermentation substrates.

    The basic substrate for citric acid fermentation in plants using the surface method of fermentation is beet or cane molasses. Plants using submerged fermentation can use not only beet or cane molasses, but a substrate of higher purity such as hydrolysed starch, technical and pure glucose, refined or raw sugar, purified and condensed beet or cane juice. This is because use of a pure substrate may result in increases in yield, or reduction in fermentation time.

Molasses

Molasses is a widely used substrate, coming in a variety of qualities. High quality molasses is usually demanded for citric acid production while poorer quality molasses is used mainly in the production of low value products such as alcohol, where the producer micro-organism has a much greater tolerance to impurities in the medium. Cane and beet molasses are not identical in composition; often one type will be preferred to the other. They are sometimes mixed to take advantage of the additional nutrients arising from the differences in composition. Besides substrate type (sugar beet, sugar cane), the chemical composition of molasses depends on many factors such as soil and climate conditions, fertilisation type, crop method, time and conditions of storage, production technology, technical equipment of plant, etc.

Beet molasses

Beet molasses consists of about 65–80 per cent dry substance and 20–25 per cent water. The main ingredient of molasses is sucrose, 44–54 per cent by weight. Other sugars (carbohydrates) which can be found in higher amounts are inverted sugar 0.4–1.5 per cent, raffinose 0.5–2.0 per cent and kestose and neokestose 0.6–1.6 per cent. Raffinose is a natural part of sugar beet, while kestose is the result of microbial action during sugar beet treatment. Other sugars in molasses are arabinose, xylose and mannose in amounts of 0.5–1.5 per cent. All sugars (except sucrose) are included in the non-nitrogen organic substances of molasses. Products of chemical and thermal sugar decomposition (melanoidines, caramel) and organic acids also belong to this group. Caramel consists of sugar anhydride and colouring matters; melanoidines are made in hot solution as the result of a reaction between reducing sugars and amino acids. In addition to the non-volatile dark coloured compounds, there are about 40 volatile compounds as aliphatic aldehyde, methylglyoxal, diacetyl, acetoin, acetone, oxymethylfurfurol and others.

The nonvolatile organic acids present in molasses are glutaric, malonic, succinic, aconitic, malic and lactic acid; the remainder are oxalic, citric and tartaric acid. These can all react with calcium to form insoluble salts that can influence the precipitation and recovery of the citric acid crystals. Molasses contain such volatile acids as formic, acetic, propionic, butyric and valeric acid. Almost all organic acids, volatile and nonvolatile, are potassium or calcium salts.

The colour of molasses ranges between 1.2 and 4.6 cm^3 of 0.1 N iodine solution (to which should be added 94 cm^3 of water to get the colour identical to that of 2 per cent molasses solution). Molasses containing higher amounts (over 1 per cent) of volatile acids are normally too dark to be used as feedstock for the citric acid fermentation, though the exact relationship between content of these substances and fermentation yield has not been established.

Other ingredients of molasses that have a negative influence on colour and thus fermentation yield are colloidal substances. Beet molasses contains about 4–6 per cent of colloids, whose chemical constitution has only recently been documented. Mostly, they are high molecular coloured complexes.

Some of these colloids (of negative potential) can be removed from solution by acid coagulation (pH 3.2, molasses dilution 20–30 per cent, temperature 80°C) and colloids of positive potential by alkaline coagulation (pH over 8.0). Nitrogen compounds contained in molasses are mostly betaine (about 60–70 per cent of total nitrogen), amino acids (20–30 per cent of nitrogen), protein (3–4 per cent of nitrogen) and traces of nitrogen in ammonium nitrate and amide. Betaine comes from beet and is not used by micro-organisms as a nitrogen source. It is not known to influence the fermentation. The amino acids content in molasses depends on the soil and climate conditions and beet cultivation. Amino acid content of beer-molasses is shown in Table 21.15.

Table 21.15. Amino acid content of beet molasses.

Amino acid	Content (% of molasses)
Leucine + isoleucine	1.7–2.9
Phenylalanine	Trace

(Contd ...)

Amino acid	Content (% of molasses)
Valine + methionine + tryptophan	0.4–1.3
Tyrosine	0.6-0.8
Proline	Trace
Alanine	1.2–2.3
Threonine + glycine	0.2–0.8
Glutamic acid	1.3–1.8
Serine	1.7–2.5
Aspartic acid	0.3–0.5
Arginine + histidine + lysine	Trace
Cysteine	Trace

The content of mineral substances in beet molasses amounts to 8.5–14.0 per cent. The main ingredient of the mineral ash is K_2O (60–70 per cent of the total), CaO (4.5–7.0 per cent) and MgO (about 1 per cent). The level of P_2O_5 in ash is normally very low (0.2–0.6 per cent), because over 90 per cent of phosphorus contained in beet is removed in the sugar extraction process. If the method of juice alkalisation by Na_3PO_4 (pH 8.3–8.5) is used in the sugar production, the contents of P_2O_5 in molasses ash can reach 1.2–2.0 per cent. There are also many other elements, so-called microelements, which have a great effect on the citric acid fermentation process. The amount of particular microelements in different molasses can range widely as indicated in Table 21.16.

Table 21.16. Content of microelements in beet molasses.

Microelement	Content (mg/100 g of molasses)
Aluminium	9.3–60.0
Strontium	4.6–59.4
Chromium	6.6–54.7
Iron	8.3–26.6
Copper	0.0–9.8
Magnesium	5.7–8.6
Manganese	1.4–7.6
Zinc	2.0–3.3
Titanium	0.21–0.70
Nickel	0.16–0.76
Cobalt	0.10–0.76
Molybdenum	0.10–0.12
Lead	0.21–0.61
Boron	0.20–0.42

Another important ingredient of molasses is vitamins, especially those that are known to stimulate microbial activity.

The content of vitamins (mg/100 g) in beet and cane molasses is shown in Tables 21.17 and 21.18 respectively.

Table 21.17. Content of vitamins in beet molasses.

Vitamin	Content (mg/100 g)
Inositol	90.0–120.0
Nicotinic acid	3.90–5.20
Pantothenic acid	0.06–0.25
Folic acid	0.01–0.03
Biotin	0.0035–0.0060
Thiamine	0.18–0.26
Riboflavine	0.02–0.08
Pyridoxine	0.30–0.45

Table 21.18. Content of vitamins in cane molasses.

Vitamin	Content (mg/100 g)
Thiamine	0.16
Riboflavine	0.30
Pyridoxine	1.15
Nicotinic acid	2.10
Pantothenic acid	3.60
Folic acid	0.06
Biotin	0.13
Inositol	158.0

The pH of molasses depends on the sugar extraction technology. It was considered that a neutral, or slightly alkaline molasses gave the best citric acid yields. However, a fermentation technology to tolerate the slightly acidic molasses produced in modern refineries has been developed. Today, it is considered that for citric acid fermentation the buffering capacity of the medium is more important than the pH value of the molasses. It is defined as the amount of 1N solution of sulphuric acid (in cm^3) used to reduce pH from 5.0 to 3.0 in 100 g molasses solution diluted in 1:1 ratio with water and acidified to pH 5.0. The buffer capacity of beet molasses usually ranges from 60 to 95 cm^3. Citric acid production needs molasses with low buffer ability, to make possible the required rapid fall of medium pH during fermentation.

Cane molasses

Cane molasses differs from beet molasses in its chemical composition. It contains less sucrose and more inverted sugar, has lower content of nitrogen and raffinose, more intensive colour and lower buffer capacity. Cane molasses of raw sugar conversion also differs from beet molasses and even from blackstrap cane molasses. The composition of cane molasses is shown in Table 21.19. Beet and cane molasses can also contain other substances which appear in small amounts, but are often crucial in deciding whether the molasses are suitable for use in citric acid biosynthesis. These are pesticides, fungicides and herbicides used in beet and cane cultivation and also substances used for defoaming in sugar production process. All have mostly toxic properties and negatively affect molasses usability.

Table 21.19. Composition of cane molasses.

Ingredient	Content (%)
Dry substances	80.0
Saccharose	42.0
Inverted sugar	20.0
Organic non-sugars	10.0
Ash	8.0
Total nitrogen	0.5–1.6
Amine nitrogen	0.2–0.5
Colloids	2.0–8.0
Volatile acids	0.6–0.9

It is considered that the best molasses for citric acid fermentation can be, as a rule of thumb, characterised as given in Table 21.20. According to all cited requirements, beet molasses is more suitable for citric acid fermentation than cane molasses. It is especially relevant in submerged fermentation where the quality of the substrate is more important for productivity and fermentation yield.

Table 21.20. Alternative analysis of cane molasses sample.

Ingredient	Content (%)
Dry substance	80
Sucrose	44
Invert sugar	1
Raffinose	2
Total nitrogen	0.2
Mineral salts	10
K_2O	3
CaO	2
MgO	1
SO_2	0.01
pH value	6.5

The microflora of molasses can be an agent of negative influence on yield and productivity of fermentation. Molasses will always contain a certain number and type of micro-organisms, sometimes the count can be higher than 10,000 per g of molasses. The most common micro-organism in molasses is sporulating rods of *Bacillus* species (over 90 per cent of total molasses microflora), bacteria producing acids and gases (*E. coli*, *Pseudomonas* and others), heterofermentative lactic acid bacteria (*Leuconostoc mesenteroides*), sometimes yeasts of *Candida* species, and very rarely, moulds of *Penicillium*, *Aspergillus* and other species. Bacteria of *Bacillus* species appear in molasses because their spores are present in beet and are unaffected by high temperatures, even 125°C (*Bacillus subtilis*). They are destructive because some of them (*B. megaterium*, *B. mesentericus*) are able to reduce nitrates to nitrites. Strains of *Aspergillus niger* can be very sensitive to nitrites (a NO_2 concentration in medium of 0.05 per cent will retard growth and cut the citric acid production by 50 per cent).

The greatest antagonists of *Aspergillus niger* among non-sporulating bacteria are *E. coli* and *Pseudomonas*. They grow very quickly in many media over a wide temperature range, decomposing sugar in solution to unwanted acids, alcohol and gases, and are able to reduce nitrates to nitrites. Bacteria of *Leuconostoc* species convert sucrose to dextran. They also produce unwanted volatile acids such as formic, acetic and propionic acid. Yeasts of *Candida* species can propagate over a wide range of temperature (5°–55°C) and pH value of medium (2–8). They can be very undesirable to *Aspergillus niger* strains, especially in submerged fermentation, where they can stop citric acid biosynthesis.

Treatment of molasses for citric acid production

Due to the varying chemical composition of molasses it is always required to evaluate any new delivery in a scaled down version of the citric acid production vessels. Even very good molasses is no guarantee for high yields of citric acid biosynthesis without special pretreatment. The basic operation in molasses preparation is a treatment for heavy metal ions removal. Potassium ferrocyanide or other complex compounds are commonly used.

Potassium ferrocyanide reacts with many heavy metals, mostly causing their precipitation. It was noted that for 21 microelements found in molasses, potassium ferrocyanide reacts with 18 of them. Potassium ferrocyanide removes not only metals of negative influence but also some of the microelements necessary for mycelium growth. Therefore its addition to molasses has to be strictly regulated. The optimum amount of ferrocyanide depends on molasses type and ranges from 200 to 1000 mg/dm^3 of medium (about 300 g of molasses); of the metals 80-85 per cent of the total is complexed as precipitate, 7–14 per cent is complexed in solution and 7–10 per cent is in elemental free state. At the optimum dose level of ferrocyanide, the part in elemental state is usually constant and ranges between 50 and 100 mg/dm^3, depending on strain and fermentation type. This has been used to develop a quick method of optimal ferrocyanide dosage in molasses media. Ferrocyanide is normally added before sterilisation. However, it can also be partially added before and after sterilisation or the total amount can be added after sterilisation.

Another compound complexing with heavy metals is the sodium salt of ethylene diamineacetic acid (EDTA). This compound reacts with metals of I and II valency at pH 7.0, with metals of III valency at pH 3–5 and with multivalency metals at pH 1. Ca and Mg ions give Trilon B soluble salts and they are not removed from solution. Other heavy metal complexing compounds can also be used, e.g. sodium polyphosphates, potassium rhodanate, 2,4-dinitrophenols and 8-oxyquinoline. Molasses media are sometimes purified by ionites, especially on cation exchanger. Not all microelements should be removed during this process, as some of them are necessary for growth of the *Aspergillus niger* mycelium.

To protect the fermentation process from unwanted micro-organisms, the molasses must be sterilised. The most economical method is steam sterilisation. For sporulating bacteria a temperature of 130°C or above for 30 minutes is recommended. However, steam sterilisation of the medium may not be sufficient to ensure total sterility because some micro-organisms can enter the fermentation broth via addition ports or from the air. Because of this, other sterilising agents such as formaline (at 0.006–0.01 per cent) (in particular for the surface fermentation) and furan derivatives are used.

Sulphamide preparations do not totally destroy the bacteria, but antibiotics, though they do not have any negative influences, are too expensive. Applying chemical sterilising agents enables softening of sharp thermal sterilisation conditions that have a negative effect on molasses quality. Other methods of sterilisation tested are UV and gamma radiation, ultrasound and ultrafiltration. They are not used in practice as they are cost-prohibitive compared with steam sterilisation.

In tropical countries where date production is considerable, date syrup is a major product. The chemical composition of this material differs from that of sugar beet molasses, but when mixed with an equal volume of beet molasses it gives the same yield of citric acid as for beet molasses based on the amount of sugar converted. Molasses from the starch industry (hydrol molasses) is also widely used in citric acid fermentation.

Refined or Raw Sucrose

Refined sugar of beet or cane is almost pure sucrose which *Aspergillus niger* strains ferment very well. This sugar is a very good substrate for the submerged fermentation because in surface fermentation, the rate of diffusion of acid in sugar solutions is too low. Preparation of a refined sugar solution as a fermentation medium is based on its diluting with water to a concentration of 15–22 per cent, adding necessary nutrients (NH_4NO_3, KH_2PO_4, $MgSO_4$) and acidifying with hydrochloric or sulphuric acid to pH 2.6–3.0. Normally the batch medium is sterilised in the fermentation vessel. In this case, all the ingredients of the fermentation medium are added straight into the bioreactor or are prepared separately by diluting in hot water (85°–95°C) and then pumped into the bioreactor. In this case, sugar is diluted to 50–60 per cent concentration and pumped into the fermenter that has had an exact amount of sterile water added, resulting in a total sugar concentration of 15–22 per cent.

Sterilisation in the fermenter lasts about 0.5–1 hour at 110°–120°C. The solution is then cooled to 32°–35°C with continuous stirring and aeration before the inoculum of *Aspergillus niger* spores or mycelium is added. The use of continuous sterilisers, where the sugar solution is sterilised separately from the other ingredients, is becoming more common.

Syrups

Syrups of beet or cane sugar can also be used as basic substrate for the submerged citric acid fermentation. The great advantage with this substrate is its purity; however, the quality of the syrups deteriorates rapidly during storage. Because of this they can only be used during the sugar campaign season and only if the citric acid plant is not too far from the sugar factory because of the large transport costs.

Preparation of the syrups for fermentation entails dilution with water to a sugar concentration of 15–20 per cent, addition of necessary nutrients (NH_4NO_3, KH_2PO_4, $MgSO_4$, $(NH_4)_2C_2O_4$), acidification with hydrochloric or sulphuric acid to pH 4–5 and sterilisation at 121°C for 0.5–1 hour.

Starch

Starch can be an attractive feed stock for many fermentation processes. It can be used directly by many micro-organisms and is frequently incorporated into fermentation media as a partial ingredient. Starch is widely used as the principal substrate for the production of amylases and amyloses in the food and brewing industries. The production of citric acid from sources of starch such as corn, wheat, tapioca and potato is widely used.

The suitability of these substrates for citric acid fermentation depends on their purity and method of hydrolysis. Acid hydrolysis, enzymatic hydrolysis, or a combination of the two, are used. Preparation of starch substrates for fermentation is based on their enzymatic liquefaction and saccharification to a defined hydrolysis level. Additional nutrients are added, depending on which starch is used. The pH is adjusted to 3–4 using hydrochloric or sulphuric acid and the medium is sterilised at 121°C for 0.5–1 hour.

Good citric acid yields have been obtained using pure starch (potatoes, wheat or maize), hydrolysed only to 10–15 DE with α-amylase. This was possible, as the applied *Aspergillus niger* strain had the ability to produce its own amylolytic enzymes which helped in the saccharification of the starch to available sugars. Dextrose syrup, obtained by enzymatic hydrolysis of starch, is now employed as a basic substrate for citric acid biosynthesis in laboratory and industrial scale. In this case it is especially important to restrict the amount of heavy metals below critical levels; heavy metals should therefore be removed by ion-exchange.

When using an *Aspergillus niger* strain resistant to higher concentrations of heavy metals, practically the same yield may be obtained on decationised and non-decationised dextrose syrup.

Hydrol

This is a paramolasses obtained as a by-product during crystalline glucose production from starch. Because of the high glucose content (40–45 per cent) and high purity coefficient it is a very good substrate for citric acid production. Preparation of hydrol for fermentation involves dilution to a sugar concentration of 15–18 per cent, addition of necessary nutrients and adjustment of pH with hydrochloric or sulphuric acid to 3.0-4.0. The solution is sterilised at 121°C for 0.5 hour and cooled to 32°–35°C.

Alkanes

The low price of alkanes, coupled with the ability of many organisms to utilise them, produced major changes in the fermentation industry during the 1960s and 1970s. Citric acid production, using *Candida lipolytica*, is a typical example and has been the subject of many patents. However, there are few industrial citric acid processes that are based on alkanes. There are two main reasons for this. Firstly, in these processes isocitric acid would also be produced at concentrations that would cause product recovery problems, as well as reduced citric acid yields. Secondly, a fourfold increase in price since 1973 no longer makes alkanes a cheap substrate.

Oils and Fats

Oils and fats are also being increasingly used as substrates in many fermentations. The oils should be liquid at the temperature of fermentation; the concentration of the oils may be up to 10 per cent but there is no reason to believe that concentrations up to 30 per cent may not be used. The prices of oils and fats vary according to their fatty acid composition, and often are very cheap. The price of the cheapest oils is such that, because of their high carbon content, they are not much more expensive than raw sugar. For citric acid production, oils are now being used as principal carbon source in a manner analogous to the previous use of alkanes. With palm oil as carbon source, a yield of citric acid of 145 per cent using a mutant of *Candida lipolytica* has been reported.

There are examples of oil being added in small concentrations to *Aspergillus niger* fermentation and even being used as a sole carbon source for *Aspergillus niger* fermentation. It was found that citric acid could be produced on these substrates with good yield. In particular with an initial 8 per cent concentration of vegetable oil, a yield of 104 per cent was obtained.

These oils and fats may replace alkanes in several fermentations, but it is unlikely that they will remain at their current low prices.

Cellulose

Cellulose is the major renewable form of carbohydrate in the world: about 10^{11} tons are synthesised annually and much of this is waste. To use it as fermentation feedstock, it must be first hydrolysed to starch and then to sugar, either chemically or by cellulases. The technology and economics of these processes are constantly being improved, but it is still not apparent when the production of sugar syrups by this route is going to become profitable. In the long-term, cellulose could become a major resource of the fermentation industry in general, including citric acid fermentation.

Other Medium Ingredients

Other nutrients

Other substances are used as sources of nitrogen, phosphorus and micro and macroelements. Organic compounds (ammonia, amino acids) or non-organic compounds (ammonia salt, nitrates) can be used as nitrogen source. The most commonly use phosphorus source is phosphoric acid or its salts. Whenever high purity carbon substrates (refined sugar and starch) are used, ammonium nitrate or ammonium sulphate will be used as nitrogen source and monopotassium phosphate as phosphorus source.

When using molasses, additional nitrogen is rarely required, as it will contain sufficient amounts of organic and inorganic nitrogen compounds to support the metabolic growth process. If the nitrogen level becomes too high, some of the sugar is converted into production of excess biomass and not citric acid. The most important microelements are magnesium, sulphur, zinc, iron, copper and manganese. They are very seldom added to the medium. In complex media the level of trace metals will normally be too high, and the main concern is simply to remove them. This is very different from academic research into citric acid fermentation. Here, a refined sugar is invariably used as the carbon source and much work has been done on the level of nutrients, in particular trace metals required for optimal acid yields and the role of individual metal ions.

Water

Water used for diluting basic substrates should be at least of drinking water quality. There should not be organic compounds and products of their decomposition (NH_3, NO_2^-, NO_3^-, and H_2S) and the level of trace metals must be controlled. All the water must be sterilised to remove contaminating microorganisms.

To sum up, citric acid is a bulk product, with the substrate cost being a major part of the plant operating cost. In terms of bulk, the carbon source is the most important substrate. The efficiency of its conversion to citric acid will determine the profitability of the fermentation process. For this reason, the carbon source is also the most important substrate for process economics. Most processes are based on molasses, although the use of cleaner sources is gaining ground. Whatever the source, its cost and preparation in order to permit optimal fermentation conditions are two important aspects of the technology in citric acid production.

Chapter 22

Amino Acids

INTRODUCTION

Amino acids are important substances which create life itself and are the oldest nutrients that have existed on earth. They have been used as the source of life over the period from primordial life to the present stage of evolution marked by the appearance of man. In 1806 an amino acid was first discovered from asparagus shoots in France, and was named asparagine. After this, cysteine, glycine and leucine were found from urinary calculus, gelatin and muscles/wool, respectively. All the protein-constituting amino acids were discovered by 1935.

In 1866 glutamate, which is familiar to us, was isolated by Ritthausen (Germany) from gluten, a wheat protein. In 1908, Dr. Kikunae Ikeda (Japan) discovered that glutamate is the *Umami* component of sea tangle. After amino acids were found to be responsible for the secret of deliciousness, the various properties of amino acids were studied in Japan in great depth.

Many theories have been presented to explain the origin of life. Some claim that life is of extraterrestrial origin, some believe that life began in the atmosphere, and some hold that the sea is the cradle of life. In all cases, however, amino acids are said to be the source of life. Some meteorites which collided with the earth after a long journey from the remotest corner of the universe contain amino acids. Trace amounts of glycine, alanine, glutamate and β-alanine were detected in a meteorite that struck Murchison (Australia) in 1969. The amino acids in meteorites are considered a trace of life elsewhere in the universe. A trilobite fossil dating back to 500 million years ago was found to contain amino acids such as alanine. Science continues its search for an answer to the intriguing mystery of the origin of life by studying the amino acids detected in fossils and meteorites.

Amino acids are very small biomolecules with an average molecular weight of about 135 daltons. These organic acids exist naturally in a zwitterion state where the carboxylic acid moiety is ionised and the basic amino group is protonated. The entire class of amino acids has a common backbone of an organic carboxylic acid group and an amino group attached to a saturated carbon atom. The simplest member of this group is glycine, where the saturated carbon atom is unsubstituted, rendering it optically inactive.

The rest of the 20 most common amino acids are optically active, existing as both D and L stereoisomers. Naturally occurring amino acids that are incorporated into proteins are, for the most part, the levorotary (L) isomer. Substituents on the alpha (or saturated) carbon atom vary from lower alkyl groups to aromatic amines and alcohols. There are also acidic and basic side chains, as well as thiol chains that can be oxidised to dithiol linkages between two similar amino acids.

Amino acids are the principal building blocks of proteins and enzymes. They are incorporated into proteins by transfer RNA according to the genetic code, while messenger RNA is being decoded by ribosomes. During and after the final assembly of a protein, the amino acid content dictates the spatial and biochemical properties of the protein or enzyme.

The amino acid backbone determines the primary sequence of a protein, but the nature of the side chains determines the protein's properties. Amino acid side chains can be polar, non-polar, or practically neutral. Polar side chains tend to be present on the surface of a protein where they can interact with the aqueous environment found in cells. On the other hand, non-polar amino acids tend to reside within the centre of the protein where they can interact with similar non-polar neighbours. This can create a hydrophobic region within an enzyme where chemical reactions can be conducted in a non-polar atmosphere. Likewise, enzymes can also have polar amino acid substituents within the active site that provide a polar region in which to conduct biochemical synthesis.

Amino acids are the 'building blocks' of the body. Besides building cells and repairing tissue, they form antibodies to combat invading bacteria and viruses; they are part of the enzyme and hormonal system; they build nucleoproteins (RNA and DNA); they carry oxygen throughout the body and participate in muscle activity. About 500 kinds of amino acids have been discovered in nature.

Monosodium L-glutamate (MSG) was found by Ikeda in 1908 as a flavouring component of *konbu*, or sea tangle. This was the start of the later development of the amino acid industry. Initially, MSG was produced industrially by extraction from a protein hydrolysate, more specifically, first from wheat gluten hydrolysate with hydrochloric acid, and then from defatted soyabean hydrolysate or by conversion from pyrrolidone-5-carboxylic acid in beet molasses, for use as a seasoning agent. This latter process was not sufficient to meet the increasing demand because it involved the protein of by-products disposal, requiring the development of new production processes. Patent applications filed around that time related to chemical synthesis of MSG from succinate semialdehyde or cyclopentane. In 1956, Kinoshita discovered a microbial process for L-glutamic acid production by direct fermentation of a micro-organism (*Corynebacterium glutamicum*) from sugar and ammonia. Consequently, industrial production of MSG as a seasoning was rapidly enlarged, and at the same time, a new industry of amino acid production by fermentation of micro-organisms emerged. In 1958, Kinosnita, Nakayama and Kitada found that an auxotrophic mutant of *C. glutamicum* requiring homoserine accumulated L-lysine in a medium, which enabled industrial production of L-lysine by fermentation. Establishing the basis for the development of the amino acid fermentation industry, this technology suggested the possibility of producing various other amino acids by auxotrophic mutants and also the importance of research in fermentative production of biological components with regulatory mutants. Since then, direct fermentation of various amino acids has been broadly studied.

Reduction of the cost of amino acids, owing to the development of fermentation techniques together with the establishment of their production processes, facilitated extended application of amino acids to uses other than as a seasoning. Particularly, L-lysine, an essential amino acid that is lacking in several food proteins, has been enjoying remarkably increased demand as a feed additive. Most of the amino acids produced in large quantities are still manufactured by fermentation, except for glycine, which does not have optical isomers, and methionine, which has a similar effect as a feed additive in both L- and DL-forms. In addition to being used as a seasoning agent and a feed additive, amino acids are currently used widely as a raw material for the sweetener Aspartame (*N*-L-α-aspartyl-L-phenylalanine 1-methyl ester), for pharmaceuticals and agrichemicals, for infusion and oral nutrition, for surfactants, and so forth, based on their reactivities and nutritional, pharmacological and flavouring effects.

In connection with amino acid fermentation, many reports have been published on the physiological properties of amino acid-producing micro-organisms. The following discussions stress problems from the standpoint of practically manufacturing amino acids on an industrial scale.

FERMENTATION PROCESSES

Amino acid fermentation may be defined in two ways. One is a definition in the narrow sense and refers to direct accumulation of amino acids in a medium containing a sugar, ammonia and other nutrients, and the other is a broad definition that covers the fermentation process involving the addition of specific precursors and amino acid production by reaction using enzymatic functions of micro-organisms. Here, mainly direct fermentation of the former type is discussed.

Fermentation processes generally have a number of advantages and benefits that accrue to the user of the process. On the other hand, they also have drawbacks. Both are summarise as follows:

Benefits and Problems

Benefits

1. Mild conditions are used both in fermentation and in product recovery; hence, little product degradation takes place.
2. Fermentation requires relatively less complex operation.
3. Once the plant is built and operation has begun, there are relatively low maintenance costs.
4. Only L-form amino acids are obtained.

Problems

1. Operations provide low product concentrations compared with chemical synthesis processes and require large volumes of water, large fermenter capacity and comparatively high capital investment.
2. The requirements for strict sterility add to capital costs and operation costs.
3. Large amounts of energy for oxygen transfer and mixing are required.
4. Product recovery may be complex, difficult and expensive.
5. The process time necessary to reach maximum concentrations of the desired product is usually comparatively long.

The aforementioned narrow-sense definition of direct fermentation of amino acids includes three types of fermentation: batch-type, fed-batch-type, and continuous.

Batch Fermentation

Industrial fermentation is mostly performed using batch processes. In a batch process, a large volume of a medium containing nutrients and substrate material is inoculated with a viable culture of one or more appropriate micro-organisms. Microbial growth and biochemical synthesis are allowed to proceed until an optimum yield of metabolite or a desired biochemical transformation has been obtained. Although this process is the basic form of fermentation, it is not frequently practiced on an industrial scale because productivity is limited by the amount and nature of the nutrients present at the time of inoculation. In most amino acid fermentation, enhanced product concentration is important to improve production efficiency and requires more advanced fermentation processes.

Fed-Batch Fermentation

Fed-batch fermentation types are classified in Table 22.1. This fermentation method is aimed at efficiently carrying out fermentation and is characterised by a low concentration of components in the initial medium to minimise metabolic regulation. At the time of inoculation the medium promotes initial growth of microbes; subsequent supplies of more raw materials drive the desirable increase in metabolite biosynthesis. Feeding is effected either intermittently or continuously. Industrial fermentation of most amino acids is accomplished with this method.

Table 22.1. Classification of fed-batch microbial reaction processes.

Case 1 (nonfeedback regulation)
Constant feeding-rate method
Exponential feeding method
Optimised feeding method
Others (intermittent feeding, etc.)
Case 2 (feedback regulation)
Indirect control
Direct control
Constant control
Programme control
Others

Fed-batch fermentation requires feeding equipment in addition to the equipment required for batch fermentation and therefore leads to higher fixed costs (Fig. 22.1).

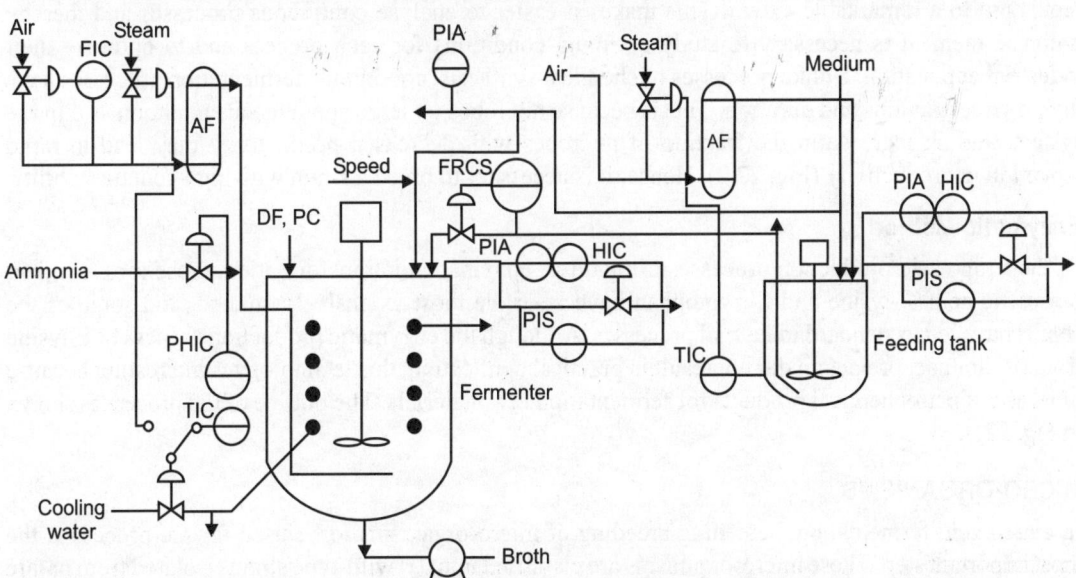

Fig. 22.1. Typical system for fed-batch fermentation. AF, air filter; DF, defoamer; PC, penicillin; FIC, flow indication control; PHIC, pH indication control; TIC, temperature indication control; PIS, pressure indication sum; PIA, pressure indication alarm; HIC, highest indication control; FRCS, flow record control sum.

However, the process can provide improved productivity as a whole because of the enhanced yield and reduced fermentation time. Actual product cost depends on the cost of the carbon source or specific precursors that are used for feeding. The nitrogen source is supplied generally through pH control with ammonia. This process is of particular importance in industrial operations where the reaction of the microbial catalyst does not last long; hence, continuous fermentation cannot be practiced, unlike in the case of L-glutamic acid fermentation from cane molasses using penicillin.

Continuous Fermentation

In continuous fermentation, a complete medium is fed to a fermenter after an appropriate period of batch fermentation, and the same quantity of broth is continuously taken from the fermenter to maintain the fermentation broth at a fixed volume. This may be performed either by the chemostat method using a substrate or limiting substance, or by the turbidostat method in which the cell level is adjusted to maintain constant cell mass. Because the continuous fermentation process allows improvement of productivity compared with the ordinary fermenter, the initial investment in equipment is small relative to the production volume, and operation cost is low. However, one drawback is that it is not suitable for small-scale production, and the challenges of sterile operation and equipment maintenance are more necessary than they are for batch and fed-batch fermentation. This process shifts from batch fermentation to continuous fermentation when productivity per unit time in the former is relatively high. There are many reports analysing the steady-state condition in continuous fermentation. Most of them relate to cell culture, but a few reports are available specifically on amino acid fermentation. One of the reasons may be that studies on amino acid fermentation have been mainly directed to the influence of metabolic regulation, as in the case of the penicillin addition method in glutamic acid fermentation, or because some amino acid processes have a distinct growth phase and production phase, and continuous culture cannot be used. Many of the microbial strains used in amino acid fermentation are released from metabolic regulation to a remarkable extent. This makes it easier to analyse continuous processes and thereby optimise them. It is necessary to study optimum conditions for each process and to optimise their industrial application. Unlike processes of chemical synthesis, continuous fermentation processes have their own restrictions and duration. This is because microbes undergo spontaneous mutation within the system, and an increase in the fraction of microbes with decreased productivity may lead to rapid reduction in productivity (Fig. 22.2). Hence, it is necessary to breed a strain with high genetic stability.

Enzymatic Method

Of the amino acid production processes using direct enzymatic biotransformation, those for L-alanine, L-aspartic acid, L-lysine and L-tryptophan have been the most extensively studied, and some of the results have led to standard industrial processes. Although the enzymatic production process of L-lysine from DL-aminocaprolactam did not result in practical application, this technology is interesting because of its use of petrochemical products for fermentation raw materials. The outline of the process is shown in Fig. 22.3.

MICRO-ORGANISMS

In amino acid fermentation, screening/breeding of micro-organisms to be used for the process is the most important step. These micro-organisms are classified into: (i) wild-type strains isolated from nature to meet a specific purpose, (ii) mutants that provide the desired properties that are developed by spontaneous or artificial mutation of wild-type strains, and (iii) recombinant strains bred or constructed through genetic recombination technologies.

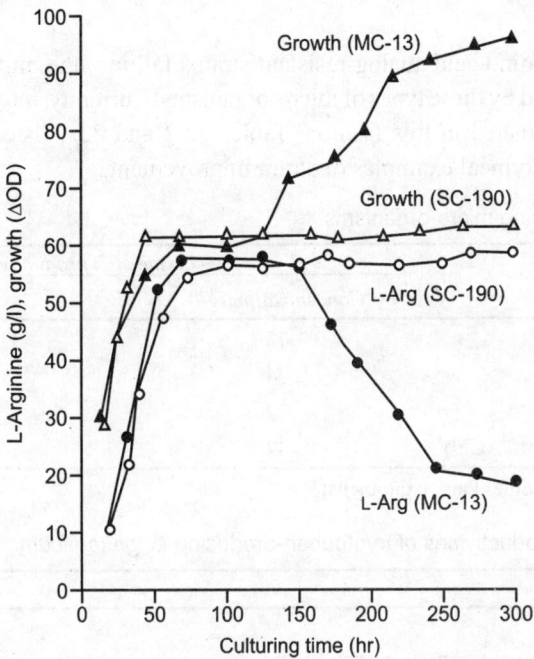

Fig. 22.2. Comparison of L-arginine continuous culture profile of MC-13 and SC-190.

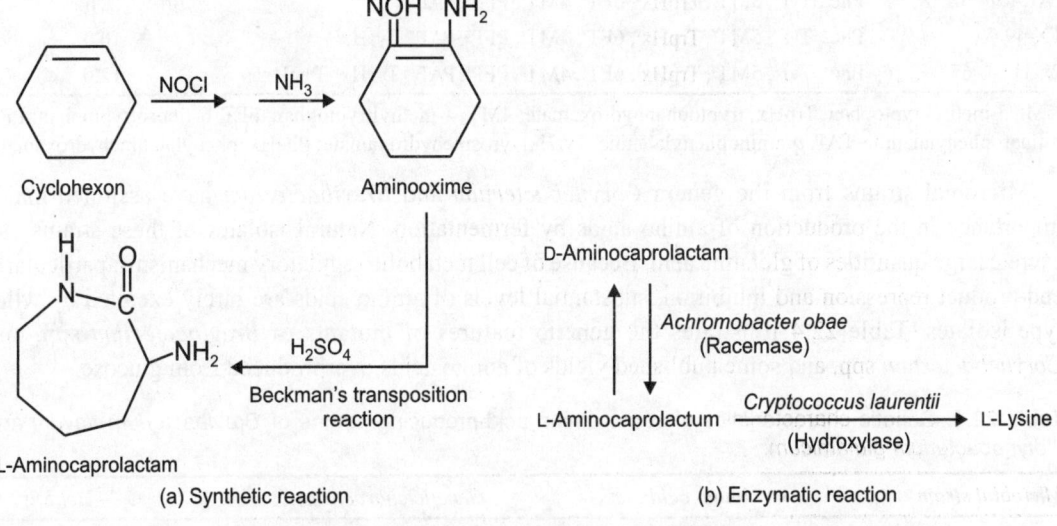

Fig. 22.3. L-Lysine production by a combination of synthetic and enzymatic reactions.

Wild-Type Strains

Micro-organisms suitable for the purpose are selected from nature. They are cultured under adjusted fermentation conditions so as to produce excess amounts of the desired products. Typical examples are *C. glutamicum* and *Brevibacterium flavum* used for L-glutamic acid fermentation.

Mutant Strains

Auxotrophic strains and amino acid analog-resistant strains fall into the mutant strain category. Most amino acids can be produced by these types of micro-organisms. Currently, most fermentative production of amino acids is accomplished in this fashion. Tables 22.2 and 22.3 listed L-lysine producers and L-tryptophan producers as typical examples of strain improvement.

Table 22.2. L-Lysine-producing micro-organisms.

Micro-organisms[a]	L-Lysine HCl productivities	
	Concentration (g/l)	Yield (%)
C. glutamicum (Hse⁻)	13	13
B. flavum (Thr⁻, Met⁻)	34	34
B. flavum (AEC^r)	32	32
C. glutemicum (Hse⁻, Leu⁻, Pant⁻, ACE^r)	42	42

[a]AEC, S-(2-aminoethyl)-L-cysteine; Pant, pantothenate.

Table 22.3. Isolation and productivities of tryptophan-producing *C. glutamicum*.

Strains	Phenotype[a]	Production of L-Trp (g/l)
KY 9456	Phe⁻, Tyr⁻	0.15
MT-11	Phe⁻, Tyr⁻, 5MT^r, TrpHx^r, 6FT^r, 4MT^r	4.9
PFP-2-32	Phe⁻, Tyr⁻, 5MT^r, TrpHx^r, 6FT^r, 4MT^r, PFP^r	5.7
PAP-136-50	Phe⁻, Tyr⁻, 5MT^r, TrpHx^r, 6FT^r, 4MT^r, PFP^r, PAP^r	7.1
TX-49	Phe⁻, Tyr⁻, 5MT^r, TrpHx^r, 6FT^r, 4MT^r, PFP^r, PAP^r, TyrHx^r	10.0
Px-115-L-67	Phe⁻, Tyr⁻, 5MT^r, TrpHx^r, 6FT^r, 4MT^r, PFP^r, PAP^r, TyrHx^r, PheHx^r	12.0

[a]5Mt, 5-methyltryptophan; TrpHx, tryptophanhydroxamate; 4MT; 4-methyltryptophan; 6FT, 6-fluorotryptophan; PFP, p-fluorophenylalanine; PAP, p-aminophenylalanine; TyrHx, tyrosinehydroxamate; PheHx, phenylalaninehydroxamate.

Microbial strains from the genera *Corynebacterium* and *Brevibacterium* have assumed major importance in the production of amino acids by fermentation. Natural isolates of these strains can excrete large quantities of glutamic acid. Because of cell metabolic regulatory mechanisms, particularly end-product repression and inhibition, substantial levels of amino acids are rarely excreted by wild-type isolates. Table 22.4 illustrates the genetic features of mutants of *Brevibacterium* spp. and *Corynebacterium* spp. and some published yields of amino acids overproduced from glucose.

Table 22.4. Genetic characteristics of some amino acid-producing strains of *Brevibacterium flavum* and *Corynebacterium glutamicum*.

Microbial strain	Amino acid	Genetic characteristics	Yield (g/l⁻¹)
Brevibacterium flavum	L-Arginine	Gua⁻TA^r	35
	L-Histidine	TA^{r}SM^{r}Eth^{r}ABT^r	10
	L-Isoleucine	AHV^{r}OMT^r	15
	L-Lysine	AEC^r	57
	L-Proline	Ile⁻ SG^{r}DHP^r	29

(Contd ...)

Microbial strain	Amino acid	Genetic characteristics	Yield (g/l^{-1})
	L-Threonine	Met$^-$ AHV^r	18
Corynebacterium glutamicum	L-Glutamate	Wild type	>100
	L-Glutamine	Wild type	40
	L-Lysine	Hom$^-$ Leu$^-$ AEC^r	39
	L-Phenylalanine	Tyr$^-$ PFP^{r}PAP^r	9
	L-Tryptophan	Phe$^-$ Tyr$^-$ 5MT^{r}TrpHx^{r}6FT^r	
		4MT^{r}PFP^{r}PAP^{r}TyrHx^{r}PheHx^r	12
	L-Tyrosine	Phe$^-$ PFP^{r}PAP^{r}PAT^{r}TyrHx^r	18

Resistance abbreviations: r, resistant; ABT, 2-aminobenzthiazole; AEC, S-(β-aminoethyl)-L-cysteine; AHV, α-amino-β-hydroxyvaleric acid; DHP, 3,4-dehydroproline; Eth, ethionine; 6FT, 6-fluorortryptophan; 4MT, 4-methyltryptophan; 5MT, 5-methyltryptophan; OMT, O-methylthreonine; PAP, *p*-aminophenylalanine; PheHx, phenylalanine hydroxamate; SG, sulphaguanidine; TA, 2-thiazolalanine; TyrHx, tyrosine hydroxamate; TrpHx; tryptophan hydroxamate.

Auxotroph abbreviations: −, auxotroph; Ile, isoleucine; Met, methionine; Hom, homoserine; Leu, leucine; Phe, phenylalanine; Tyr, tyrosine; Gua, guanine.

PRODUCTION METHODS AND TOOLS

Some amino acids are chemically synthesised, such as glycine, which has no stereochemical centre or D,L-methionine. This latter sulphur-containing amino acid can be added to feed as a racemic mixture, since animals contain a D-amino acid oxidase which, together with a transaminase activity, converts D-methionine to the nutritively effective L-form. The classical procedure of amino acid isolation from acid hydrolysates of proteins is still in use for selected amino acids with a low market volume, e.g. L-cysteine. Other methods in use are those of precursor conversion with bacteria or enzymatic synthesis. However, for L-amino acids required in large volumes, fermentation production with bacteria is the method of choice.

Classical Strain Development

However, bacteria do not normally excrete amino acids in significant amounts because regulatory mechanisms control the amino acid synthesis in an economical way. Therefore, mutants have to be generated which over-synthesise the respective amino acid. A great number of amino-acid-producing bacteria have been derived by mutagenesis and screening programmes. This has involved the consecutive application of:

1. Undirected mutagenesis.
2. Selection for a specific phenotype.
3. Selection of the mutant with the best amino acid accumulation.

Taking the best resulting strain, the entire procedure was repeated over several additional rounds to increase the productivity each time and eventually, resulted in an industrial producer. Due to this optimisation over several decades, together with the accompanying process adaptation, excellent high-performance strains are now available. They certainly carry a variety of unknown mutations also decisive for their production properties, as will become evident from the examples described.

Application of Recombinant Techniques

In conjunction with this classical technique for strain development, recombinant DNA techniques are also applied, which serve:

1. To rapidly develop new producers by increasing limiting enzyme activities.
2. To analyse mechanisms of flux control.
3. To combine this knowledge with classically obtained strains for their further development.

Intracellular Flux Analysis

An exciting new approach in strain development combining both the genetic and classical procedure is the reliable quantification of the carbon fluxes in the living cell. A great deal of progress has been made here recently in developing to a high level of sophistication the old isotope labelling technique. In particular, with ^{13}C-NMR spectroscopy the intracellular fluxes were quantified to extreme high resolution. For instance, in *C. glutamicum* it has even been possible to quantify the exchange flux rates as are present in the pentose phosphate pathway. Such flux identifications are of major assistance in selecting the reactions in the central metabolism to be modified by genetic engineering.

Functional Genomics

Another tool whose potential is only now being exploited is the genome analysis of producer strains. The availability of the entire sequence of the chromosomes from *C. glutamicum* and *E. coli* opens up exciting possibilities to compare mutants and to uncover new mutations essential for high overproduction of metabolites. For instance, RNA analysis using chip technology will make it possible to detect whether a specific gene is altered in its expression for producers of different efficiency. New mutations and genes might thus be discovered which are not directly concerned with carbon fluxes, but rather with total cell control or are involved in energy metabolism. Chip technology will also make it possible to use genome analysis as a tool to qualify individual fermentations, thus resulting in still further improvements and consolidations of the production processes.

L-GLUTAMATE

L-Glutamate was the first amino acid to be produced. The very successful production still exclusively uses the original bacterium *C. glutamicum*. As metabolic pathways *C. glutamicum* uses glycolysis, the pentose phosphate pathway and the citric acid cycle to generate precursor metabolites and reduced pyridine nucleotides. However, this bacterium displays a special feature in the anaplerotic reactions of the citric acid cycle (Fig. 22.4). Since L-glutamate is directly derived from α-ketoglutarate, a high capability for replenishing the citric acid cycle is, of course, a prerequisite for high glutamate production. It was originally assumed that only the phosphoenolpyruvate carboxylase is present as a carboxylating enzyme within the anaplerotic reactions. However, molecular research in close conjunction with ^{13}C-labelling studies and flux analysis showed that an additional carboxylating reaction must be present. The pursuit of this enzyme activity resulted in the detection of pyruvate carboxylase activity, PyrC and the cloning of its gene. This carboxylase was not detected by the original enzyme measurements since it is very unstable in crude extracts. Its detection requires an *in situ* enzyme assay using carefully permeabilised cells. Therefore, *C. glutamicum* has the pyruvate dehydrogenase (PyrDH) shuffling acetyl-CoA into the citric acid cycle but two enzymes supplying oxaloacetate: pyruvate carboxylase (PyrC) together with a phosphoenolpyruvate carboxylase (PEPC) (Fig. 22.4). The successful cloning of both genes together with mutant studies showed that both carboxylases can basically replace each other to ensure conversion of glucose-derived C3-units to oxaloacetate. This is different from *E. coli*, which has exclusively the phosphoenolpyruvate carboxylase serving this purpose, or *Bacillus subtilis*, where only the pyruvate carboxylase is present. Since *C. glutamicum* possesses both enzymes, it has an enormous flexibility for replenishing citric acid cycle intermediates upon their withdrawal.

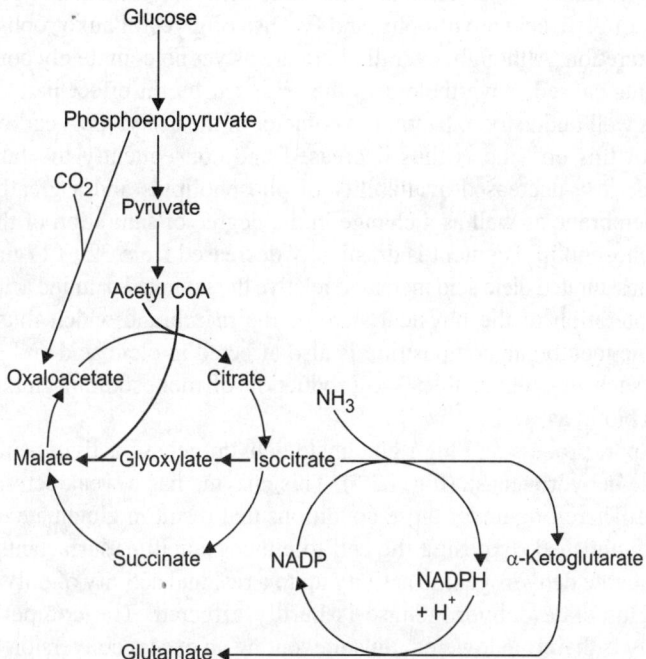

Fig. 22.4. Metabolic pathway for production of glutamic acid from glucose.

The reductive amination of α-ketoglutarate to yield L-glutamate is catalysed by glutamate dehydrogenase. The enzyme is a multimer, each subunit having a molecular weight of 49,100. It has a high specific activity of 1.8 mmol min^{-1} mg protein and L-glutamate is present in the cell in a rather high concentration of about 150 mM. In the case of other amino acids, in contrast, the intracellular concentrations are usually below 10 mM. The high concentration serves to ensure the supply of L-glutamate directly required for cell synthesis and also for the supply of amino groups via transaminase reactions for a variety of cellular reactions. As much as 70 per cent of the amino groups in cell material stems from L-glutamate.

Production Strains

For the biotechnological production of L-glutamate the intracellularly synthesised amino acid must be released from the cell. This is, of course, usually not the case since the charged L-glutamate is retained by the cytoplasmic membrane, otherwise the cell would not be viable. However, as shown by the special circumstances in discovering *C. glutamicum*, L-glutamate is already excreted when biotin is limiting. This striking fact is based on two essential characteristics:

1.   A carrier is present mediating the active excretion of L-glutamate.
2.   The lipid environment of this carrier triggers its activity.

A specific carrier is required since otherwise, in addition to the charged L-glutamate, other metabolites and ions would also leak from the cell. Moreover, only an active export enables the energy-dependent 'uphill' transport of L-glutamate from inside the cell (0.15 M) towards the very high concentrations obtained in fermentation broths (more than 1 M). However, for practical purpose, the triggering of active export by the appropriate molecular environment of the cytoplasmic membrane is important. The switches for tuning this environment and thus eliciting glutamate export are surprisingly diverse: (i) growth under biotin limitation, (ii) addition of local anaesthetics, (iii) addition of penicillin, (iv) addition of surfactants, (v) use of oleic acid auxotrophs, and (vi) use of glycerol auxotrophs. All of these means trigger L-glutamate excretion. Although, overall, there are as yet no completely conclusive ideas on the molecular changes thus caused, nevertheless in the classical biotin effect part of the causal link to glutamate excretion is well understood. Biotin is a cofactor of the acetyl-CoA carboxylase. With limited supply, the activity of this enzyme is thus decreased and consequently the fatty acid synthesis is diminished. This leads to a decreased availability of phospholipids and a greatly decreased lipid to protein ratio in the membrane as well as a change in the degree of saturation of the fatty acids. Under biotin limitation the phospholipid content is drastically decreased from 32 to 17 nmol mg^{-1} dry weight and the content of the unsaturated oleic acid increased relative the saturated palmitic acid by 45 per cent. This represents a severe alteration of the physical state of the membrane which thus dramatically alters L-glutamate efflux. The membrane composition is also affected in oleic acid and glycerol auxotrophic mutants. The use of such mutants enables the production of monosodium glutamate from substrate which may be rich in biotin as well.

Apart from the export process and high glutamate dehydrogenase activity, another key reaction is that of α-ketoglutarate dehydrogenase (Fig. 22.4). This enzyme has a weak activity in *C. glutamicum* and it is also unstable. Therefore, under those conditions that result in glutamate efflux, the activity of this enzyme in also diminished. Exposing the cell to either penicillin, surfactants or biotin-limitation reduces the α-ketoglutarate dehydrogenase activity up to a residual activity of only 10 per cent, whereas the activity of the glutamate dehydrogenase is hardly affected. The competing α-ketoglutarate dehydrogenase activity is therefore lowered, thus preventing an excess conversion of α-ketoglutarate to succinyl-CoA and therefore favouring its conversion to L-glutamate.

Production Process

The most relevant factors influencing L-glutamate formation are the ammonium concentration, the dissolved O_2 concentration and the pH. Although, in total, a large amount of ammonium is necessary for sugar conversion to L-glutamate, a high concentration is inhibitory to growth as well to the production of L-glutamate. Therefore, ammonium is added in a low concentration at the beginning of the fermentation and is then added continuously during the course of the fermentation. The oxygen concentration is controlled, since under conditions of insufficient oxygen, the production of L-glutamate is poor and lactic acid as well as succinic acid accumulates, whereas with an excess oxygen supply the amount of α-ketoglutarate as a by-product accumulates. A flow diagram of the process is shown in Fig. 22.5.

For the actual fermentation the production strains are grown in fermenters as large as 500 m^3. After precultivation, the onset of L-glutamate excretion is controlled by the addition of surfactants like polyoxyethylene sorbitan monopalmitate (Tween 40). Yields of 60–70 per cent L-glutamate, based on the glucose used, have been reported. At the end of the fermentation the broth contains L-glutamate in the form of its ammonium salt. In a typical downstream process, the cells are separated and the broth is passed through a basic anion exchange resin. L-Glutamate anions will be bound to the resin and ammonia will be released. This ammonia can be recovered via distillation and reused in the fermentation. Elution is performed with NaOH to directly form MSG in the solution and to regenerate the basic anion exchanger. From the eluates, MSG may be crystallised directly followed by further conditioning steps like decolourisation and sieving to yield a food-grade quality.

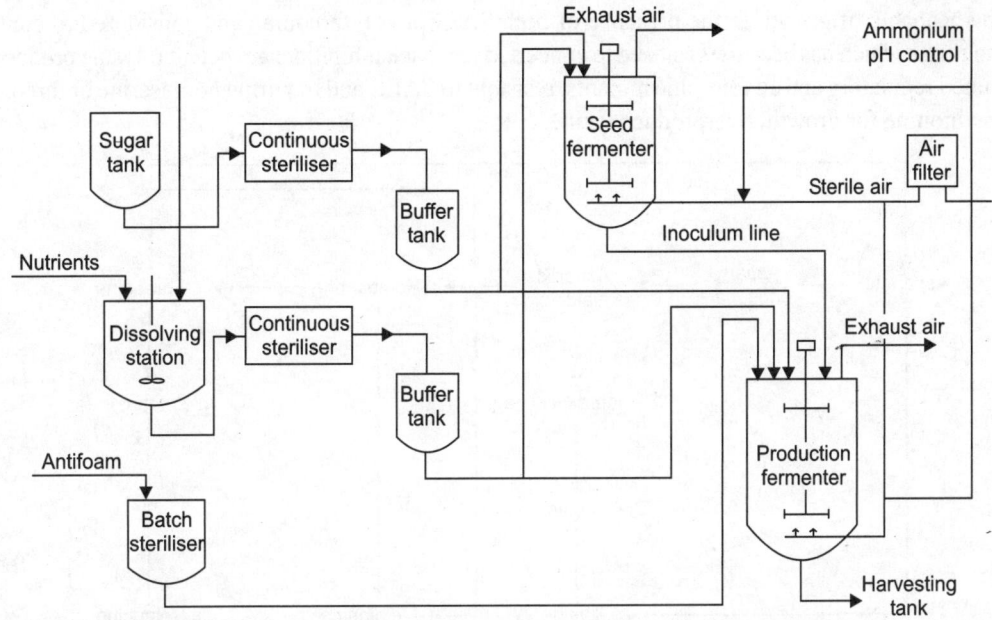

Fig. 22.5. A scheme of the material flow in an L-glutamate production plant.

The monoamide of glutamic acid, an amino acid occurring in proteins, is an important carrier of urinary ammonia and is broken down in the kidney by the enzyme glutaminase. It is useful in treatment of alcoholism by reducing the desire to drink and may be helpful in the improvement of Autism and mental retardation in children. It is reported to show improvement in mental functions such as memory and dexterity and aids peptic ulcer healing due to antacid quality. It crosses the blood brain barriers and participates in nucleonic acid synthesis. Gluatamine converts to glutamic acid, the negatively charged amino acid found on the surface of proteins. Considered to be nature's 'Brain food' by improving mental capacities; it helps speed the healing of ulcers; gives a 'lift' from fatigue; helps control alcoholism, schizophrenia and the craving for sugar.

LYSINE PRODUCTION

Lysine, an amino acid which is essential for animal and human nutrition, is lacking in cereals. The amino acid is produced predominantly by direct fermentation using an auxotrophic mutant of *Corynebacterium glutamicum*. Recently, a second fermentation process, involving a regulatory mutant of *Brevibacterium flavum* and a biotransformation process, involving conversion of chemically-synthesised α-aminocaprolactam to L-lysine, have been commercialised.

The pathway for biosynthesis of lysine by *C. glutamicum* and *B. flavum* is illustrated in Fig. 22.6. The first enzyme, aspartokinase, is regulated by concerted feedback inhibition by L-threonine and L-lysine. L-Threonine causes feedback inhibition of homoserine dehydrogenase, while L-methionine represses synthesis of this enzyme. Hence, a homoserine auxotroph or a threonine–methionine double auxotroph of *C. glutamicum* diminishes the intracellular pool of threonine and reduces its marked feedback inhibitory effect on aspartokinase and promotes good lysine production. S-(2-aminoethyl)-L-cysteine, a lysine analogue (SAEC) which behaves as false feedback inhibitor of aspartokinase, inhibits growth of *B. flavum*. Growth inhibition is markedly enhanced by L-threonine and is reversed by L-lysine. Some mutants, capable of growth in the presence of both SAEC and L-threonine and considered to contain aspartokinase which has been desensitised to concerted feedback inhibition, are potent L-lysine producers. Combined regulatory and auxotrophic mutants, resistant to SAEC and requiring homoserine or threonine and methionine for growth, overproduce lysine.

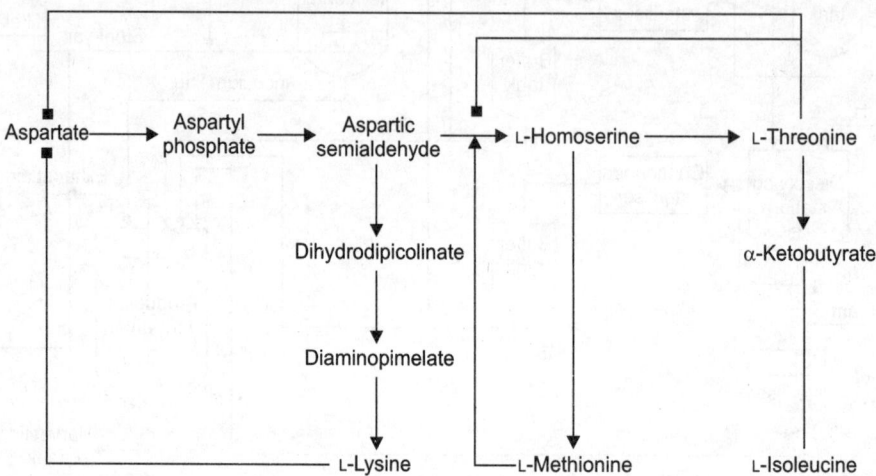

Fig. 22.6. Metabolic pathway for lysine biosynthesis in *Corynebacterium glutamicum* and *Brevibacterium flavum*. ■, inhibition; ▲, repression.

Biosynthesis of asparate for lysine production is from the oxaloacetate component of the Krebs cycle. The predominant anaplerotic reaction is considered to be the phosphoenolpyruvate carboxylation system rather than the glyoxylate cycle. Incorporation of excess biotin into the medium inhibits undesirable glutamate overproduction.

An example of a fermentation profile for production of lysine by a homoserine auxotroph is illustrated in Fig. 22.7.

D,L-α-Aminocaprolactam, chemically synthesised from cyclohexane, is the raw material for production of L-lysine by biotransformation. Acetone-dried cells of *Cryptococcus laurentii*, which contain the enzyme L-α-aminocaprolactam hydrolase, convert L-aminocaprolactam to L-lysine, while acetone dried cells of *Achromobacter obae* contain a racemase to convert D-α-aminocaprolactam to the L-form (Fig. 22.8).

Found in abundance in muscle tissue, connective tissue and collagen. The main sources of this amino acid are most kinds of nuts, seeds, vegetables and subacid fruits. It is essential for optimal growth in human infants, and for maintenance of nitrogen equilibrium in adults. Lack of adequate lysine in the diet may cause headaches, dizziness, nausea and incipient anaemia.

Lysine upsets in the body have also been associated with pneumonia, nephrosis and acidosis, as well as malnutrition and rickets in children. It is considered a natural remedy for cold, sores, shingles and genital herpes. Lysine also influences the female reproductive cycle. Some other functions are as below:

1. It insures the adequate absorption of calcium.
2. Helps form collagen (which makes up bone cartilage and connective tissues).
3. Aids in the production of antibodies, hormones and enzymes.
4. Reported to inhibit growth and replication of herpes simplex and epstein barr viruses. Its use along with vitamin C, zinc and vitamin A helps eliminate virus infections. Vitamin C protects

this amino acid while in the body so that lysine plus vitamin C has a much stronger anti-virus effect than if either is used separately.

5. Stimulates secretion of gastric juices.

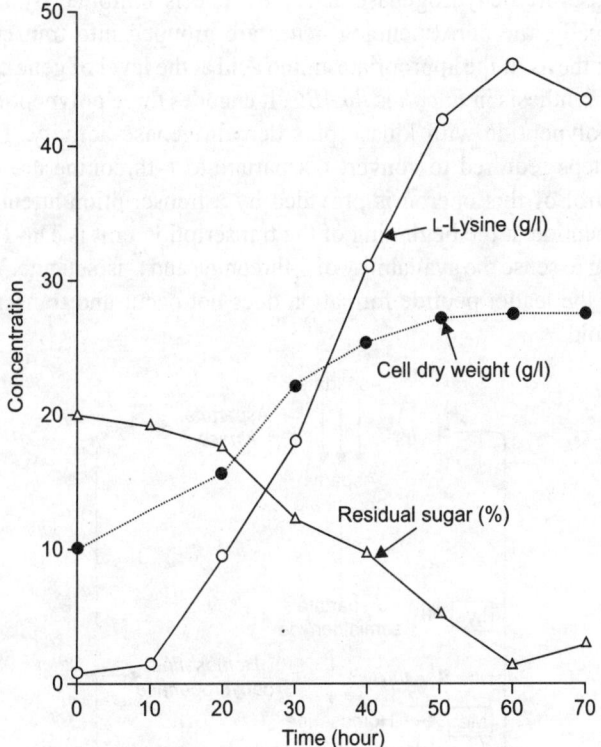

Fig. 22.7. Time course of a lysine fermentation.

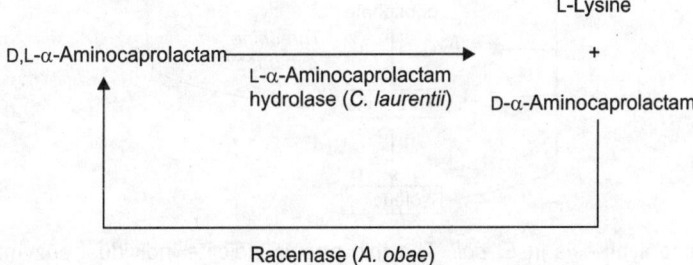

Fig. 22.8. Conversion of D,L-α-aminocaprolactam to L-lysine by biotransformation.

L-THREONINE

The commercial production of L-threonine is possible with either *E. coli* or *C. glutamicum* mutants. However, the production figures of selected *E. coli* strains are superior. The synthesis of L-threonine proceeds via a short pathway comprising only five steps (Fig. 22.9). As already mentioned, the first steps are shared with that of L-lysine and L-methionine synthesis. Furthermore, L-threonine is also an intermediate in the L-isoleucine synthesis. This naturally requires special metabolic regulation. In *C. glutamicum* this was solved in such a way that the sole aspartate kinase present was only inhibited by the joint presence of L-lysine and L-threonine, one by L-lysine and one by L-methionine. There are furthermore two homoserine dehydrogenase activities: one is inhibited by L-threonine and one by L-methionine. Additionally, the corresponding genes are grouped into transcriptional units, thereby ensuring a balanced synthesis of the appropriate amino acid at the level of gene expression. The relevant operon for L-threonine synthesis in *E. coli* is *thrABC*. It encodes three polypeptides, with *thrA* encoding an apparently fused polypeptide with kinase plus dehydrogenase activity. Therefore, four enzyme activities of the five steps required to convert L-aspartate to L-threonine are encoded by *thrABC*. A strong expression control of this operon is provided by a transcription attenuation mechanism. The corresponding leader peptide at the beginning of the transcription unit is Thr-Thr-Ile-Thr-Thr-Thr-Ile-Thr-Ile-Thr-Thr, serving to sense the availability of L-threonine and L-isoleucine. When the corresponding tRNAs are uncharged, the leader peptide formation does not occur and transcription of the operon is increased at least ten-fold.

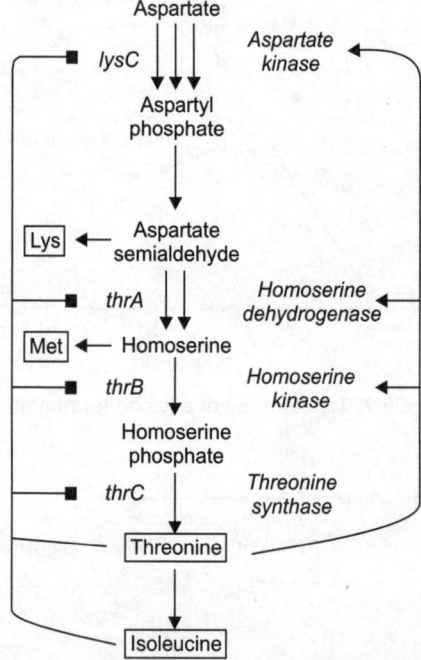

Fig. 22.9. L-Threonine synthesis in *E. coli*. The thin arrows indicate individual enzyme activities and the genes *thrABC* constitute an operon. Only the regulation of genes and enzymes by L-threonine and L-isoleucine is shown, where the square ends indicate gene repression and the arrowhead ends enzyme activity inhibition.

Production Strains

Based on this regulation there is a clear focus on two major targets for the design of a production strain: the prevention of L-isoleucine formation and stable high-level expression of *thrABC*. Therefore, in one of the first steps of strain development, chromosomal mutations were introduced to give an isoleucine leaky strain (Fig. 22.10). The isoleucine mutation is a very specific and important one. L-Isoleucine is required for growth only a low L-threonine concentrations but, at high concentrations of L-threonine, growth is independent of L-isoleucine. The mutation therefore has several advantageous consequences. In the first place, it prevents an excess formation of the undesired by-product L-isoleucine. Additionally, it prevents the L-isoleucine-dependent premature termination of the *thrABC* transcription due to limiting tRNA^{Ile}. A high transcription rate is, of course, required to have high specific enzyme activities.

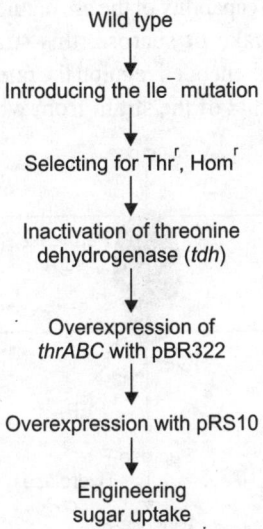

Fig. 22.10. Relevant steps in the development of an *E. coli* strain suitable for L-threonine production involving undirected mutagenesis, gene inactivation and use of different plasmids.

Another consequence of the isoleucine mutation is more subtle. It relates to the stability of the plasmid-containing producer strain in the various precultivation steps. Starting from a single clone, a preculture is inoculated for each production run and is then enlarged in several stages. This means that the clone is fermented for about 25 generations so that there is a great danger of the plasmid containing the *thrABC* operon being lost. This would of course be a complete disaster if it happened in the final production stage. In the presence of the isoleucine leaky mutation, however, cells that have lost the plasmid now are clearly disadvantaged when not supplied with L-isoleucine. Their further proliferation is halted, thereby stabilising a culture where almost all the cells that are growing contain the plasmid. Further engineering during strain evolution involved the introduction of resistance to L-threonine and L-homoserine. Subsequently, *tdh*, which encodes threonine dehydrogenase, was inactivated thus preventing threonine degradation. To obtain very high activities of the *thrABC*-encoding enzymes, the operon was cloned from a strain whose kinase and dehydrogenase activities are resistant to L-threonine inhibition. In addition, the transcription attenuator region was deleted. In fermentations the operon engineered in this way was successfully used with pBR322 as a vector, but a further improvement was obtained by replacing this plasmid by a pRS1010 derivative, resulting in an even more stable high-level expression.

Substrate uptake

Since the cost of the sugar source has a decisive influence on the price of the amino acid produced it is essential to be able to switch between glucose and sucrose as substrates. However, only a few of the *E. coli* strains can use sucrose. Two different sucrose-utilising systems of *E. coli* are available to engineer sugar utilisation in L-threonine producing strains (Fig. 22.11). One of them is represented by the *scr* regulon, where the actual translocator consists of a phosphoenolpyruvate: sugar phosphotransferase system (PTS). Introduction of the *scr* genes into a glucose-utilising *E. coli* strain results in the uptake and phosphorylation of sucrose. Due to subsequent hydrolase and fructokinase activities the sugar is then channelled into the central metabolism. An alternative sucrose utilisation system is provided by the *csc* regulon of some *E. coli* strains. In this case, sucrose is translocated by the *cscB* encoded translocator is symport with protons. Using transposition the sucrose-utilisation capability of the *csc* regulon was introduced into a glucose-utilising strain. Although originally without uptake of sucrose, this strain now imported sucrose at a rate of 9 pmol min^{-1}·mg dry wt. With the plasmid-encoded regulon the rate obtained was 43 pmol min^{-1} mg cell dry weight, which was almost identical to that of the strain from which the *csc* regulon had been isolated.

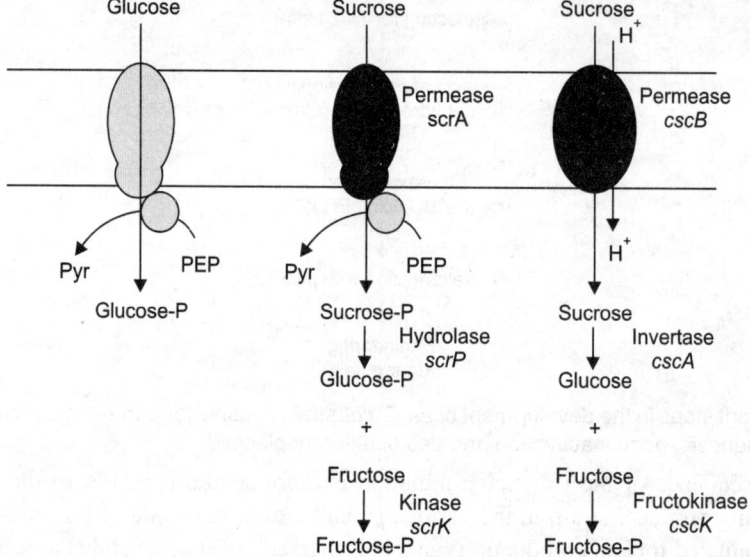

Fig. 22.11. Mechanisms of sugar uptake and phosphorylation in *E. coli*. Translocation is coupled by phosphorylation, as is the case for the phosphotransferase system (left and middle) or occurs in symport with protons without phosphorylation (right). The phosphotransferase translocating sucrose (middle) shares one of the phosphoryl transfer domains with a component of the phosphotransferase translocating glucose. Pyr, pyruvate; PEP, phosphoenolpyruvate.

Production Process

The fermentation of the engineered L-threonine producer is in a simple mineral salts medium with either glucose or sucrose as the substrate with addition of a small amount of a complex medium component like yeast extract. After the inoculation and consumption of the initially provided sugar, continuous feeding of sugar begins. Additionally, ammonia has to be fed in the form of gas or as NH_4OH which is regulated via pH control. Thus the feeding strategy in the case of L-threonine fermentation is quite easy compared to L-lysine fermentation where the accumulation of the basic product requires the feeding of sulphate as the counter-ion. At the end of the fermentation, L-threonine is present in concentrations of about 85 g l^{-1} with a conversion yield of up to 60 per cent based on the carbon source used. Such fermentations with high yields show quite low by-product levels. This is an advantage for downstream processing. Crystallisation of L-threonine is easy due to its low solubility (about 90 g l^{-1} in water) and the low salt concentration present. A process is described where the cells are initially coagulated by a heat- or pH-treatment step, followed by filtration. Subsequently, the broth is concentrated and crystallisation initiated by cooling. The separation and drying of the crystals leads to an isolation yield of 80 to 90 per cent with the L-threonine having a purity of more than 90 per cent. A recrystallisation step may be required for high-purity L-threonine. This is a naturally occurring amino acid, essential for human metabolism. It is found in various types of milk and is a major constituent in cow's milk. Other sources are nuts, seeds, carrots and green vegetables. Without threonine, a child's development will be incomplete and there will be malfunctioning of the brain. This amino acid has a powerful anti-convulsive effect and rises to three times its normal value at pregnancy. Some important functions in the human body are:

1. It acts as a lipotropic factor.
2. It has been recently found to increase brain glycine content, greatly reducing ALS symptoms (Amylotrophic Lateral Sclerosis or 'Lue Gehrig's disease').
3. It is an amino acid alcohol involved in porphyrin metabolism.
4. It is an important constituent of collagen, Elastin and enamel protein.
5. It helps prevention of fat build-up in the liver.
6. Helps the digestive and intestinal tracts to function more smoothly.
7. Assists metabolism and assimilation.

L-PHENYLALANINE

L-Phenylalanine can be produced with *E. coli* or *C. glutamicum*. The pathway for L-phenylalanine synthesis is shared in part with that of L-tyrosine and L-tryptophan. These three aromatic amino acids have in common the condensation of erythrose 4-phosphate and phosphoenolpyruvate to deoxyarabino-heptulosonate phosphate (DAHP) with further conversion in six steps up to chorismate. L-Phenylalanine is then finally made in three further steps (Fig. 22.12).

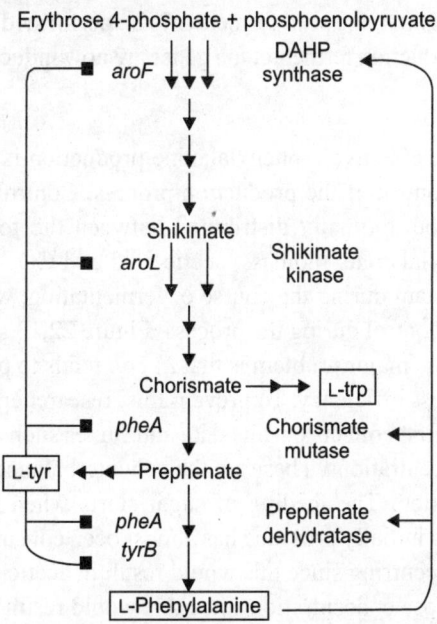

Fig. 22.12. Simplified pathway of L-phenylalanine synthesis and the relevant regulation by L-phenylalanine and L-tyrosine (L-tyr) with feedback control of enzyme activity (arrowhead ends) and gene repression (square ends).

There are three DAHP synthase enzymes in *E. coli* encoded by *aroF, aroG* and *aroH*. These enzymes play a key role in flux control. Their regulation of catalytic activity, in each case by one of the three aromatic amino acids, recalls the specific regulation of aspartate kinase in the synthesis of threonine. About 80 per cent of the total DAHP-synthase activity is contributed by the *aroG*-encoded enzyme. Increased flux towards L-phenylalanine can be obtained by over-expression of either *aroF* or *aroG* encoding feedback-resistant enzymes. Furthermore, *pheA* overexpression is essential. This gene encodes the bifunctional corismate mutase-prephenate dehydratase. A second chorismate activity is present as a bifunctional chorismate mutase-prephenate dehydrogenase. The *pheA*-encoded enzyme activities are inhibited by L-phenylalanine and *pheA* expression is dependent on the level of tRNA^{Phe}.

Production Strains

Producer strains have a DAHP activity that is resistant to feedback inhibition and which is encoded either by *aroF* or *aroG* and a feedback-resistant chorismate mutase-prephenate dehydratase. As a rule, the producers are L-tyrosine auxotrophic mutants. There are very good reasons for this, one of which is that the enzymes of the common pathway from DAHP to prephenate are no longer regulated by L-tyrosine and enzyme activities are no longer feedback-inhibited. Another reason is that in this way tyrosine accumulation is prevented, which would otherwise undoubtedly result as a by-product since there are only two additional steps from prephenate to L-tyrosine. An essential aspect is that due to the auxotrophy, a beneficial growth limitation is possible by appropriate tyrosine feeding. In some *E. coli* strains, the temperature-sensitive cI$_{857}$ repressor of bacteriophage λ has been used together with the λP$_L$ promoter to enable inducible expression of key genes *pheA* and *aroF*. This enables extremely high enzyme activities to be adjusted solely in the actual production runs thus eliminating the inherent problems of strain stability due to the resulting high metabolite concentrations or side activities of the enzymes. It enables the precultivation steps up to the seed fermenter to be performed with low expression of the key genes but in the actual large production fermenter the genes are now induced to a high level of expression.

Production Process

As with the other amino acids, effective L-phenylalanine production is the joint result of engineering the cellular metabolism and control of the production process. Control is necessary for two reasons. First, the carbon flux has to be optimally distributed between the four major products of glucose conversion, which are L-phenylalanine, biomass, acetic acid and CO_2. The second reason is that the cellular physiology is not constant during the course of fermentation, which correspondingly requires an adaptation of fermentation control during the process. Figure 22.13 shows the typical time curve of L-phenylalanine production. The major problem is that *E. coli* tends to produce acetic acid which has a strong negative effect on process efficiency. To prevent this, researchers have developed an ingenious sugar-feeding strategy, which first collects on-line data and fluxes such as oxygen concentration, sugar consumption and biomass concentrations. These are then counterbalanced during the process to control the optimum sugar concentration. The feeding of sugar starts when the cells enter Stage 2 of the fermentation where the glucose initially provided has almost been consumed. The trick is to prevent too high a glucose concentration occurring since this would result in acetic acid formation and at the same time, to prevent too low a glucose concentration since this would result in an excess of CO_2 evolution. Thus the feeding rate is a compromise where the process is run at the highest possible feeding rate which still provides a sufficiently strong limitation to prevent acetic acid excretion. When the L-tyrosine initially present has been consumed, the cells proceed to Stage 3. As already mentioned, almost all L-phenylalanine producers cannot synthesise tyrosine. The L-tyrosine concentration selected at the start of the culture therefore fixes the minimum amount of biomass necessary to efficiently metabolise the predetermined amount of glucose. In Stage 3, the metabolic capacity of the cells decreases which brings about a consequent decrease of the glucose feeding rate. At the end of Stage 3, acetic acid excretion begins and the cells enter Stage 4 where no further L-phenylalanine accumulation occurs and the process is eventually terminated. This example of amino acid production shows that by the sophisticated application of feeding strategies with adaptive control a very high L-phenylalanine concentration can be achieved with a high yield within 2.5 days. Values of 50.8 gram phenylalanine per litre with a yield of 27.5 per cent of carbon used have been reported.

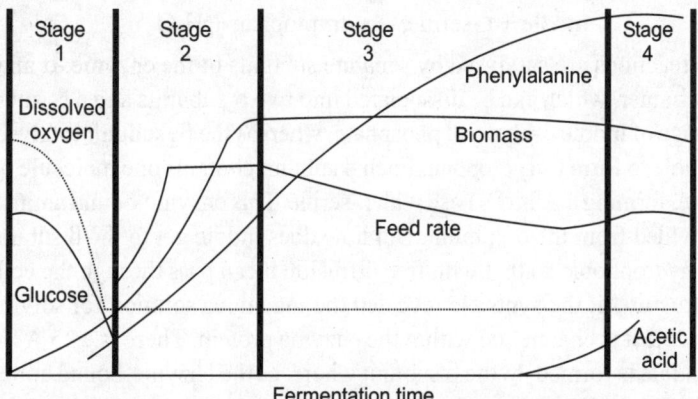

Fig. 22.13. The four stages of L-phenylalanine production characterised by different physiology requiring different process control regimes to give the highest yields in shortest times.

It is the most common aromatic amino acid found in proteins and is one of the amino acids in the dipeptide sweetener Aspartame. This amino acid is essential for the production of the hormone adrenaline, and production of the thyroid secretion and the hair and skin pigment, melanin. It is effective in weight control because of its effect on the thyroid. Its use before meals suppresses the appetite substantially. Patients taking half a teaspoon of the powder 30 minutes before each meal, lose from a quarter to half a pound a day.

It is also essential for the efficient functioning of kidneys and bladder. Major source are nuts, seeds, carrots, parsley and tomatoes. An important recently discovered therapeutic use of phenylalanine is its ability to overcome most conditions of lethargy through stimulation of adrenaline. Some other functions of phenylalanine are:

1. It is essential for optimal growth in infants, and for nitrogen equilibrium in human adults.
2. It is used by the brain to produce Norepinephrine, a chemical that transmits signals between nerve cells and the brain.
3. It keeps one awake and alert.
4. Reduces hunger pangs (may be useful in appetite control by stimulating CCK, Chaleceptokinin enzyme, secretion).
5. Functions as an antidepressant and helps improve memory.
6. Gives rise to tyrosine and increases blood pressure in hypotension.

L-TRYPTOPHAN

L-Tryptophan is a high-price amino acid which still has a rather low market volume. Effective production processes are available with mutants of different bacteria, including *Bacillus subtilis*. However, cellular synthesis is no longer performed due to originally not realised impurities in the final product used for medical purposes. These impurities arose during the isolation of L-tryptophan from a chemical reaction with traces of acetaldehyde at low pH. An alternative process is the enzymatic synthesis of L-tryptophan from precursors. The current enzymatic production process uses the activity of the biosynthetic tryptophan synthase (Fig. 22.14). This enzyme catalyses the last step in the tryptophan synthesis, which consists in fact of two partial reactions:

$$\text{Indole 3-glycerol phosphate} \rightarrow \text{Indole} + \text{glyceraldehyde 3-phosphate}$$

$$\text{Indole} + \text{L-serine} \rightarrow \text{L-tryptophan} + H_2O$$

These separate reactions are catalysed by separate subunits of the enzyme: α and β. The enzyme of *E. coli* is an $\alpha_2\beta_2$ tetramer, which can be dissociated into two α subunits and a β_2 subunit. The α subunit catalyses the cleavage of indole 3-glycerol phosphate, whereas the β_2 subunit catalyses the condensation of L-serine with indole to form L-tryptophan. Each β subunit contains one molecule of covalently bound pyridoxal phosphate, forming a Schiff's base with L-serine. This enzyme-bound aminoacrylate is attacked when indole is provided from the α subunit. But how does indole get to the β subunit? The problem is that indole is very hydrophobic so that with free diffusion it can pass through the cell membrane and be lost. The crystal structure of the synthase revealed the ingenious solution for solving this problem. To prevent a loss of indole it is channelled within the enzyme protein. There is a 25 Å long tunnel from the α subunit, where indole is formed, to the β subunit where, as the enzyme-bound aminoacrylate, L-serine is ready to accept the indole. Furthermore, within the native tetramer both partial reactions are coordinated. Only when L-serine, as aminoacrylate, is ready to accept the indole, does indole 3-glycerol phosphate conversion occur at the β subunit. Tryptophan synthase is thus an example of how an enzyme complex is used as sophisticated device to handle a reactive and diffusible intermediate within the cell.

Production from Precursors

The process of L-tryptophan production with this enzyme is based on *E. coli* cells which have a high tryptophan synthase activity. The α and β subunits encoding genes *trpA* and *trpB*, respectively, are located on the *trpEDCBA* operon which is regulated by repression and attenuation. In the *E. coli* mutant used, the repressor of that operon has been deleted as is part of the attenuator region together with the first structural genes of the operon. In the resulting strain, about 10 per cent of the total protein is tryptophan synthase with an excess of the β subunit. Although indole is not the true substrate of the enzyme (Fig. 22.14), with a sufficiently high concentration the enzyme will react with it. Indole is available from the petrochemical industry as a comparably cheap educt, whereas the second educt, L-serine, is recovered from molasses during sugar refinement using ion exclusion chromatography and further purification steps (Fig. 22.15). The resulting L-serine is fed to the previously cultivated *E. coli* cells and indole is added continuously at a concentration adjusted to 10 mM, which is controlled on-line. This type of process ensures an almost quantitative conversion of indole to yield L-tryptophan with a space-time yield of about 75 g per litre a day.

Further processing of the L-tryptophan solution can be taken from Fig. 22.15 leading to a pyrogen-free pharmaceutical product of the highest quality.

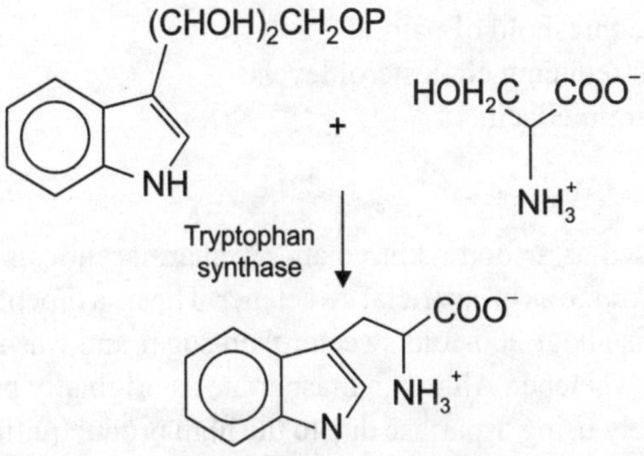

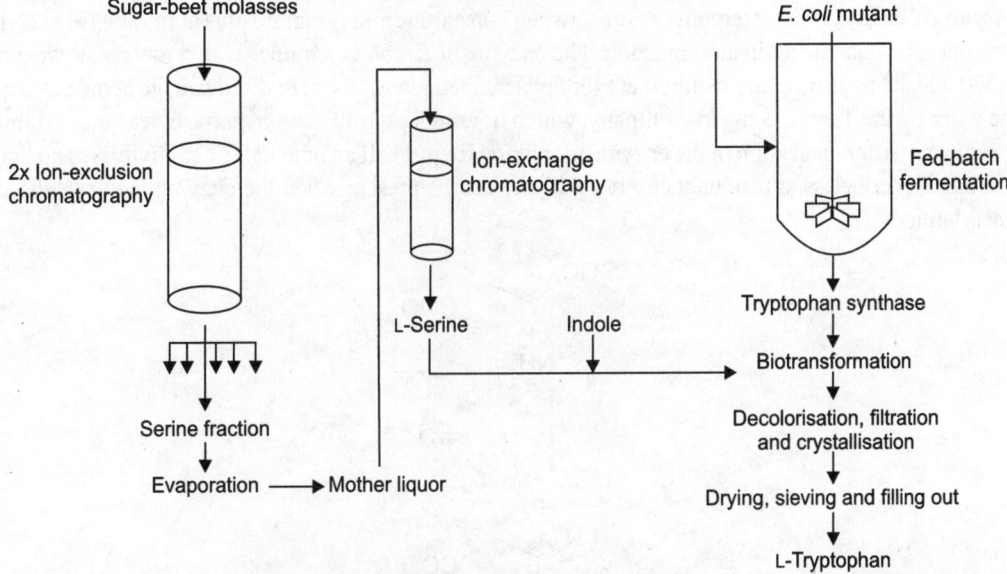

Fig. 22.14. The tryptophan synthase uses *in vivo* indole 3-glycerol phosphate plus L-serine and in the production process indole plus L-serine.

Fig. 22.15. Production plant to fractionate molasses by ion-exclusion chromatography, with isolation of L-serine. An *E. coli* mutant overexpressing tryptophan synthase is pregrown and subsequently mixed with L-serine plus indole to convert these substrate to L-tryptophan.

Of all the essential amino acids, tryptophan is the one that is most investigated by nutrition researchers. Lack of tryptophan causes symptoms similar to those of vitamin A deficiency. Major sources of this amino acid are nuts, and most vegetables. As a natural relaxant:

1. It helps alleviate insomnia by inducing normal sleep (produces serotonin, which induces sleep; has a Serotonengenic effect).
2. Reported useful in the management of depression and schizophrenia.
3. Helps in the treatment of migraine headaches.
4. Helps the immune system.
5. Helps reduce the risk of artery and heart spasms.
6. Vasoconstrictor, which appears to aid in blood clotting mechanism.

7. Aids in elevating the threshold of pain.
8. Works with lysine in reducing cholesterol levels.
9. Precursor of the vitamin Niacin.

L-ASPARTATE

L-Aspartic acid is widely used as a food additive and in pharmaceuticals. Demand increased rapidly with the introduction of aspartame as an artificial sweetener. This is a dipeptide consisting of L-aspartate and L-phenylalanine which is about 200-fold sweeter than sugar and was successfully introduced into the market as a low-calorie sweetener. Although L-aspartate as originally produced fermentatively, it is currently produced exclusively using aspartase due to the high productivities and the cost effectiveness of the process. In fact, the use of aspartase to make L-aspartate represents one of the highest productivities known for an enzyme used in biotechnology. The method developed allows reuse of the enzyme to the extent that over 2,20,000 kg of product can be produced per kg of enzyme.

Aspartase catalyses the interconversion between L-aspartate and fumarate plus ammonia (Fig. 22.16). The reaction favours the amination reaction. The enzyme of *E. coli* is tetramer with a molecular weight of 1,96,000 which has an absolute requirement for divalent metal ions. A severe disadvantage at the beginning of the work by the Tanabe Seiyaku company, which now successfully uses aspartase, was the instability of the enzyme. After incubation of the enzyme in solution for just half an hour at 50°C, activity was no longer detectable. Nevertheless, a residual activity of 10 per cent is present when the enzyme is immobilised in polyacrylamide.

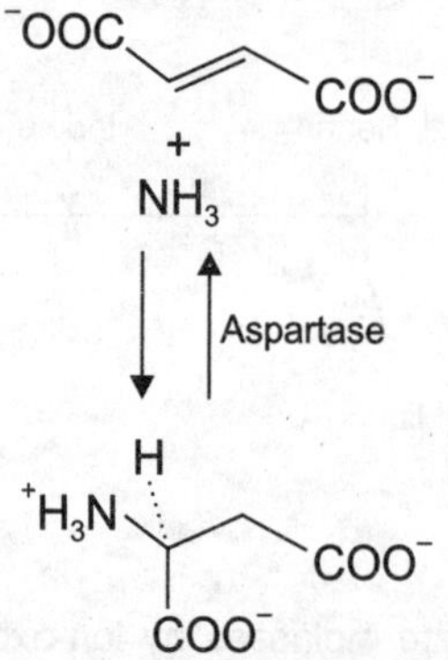

Fig. 22.16. Fumarate and ammonium serve as substrates for the aspartase.

Such a physical confinement of cells in space turned out to be the method of choice. Table 22.5 shows that with the natural polymer k-carrageenan, resulting from a screening of different polymers and use of appropriate cross-lining exceptional improvements are obtained in the relative productivity as well as in the stability of the catalyst. The final material has a half-life of almost two years. This represents almost unimaginable progress in comparison to the initial situation where enzyme in free solution only had a half-life measured in minutes. An initial disadvantage of the original cells used, was their fumarase activity which results in the partial conversion of fumarate to L-malic acid.

To solve this problem a heat treatment step of the cells is used which eliminates the fumarase activity almost completely. Using such conditioned cells and starting with 1 M ammonium fumarate, the final product solution contains 987 mM L-aspartate, 10.7 mM non-reacted fumarate and only trace quantities of L-malic acid of 1.9 mM.

For the production process the immobilised cells are packed into a column designed as a multistage system. The stages introduced, consisting of horizontal tubes, serve two purposes. On the one hand, they allow effective cooling to prevent decay of the catalytic activity since the aspartase reaction is exergonic. About 6 kcal heat mol^{-1} substrate evolves in the actual large-scale production process which is very close to that calculated from the standard free energy change of the aspartase reaction of 4 kcal mol^{-1}. On the other hand, the flow properties of the column are increased. Any compacting of the bed over time is prevented and the preferred plug-flow characteristics are obtained. With such a column, flow rates of two column volumes per hour are possible. The continuous process enables full automation and control to achieve an optimum throughput with the highest product quality. Yet another advantage of such a controlled continuous process is its reduced waste production. A typical volumetric activity is about 200 mmol hr^{-1} g cells. Assuming a 1000 litre column, the yield of L-aspartate is 3.4 T per day which is 100 T per month. The final product is eventually purified by crystallisation.

Table 22.5. Comparison of immobilised *E. coli* cells used for production of L-aspartate.

Immobilisation method	Aspartase activity (U/g cells)	Half-life (days)	Relative productivity (%)[a]
Polyacrylamide	18850	120	100
Carrageenan	56340	70	174
Carrageenan (GA)[b]	37460	240	397
Carrageenan (GA + HA)[b]	49400	680	1498

Notes: [a]Considers the activity, decay constant and operation period. [b]GA = glutaraldehyde, HA = hexamethylene diamine.

Aspartic acid is a non-essential, natural dibasic amino acid, involved in transamination reactions, the ornithine cycle, and the formation of carnosine, anserine, purines and pyrimidines. It has a protective function over the liver and helps in detoxification of ammonia. Besides, it also promotes mineral uptake in the intestinal tract and is part of the sweetener Aspartain that is a dypeptide of the amino acids, aspartic acid and phenylalanine.

Aspartic acid is an important intermediate in the citric acid cycle. It aids in the expulsion of harmful ammonia from the body. When ammonia enters the circulatory system it acts as a highly toxic substance which can be harmful to the central nervous system. Recent studies have shown that aspartic acid may increase resistance to fatigue and increase endurance. Asparagine is the amide derivative of aspartic acid. Production of amino acids by fermentation is given in Table 22.6 and enzymatic production of amino acids is given in Table 22.7.

Table 22.6. Production of amino acids by fermentation.

Amino acid	Strain used	Genetic characteristics	Yield (g/l)	Carbon source
D,L-Alanine	*Microbacterium ammoniaphilum*	ArgHx^r	60	Glucose
L-Alanine	*Pseudomonas* no. 483	Wild type	17.5	Glucose
L-Arginine	*Serratia marcescens* AT 428 (*aru argR2 argA2*)	Transduction Canavanine^r	50	Glucose

(Contd ...)

Amino acid	Strain used	Genetic characteristics	Yield (g/l)	Carbon source
L-Aspartic acid	Escherichia coli K1-1023*		56	Fumaric acid
L-Glutamic acid	Corynebacterium glutamicum	Wild type	100	Glucose
	Brevibacterium flavum		98	Acetate
	Arthrobacter paraffineus		82	n-Alkanes
L-Glutamine	Corynebacterium glutamicum	Wild type of glutamic acid producer	58	Glucose, with high biotin and NH$_4$Cl content
L-Histidine	Serratia marcescens L 120 (pSH 368)	rDNA	40	Sucrose
L-Isoleucine	B. flavum	Eth^r	30	Acetate
L-Leucine	Brevibacterium lactofermentum	Ile$^-$ Met$^-$ TA^r	28	Glucose
L-Lysine	B. lactofermentum AJ 11204	AEC^{r}Ala$^-$ CCL^{r}ML^{r}FP^s	70	Glucose
	B. flavum	Hom^{leaky} Thre$^-$	75	Acetate
L-Methionine	C. glutamicum KY 9276	Thr Eth^r MetHx^r	2	Glucose
L-Ornithine	C. glutamicum	Arg$^-$	26	Glucose
L- Phenylalanine	B. lactofermentum	5MT^{r}PFP^{r}Decr Tyr^{r}Met$^-$	25	Glucose
L-Proline	C. acetoacidophilum	Uncharacterised mutant	108	Glucose + Glutamic acid
L-Serine	B. lactofermentum	SG^r	4.5	Glucose
L- Threonine	E. coli VL 344 (pYN7)	rDNA	55	Sucrose
L- Tryptophan	E. coli JP 4114	rDNA	23.5	Glucose
L- Tyrosine	C. glutamicum Pr-20	Phe$^-$ PFP^r P AP^r PAT^r TyrHx^r	18	Glucose
L-Valine	Brevibacterium lactofermentum No. 487	TA^r	31	Glucose

*Technique used for the production of L-aspartic acid between 1960 and 1973. Resistance: AEC S-(β-Aminoethyl)-L-cysteine; ArgHx Arginine hydroxamate; CCL, α-Chlorcaprolactam; Dec, Decoyinine; Eth Ethionine; FP, β-Fluoropyruvate; MetHx Methionine hydroxamate; ML, γ-Methyl-L-lysine; 5 MT 5-Methyltryptophan; PAP p-Amino-phenylalanine; PAT p-Aminotyrosine; PFP p-Fluorophenylalanine; SG Sulphaguanidine; TA 2-Thiazolalanine; TyrHx Tyrosine hydroxamate. Auxotrophs: Ala, alanine; arg, arginine; hom, homoserine; ile, isoleucine; met, methionine; phe, phenylalanine; thr, threonine; tyr, tyrosine. aru: block in arginine degradation; argR: biosynthetic enzyme is derepressed; argA: N-acetylglutamate synthesis is insensitive to feedback inhibition by arginine.

Table 22.7. Enzymatic production of amino acids.

Amino acid	Enzyme	Enzyme-producing micro-organism	Reaction	Yield (g/l)	Efficiency (%)
L-Alanine	Aspartate decarboxylase (RC)	Pseudomonas dacunhae	L-Aspartate→L-Alanine + CO_2	600	100
L-Aspartic acid	Aspartase (IC)	Escherichia coli	Fumarate + NH_4^+ → L-Aspartic acid	560	99
L-Cysteine	Cysteine desulphydrase (RC)	Bacillus sphaericus	β-Chloro-L-alanine + Na_2S → L-Cysteine + NaCl + NaOH	70	80–85
L-DOPA (L-3,4-Di-hydroxyphenyl-alanine)	Tyrosinase (RC)	Erwinia herbicola	Pyrocatechol + Pyruvate + NH_4^+ → L-DOPA + H_2O	59	95
L-Leucine	L-Leucine dehydrogenase (EMR)	Bacillus sphaericus	α-Ketoisocapronic acid + NH_4^+ + NADH-L-Leucine + H_2O + NAD^+	42 $g \cdot l^{-1} d^{-1}$	max. 99.7
L-Lysine	D-Amino-caprolactam racemase, L-Amino-caprolactam hydrolase (RC)	Achromobacter obae, Cryptococcus laurentii	DL-Aminocaprolactam + H_2O → L-Lysine	100	100
L-Phenyl-alanine	L-Phenylalanine dehydrogenase (ER)	Brevibacterium sp.	Phenylpyruvate + NH_4^+ → L-Phenylalanine+ H_2O	37 $g \cdot l^{-1} d^{-1}$	
	Acetamidocinnamate amidohydrolase (RC)	Bacillus sphaericus	Acetamido cinnamic acid → L-Phenylalanine	8	94
	Phenylalanine ammonia lyase (RC)	Rhodotorula glutinis	trans-Cinnamic acid + NH_4^+ → L-Phenylalanine	18	70
	Aspartate phenylalanine transaminase (EMR)	E. coli	L-Aspartate + Phenylpyruvate → L-Phenylalanine + Oxalacetate	30	98
	D-Hydroxyisocaproate dehydrogenase	Lactobacillus casei	D,L-Phenyllactate → Phenylpyruvate		
	L-Hydroxyisocaproate dehydrogenase	Lactobacillus confusus			
	L-Phenylalanine dehydrogenase (EMR)	Rhodococcus sp.	Phenylpyruvate + NH_4^+ → L-Phenylalanine + H_2O	28 $g \cdot l^{-1} d^{-1}$	

(Contd...)

Amino acid	Enzyme	Enzyme-producing micro-organism	Reaction	Yield (g/l)	Efficiency (%)
L-Serine	Serine hydroxymethyl transferase (CCE)	*Klebsiella aerogenes*	Glycine + HCHO → L-Serine	450	88
L-Tryptophan	Serine hydroxymethyl transferase	*Klebsiella aerogenes*	Glycine + HCHO → L-Serine	200	95 based on indole
	Tryptophanase (ER)	*E. coli*	L-Serine + Indole → L-Tryptophan + H_2O		
L-Tyrosine	Serine hydroxymethyl transferase	*Klebsiella aerogenes*	Glycine + HCHO → L-Serine		
	β-Tyrosinase (RC)	*Erwinia herbicola*	L-Serine + Phenol → L-Tyrosine + H_2O	26	61 based on glycine

EMR, enzyme/membrane reactor; IC, immobilised cells; RC, resting cells; CCE, crude cell extract.

OTHER AMINO ACIDS

Methionine

This is a vital sulphur bearing compound which helps dissolve cholesterol and assimilates fat. It is required by haemoglobin, the pancreas, the lymph and the spleen. It is necessary to maintain normal body weight and also helps maintain the proper nitrogen balance in the body.

Rich sources of methionine are Brazil nut, Hazel nut, and other nuts. It is also found in Brussel sprouts, cabbage, cauliflower, pineapples and apples. Its deficiency can lead to chronic rheumatic fever in children, hardening of the liver (cirrhosis) and nephritis of the kidneys. Studies show that methionine and chorine prevent tumours and proliferation. It prevents deposits and cohesion of fats in the liver and gives rise to taurine (an important inhibitory neuro-modulator in the brain). The sulphur it provides has the following benefits:

1. Prevents disorders of the hair, skin and nail.
2. Helps lower cholesterol levels by increasing the liver's production of lecithin.
3. Reduces liver fat and protects the kidneys.
4. Acts as a natural chelating agent for heavy metals.
5. Regulates the formation of ammonia and creates ammonia-free urine which reduces bladder irritation.
6. Influences hair follicles and promotes hair growth.

Valine

Valine is an essential body growth factor, particularly for mammary glands and ovaries. Valine is directly linked with the nervous system. It is essential for the prevention of nervous and digestive disorders.

Major sources are almonds, apples and most vegetables. Lack of this amino acid makes a person sensitive to touch and sound. Valine is a hydrophobic aliphatic amino acid used to hold proteins together. It promotes mental vigour, muscle coordination and calm emotions and is required in the precursors of cholesterol.

Leucine and Isoleucine

Leucine and isoleucine are hydrophobic amino acids used almost exclusively in protein and enzyme construction. They provide ingredients for the manufacturing of other essential biochemical components in the body, some of which are utilised for the production of energy, stimulants to the upper brain and helping one to be more alert. They are essential for optimal growth in infants, and for nitrogen equilibrium in adults. Rich sources are sunflower seeds, all nuts, except cashew nuts, avacados and olives.

Leucine (and isoleucine) are metabolised along the same pathways as fat. It is a precursor of cholesterol and is involved in the role of energy release during any work of the muscles.

Arginine

This amino acid is often used at the active sites of enzymes. It occurs in proteins; and is involved in the urea cycle, which converts ammonia to urea. This is called the 'fatherhood' amino acid as it comprises 80 per cent of all male reproductive cells. It is essential for normal growth. Serious lack of this amino acid reduces the sex instinct, causing impotence. It is found in most vegetables, especially, green and root vegetables. Same of its features are given below:

1. Induces growth hormone release from the pituitary gland.

2. Is a major component of seminal fluid.
3. Is helpful in burn treatment, elevated ammonia levels and cirrhosis of the liver.
4. Stimulates immune response by enhancing the production of t-cells.
5. Has protective effect of toxicity of hydrocarbons and intravenous diuretics.

Tyrosine

This can be called an anti-stress amino acid. Tyrosine is also beneficial for depression, nervousness, irritability and despondency. Research has established this amino acid to be effective in the management and control of depression in conjunction with glutamine, tryptophan, niacin and vitamin B6. It is also helpful in the treatment of allergies and high blood pressure.

It is a naturally occurring amino acid present in most proteins. Tyrosine is a product of Phenylalanine metabolism and a precursor of thyroid hormones, catecholamines and melanin. It is a hydroxyl-phenyl amino acid that is used to build neurotransmitters and hormones. It transmits nerve impulses to the brain, helps overcome depression, improves memory, increases mental alertness and promotes the healthy functioning of the thyroid, adrenal and pituitary glands. Along with phenylalanine it is a useful anti depressant due to increased production of tacolamine and is reported to stabilise blood pressure by lowering energy in some cases and elevating it in others.

Tyrosine is involved in tissue pigmentation and is important in the formation of thyroid hormone.

Glycine

Glycine is the simplest amino acid, occurring as a constituent of proteins and functioning as an inhibitory neurotransmitter in the central nervous system. It helps trigger the release of oxygen to the energy requiring cell-making process and is important in the manufacturing of hormones responsible for a strong immune system.

Glycine is used as a gastric antacid and dietary supplement, and in the treatment of various myopathies. It is the simplest and sweetest of amino acids and can be used as a sweetener in herbal beverages. It is reported useful in degenerative diseases such as muscular dystrophy (MD) and detoxifies benzoic acid (a common food additive) and aromatic hydrocarbons in the liver. Glycine is also involved in synthesis of nucleic acids and bioacids and may be useful in conditions characterised by abnormal nerve firing such as epilepsy, inhibition of tripeptides glutathione and GTF.

It is one of the amino acids in the tripeptides glutathione and GTF. Low brain concentrations of glycine have recently been found in ALS.

Serine

This non-essential amino acid alcohol is found in the active site of serine proteases. Serine is a storage source of glucose by the liver and muscles and helps strengthen the immune system by providing antibodies. It synthesises fatty acid sheath around nerve fibres.

Taurine

This mercaptan-containing amino acid is involved in bile acid biochemistry. It helps stabilise the excitability of membranes which is very important in the control of epileptic seizures. Taurine and sulphur are considered to be factors necessary for the control of many biochemical changes that take place in the ageing process; it also aids in the clearing of free radical wastes. Taurine is a crystallised acid, ethylamine sulphonic acid, from the bile; found also in small quantities in lung and muscle tissue.

Some of its features are the following:
1. Low levels seen in newborn infants fed low Taurine diets.
2. Associated with retinal degenerations.
3. The role of Taurine as a nutrient is to protect the cell membranes by attenuating such toxic compounds as oxidants, secondary bioacids and antibiotics.
4. Recommended for children on long-term parenteral nutrition.
5. Helpful in balancing calcium and potassium flux in heart muscle.
6. Helps patients suffering from congenitive heart failure by alleviating their physical signs and symptoms.
7. Increases left ventricular performance without any significant changes in atrial pressure.
8. Often times considered a neuro modulator.
9. Helpful in treating some types of epilepsy.
10. Does not readily pass across the blood brain barrier because of its two polar and non fat-soluble nature.

Cystine

Cysteine is the thiol containing amino acid involved in active sites and protein tertiary structure determination. Cystine is the oxidation product of cysteine that holds proteins together. An essential, sulphur-containing amino acid, produced by digestion or acid hydrolysis of proteins, it is sometimes found in the urine and kidneys, and is readily reduced to two molecules of Cysteine. It provides resistance by building up white-cell activity. It is an indispensable amino acid. It is one of the mainstays of health as it is essential for the proper formation of skin and helps one recover from surgery. It promotes the formation of carolene which helps hair growth. It is used in the treatment of skin diseases, for low white blood-cells counts and for some cases of anaemia. Cystine's functions and features are as follows:
1. Acts as an antioxidant and is a powerful aid to the body in protecting against radiation and pollution.
2. Can help slow down the ageing process, deactivate free radicals, neutralise toxins.
3. Aids in protein synthesis and presents cellular change.
4. Is necessary for the formation of the skin, which aids in the recovery from burns and surgical operations. Hair and skin are made up 10–14 per cent cystine.
5. Reported helpful in dermatological conditions.
6. Promotes faster recovery of tissue after surgery.
7. Part of the insulin molecule.
8. Found high in hair (sulphur bonds).

Histidine

Histidine is the amino acid responsible for histamine biosynthesis. Histidine is found abundantly in haemoglobin and has been used in the treatment of rheumatoid arthritis, allergic diseases, ulcers and anemia. Deficiency can cause poor hearing. Histidine is not listed as essential for adults, but is very essential for infants.

It is an amino acid obtainable from many proteins by the action of sulphuric acid and water; and it is essential for optimal growth in infants. Decarboxylation results in formation of histamine. Release of histamines from body stores are required for sexual arousal. It is also reported to be useful in alleviating pain associated with rheumatoid arthritis.

Proline

This cyclic aliphatic amino acid used in the synthesis of collagen. Is extremely important as an anti-hypotensive agent in lowering high blood pressure; in repairing muscle and tendon damage; and in promoting skin flexibility in relation to ageing and sun exposure.

Alanine

It is the second simplest amino acid, but used mostly in proteins. Beta-alanine is the only naturally occurring *beta* amino acid. Alanine is an important source of energy for muscle tissue, the brain and central nervous system. It strengthens the immune system by producing antibodies and helps in the metabolism of sugars and organic acids.

Chapter 23

Vinegar

INTRODUCTION

Vinegar is an acidic liquid processed from the fermentation of ethanol in a process that yields its key ingredient, acetic acid (also called ethanoic acid). It also may come in a diluted form. The acetic acid concentration typically ranges from 4 to 8 per cent by volume for table vinegar (typically 5 per cent) and higher concentration for pickling (up to 18 per cent). Natural vinegars also contain small amounts of tartaric acid, citric acid and other acids. Vinegar has been used since ancient times and is an important element in European, Asian and other traditional cuisines of the world.

Vinegar has a density of approximately 0.96 g/ml. The density level depends on the acidity of the vinegar. Household vinegar used for cooking is 1.05 g/ml.

KINDS OF VINEGAR

Vinegars may be classified on the basis of the materials from which they have been made: (i) those from the juices of fruits, e.g. apples, grapes, oranges, pears, berries, etc. (ii) those from starchy vegetables, e.g. potatoes or sweet potatoes, whose starch must first be hydrolysed to sugars, (iii) those from malted cereals, such as barley, rye, wheat, and corn, (iv) those from sugars, such as sirups, molasses, honey, maple skimmings, etc. and (v) those from spirits or alcohol, e.g. from waste alcoholic liquor (beer) from yeast manufacture or from dilute, denatured ethyl alcohol. Anything, in fact, that contains enough sugar or alcohol and is in no way objectionable as food may be used to make vinegar. The base materials for the production of vinegar are shown in Table 23.1. The vinegar usually derives its descriptive name from the material from which it was made: cider vinegar from apple juice, alegar from ale, malt vinegar from malted grains, spirit vinegar from alcohol, etc. In the United States most table vinegar is cider vinegar, and therefore the term vinegar by itself usually means cider vinegar. Vinegar from grapes (wine) is most popular in France, and vinegar from malt liquors (alegar) in the British Isles.

Table 23.1. Base materials for the production of vinegar.

Apple	Palm sap
Banana (and skins)	Peach
Cashew apples	Pear
Cocoa sweatings	Persimmon

(Contd ...)

Coconut water	Pineapple
Coffee pulp	Prickly pear
Dates	Prune
Ethanol	Rice
Honey	Sugar cane
Jackfruit	Sweet potato
Jamun	Tamarind
Kiwi fruit	Tea
Malted barley	Tomato
Mango	Watermelon
Maple products	Whey
Molasses	Wine
Orange	

Fermentation

As has been indicated, the manufacture of vinegar from saccharine materials involves two steps: (i) the fermentation of sugar to ethyl alcohol, and (ii) the oxidation of alcohol to acetic acid. The first step is an anaerobic process carried out by yeasts, either those naturally present in the raw material or, preferably, added cultures of high-alcohol-producing strains of *Saccharomyces cerevisiae* var. *ellipsoideuis*. A simplified equation for the process is:

$$C_6H_{12}O_6 \longrightarrow 2CO_2 + 2C_2H_5OH$$
$$\text{glucose} \qquad\qquad\qquad \text{alcohol}$$

Actually a series of intermediate reactions takes place, and small amounts of other final products are produced, such as glycerol and acetic acid. Also, there are small amounts of other substances, produced from compounds other than sugar, including succinic acid and amyl alcohol.

The second step, oxidation of the alcohol to acetic acid, is an aerobic reaction carried out by the acetic acid bacterial (Fig. 23.1).

$$C_2H_5OH + O_2 \longrightarrow CH_3COOH + H_2O$$
$$\text{alcohol} \quad \text{oxygen} \qquad \text{acetic acid} \quad \text{water}$$

Acetaldehyde is an intermediate compound in this reaction. Among the final products are small amounts of aldehydes, esters, acetoin, etc.

Scientists have found three groups of *Acetobacter* with a total of nine subspecies. The genus *Gluconobacter* contained species capable of oxidizing ethanol to acetic acid. Further a Family called Acetobacteriaceae with two genera, *Acetobacter* and *Gluconobacter* have been suggested. The later species are differentiated from *Acetobacter* by their inability to oxidise acetic or lactic acid to carbon dioxide. *Acetobacter* is currently described as containing species which can oxidise acetic or lactic acid to carbon dioxide. Many 'acetic acid bacteria' are now classified in the genus *Gluconobacter*. Although the majority of the vinegar fermentation 'work' may be done by *Gluconobacter* sp., the cultures actually used commercially are not pure but rather are a mixture of strains that have been adapted to the fermentation.

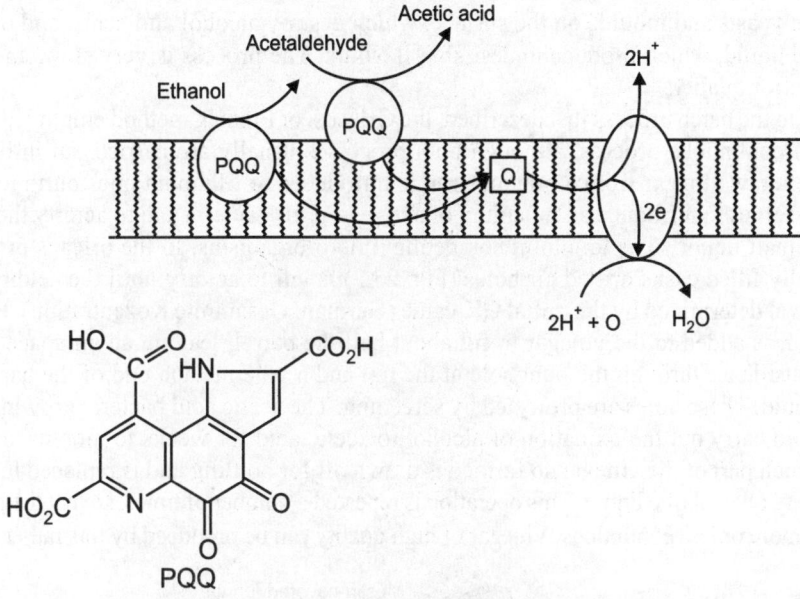

Fig. 23.1. Oxidation of ethanol by acetic acid bacteria.

Methods of Manufacture

The ways of making vinegar may be divided into the 'slow' methods, such as the home, or 'let-alone', method and the French, or Orleans, method, and 'quick' methods, such as the generator process or the fogging procedure. In slow methods the alcoholic liquid is not moved during acetification, while in quick methods the alcoholic liquid is in motion. For the most part the slow methods utilise fermented fruit juices or malt liquors for acetic acid production, whereas the quick methods are applied mostly to the production of vinegar from spirits (alcohol). Fruit or malt liquors are well supplied with food for the vinegar bacteria, but to maintain active vinegar bacteria in generator methods using alcohol, denatured with ethyl acetate or vinegar, it must be supplemented with a 'vinegar food', which is a combination of organic and inorganic compounds that varies with the compounder. Combinations of substances such as dibasic ammonium phosphate, urea, asparagine, peptones, yeast extract, glucose, malt, starch, dextrins, salts, and other substances have been reported in use.

Slow methods

In the home, or let-alone, method, a fruit juice such as apple juice is allowed to undergo a spontaneous alcoholic fermentation, preferably to about 11 to 13 per cent of alcohol, by yeasts originally present, after which a barrel is partially filled with the fermented juice and placed on its side with the bunghole upward and open. Then the alcoholic solution is allowed to undergo an acetic acid fermentation, called acetification, carried out by vinegar bacteria naturally present until vinegar is produced. A film of vinegar bacteria called 'mother of vinegar' should grow on the surface of the liquid and oxidise the alcohol to acetic acid. Unfortunately, the yield may be low because of a poor yield of alcohol during the yeast fermentation, because of the absence of productive strains of vinegar bacteria, because of the oxidation of acetic acid by the vinegar bacteria if there is a shortage of alcohol, or because of the competitive growth of film yeasts and moulds on the surface, which destroy alcohol and acids, and of undesirable bacteria in the liquid, which produce undesirable flavours. The process is very slow, and the product often is of inferior quality.

In contrast to the batch process just described, the Orleans, or French, method employed considerably in Europe is a continuous process, although both processes usually are carried out in barrels. In the Orleans process raw vinegar from a previous run is introduced to fill about one-fourth to one-third of the barrel and serves to introduce an inoculum of active vinegar bacteria and to acidify the added wine, hard cider, or malt liquor so as to inhibit competing micro-organisms. In the orleans process vinegar stock is partially filled casks drilled air holes (Fig. 23.2) is left to acidify until the acidity reaches the appropriate level determined by the initial GK value (German: Gesammte Kozentration). Enough of the alcoholic liquor is added to the vinegar to fill about half the barrel, leaving an air space above that is open to the outside air through the bunghole at the top and a hole in each end of the barrel above the level of the liquid. These holes are protected by screening. The acetic acid bacteria growing in a film on top of the liquid carry out the oxidation of alcohol to acetic acid for weeks to months at about 21° to 29°C, after which part of the vinegar so formed is drawn off for bottling and is replaced in the barrel by an equal quantity of alcoholic liquor. This operation is repeated a number of times, so that the process in this way becomes more or less continuous. Vinegar of high quality can be produced by this rather slow process.

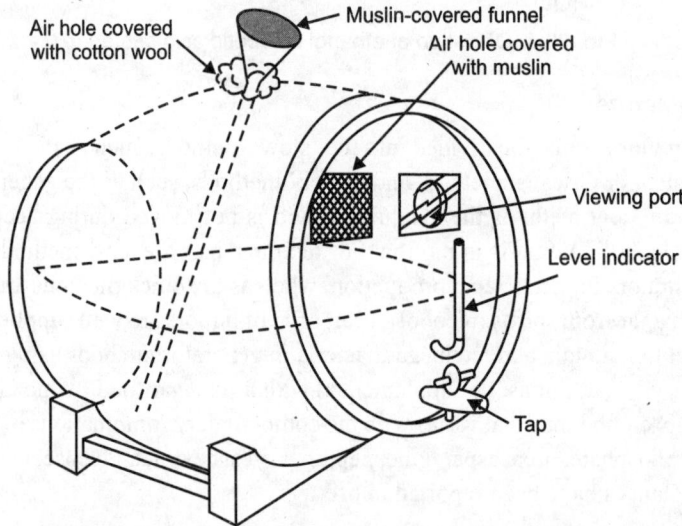

Fig. 23.2. The orleans process of vinegar manufacture.

One difficulty in this method is the dropping of the gelatinous film of vinegar bacteria and the resulting retardation of acetification. To avoid this difficulty a raft or floating framework sometimes is provided to support the film. It is claimed that too heavy a bacterial film will result in reduced acetification.

Quick methods

As has been indicated, quick methods of vinegar manufacture involve the movement of the alcoholic liquid during the process of acetification. Most commonly this liquid is trickled down over surfaces on which films of the vinegar bacteria have grown and to which a plentiful supply of air is provided.

The generator method is the one in common use at present. The simple generator is a cylindrical tank that comes in different sizes and usually is made of wood. The interior is divided into three parts:

an upper section, where the alcoholic liquid is introduced; the large middle section, where the liquid is allowed to trickle down over beechwood shavings, corncobs, rattan shavings, charcoal, coke, pomace, or some other material that will give a large total surface yet not settle into a compact mass; and the bottom section, where the vinegar collects. The alcoholic liquid is fed in at the top through an automatic feed trough or a sprinkling device (sparger) and trickled down over the shavings or other material on which has developed a slimy growth of acetic acid bacteria, which oxidise the alcohol to acetic acid. Air enters through the false bottom of the middle section and, on becoming warm, rises, to be vented above. Since the oxidation process here releases considerable heat, it usually is necessary to control the temperature so that it does not rise much above 29° to 30°C. This can be done by using cooling coils, by adjusting the rate of feeding air and alcoholic liquid, and by cooling the alcoholic liquid before it enters the generator or by cooling the partially acetified liquid that is returned to the top from the bottom section of the tank for further action. In starting a new generator, the slime of vinegar bacteria must be established before vinegar can be made. First, the middle section of the tank is filled with raw vinegar that contains active vinegar bacteria to inoculate the shavings with the desired bacteria, or this material is circulated through the generator. Then an alcoholic liquid, acidified with vinegar, is slowly trickled through the generator to build up bacterial growth on the shavings and then is recirculated. Some makers acidify all the alcoholic liquid with vinegar before introducing it into the generator or leave some vinegar to acidify the new lot of liquid.

The vinegar may be made by one run of the alcoholic liquid through the generator, or the vinegar collected at the bottom may be recirculated through the generator if insufficient acid has been produced at first or too much alcohol is left. Sometimes generators are operated in tandem, the liquid from the first tank going through second or even a third generator.

The vinegar generator (Fig. 23.3) is a large, cylindrical, airtight tank equipped with a sparger (sprinkler) at the top, cooling coils about the lower part of the middle section containing the shavings, and facilities for the recirculation of the vinegar from the bottom collection chamber through the system. Modern types of these generators are equipped with automatic controls for feeding the alcoholic liquid, for introducing filtered air, for controlling temperature, and for recirculating the liquid collected at the bottom. These generators give high yields of acetic acid and leave little residue of alcohol.

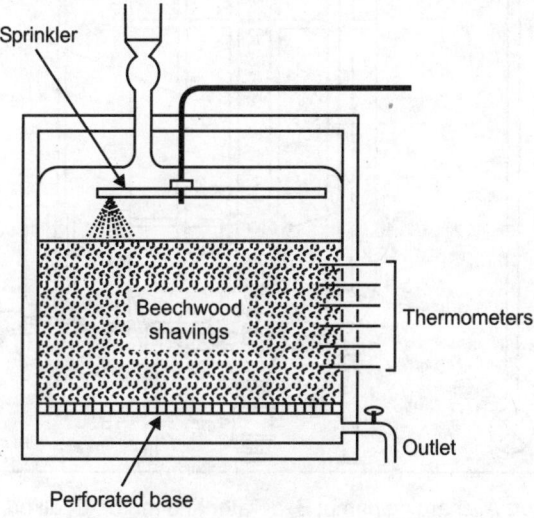

Fig. 23.3. A vinegar generator.

In the Mackin process, a fog or fine mist of a mixture of vinegar bacteria and nutrient alcohol solution is sprayed through jet nozzles into a chamber. The mist is kept in circulation by filtered air for a while and then is allowed to fall to the bottom for collection, to be cooled, reatomised, and returned to the chamber. This process is continued until oxidation of the alcohol is almost complete.

The dipping generator consists of a tank containing a basket filled with beechwood shavings that can be raised out of or lowered into dilute alcohol solution in the lower part of the tank. While the basket is out of the liquid, aeration permits rapid acetification by vinegar bacteria on the shavings, and lowering the basket into the liquid adds more culture medium and removes some of the acetic acid made.

Submerged method

In submerged fermentation a stirred medium containing 8 to 12 per cent alcohol (hard cider, wine, fermented malt mash or spirits) is inoculated with *Acetobacter acetigenum* and is held at 24° to 29°C with controlled aeration by means of finely divided air. Later, Hromatka described the use of a pure culture of *Gluconobacter oxydans* in a submerged vinegar fermentation. The frings acetator, shown in Fig. 23.4, is an example of equipment for this method, which uses a patented self-printing aerator to achieve very efficient oxygen transfer.

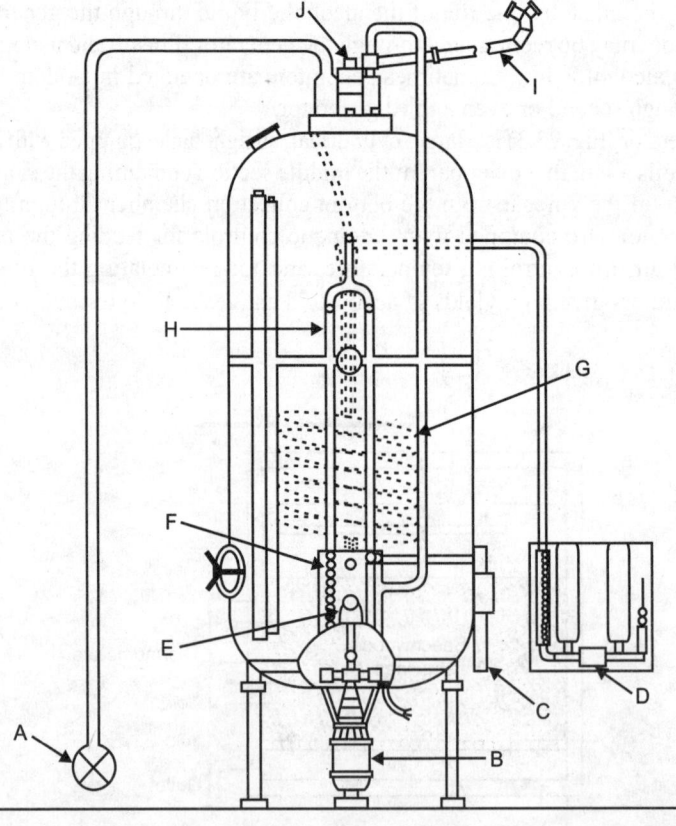

Fig. 23.4. The frings acetator. A, charging pump; B, aerator and motor; C, alkograph; D, cooling water valve; E, thermostat controlling D; F, rotameter; G, cooling coil; H, air line; I, air exhaust line; J, defoamer.

Submerged culture is very efficient and rapid, a semicontinuous run normally takes 24–48 hours. It does however require far more careful control than simpler processes. The acetic acid bacteria are very susceptible to interruptions to the air supply, indicating that, in order to survive suspended in a medium with a pH of 2.5 and 10–14 per cent acidity, the bacteria need a constant supply of energy from respiration. A stoppage of only one minute in a stock with a GK of 11.35 is enough to completely arrest acetification which will not resume when aeration is resumed.

Another possible cause of fermentation failure in submerged acetification is phage infection. The presence of bacteriophage particles has been demonstrated in disturbed vinegar fermentations both in submerged acetifiers and the quick vinegar process. The performance of quick vinegar generators appears to be less affected as their acetification rate may slow but rarely stops. This is probably due to the greater heterogeneity of the culture present which allows organisms of different phage susceptibility to take over in the event of phase attack.

Where legal definitions of vinegar exist, it is specified as a fermentation product. 'Artificial vinegars' made by diluting and colouring acetic acid are thus excluded and, in the UK, have to be known rather laboriously as 'non-brewed condiment'. Although vinegar can be made up to 14 per cent acidity, it is usually diluted down to an appropriate strength for bottling. The minimum acetic acid content is usually prescribed to be something between 4 and 6 per cent w/v, but higher strength vinegars are available for pickling.

Finishing

The composition of vinegar depends, of course, on the material from which it was made. Vinegars from fruits and malt liquors carry flavours characteristic of these materials. The method of manufacture also influences the character of the product. Vinegars made by slow methods are less harsh than those made by quick methods because of the ageing undergone during the long time of preparation. Quickly made vinegars, when aged in tanks or barrels, improve in body, taste and bouquet. Filtration and 'fining', which is clarification by the settling out of added suspended materials, are employed to clarify the vinegar, which should be very clear. Most market vinegar now is pasteurised in bulk or in the bottles. Times and temperatures vary, but heating at 60° to 66°C for a few seconds is an example.

The strength of the vinegar is expressed in grains, that is, ten times the number of grams of acetic acid per 100 ml of vinegar. Thus 40 grain vinegar contains 4 gram of acetic acid per 100 ml of vinegar at 20°C.

Vinegar Defects and Diseases

As in wines, metals and their salts may cause cloudiness and discolouration of vinegar. Ferrous iron may be oxidised to ferric iron and combine with tannins, phosphates or proteins to produce a haze. Cloudiness also may be caused by salts of tin or copper. Iron acting on tannin or oxidase activity may be responsible for the darkening of vinegar.

Malt Vinegar

Malting of barley and ensuing mashing and fermentation are exactly analogous to the approaches for beer. However, of course, no hops are used in the boiling stage. Adjuncts such as corn or rice may be used. The alcoholic solution obtained is separated from the yeast and inoculated with Acetobacter. Such vinegar must contain at least 4 per cent w/v acetic acid.

Distilled malt vinegar (colourless) is made by the distillation of malt vinegar and is used, for example, in the pickling of onions.

Wine Vinegar

This is the main vinegar on the continent of Europe, and is made from low alcohol wines (7–9 per cent) or from those with too high volatile acidity. Any wines that have too high an alcohol content must be diluted; otherwise, the acetobacter will be inhibited. Too high a sulphur dioxide level or sediment level will also be a problem. When produced on a small scale, the wine is mixed in small wooden barrels with mother vinegar. The barrel must contain air so it is not filled completely. The process halts naturally when the acetic acid content reaches 7–8 per cent w/v. The product will contain elevated levels of acetaldehyde and ethyl acetate when compared with the parent wine. Some of the vinegar will now be drawn off for use and replaced with fresh wine. Production on a larger scale is subject to EU regulations, with the stipulation that the total acid developed must be greater than 6 per cent w/v and the maximum surviving ethanol being less than 1.5 per cent v/v.

Other Vinegars

Cider vinegar is produced from hard cider or apple wine, has a yellow hue and may be coloured further with caramel. Such ciders tend to have a relatively low acidity. Vinegars may be made from a range of other fermented fruits, taking on some of the character of the original base.

Rice vinegar derives from the acetification of sake or its co-products. When compared with cider vinegar, rice vinegar tends to have a fairly low acidity and has a light and delicate flavour highly favoured for oriental cooking because of its low impact on the flavour imparted by the other materials in the dish.

Molasses has been used as a base for vinegar production (though not extensively) as a mechanism for dealing with by-products of the sugar industry. Mead has been employed as a vinegar base, too.

Spirit vinegar, sometimes called white distilled vinegar, is derived from alcohol obtained by the distillations of fermented sugar solutions. If legally permitted, synthetic ethanol is used, diluted to 10–14 per cent ABV. It is colourless of course, but may be darkened by the addition of caramel. As is to be expected, this is the cheapest vinegar to produce and, accordingly, is the one that is most widespread, for general use and, when diluted to 4–5 per cent for use in pickling.

Chemical Synthesis of Vinegar

Acetic acid can be produced by the catalytic oxidation of acetaldehyde, which in turn is produced by the catalytic hydration of acetylene or by the catalytic dehydrogenation of ethanol. The undesirable formic acid and formaldehyde are eliminated by distillation. The acetic acid is purified before diluting to 60–80 per cent by volume to obtain the vinegar essence. This in turn is diluted to 4–5 per cent in the generation of food grade 'vinegar'. Sugar, salt and colour may be added. In the United Kingdom, such a product must be labelled 'non-brewed condiment'.

Balsamic

At the other end of the quality spectrum is balsamic vinegar. It has been produced for hundreds of years in Northern Italy, notably the provinces of Modina and Reggio Emilia. The base material is grape must, preferably Trebbiano. Alcoholic fermentation is effected about 24 hours after pressing, with must gently boiled until it is reduce to a third or a half by volume. This leads to a high sugar concentration of about 30 per cent. The alcoholic fermentation and the acetification occur together very slowly. The relevant organisms are yeasts *Saccharomyces* and *Zygosaccharomyces* and bacteria *Acetobacter* and *Gluconobacter*. In the process, a series of chemical transformations alongside the slow microbial action leads to a flavoursome and complex mix of alcohols, aldehydes and organic acids.

The process is performed in a series of decreasingly sized barrels made of various types of wood. They are located in efficiently ventilated areas that are hot and dry in the summer months but cool in winter. Each year a portion from the smallest barrel is removed for consumption to be replaced by an equivalent amount from the next sized barrel, which in turn has its volume restored from the next barrel, and so on. The largest barrel is made up to volume using that season's boiled must. The finished product is dark brown, syrupy, sweet, sour (6–18 per cent acetic acid by weight) and with a pleasant aroma. This patient process takes at least a dozen years, with some products emerging for sale after as many as 50 years. Yields are perforce low (less than 1 l of vinegar from 100 kg of fresh must). The chemical composition and major volatile components of the main vinegars are shown in Tables 23.2 and 23.3, respectively.

Table 23.2. Chemical composition of vinegars.

Parameter	Balsamic	Cider	Malt	Wine	Synthetic
Specific gravity	1.042–1.361	1.013–1.024	1.013–1.022	1.013–1.02	1.007–1.022
Total solids (g l^{-1})	337–874	19–35	3.0–28.4	8.7–24.9	1.0–4.5
Total acidity (as acetic acid, %)	6.2–14.9	3.9–9.0	4.3–5.9	5.9–9.2	4.1–5.3
Sugars (g l^{-1})	351–690	1.5–7.0	–	0–6.2	–

Table 23.3. Volatile components in vinegars.

Volatile	Balsamic	Cider	Malt	Wine
Acetaldehyde	√	√	√	√
Acetone	√		√	√
Benzaldehyde		√	√	
2,3-Butanediol	√			√
2,3-Butanedione	√			
2-Butanone	√			
γ-Butyrolactone				√
Diethyl succinate		√		
Ethanol	√	√	√	√
Ethyl acetate	√	√	√	√
Ethyl formate	√	√	√	√
Ethyl lactate		√		
Furan	√			
Furfural	√			
3-Hydroxy-2-butanone	√			√
Isobutanal	√			
Isobutyl acetate			√	√
Isobutyl formate			√	√
Isopentyl acetate			√	√
Isopentyl formate			√	
Isovaleraldehyde				√
Methyl acetate	√			

(Contd ...)

Volatile	Balsamic	Cider	Malt	Wine
2-Methylbutanal	√			
2-Methyl-1-butanol		√	√	√
3-Methyl-1-butanol	√	√	√	√
2-Methyl-1-propanol		√	√	√
2- Methyl-3-butene-2-ol			√	
2-Pentanone		√	√	√
2-Pentanol		√		
3-Pentanol		√		
Phenylacetaldehyde		√		
Propionaldehyde		√		
2,4,5-Trimethyl-1,3-dioxolane	√			

Microbial defects

Defects caused by micro-organisms may result in inferior materials from which the vinegar is made or in inferiority of the condiment itself. Wine and hard cider, for example, are subject to the troubles listed in the discussion of diseases of wine. *Lactobacillus* and *Leuconostoc* species in fruit juice not only may be responsible for off-flavours, e.g. the 'mousy' taste, but also may produce enough acetic acid to interfere with the alcoholic fermentation by yeasts. Under anaerobic conditions butyric acid bacteria may produce their undesirable acid. These difficulties may be reduced by the addition of sulphur dioxide to the juices, but this chemical is inhibitory to the vinegar bacteria.

The defects of vinegar itself are confined for the most part to the production of excessive sliminess in the mass of vinegar bacteria and the destruction of acetic acid in the product. It has been mentioned that an especially heavy, thick, slimy film of bacteria in the slow process of vinegar manufacture reduces the rate of acetification. Excessive sliminess is much more harmful, however, in the generator process, for it interferes with aeration. Sliminess is favoured by an alcoholic liquid that is a good culture medium, e.g. cider, wine, or a medium to which too much rich vinegar food has been added, but is not ordinarily troublesome in the acetification of a poor medium like that used in making vinegar from spirits (alcohol). Several species of vinegar bacteria can cause sliminess (cellulose), but *Acetobacter aceti* subsp, *xylinum** is probably the most important one. Oxidation of acetic acid in vinegar to carbon dioxide and water can be brought about by the acetic acid bacteria themselves during the vinegar-making process if there is a shortage of alcohol or an excessive amount of aeration. Other organisms that can oxidise acetic acid under aerobic conditions are the film yeasts ('wine flowers'), moulds and algae.

Chapter 24

Fermentation Alcohol and Algae for Biofuels

INTRODUCTION

The search for alternative fuel is not new. The major reason to introduce alternative fuels during World War II or after the oil crisis in 1973 was the concern about the extent of petroleum reserves or greater dependence on oil producing countries. To avoid the problems of petroleum reserves crunch and over dependence in future, the attempts were shifted to produce usable fuels from petroleum to other fossils energy sources such as coal, biomass and natural gas. In late seventies due to environmental awareness and problems created by the extensive fossil fuels usage, the emphasis of fuel production and utilisation was shifted to develop efficient technologies for production of clean conventional fuels and fuel additives to decrease the pollutants formation and release.

Each crisis in energy and fuels forced a relook at alternative feed stocks and fuels. In this context the attempts were shifted to process more widely available coal, biomass feed stocks. The commercial processing of these resources and natural gas was fuel grade alcohols as alternative fuels and conventional fuels via synthesis gas production and conversion. Fuel alcohols have more environmental friendly characteristics than the conventional fuels. Because of these fuel properties and abundance of their resource base added the blending concept of oxygenates to the conventional fuel. A number of field trials and testing are continuing in many parts of the world. Among the fuel alcohols, methanol and ethanol are prominent candidates to use as alternative fuels or blending with conventional fuels or as precursors for fuel additives to conventional fuels. Ethanol and methanol have superior fuel properties in comparison to petroleum products as motor fuels because of their wide flammability limits, high flame speeds and low flame luminosinosity.

Methanol can be efficiently produced from the most difficult to process fuel feedstock for conventional fuels and easily processable natural gas. Ethanol in general predominantly produced by conversion of biomass with fermentation techniques. At present corn and sugar industries are the major feedstock sources for production of ethanol apart from the high starch containing biomass and ethylene derived from petroleum sources. Some extent, higher alcohols were also proposed as oxygenated alternative fuels or fuel blends because of their advantageous fuel properties. The comparative fuel properties of alcohols and gasoline are shown in Table 24.1.

In the past, alcohol has been used as fuel at various times particularly when petroleum was not known or in short supply, alcohols (C1 to C4) became popular in 1820's when it replaced fish and whale oil as fuel for lighting. Kerosene then replaced alcohol around 1880 because of its sooty flame, which gave more light during the middle of the last century, wood was distilled in the provinces of France to give methanol, which was burned in Paris for heating, lighting and cooking. During the World Wars I and II, there was gasoline shortage in many European countries, vehicles of all sorts used wood burner to distil wood chips to make methanol vapours that could power the engines. There were 9,000 such cars in Europe in 1938. Today, most racing cars are designed to use the more thermally efficient methanol rather than gasoline.

Table 24.1. Comparison of fuel properties of alcohols and gasoline.

Property	Methanol	Ethanol	Isopropyl alcohol	Tert-butyl alcohol	Gasoline
Chemical formula	CH_3OH	C_2H_5OH	$(CH_3)_2CHOH$	$(CH_3)_3COH$	C_4 to C_{12}
Molecular weight	32.04	46.07	60.09	74.12	100–105
Composition, weight %					
Carbon	37.5	52.2	60.0	64.8	85–88
Hydrogen	12.6	13.1	13.4	13.6	12–15
Oxygen	49.9	34.7	26.6	21.6	0
Specific gravity, 60°F	0.796	0.794	0.789	0.791	0.72–0.78
Density, lb/gal @ 60°F	6.63	6.61	6.57	6.59	6.0–6.5
Boiling temperature, °F	149	172	180	181	80–437
Reid vapour pressure, psi	4.6	2.3	1.8	1.8	8–15
Water solubility, @ 70°F					
Fuel in water, volume %	100	100	100	100	Negligible
Water in fuel, volume %	100	100	100	100	Negligible
Viscosity, centipoise @ 68°F	0.59	1.19	2.38	4.2@78°F	0.37–0.44
Flash point, closed cup, °F	52	55	53	52	–45
Autoignition, temperature, °F	867	793	750	892	495
Flammability limits, volume %					
Lower	7.3	4.3	2.0	2.4	1.4
Higher	36.0	19.0	12.0	8.0	7.6
Latent heat of vapourisation, Btu/gal @ 60°F	3340	2378	2100	1700	~900
Heating value, lower (liquid fuel-water vapour) Btu/gal @ 60°F	56800	76000	87400	94100	109000–1190000
Stoichiometric air-fuel, weight	6.45	9.00	10.3	11.1	14.7
Ratio moles product/ moles $O_2 + N_2$	1.21	1.12	1.10	1.10	1.08

ALCOHOLS AS ALTERNATIVE FUELS

A number of alcohols produced by synthesis gas conversion and fermentation of biomass proposed as efficient alternative transportation fuels. Methanol and ethanol are the prominent candidates in the proposed oxygenates because of their promising fuel characteristics and huge raw material base with commercial technologies.The fuel characteristics of methanol and ethanol is given in Table 24.2. Methanol and ethanol are suitable as alternative fuels for automobiles, their major advantage over hydrocarbon fuels derived from crude oil is that they can be readily made from resources that are fairly, evenly distributed over the globe, unlike crude oil where over 50 per cent is located in the Middle East. With these fuels, it is possible to achieve lower exhaust emissions of hydrocarbons along with the reduced photochemical 'Smog-forming' activity. Essentially, these fuels can be attractive as alternative fuel in areas where there is severe atmospheric pollution.

Methanol

Methanol is predominantly produced from synthesis gas. A number of experimental trials have been conducted by using methanol as a potential alternative fuel (Table 24.2). The high consumption and high engine adaptation costs are a disadvantage currently. However, the introduction of methanol fuel is being considered once more in California to control ozone formation. The fuel properties of methanol and ethanol are given in Table 24.2.

Table 24.2. Fuel properties of methanol and ethanol.

Properties	Methanol	Ethanol
Molecular weight	32.04	46.07
Specific gravity	0.783	0.789
Boiling point °C	+65.0	+78.32
Melting point °C	−182.5	−114.1
Calorific value, kcal/kg	5300	6600–7300
O_2 required for combustion kg/kg fuel	1.5	2.08
Chemical composition, kg/kg fuel		
Carbon	0.38	0.52
Hydrogen	0.12	0.13
Oxygen	0.50	0.35
Stoichiometric air-fuel ratio, kg air/kg fuel	6.4	9.0
Air required for combustion, kg/kg fuel	6.50	9.04
Products of combustion, kg/kg fuel	$CO_2 = 1.3$	$CO_2 = 1.90$
	$H_2O = 1.1$	$H_2O = 1.17$
	$N_2 = 5.0$	$N_2 = 6.95$
Latent heat values, kilo joules/litre	931	663
Research octane number	112	111
Motor octane number	91	94

Methanol as a transportation fuel

The potential of methanol as fuel for automobile has been recognised for quite some time. The interest has renewed due to clean air act regulation. Methanol is a fairly volatile liquid. It has low volatility, a little higher density and about half the heating value per gallon as compared to iso-octane which is 100 octane gasoline reference fuel. An appreciable experience exists with automobile propulsion system. Methanol is used preferentially, in high performance racing car because it is safe and has octane rating.

The use of 100 per cent methanol has the potential of much larger consumption as gasoline replacement than as blended product. However methanol-gasoline blend has the significant advantage of not requiring major changes in storage and distribution facilities. The use of neat methanol as a motor vehicle fuel will be extremely advantageous if two of the major problems with neat methanol like cold starting and formaldehyde emission can be overcome. One of the ways that offers promise to overcome the problems is the use of an engine that injects fuel directly into the combustion chamber. Methanol for direct combustion would compete with gasoline, low sulphur fuel oil, solvent refined coal, or coal with stroke gas cleanup.

Methanol as a utility fuel

Methanol can be fired in conventional boilers, Vulcon Cincinnati and New Orleans Public Service carried out demonstration firing tests which were successful, with methanol fuel NO_x emission were lower than the other fuels. Overall thermal efficiency of boilers should be unaffected by a switch from natural gas to methanol. Although methanol has a high latent heat of vapourisation about 500 Btu/lb or equivalent to 5 per cent of the gross heating value.

Methanol—fuel for fuel cells

Methanol has a unique characteristic, which is not found in gasoline, or heavier petroleum based fuel. This special characteristic is its suitability to use as a fuel in fuel cell and facile generation of hydrogen fuel for fuel cells. Fuel cells are the promising new generation high efficiency power producing electrochemical devices, which may replace the current engine based technologies. Next to hydrogen, methanol has received the most attention for potential use as a fuel for fuel cells. It has a high theoretical potential (1.2 V) and high energy density (2.75 kWh/lb fuel).

Ethanol

Ethanol, also called ethyl alcohol, pure alcohol, grain alcohol, or drinking alcohol, is a volatile, flammable, colourless liquid. It is a psychoactive drug, best known as the type of alcohol found in alcoholic beverages and in modern thermometers. Ethanol is one of the oldest recreational drugs known to man. In common usage, it is often referred to simply as alcohol or spirits.

Ethanol is a straight-chain alcohol, and its molecular formula is C_2H_5OH. Its empirical formula is C_2H_6O. An alternative notation is $CH_3–CH_2–OH$, which indicates that the carbon of a methyl group (CH_3^-) is attached to the carbon of a methylene group $(–CH_2–)$, which is attached to the oxygen of a hydroxyl group $(–OH)$. It is a constitutional isomer of dimethyl ether. Ethanol is often abbreviated as EtOH, using the common organic chemistry notation of representing the ethyl group (C_2H_5) with Et. The fermentation of sugar into ethanol is one of the earliest organic reactions employed by humanity. The intoxicating effects of ethanol consumption have been known since ancient times. In modern times, ethanol intended for industrial use is also produced from by-products of petroleum refining.

Ethanol has widespread use as a solvent of substances intended for human contact or consumption, including scents, flavourings, colourings and medicines. In chemistry, it is both an essential solvent and a feedstock for the synthesis of other products. It has a long history as a fuel for heat and light and also as a fuel for internal combustion engines.

For a long time ethanol is promoted as alternative transportation fuel in different parts of the world where ethanol is produced extensively from biomass. The use of ethanol as an alternative fuel has been put into practice in Brazil (85 per cent ethanol). Both pure ethanol fuel and a 25 per cent blend in gasoline have been marketed. Ethanol is produced mostly from biomass and could therefore potentially help to reduce carbon dioxide emissions because of a closed carbon dioxide cycle.

On the other hand, catalytic exhaust gas treatment is also required even when ethanol is used because of other emissions (CO, HC, NO_x and aldehyde). From the viewpoint of technical application the use of ethanol is somewhat less problematic than that of methanol. However the high production costs and the huge cultivation area for biomass have kept its use as a fuel within narrow limits.

Ethanol fuel

Ethanol fuel is ethanol (ethyl alcohol), the same type of alcohol found in alcoholic beverages. It can be used as a fuel, mainly as a biofuel alternative to gasoline, and is widely used by flex-fuel light vehicles in Brazil, and as an oxygenate to gasoline in the United States. Together, both countries were responsible for 89 per cent of the world's ethanol fuel production in 2008. Because it is easy to manufacture and process and can be made from very common crops such as sugar cane and corn, in several countries ethanol fuel is increasingly being blended as gasohol or used as an oxygenate in gasoline. Bioethanol, unlike petroleum, is a renewable resource that can be produced from agricultural feedstocks.

Anhydrous ethanol (ethanol with less than 1 per cent water) can be blended with gasoline in varying quantities up to pure ethanol (E100), and most modern gasoline engines will operate well with mixtures of 10 per cent ethanol (E10). Most cars on the road today in the US can run on blends of up to 10 per cent ethanol, and the use of 10 per cent ethanol gasoline is mandated in some cities where harmful levels of auto emissions are possible.

Ethanol can be mass-produced by fermentation of sugar or by hydration of ethylene (ethene $CH_2 = CH_2$) from petroleum and other sources. Current interest in ethanol mainly lies in bio-ethanol, produced from the starch or sugar in a wide variety of crops, but there has been considerable debate about how useful bio-ethanol will be in replacing fossil fuels in vehicles. Concerns relate to the large amount of arable land required for crops, as well as the energy and pollution balance of the whole cycle of ethanol production. Recent developments with cellulosic ethanol production and commercialisation may allay some of these concerns.

According to the International Energy Agency, cellulosic ethanol could allow ethanol fuels to play a much bigger role in the future than previously thought. Cellulosic ethanol offers promise as resistant cellulose fibres, a major and universal component in plant cells walls, can be used to generate ethanol.

Sources

Ethanol is a 'renewable' because it is primarily the result of conversion of the sun's energy into usable energy. Creation of ethanol starts with photosynthesis causing the feedstocks such as switchgrass, sugar cane or corn to grow. These feedstocks are processed into ethanol.

Bio-ethanol is usually obtained from the conversion of carbon based feedstock. Agricultural feedstocks are considered renewable because they get energy from the sun using photosynthesis, provided that all minerals required for growth (such as nitrogen and phosphorus) are returned to the land. Ethanol can be produced from a variety of feedstocks such as sugar cane, bagasse, miscanthus, sugar beet, sorghum, grain sorghum, switchgrass, barley, hemp, kenaf, potatoes, sweet potatoes, cassava, sunflower, fruit, molasses, corn, stover, grain, wheat, straw, cotton, other biomass, as well as many types of cellulose waste and harvestings, whichever has the best well-to-wheel assessment.

An alternative process to produce bio-ethanol from algae is being developed by the company Algenol. Rather than grow algae and then harvest and ferment it the algae grow in sunlight and produce ethanol directly which is removed without killing the algae. It is claimed the process can produce 6000 gallons per acre per year compared with 400 gallons for corn production.

Currently, the first generation processes for the production of ethanol from corn use only a small part of the corn plant: the corn kernels are taken from the corn plant and only the starch, which represents about 50 per cent of the dry kernel mass, is transformed into ethanol. Two types of second generation processes are under development. The first type uses enzymes and yeast to convert the plant cellulose into ethanol while the second type uses pyrolysis to convert the whole plant to either a liquid bio-oil or a syngas. Second generation processes can also be used with plants such as grasses, wood or agricultural waste material such as straw.

Production process

The basic steps for large scale production of ethanol are: microbial (yeast) fermentation of sugars, distillation, dehydration (requirements vary) and denaturing (optional). Prior to fermentation, some crops require saccharification or hydrolysis of carbohydrates such as cellulose and starch into sugars. Saccharification of cellulose is called cellulolysis. Enzymes are used to convert starch into sugar.

Fermentation

Ethanol is produced by microbial fermentation of the sugar. Microbial fermentation will currently only work directly with sugars. Two major components of plants, starch and cellulose, are both made up of sugars, and can in principle be converted to sugars for fermentation. Currently, only the sugar (e.g. sugar cane) and starch (e.g. corn) portions can be economically converted. However, there is much activity in the area of cellulosic ethanol, where the cellulose part of a plant is broken down to sugars and subsequently converted to ethanol.

Distillation

For the ethanol to be usable as a fuel, water must be removed. Most of the water is removed by distillation, but the purity is limited to 95–96 per cent due to the formation of a low-boiling water-ethanol azeotrope. The 95.6 per cent m/m (96.5 per cent v/v) ethanol, 4.4 per cent m/m (3.5 per cent v/v) water mixture may be used as a fuel alone, but unlike anhydrous ethanol, is immiscible in gasoline, so the water fraction is typically removed in further treatment in order to burn with in combination with gasoline in gasoline engines.

Dehydration

There are basically five dehydration processes to remove the water from an azeotropic ethanol/water mixture. The first process, used in many early fuel ethanol plants, is called azeotropic distillation and consists of adding benzene or cyclohexane to the mixture. When these components are added to the mixture, it forms an heterogeneous azeotropic mixture in vapour-liquid-liquid equilibrium, which when distilled produces anhydrous ethanol in the column bottom and a vapour mixture of water and cyclohexane/benzene. When condensed, this becomes a two-phase liquid mixture. Another early method, called extractive distillation, consists of adding a ternary component which will increase ethanol relative volatility. When the ternary mixture is distilled, it will produce anhydrous ethanol on the top stream of the column.

With increasing attention being paid to saving energy, many methods have been proposed that avoid distillation all together for dehydration. Of these methods, a third method has emerged and has been adopted by the majority of modern ethanol plants. This new process uses molecular sieves to remove water from fuel ethanol. In this process, ethanol vapour under pressure passes through a bed of molecular sieve beads. The bead's pores are sized to allow absorption of water while excluding ethanol. After a period of time, the bed is regenerated under vacuum to remove the absorbed water. Two beds are used so that one is available to absorb water while the other is being regenerated. This dehydration technology can account for energy saving of 3000 Btus/gallon compared to earlier azeotropic distillation.

BLENDING OF ALCOHOLS WITH GASOLINE/DIESEL

A number of alcohols derived from biomass and fossils fuels sources have been tested in different applications as blending components for transportation fuels. The characteristic of alcohol blends with traditional fuel are discussed below.

Alcohol-Gasoline Blends

Gasohol is ten to twenty per cent of ethanol in 80–90 per cent with lead free gasoline by volume. Gasohol can be used in existing engines with no modifications. Alcohol acts as an octane booster to replace tetraethyl lead in gasoline. Other technical advantages are small. Only alcohol of very low water content is suitable for blending. Alcohol and gasoline separate in the presence of water and the water tolerance of the blend becomes more critical at low temperatures. Methanol is slightly more tolerant of moisture in the blend than ethanol. M-85 (85 per cent methanol, 15 per cent gasoline is the form in which methanol fuel is generally expected to be sold and used by flexible fuel vehicles.

Alcohol Diesel Fuel Blends

Ten per cent of ethanol can be mixed with diesel fuel, again if both the alcohol and the diesel fuel are very low in water content. As in the blend with gasoline, the diesohol evaporates more easily than either of its parent materials. This property will cause vapour lock on the suction side of the fuel pump. This can be prevented by pressurising the fuel tank.

Straight Alcohol

Of great significance is the fact that straight alcohol fuel may contain as much as 20 per cent water without any loss of power or efficiency in the engine. Some engines can be modified to run on straight ethanol, giving the same mileage and overall performances as gasoline engine. The most advanced alcohol engines are high compression, fuel injected, spark ignition type. On the basis of experimentation conducted by the Indian Institute of Petroleum, Dehradun, a minimum of 10 per cent ethanol blending for petrol and 15 per cent ethanol blending for diesel has been considered for working out the alcohol requirement for use in blending with fuel in road transport.

ETHANOL AND BIOTECH

The production of industrial, potable and anhydrous alcohol from molasses, cane juice and other raw materials by fermentation and distillation process is of significant social and economical value in India. Ethyl alcohol blending in petrol and diesel as oxygenator and fuel is of immense value to lower oil dependence, reduce vehicular pollution (HC, NO_x, CO, VOCs) and improve rural economy in India. Use of ethyl alcohol @ 10 per cent and more in petrol has been very successful in Brazil, USA, Canada, Sweden, etc. In India, technical studies and large-scale trials have concluded that ethyl alcohol blending in petrol is technoeconomical. Further, studies on ethyl alcohol blending in diesel are in progress.

Further with adoption of an appropriate technology based on latest biotechnology developments, it should be possible to technoeconomically produce ethyl alcohol from available molasses, cane juice and alternate raw materials to meet the entire requirements of ethyl alcohol for industrial, chemicals, potable and blending in petrol and even in diesel in India (Fig. 24.1).

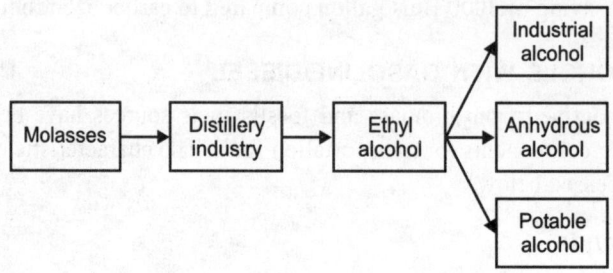

Fig. 24.1. Molasses to ethanol.

The alcoholic fermentation of molasses and alternate raw materials results in discharge of large volume of nontoxic liquid and solid effluents of high BOD/COD causing pollution. The reduction of effluent volumes, recycling and converting into biofuel as an energy source offers promising technology development for a 'zero pollution' system. The alternate source of raw material for ethanol are listed in Table 24.3.

Table 24.3. Alternate source of raw material for ethanol.

Crop	Alcohol yields (l/mt)	Crop yield (mt/hectare)	Alcohol production (l/hectare)
Sugar cane	70	56.04	3923
Cassava	180	8.75	1575
Sugar beet	110	30.21	3323
Sweet sorghum	60	1.32	80
Molasses	220	–	–
Wheat	340	1.78	605
Maise (corn)	360	3.27	1177
Barley	250	1.76	440
Potatoes	110	15.50	1705
Sweet potatoes	125	8.36	1045
Rice	430	2.67	1127

The section covers adaptation of an 'Integrated technology' for manufacture of ethyl alcohol with zero pollution, providing alcohol for industrial, chemical, potable and anhydrous alcohol (gasohol) (Fig. 24.2).

An Integrated Crest Technology

Use of suitable yeast strain (high alcohol)

Own propagation.

Propagation of yeast under optimal conditions

1. Update laboratory systems.
2. Design equipments.

3. Optimise sterilisation of media.
4. Use spent lees for molasses dilution.
5. Adopt CIP system.
6. Use optimum dosage of nutrients.
7. Improve aeration system.
8. Adopt microbial air filters system.
9. Use contamination-free water.
10. Use decontaminants.
11. Maintain optimum temperature.
12. Use indicator/control equipments.
13. Data logging and MIS.

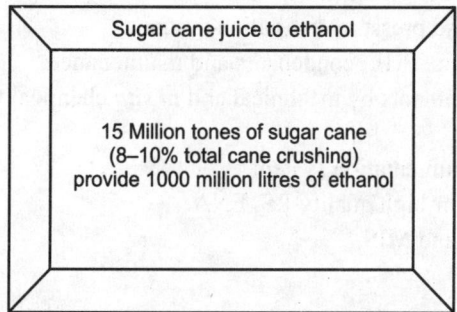

Fig. 24.2. Sugar cane juice to ethanol.

Fermentation under optimal conditions

1. Prefermentor, fermentor and other equipment's design.
2. Clean and sterilise equipments and pipelines.
3. Use weighed quantity of raw materials based on TRS/FS.
4. Use predetermined nutrients and decontaminates.
5. Recycle spent lees spent wash/condensate for molasses dilution.
6. Adopt molasses wort diluter with on line sampler.
7. Use feed rotameters.
8. Adopt fermentor wort cooling by PHE/recirculation pumps.
9. Adopt CIP system.
10. Use anti algae and anti scaling agents in cooling tower water.
11. Use temperature recorder.
12. Use sterilised antifoam and antifoaming devices.
13. Cover fermentors, recover carbon dioxide and scrub the same.
14. Use mechanical cleaning system to clean fermentors.
15. Collect sludge from the bottom of the fermentors and wash to recover alcohol, specially designed sludge-settlers.
16. Instrumentation design and adaptation.
17. Data logging system and MIS.

Preclarification or post clarification

1. Preclarification molasses without heating and acid (cold non-acid system).
2. Specially designed settlers, to remove continuously sludge from molasses wort/fermented wash.
3. Mechanical, mild steel settlers, no moving parts or centrifuges.

Distillation under optimal condition (rectified spirit, ena and anhydrous)

Basic and detailed engineering:

1. Mass balance, energy and utilities requirements.
2. Maintain and augment steam, power and water supply.
3. Design and adopt waste heat recovery systems.
4. Design and adopt reboiler systems.
5. Adopt multi column and pressure distillation systems.
6. Optimise cooling towers, PHE, condensors and maintenance.
7. Clean distillation equipments by mechnical and *in situ* chemical treatment.
8. Water management.
9. Design and adopt instrumentation system.
10. Optimise parameters for high quality RS, ENA.
11. Data logging systems and MIS.

Zero pollution system

1. Reduce effluent generation.
2. No dilution of effluent before treatment by biomethanation.
3. Recycling of effluent in the process.
4. Effective and efficient acid and biomethanation system.
5. Biodigestor—high rate, up flow, packed, high breed, top not covered but with liquid seal.
6. Effluent from biomethanation over flow (high TS, pH neutral, low ash content).
7. Multiple effect evaporators with thermal vapour recompression of moc-SS and MS.
8. Steam and power saving systems for concentrations.
9. Concentrate mix with organic residues, of high gross calorific value for straight use in fuel in boiler.
10. Condensate to be recycled for molasses dilution in fermentation house (Fig. 24.3).

Upgrade process and R&D laboratory

Human Resource Development

1. In service training.
2. Arrange refreshers course.
3. Advance training particularly to develop awareness for biotechnology developments.

Anhydrous Alcohol (AA)

Crest provides technology for manufacture of anhydrous alcohol (gashol) (Fig. 24.4).

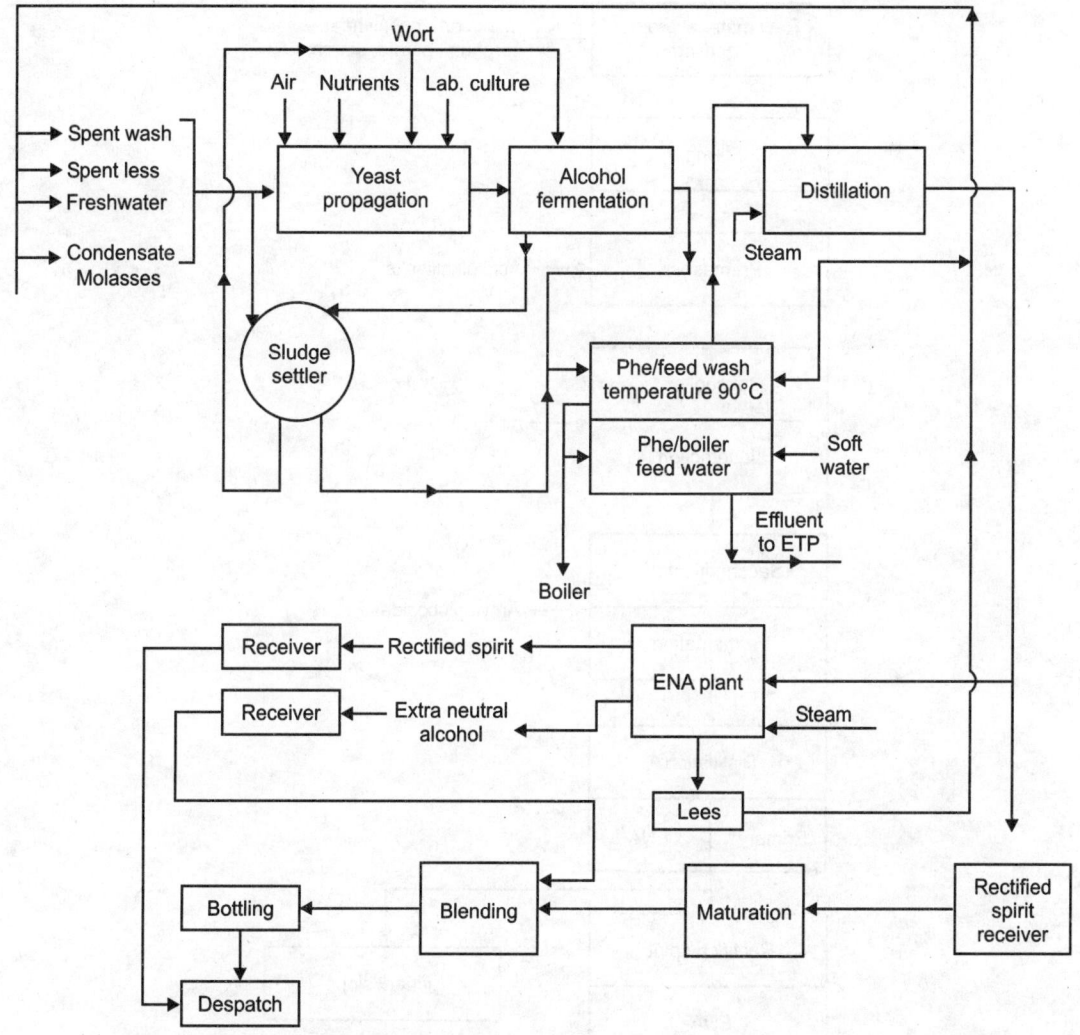

Fig. 24.3. Process flow diagram for improved fermentation and distillation system for distillery.

Azeotropic distillation

An entrainer—benzene/cyclohexane is added to the rectified spirit and it is distilled employing dehydration, recovery columns and decanter.

Performance

Rectified spirit (94.5 – 95.0%)	1065 ~ 1070 l/Kl AA
Steam	1.7 ~ 1.9 m^3/Kl AA
Power	60 Kw ~ 65 Kw/Kl AA
Cooling water (make up)	4 ~ 5m^3/AA
Entrainer	1.8 ~ 2.0 kg/Kl AA

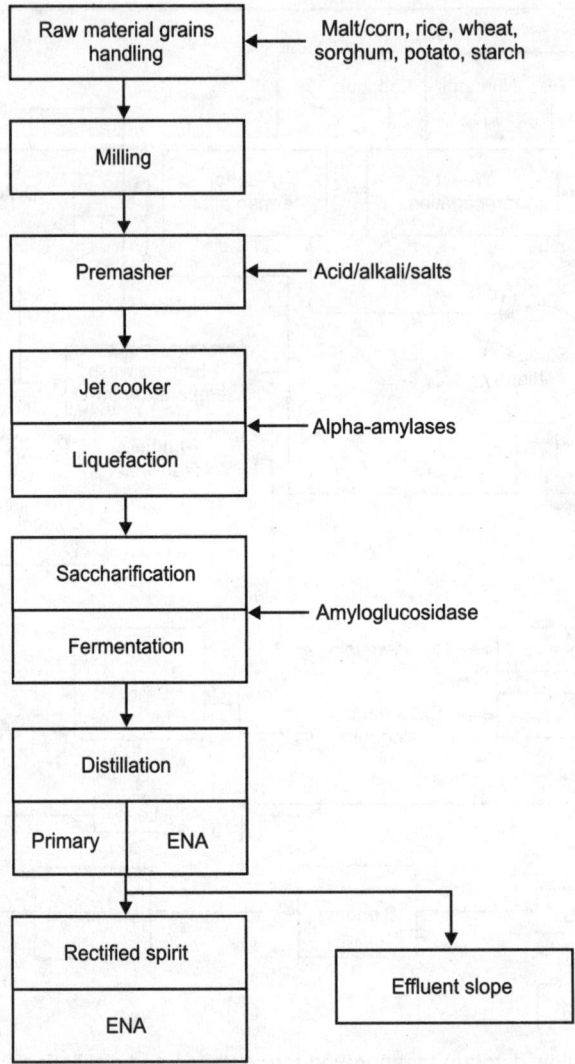

Fig. 24.4. Schematic flow sheet for malt/grain alcohol manufacturing.

Molecular sieve technology

Rectified spirit vapours are fed to one molecular sieve column (synthetic zeolites). Anhydrous alcohol is condensed as final product. Simultaneously, second molecular sieve column at low pressure is regenerated using part of anhydrous alcohol vapours employing vacuum pump. The lean alcohol (containing 69 per cent alcohol + 31 per cent water) is condensed and redistilled to 94.5–95 per cent concentration in main column.

Performance

Rectified spirit	1055–1066 l/Kl AA
Steam (6 kg/cm^2)	0. 50 ~ 0.60 MT/Kl AA

Power	10 ~ 15 Kw/Kl AA
(3 Phase)	
Cooling water	2.4–2.5 m³/Kl AA
(32°C)	
Air	4.8–5.0 Nm³/Kl AA
(5 kg/cm²)	
Entrainer	10 years life
(Sieve replacement)	

Membrane technology: pervapouration

Pervapouration is one of the most advanced technology for manufacture of anhydrous alcohol. Crest and Frings, Germany are working on technoeconomics of adopting this technology in Indian conditions. Membrane technology will enable the existing alcohol plant to increase overall recovery by 10 per cent and 60 per cent in capacity with the existing installation (Fig. 24.5).

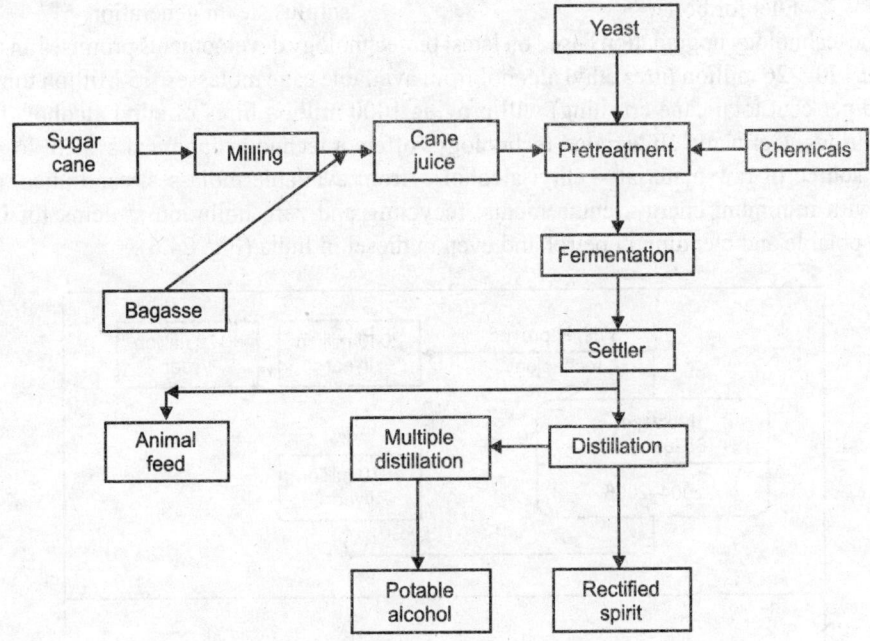

Fig. 24.5. Flow diagram for alcohol from sugar cane juice.

Fermentation

By upgradation of the fermentation and adaptation of Crest technology, it is possible to achieve:

Alcohol % wash	7.5–9.0%
Fermentation efficiency	87–90%
Time cycle	12–16 hours.
Recycle	Spent lees, spent wash and condensate for molasses dilution.

Distillation

Similarly, by adapting improved distillation system it is possible to obtain:

Distillation efficiency	97–98%
Steam consumption	2.0–2.3 kg/l alcohol
Effluent generation	10 l/l alcohol

Zero pollution system

Crest has developed an integrated system for zero pollution to achieve:

Reduced effluent generation	10 l/l alcohol
Acid phase	control vfa
Bio methane phase	45 m^3 gas/m^3 effluent
Multiple effect evapouration	45–55 per cent concentrate
Condensate	recycle
Mix fuel	3000 kcal
Fuel for boiler	surplus steam generation

Thus, the technology upgradation based on latest biotechnology developments promises an additional recovery of 170–226 million litres ethyl alcohol from available cane molasses. 15 Million tons of sugar cane (8–10 per cent total cane crushing) will provide 1000 million litres of ethyl alcohol. The Crest, India and Frings, Germany: 'Integrated technology' offers a techno economical system to produce a renewable source of raw material—ethyl alcohol—from available molasses, cane juice, other raw materials with minimum energy requirements, recycling and zero pollution systems for industrial, chemicals, potable and blending in petrol and even in diesel in India (Fig. 24.6).

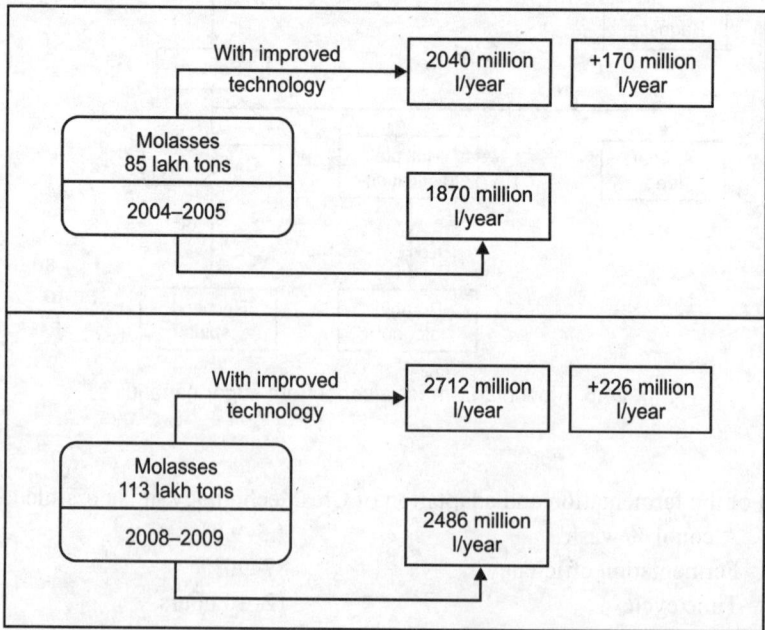

Fig. 24.6. Technology upgradation based on latest biotechnology developments premisses.

MAXIMISATION OF ETHANOL PRODUCTION FOR ANHYDROUS ALCOHOL

Production of anhydrous alcohol for the purpose of blending it with petrol is only now being given due credit and attention in India. Besides minimising pollution and saving foreign exchange it will solve problem of piling of sugar in godowns to some extent. Molasses alone will not be sufficient to meet India's requirement of ethanol for industrial chemicals portable and fuel ethanol purpose. Attention is therefore, drawn to the possibility of using secondary cane juice for production of ethanol. Techniques are economical and have a place in future development in India.

Ethanol has been known as a fuel for many decades. Production of ethanol in the world is increasing very rapidly and has grown from only 10 billion litres in 1980, to over 55 billion litres in 2008. This major increase is on account of use of fuel ethanol as a part of motor-spirit in Brazil and the US. India is expected to have contributed 1.3 billion litres of 35 billion litrer production (3.65 per cent of world production).

As India is a agriculture based country, biofuel (ethanol) provides us with an excellent opportunity to improve our economy by cutting imports of crude oil, saving precious foreign exchange and also reducing pollution. Fuel ethanol is used in petrol as an oxygenate which reduces emission of carbon monoxide in exhaust gases of vehicles.

There are many other compounds which can be used in petrol as an oxygenate — tetraethyl lead, methyl tetrabutyl ether (MTBE), etc. but use of these compounds creates some problem. Tetraethyl lead emits poisonous and dangerous fumes containing lead, which are suspected to cause cancer. MTBE gets settled onto surface water of lakes, dams and reservoirs, and contaminates the water. This contamination is dangerous and could be harmful to health. But use of ethanol in petrol is free from such type of contamination and cause of disease, so ethanol can be used on a large scale. To be able to achieve this, we increase the production of ethanol by using recent techniques instead of traditional ones.

Advantages of Anhydrous Alcohol

1. Does not use tetraethyl lead.
2. CO_2 emissions are 57 per cent lower than with gasoline.
3. No SO_2 emissions.
4. Ethanol vehicles do not have particulate emissions.
5. CO_2 emissions are compensated with absorption of sugar cane.

Techniques for Maximisation of Ethanol Production

The major raw material for industrial ethanol is cane molasses, a by-product of sugar factories. The recovery of alcohol/ton of molasses abroad is 270–300 litres as compared to 200 to 250 litres in India. In the Indian context, this low recovery is attributed to the nature of raw material itself, as well as its storage conditions. A typical comparison of Indian and Brazilian molasses is given in Table 24.4.

Table 24.4. Composition of molasses.

Parameters	Brazilian molasses (%)	Indian molasses (%)
Total sugar	56 ± 2	46 ± 3
Unfermentable sugar	5 ± 1	10 ± 2
Total solids	75 ± 3	72 ± 3
Ash	7 ± 2	12 ± 3
Calcium (CaO)	0.5 ± 0.1	1.6 ± 0.4
Total nitrogen	0.3–0.4	0.1–0.2

Further during the process of sugar extraction, chemical reactions at high temperature lead to the production of other undesirable products such as hydroxy-methyl furfural, caramel, etc. which are harmful to yeast fermentation. Some of the inhibitors that play a critical role in alcoholic fermentation are given in Table 24.5.

Table 24.5. Inhibitors encountered in Indian molasses.

Inhibitors	Approx conc. (%)
Caramel	3.00
Hydroxyl methyl furfural	0.05
Fatty acids	
Acetic	0.75
Butyric	0.10
Valeric	0.05
Sulphur dioxide	0.08
Pesticide residues	ppm
Heavy metals	ppm
Sugar processing chemicals (antiscalant, viscosity reducer, flocculant, whitener, mill biocides, etc.)	ppm

Different techniques for the maximisation of ethanol production are discussed below.

Yeast selection

Recent interest in ethanol as a potential fuel or fuel supplement has stimulated research into various aspects of the fermentation process. Apart from the improvements in the fermentation techniques for better efficiency of ethanol production, another equally important area is selection of highly efficient yeast for production of ethanol. Traditionally Saccharomyces organism is used for ethanol fermentation but, nowadays if we use *Zymomonas mobilis* for production of ethanol, efficiency of production will be increased.

Yeast recycling

This technique was first described by Melle Boinot in 1939 and is widely practiced in Brazil. This process involves, the use of centrifugal separators by which yeast is recovered after the completion of fermentation. The separated yeast cream is subjected to pre-treatment by lowering the pH to 3.0 by means of sulphuric acid, to reduce the bacterial contamination, and is used as such for seed in the next cycle (Fig. 24.7). The advantages of this are:

1. Saving of molasses used for yeast propagation.
2. Higher alcohol recovery.
3. Little modification needed for converting the conventional system.
4. Low BOD in effluent because of the separation of yeast.

This process of fermentation has been used in Japan. The fermentation is carried out as in a conventional batch process. However, after the completion of fermentation, 25 per cent of fermented broth is retained as seed for the next cycle. The fermenters are aerated for the first few hours. A selective biocide is incorporated in each cycle, to knock down the bacterial contamination (Fig. 24.8).

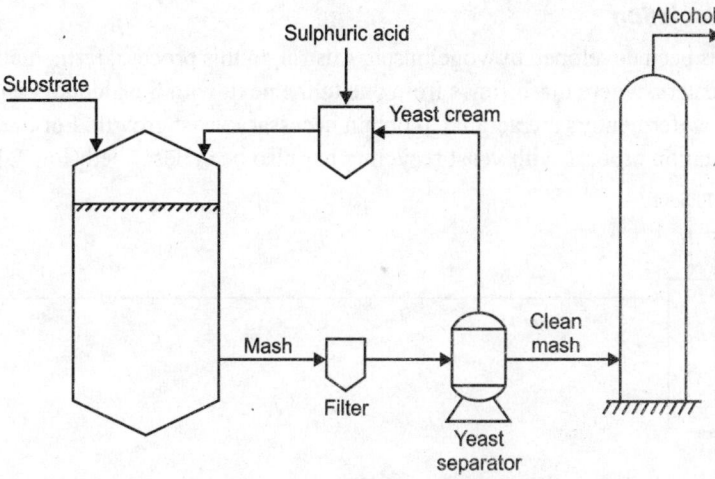

Fig. 24.7. Yeast recycling process.

This technology has been adopted by Daurala distillery which has, thereby, achieved a fermentation efficiency of 88 per cent and a steam consumption rate of 2.0 kg/l of rectified spirit. The various advantages are:

1. Yeast is reused without any mechanical device.
2. Reduction in frequency of fresh yeast propagation-saving in molasses.
3. Fermentation temperature does not exceeds $36° \pm 1°C$; low process water requirement.
4. Microbial contamination is controlled without any additional energy input.
5. Process can be easily adopted in existing plants with little modification.
6. Fermentation efficiency and alcohol recovery are significantly increased over conventional batch process.

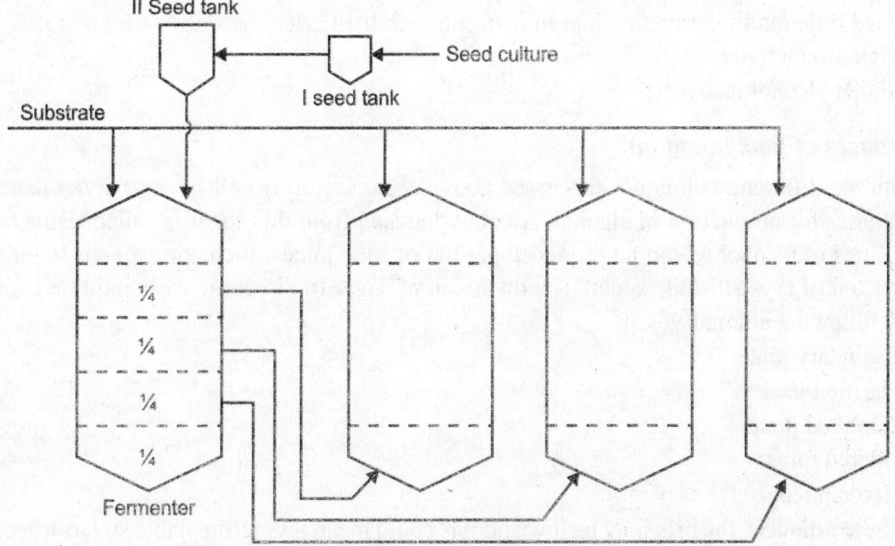

Fig. 24.8. Semi-continuous fermentation process.

Continuous fermentation

This technology has been developed by Vogelbusch, Austria. In this process, fermentation is carried out in a series of fermenters, where mash flows from one to the next, with the alcohol concentration rising in each. The first few fermenters are aerated to obtain necessary yeast growth. For higher productivity, continuous fermentation process with yeast recycling has also been described (Fig. 24.9).

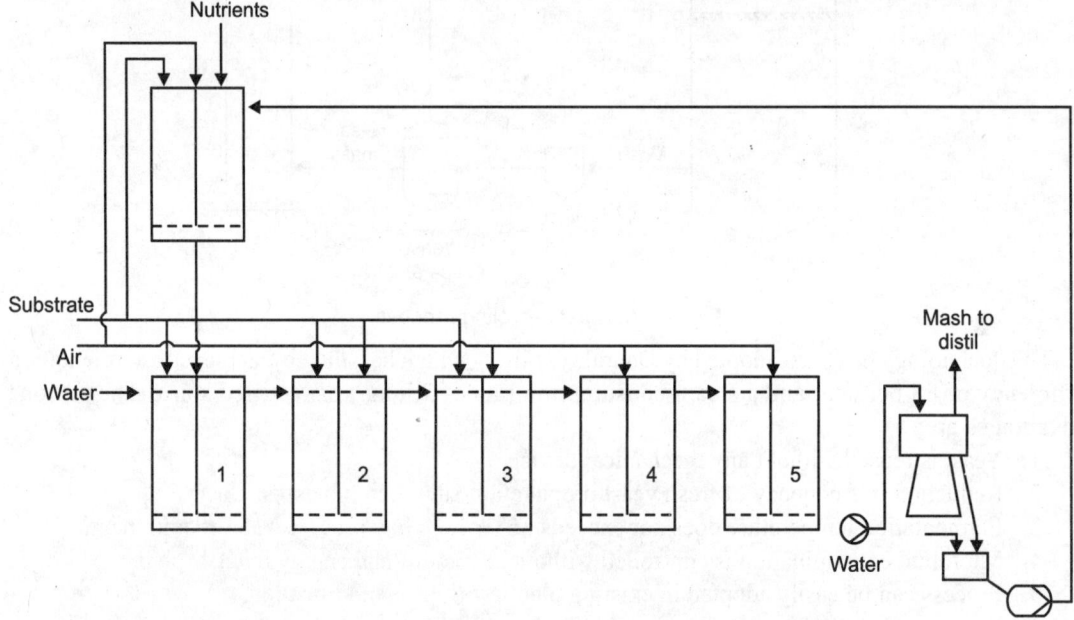

Fig. 24.9. Vogelbusch continuous fermentation process (with yeast recycling).

The various advantages are:
1. Need little modification to adopt in conventional distilleries.
2. High productivity.
3. Higher alcohol recovery.

Other aspects of maximisation

Along with the different techniques discussed above sugar factories will have to divert cane juice to their distilleries for production of alcohol. Alcohol poduced from this sugar is called 'Direct alcohol'. About 67 litres of alcohol would be produced per ton of cane juice which corresponds to 600 litres of alcohol per ton of crystallisable sugar. The diversion of sugar to direct alcohol could be chosen from one of the following alternatives:
1. Secondary juice.
2. Clarified juice.
3. Sulphited juice.
4. Filtered juice.
5. Mixed juice.

In all these products, the brix may be low and this could mean less fermentable sugars affecting both final concentration of alcohol in fermented wash and distillery capacity. In view of this, it is proposed either to preconcentrate the juice to obtain desired brix or mix molasses to such an extent so as to adjust desired brix. Each of above mentioned possibilities would be discussed.

Secondary juice

Juice drawn from the mills need to be screened and treated so as to avoid the problems to be encountered subsequently with the fermentation and centrifuging.

Clarified juice

Clarified juice is free of suspended particles, but it has following defects when considered for distillery:
1. It is hot hence it requires to be cooled.
2. The pH needs adjustment for fermentation.
3. It usually contains sulphites.

A disadvantage of sending clarified juice to the distillery with factories working with sulphitation process will be deterioration in the quality of alcohol produced due to presence of SO_2, which forms mercaptans and other impurities.

Sulphited juice

The advantages of sulphited juice from the point of view of distillery would be its low pH and the sterilising action of the SO_2. However, the alcohol produced will have more by-products including glycerine and the quality of alcohol would be bad.

Filtrate juice

It is well known that the return of the filtrate to the clarification system of sugar manufacturing process not only affects the clarification but also the quality of sugar. This filtrate is dirty. It needs to be settled and cooled further before it is used for fermentation.

Mixed juice

This will be an ideal culture for yeast with regard to physical and chemical parameters such as pH, temperature, fermentable, protein, vitamins, mineral salts, etc. however, it will be necessary to have fine screening (less than 60 mesh) to prevent problem with yeast separator. It needs thermic treatment too.

Juice treatment

The direct fermentation of juice (mixed juice and secondary juice) without treatment poses some problems in relation to the equipment wear down, consumption of chemicals, activities of contaminant micro-organisms, etc. After experimenting with various systems of juice treatment, the one which is being practiced by industries in Brazil, consists of screening, chemical and thermic treatment, decantation, filtration and concentration of the juice.

Economical aspects

As India has very large area under sugar cultivation, we can also follow the Brazilian route (i.e. using ethanol as motor fuel) of ethanol production. It has been observed that upto 5 per cent of the ethanol can be blended with petrol without any modification in the carburettor or the engine, provided ethanol is anhydrous, while upto 10 per cent of ethanol can be blended with minor adjustment in the carburettor or the engine.

Thus, the objective of this section was to provide an overview of maximisation of ethanol production by utilisation of different economical techniques. Large financial benefits can be obtained by using blended fuels. If only 10 v/v of alcohol is used for blending in place of costly anti-knocking agents then we can save around 10 v/v of petrol/diesel of the total consumption, resulting in large saving of foreign exchange. While the generation of profits will take some time to come and need initial investment, within a very short period this investment can pay off.

BIOFUEL: AN ALTERNATIVE SOURCE OF DIESEL AND GASOLINE

As already discussed the rapid depletion in world petroleum reserve and uncertainty in petroleum supply due to political and economical reasons, as well as the sharp escalation in the petroleum prices have stimulated the search for alternative sources for petroleum based fuels specially diesel and gasoline. Biofuels are one of the most promising alternative to conventional fuels. Its proponents have predicted an age of abundance and cheap energy used in a relatively non-polluted manner. Though the existence of numerous minor market for biofuels is evident, the scale on which they are conducted is small compared to that of other fuels. The level of research proposed for bioenergy cannot be justified by such markets. Instead a real promise of products which will substitute (on a large scale) conventional fuels particularly petroleum is needed.

Sources of Biofuels

The difference sources of biofuels has been outlined in Fig. 24.10.

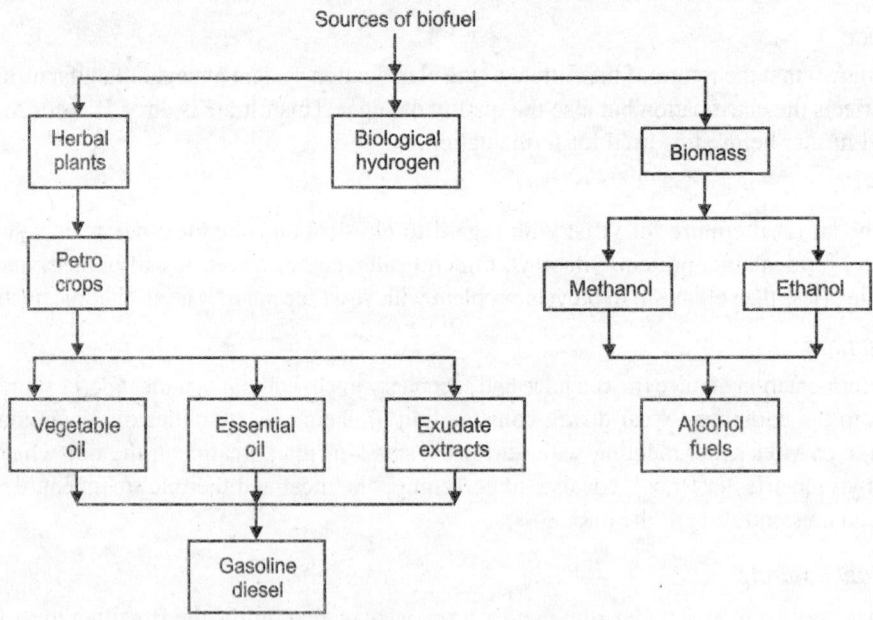

Fig. 24.10. Different sources of biofuel.

Herbal Plants

Plant science had a remarkable effect on the yields, geographic distribution and crop hardiness of many of the species yielding oil-like materials. Plants are complex mixture of different substances, some of which are of high calorific value such as fats and oils. Others are intermediate in energy content, e.g.

sugar, polysaccharides and protein. The plant oil have been used a very long time for food, fuels and other uses. At one time most of the lamp oil in Europe was produced from oil-seed (spirit lamp) e.g. rape seed because its characteristics were comparable with that of diesel.

The different herbal plants from which fuel can be extracted are described below.

Petro crops

Petro crops are plants that yield oil or hydrocarbon which can be used as substitutes for diesel, gasoline or petroleum products. After the oil crises of 1973, these plants received much attention. The material in petro crops that can be used for energy production is a complex mixture of terpenoids (mono-, sesqui di- and tri-polymeric), long chain aliphatics (waxes, wax esters, triglycerides and fatty acids) and phenolic (phenols, flavanoids and polyphenolics). Such materials are called as hydrocarbons, botano-chemical, whole plant oil, terpenoids, resins or biocrude. As long as the oxygen content of these extractives is less than 20 per cent, the material can be upgraded to gasoline, diesel fuel or chemical feedstocks. These can be accomplished by the use of conventional catalyst in fluidised bed cracking units.

Classification of petro crops

The classification of petro crops is given in Fig. 24.11.

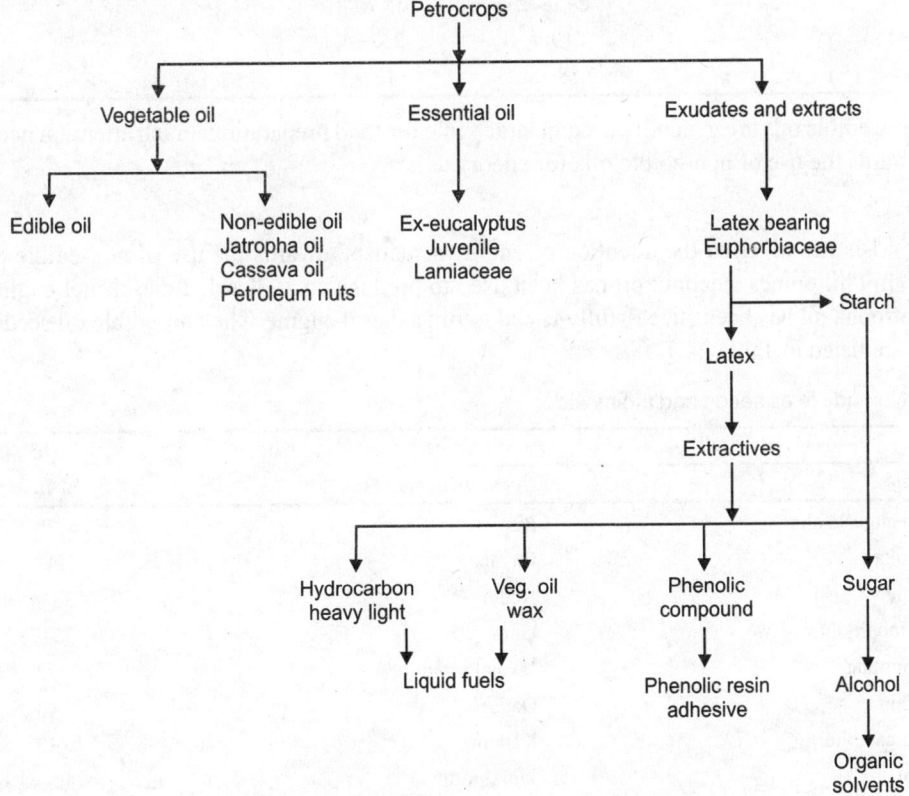

Fig. 24.11. Classification of petro crops.

Vegetable oil

A diesel engine was run on peanut oil at the Paris exposition during 1990. Recently, scientists in Australia have conducted short terms tests on vegetable oils such as sunflower, peanut, rapeseed, corn, linseed, safflower, soyabean and coconut in unmodified diesel engines. The studies involving the use of crude degummed oils showed that power output and brake thermal efficiency values are comparable to those obtained with distillate. Fuel consumption was slightly higher for seedoil, probably due to their high calorific value. The comparison of the properties of these vegetable oil with diesel is given in Table 24.6.

Table 24.6. Characteristics of some important vegetable oils and diesel.

Properties	Vegetable oils					
	Sunflower oil	*Soya oil*	*Peanut oil*	*Rapeseed oil*	*Palm oil*	*Diesel oil*
Density at 20°C (g/cm³)	0.913	0.910	–	0.906	–	0.845
Viscosity at 20°C (cp)	55.6	57.2	–	66.0	–	4.8
Heating value (MJ/l)	34.0	34.0	33.7	33.9	35.1	35.5
Flash point	–	219	237	–	–	46
Cetane no.	–	38	41	–	–	42–43

Since these edible oils are generally used in large scale for food preparation, much attention needs to be given towards the use of non-edible oils for energy use.

Non-edible oils

The energy crisis has diverted the attention of energy scientists towards the use of non-edible oil as engine fuel. In Philippines, coconut oil has been used to produce coco-diesel, a diesel fuel engine. In Thailand, Jatropha oil has been successfully tested to run a diesel engine. The non-edible oil seeds and their yields are listed in Table 24.7.

Table 24.7. Non-edible oil seeds and their yield.

Oil seeds		Oil
Botanical name	*Common name*	*% Yield*
Actinodaphne angustifolia	Pisa	75
Amoora rohituka	Rayana	47
Azadirachta indica	Neem	33–45
Calophyllum inophyllum	Undi	55–73
Canarium commune	Java almond	73
Cerbera odollam	Dadur	43
Cinnamomum camphora	Kapoor	42
Croton tiglium	Jamalgotta	30–45
Garcinia indica	Kokm	44

(Contd...)

Oil seeds		Oil
Botanical name	Common name	% Yield
Garcinia morella	Gamlog	59
Hydro carpus wightiana	Maroti	63
Jattropha curcas	Ratanjyot	46–58
Jutropha euphorbeacea	Vilayati erand	32
Juglans regia	Walnut	60–70
Madhuca butyracea	Phulwara	55–66
Mecua ferra	Nahar	70–80
Mimusops hexendra	Khirni	47
Perilla frutescens	Bhaujira	30–57
Qrbera camphora	Dadur	42
Salvadora oleaides	Pilu	40–43
Sapindus trifoliatus	Ritha	44–47
Stercutea foetide	Jangli badam	53–55

The vegetable oils which are considered most suitable for the production of effective engine fuel are:

Jojoba

It is a hardy shrub well suited for cultivation under arid conditions. Its seeds contain a liquid 'wax' that has impressive industrial potential, as substitute in sperm whale oil.

Jatropha

The plant is adaptable to marginal lands. It can grow on gravel, sandy, clayey and eroded lands. The seeds of jatropha produce a semi-drying oil. The nuts consists of 45 per cent hulls and 55 per cent kernels. The kernels yield 63.05 per cent oil (34.65 per cent on whole seed basis). It has been estimated that trees planted 2 m apart could produce 2 kg seed oil per plant per year and 2500 trees per hectare could yield 2000 kg of crude oil per hectare on 40 per cent oil basis. An advantage is that it begins to yield nuts in 4–5 months and can live for 50 years.

Petroleum nut oil

Petroleum nut (*Pittosporum resiniferun*) bears nut, which when cut and lit, burn brilliantly. The fruits are known to yield an oil which has fuel properties comparable with those of gasoline, except for the octane number, which is lower than that of gasoline and initial boiling point, which is higher than that of gasoline. However, there is no sulphur.

Other seed oils

Several other oils have been successfully road tested in diesel automobiles. Castor oil contains 90 per cent ricinoleic acid, the unsaturated long chain acid, which on cracking yields motor and diesel fuels. Availability of seeds of a number of other plants like neem (*Azadirachta indica*), and others are estimated, to be nearly 9,06,316 tons in India. These need to be looked into for their potential as source of energy oils.

Extraction of vegetable oils

The oil bearing material are first subjected to a range of preliminary process to remove foreign matter, to crack shell, remove the germ and convert the whole into a meal. The meal is then cooked and the oil removed by either low or high pressure expression by solvent extraction using trichloroethylene or hexane. The crude oil is refined by neutralisation, bleaching, deodourisation, winterisation and gum removal by filtration through suitable adsorbents.

Essential oils

Like terpenes, essential oils are highly combustible. A recent research project conducted in Japan was aimed at using eucalyptus oil/gasoline blend. According to reports from USA, eucalyptus oil gave fairly good performance as an engine oil. It is believed that blends with gasoline are highly promising. In China, juvenile shoots and leaves of *Rhododendron capitatum* have been found to give an essential oil which is a potential petro substitute. The cost of essential oil is high, therefore it is not worthwhile to use them for energy purpose. Nevertheless, there are a number of weeds, specially of lamiaceae (labiatae) groups which need investigation for possible use of energy source.

Process

Essential oils are extracted by steam distillation, enfleurage (pressing in contact with absorbent), solvent extraction and expression. Sometimes a fermentation process is used to disintegrate the biomass and release the oils.

Exudates and extracts

Exudates

Plants exudates and extracts contain latex or resins which can be processed into liquid fuel. Water and hydrocarbons have been found to be the principal component of plant latex. The hydrocarbon of plants latex are polymers of isoprene (C_5H_8), ranging from relatively large molecule (molecular wt. 5,00,000–20,00,000). Plant latex are found in special cell in a wide variety of plants. Turpentine is a highly combustible chemical consideration. At the Indian Institute of Petroleum, Dehradun latex was collected, dried and processed into petroleum like substance.

Extracts

The attention on whole plant extract as source of hydrocarbon for liquid fuels has been at its maximum during the past decade. Thousand of laticiferous and resinous plants have been examined for their potential as source of hydrocarbon.

In this direction, good amount of work has been done on gopher plant (*Euphorbia lathyris*), milk-bush (*Euphorbia tirucalli*), Euphorbia lactea, (*Calotropis procera*), *calotropis gigantea, cryptostegia grandiflora*, and species of genus *Asclepias* and *pedilanthus* and some members of compasitos family. *Euphorbia lathyris* figures as one of the most potential species for solvent extraction. Potential yield in the form L. Lathyris has been suggested as 6.5×10^4 MJ per ha per year in the form of hydrocarbon and 5.2×10^4 MJ per ha per year. The terpenoids can be converted to gasoline like substances and the sugar can be converted to alcohol. In India, National Botanical Research Institute (NBRI), Lucknow and IIP, Dehradun, have studied 386 plant species, of which 10 have been considered to offer good potential for solvent extraction. If the price of crude oil keeps on rising, there is every possibility of petroleum farming becoming a profitable venture in the next future.

Biomass

Biomass — a carbonaceous waste of various natural and human activities can be obtained from numerous sources like by-product of agricultural crops, raw material from the forest, from sugar industry and wood. The primary advantage of using biomass is that it does not add dangerous gases like carbon monoxide to the atmosphere.

Alcohol as Fuel

Ethanol and methanol are the two alcohols commonly considered for fuel use. The potential for substituting alcohol fuel for those based on petroleum is especially significant in the transportation sector.

Ethanol

Ethanol has the potential of being an alternative transport fuel. Modern vehicles can run on 20–80 per cent ethanol/petrol blend without having to modify the engines. Ethanol produced from plant material is considered to be greenhouse neutral and thus possesses great scope for reducing environmental pollution. Besides, the use of ethanol in petrol can reduce carbon monoxide emissions ranging from 10 to 30 per cent.

Production

Ethanol is produced from biomass by fermentation. The preparation of ethanol from cellulose, starch and sugar containing raw materials involves pretreatment of the raw material, hydrolysis to convert pretreated raw material to sugar, yeast fermentation to convert sugar into ethanol and purification, in which ethanol is separated from by-product and wastes. Present ethanol is produced in large scale by continuous fermentation process.

Ethanol from starch

Starchy material, e.g. grain are first cooked to a gel consistently, cooled and mixed with malt. Malt contains diastase enzyme which has the ability to convert starch to fermentable sugar (maltose). This is converted by zymase bacteria to ethanol.

$$(C_6H_{10}O_5)_n \xrightarrow{H_2O} C_{12}H_{22}O_{11} \xrightarrow{\text{Yeast enzyme}} C_6H_{22}O_6 \xrightarrow{\text{Zymase}} 2CH_3CH_2OH + 2CO_2$$

Ethyl alcohol from sugar/molasses

Fermentation of sugar by yeast, is essentially used for the manufacture of ethanol. Yeast contains the enzyme invertase and zymase. The invertase catalyses the hydrolysis of sucrose in mash to invert sugar.

$$C_{12}H_{22}O_{11} + H_2O \xrightarrow{\text{Invertase}} C_6H_{12}O_6 + C_6H_{12}O_6$$

Invert sugar are subsequently converted into about equal parts of ethyl alcohol and carbon dioxide by action of zymase enzyme.

$$C_6H_{12}O_6 \xrightarrow{\text{Zymase}} 2CH_3CH_2OH + 2CO_2$$

Microbiological aspects

Presently, large scale ethanol plants use Saccharomyces strains. Most yeast grow well on a variety of amino acids, purines and pyrimidines as the sole source of nitrogen. Biotin and pantothenate are essential for all strains of Saccharomyces. Even if sufficient nutrients such as sugar, nitrogen and vitamins are present, it is the dissolved oxygen in the solution which limit the population of yeast in the fermentation medium. Once the dissolved oxygen is depleted during fermentation the yeast population slows and eventually ceases. Anionic detergents, sorbic acid, diethyl pyrocarbonate (DEP) and the antibiotics cyclohexamide, antimycin A and nystalin completely inhibit growth of more common yeasts. In fermentation of lignocellulosic hydrolysates, acetic acid, furfural and lignin-derived phenolics are found to be inhibitory. The best ethanol yields are generally obtained at pH 4.5–4.7. In lightly buffered media, the optimum starting value is nearer pH 5.5. After fermentation is complete this falls to about pH 3.5 yeasts survive in the approximate range of pH 2.0–8.6. The temperature for growth of yeasts is about 25°C. Since yeast growth and fermentation both produce heat, cooling may be necessary to maintain the desired temperature.

Methanol

Fuel grade methanol for driving vehicles can also be obtained by fermentation process by utilising bacteria. However, commercial methanol production by these processes has not yet developed.

Production

Fermentation methanol process have not been developed, although an aerobic fermentation in which methanol forms directly from methane or natural gas by means of agent that capture methanol before being oxidised to overproducts has been reported. Conversely the biological reduction of carbon monoxide produces methane, so anaerobic process in which methanol intermediate is trapped and removed from the system are possible. However there has been little research involving these concept.

Characteristic of alcohol fuel

The characteristic of alcohol fuel and its comparison with gasoline is given in Table 24.8.

Table 24.8. Comparison of properties of ethanol, methanol and gasoline.

Property	Ethanol	Methanol	Gasoline
Density at 20°C kg/m^3	789.5	792.0	702.0
Carbon, present by weight	52.0	37.5	84.0
Hydrogen, present by weight	13.0	12.5	16.0
Boiling point °C	78.3	64.5	125.7
Viscosity at 20°C NS/m^2	12×10^{-4}	5.84×10^{-4}	5.4×10^{-4}
Spontaneous ignitions temperature °C	440	480	425–510
Heating value			
Higher, Btu/lb	20,570	9770	12,780
Lower, Btu/lb	19,080	8640	11,550
Octane quality			
Research octane number	106	110	80–95
Motor octane number	89	92	70–85

Future Prospects

Due to rapid depletion in finite source of energy such as petroleum, the need to find some promising alternative is obvious. Among the current alternatives available, vegetable oil based fuel are most important to replace diesel in future because it can be used without any major engine, vehicle or infrastructural modification in existing facilities. The potential for substituting alcohol fuel to gasoline is significant in the transportation sector. Though this fuel has been tested as engine fuel in some foreign countries, there is very little progress in India in this regard. Since there is abundant alcohol production in India it could be used as a future automobile fuel. Adequate financial support must be provided by the government for future research in the area of vegetable and alcohol based fuel to make them cost effective and improve characteristics.

Energy Equation

Ethanol has a low energy content of 26.68 million joules (MJ)/kg against 42–44 MJ/kg of gasoline and is about 40 per cent less energy efficient than gasoline. Despite the improved volumetric efficiency of the engine due to 16.5 per cent increase in the heat of vapourisation of alcohol blended fuel, alcohol still remains around 22.5 per cent less energy efficient as compared to gasoline. There was an interesting study by Pimental, Chairman, US department of energy panel a few years back in year 2003. He investigated the energy economics and environmental aspects of ethanol production from corn.

The result revealed that an acre of US corn yields about 7110 pounds of corn, which when processed yield 328 gallons of ethanol. However, planting, growing and harvesting that much corn needs about 1000 gallons of fossil fuels costing US $347/acre. Thus even before corn is converted to ethanol, it costs US $1.05/gallon of ethanol. The economics worsen at processing plants were corn is crushed, fermented and 8 per cent ethanol is separated from 92 per cent water. Additional treatment is then required to produce 99.8 per cent purity ethanol to mix with gasoline. Total energy required to process corn to one gallon of ethanol was calculated at 1,31,000 BTus against 77,000 BTus available in ethanol i.e. 70 per cent more energy is required than the energy actually available in ethanol and there is a loss of 54,000 BTus per gallon.

Environmental Issues

Ethanol blended fuel reduces carbon monoxide and other emissions and reduces greenhouse gases. However, it causes increase in acetaldehyde emissions, which react with nitrogen in the air to produce peroxy acetyl nitrate (PAN) a known carcinogen that can persist for many days in the atmosphere, especially in winter. In the United States of America, which produces ethanol from corn, an expert study indicated that corn production erodes soil about 12 times faster than the soil can be reformed and irrigating corn fields deplete groundwater 25 per cent faster than the natural recharge rate of groundwater.

The first century of the new millennium opened with the threat for the ethanol-based chemical industry as the Petroleum Ministry went ahead with initial trial of fuel ethanol. While both the ethanol based chemical industry, including the pharmaceutical industry, and the potable liquor industry are continuing their normal operations, the threat on availability and higher price of ethanol hangs on the existing ethanol user industries in India, as more and more ethanol will be diverted to the fuel ethanol programme. This scenario raises numerous questions on the economical, energy and environmental aspects.

Advantages and Disadvantages of Alcohol Fuels

Advantages of alcohol fuels

Some of the advantages are listed below:

1. For constant engine size, equal rate of fuel consumption to that of a gasoline, power is available from an engine designed for alcohol.
2. Since nitrogen oxides emitted by internal combustion engines originate from air being heated in the combustion chambers, the low temperature of alcohol flame will result in very low level of pollution.
3. When alcohol burns in lean mixture with air, the products from the fuel are nothing more carbon dioxide and moisture.
4. Since the exhaust temperature is lower, a smaller cooling system can be used.
5. The burning of alcohol forms no soot or carbon; carbon build up in an engine is eliminated.

6. The door of alcohol is not unpleasant, and a spill of this fuel would do only minor damage to environment.

7. Alcohol is sola: energy in liquid form. It can be made in large quantities from renewable sources.

8. The alcohol production from agricultural material uses non-protein biomass. All protein can be extracted for human or for livestock consumption/usage.

9. Unlike gasoline, alcohol is a pure chemical, which does not evaporate from storage as easily as gasoline and is unlikely to cause vapour lock of the fuel system.

10. Fire with alcohols does not start as easily as do gasoline fires because alcohols do not contain lighter hydrocarbon fractions. Besides, small alcohol fires can be extinguished using water.

11. Road traffic is the major source of pollution and produces substantial percentage of NO_x, hydrocarbons, CO. Today all new cars are equipped with catalytic converter which are very efficient in reducing the above pollutants by > 90 per cent in ideal conditions.

Disadvantages of alcohol fuels

Unlike petroleum product, alcohol has no lubricating property; hence additional lubricant like caster oil is required to mix with alcohol for proper engine lubrication. When ethanol burns in less quantity of air, acetic acid is formed which causes corrosion in engines. The benzol is recommended to be mixed with it to overcome this trouble. Ammonia in small quantity can prevent corrosive effect of exhaust gases. Combustion of alcohol is likely to be complete due to a wide range of fuel air ratios, which results in an explosion, with alcohol air fuel mixture found in partly empty storage tanks will probably be explosive. So special cellular fuel tank will have to be built for safety. The serious advantage in using of a carburettor which is designed for gasoline in alcohol as a fuel is the need of very high amount of heat, required to change liquid, alcohol into vapour, which is necessary for combustion. If alcohol vapourises inside the cylinder, causes a great cooling effect on air fuel mixture in that chamber due to which air fuel mixture shrinks in volume and lower the piston against which piston works.

Technical constraints and corrective action points

A fleet trial aimed at studying the fuel economy and driveability in case of ethanol blended fuel was conducted by IIP and IOC (R&D) and the results of these studies are shown below.

As blends

1. Under city driving economy loss was 1 per cent with 10 per cent ethanol blended fuel and 3.90 per cent with 20 per cent ethanol blended fuel.

2. Low octane number and high self-ignition temperature makes alcohol unsuitable for diesel engines unless the fuel or the engine is modified to watch the other.

3. Alcohol and diesel are not miscible with each other and thus cannot be used as blend.

4. In gasoline 100 per cent anhydrous alcohol would be preferred in the long run, which would make the use of blended fuel more uneconomical. A distillery producing ethanol under 1.5 per cent water content costs about three times as much as a distillery to produce alcohol of 10 per cent water by volume.

5. A long-term continued availability of alcohols will be required to overcome any meaningful alco-fuel-programme and it has to be fully commercialised to get economical advantage that will require large commercial scale experimentation with alco-fuel, which has not so far been conducted.

6. In the Indian context no experimentation whatsoever has yet been conducted for finding out operational compatibility of motor engines to alcohol/neat alcohol as an oxygenator.

7. The production rate of alcohol per ton of molasses is quite low (200 to 240 litres per ton). Efforts should be directed to improve these yields to about 300–350 litres. Steps should be taken to produce alcohol from sources other than molasses, such as food grains, wood and waste cellulosic materials. Crops with high carbohydrates such as potatoes, corn, etc. have theoretical alcohol equivalent yield in excess of 2000 litre/hectare.

Sugarcane is indeed, one of the most efficient biological converter of solar energy. Its photosynthetic efficiency is 3.8 per cent as compared to earth's average (all vegetation inclusive) of 16 per cent only. It has been estimated that 5.6 tons of molasses (approximately 50 per cent sugar) can yield 1 ton of ethanol. India being the largest sugarcane country is in a better position with an area of 8.0 million hectares under sugar cane plantation and an average yield of 82.0 tons/hectare at 1990 level besides all agricultural crops and forests can be used to make alcohol.

Efficient conversion methodologies have to be developed to convert the huge renewable biomass resources base into usable value added products and alternative fuels or conventional fuel blending components for reformulated fuels. There is an essential need to formulate the integrated research and development programmes to produce alcohol from cellulosic biomass and use the same more efficiently for various applications.

Thus, relative to gasoline and diesel, fuel alcohol offers potential advantages for vehicle manufacturer, for small spark ignition engines, for example methanol's high octane permits high compression ratios, which improve engine efficiency and fuel economy. Additional engine efficiency results from linear burning and cooler combustion. These and other factors allow the design of smaller engines without sacrificing engine performance. Alternatively a larger engine offers high power and performance than its gasoline counterpart. Improved emissions are an additional bonus. Alcohol, a renewable energy source, its production and use should not be curbed, but rather guided by a long-term perspective. The laws governing licensing policies of power alcohol distilleries should be amended in all states and union territories so as to remove any unnecessary restriction for its production and use.

UTILISATION OF ALCOHOL IN VEHICULAR ENGINES

Extensive experimental tests and computerised theorectical investigations carried out by various scientists have shown that ethyl alcohol can be utilised with great advantage in existing automobile/scooter/motorcycle engines, in the form of alcohol-gasoline blends without any major engine modifications. After extensive trials, an 'optimum' blend has been perfected which gives improved performance, lesser consumption, lesser exhaust emission, very much reduced carbon deposits, and smoother and cooler engine operation as compared to that obtained with gasoline alone. Effective additives have been developed and perfected to stabilise the 'optimum blend, denature it and give it a distinct colour and odour.

Carburation of ethyl alcohol in heavy vehicular engines powered by diesel has been found to increase their power rating by 20–50 per cent depending upon the type of combustion chamber used. Engine noise level and exhaust smoke density reduces considerably with the use of ethyl alcohol as a biofuel in these engines.

Vehicular Engines and Fuels

There are now more than two hundred million passenger cars, trucks and buses the world over using combustion engines. Of these the Spark Ignition engines, burning gasoline, are almost exclusively the power plants for passenger cars and light trucks. Diesel engines, using another petroleum product, diesel oil, power most of the trucks and buses. The total horsepower of these engines used in automobiles and trucks alone amounts to many times more than the entire installed horsepower of central power stations the world over. These engines continue to grow in numbers and it is hard to see a replacement for them in the foreseeable future. Their growing number has made modern industrial civilisation dependent on oil.

Both gasoline and diesel oil used in these vehicles are 'stored' fuels extracted from the earth. There are limited reserves of these fuel oils and economists are haunted with the knowledge that they are irreplaceable. The products of decay of prolific animal and vegetable life existing millions of years ago, the conditions that created them, no longer exist. With our present known resources and the present rate of consumption it is feared that they will not last long.

It is, therefore, necessary and desirable to search out and investigate the possibility of using 'unstored' liquid fuels which can be synthetically prepared from such renewable stores of raw materials that are available in nature in abundance.

Ethanol-based engines

Ethanol is most commonly used to power automobiles, though it may be used to power other vehicles, such as farm tractors and airplanes. Ethanol (E100) consumption in an engine is approximately 51 per cent higher than for gasoline since the energy per unit volume of ethanol is 34 per cent lower than for gasoline. However, the higher compression ratios in an ethanol-only engine allow for increased power output and better fuel economy than could be obtained with lower compression ratios. In general, ethanol-only engines are tuned to give slightly better power and torque output than gasoline-powered engines. In flexible fuel vehicles, the lower compression ratio requires tunings that give the same output when using either gasoline or hydrated ethanol. For maximum use of ethanol's benefits, a much higher compression ratio should be used, which would render that engine unsuitable for gasoline use. When ethanol fuel availability allows high-compression ethanol-only vehicles to be practical, the fuel efficiency of such engines should be equal or greater than current gasoline engines. The mileage (miles-per-gallon) is therefore usually 20–30 per cent higher than a gasoline-only engine.

A 2004 MIT study and an earlier paper published by the society of automotive engineers identify a method to exploit the characteristics of fuel ethanol substantially better than mixing it with gasoline. The method presents the possibility of leveraging the use of alcohol to achieve definite improvement over the cost-effectiveness of hybrid electric. The improvement consists of using dual-fuel direct-injection of pure alcohol (or the azeotrope or E85) and gasoline, in any ratio up to 100 per cent of either, in a turbocharged, high compression-ratio, small-displacement engine having performance similar to an engine having twice the displacement. Each fuel is carried separately, with a much smaller tank for alcohol. The high-compression (which increases efficiency) engine will run on ordinary gasoline under low-power cruise conditions. Alcohol is directly injected into the cylinders (and the gasoline injection simultaneously reduced) only when necessary to suppress 'knock' such as when significantly accelerating. Direct cylinder injection raises the already high octane rating of ethanol up to an effective 130. The calculated over-all reduction of gasoline use and CO_2 emission is 30 per cent. The consumer cost payback time shows a 4:1 improvement over turbo-diesel and a 5:1 improvement over hybrid. In addition, the problems of water absorption into pre-mixed gasoline (causing phase separation), supply issues of multiple mix ratios and cold-weather starting are avoided.

Ethanol's higher octane rating allows an increase of an engine's compression ratio for increased thermal efficiency. In one study, complex engine controls and increased exhaust gas recirculation allowed a compression ratio of 19.5 with fuels ranging from neat ethanol to E50. Thermal efficiency up to approximately that for a diesel was achieved. This would result in the MPG (miles per gallon) of a dedicated ethanol vehicle to be about the same as one burning gasoline.

Since 1989 there have also been ethanol engines based on the diesel principle operating in Sweden. They are used primarily in city buses, but also in distribution trucks, and waste collectors use this technology. The engines, made by Scania, have a modified compression ratio, and the fuel (known as ED95) used is a mix of 93.6 per cent ethanol and 3.6 per cent ignition improver, and 2.8 per cent denaturants. The ignition improver makes it possible for the fuel to ignite in the diesel combustion cycle. It is then also possible to use the energy efficiency of the diesel principle with ethanol.

Engine cold start during the winter

High ethanol blends present a problem to achieve enough vapour pressure for the fuel to evaporate and spark the ignition during cold weather (since ethanol tends to increase fuel enthalpy of vapourisation). When vapour pressure is below 45 kPa starting a cold engine becomes difficult. In order to avoid this problem at temperatures below 11°C (59°F), and to reduce ethanol higher emissions during cold weather, both the US and the European markets adopted E85 as the maximum blend to be used in their flexible fuel vehicles, and they are optimised to run at such a blend. At places with harsh cold weather, the ethanol blend in the US has a seasonal reduction to E70 for these very cold regions, though it is still sold as E85. At places where temperatures fall below –12°C (10°F) during the winter, it is recommended to install an engine heater system, both for gasoline and E85 vehicles. Sweden has a similar seasonal reduction, but the ethanol content in the blend is reduced to E75 during the winter months.

Brazilian flex fuel vehicles can operate with ethanol mixtures up to E100, which is hydrous ethanol (alcohol with up to 4 per cent water), which causes vapour pressure to drop faster as compared to E85 vehicles, and as a result, Brazilian flex vehicles are built with a small secondary gasoline reservoir located near the engine to avoid starting problems in cold weather. The cold start with pure gasoline is particularly necessary for users of Brazil's southern and central regions, where temperatures normally drop below 15°C (59°F) during the winter. An improved flex motor generation that will be launched shortly which will eliminate the need for this secondary gas storage tank.

Ethanol fuel mixtures

To avoid engine stall due to 'slugs' of water in the fuel lines interrupting fuel flow, the fuel must exist as a single phase. The fraction of water that an ethanol-gasoline fuel can contain without phase separation increases with the percentage of ethanol. This shows, for example, that E30 can have up to about 2 per cent water. If there is more than about 71 per cent ethanol, the remainder can be any proportion of water or gasoline and phase separation will not occur. However, the fuel mileage declines with increased water content. The increased solubility of water with higher ethanol content permits E30 and hydrated ethanol to be put in the same tank since any combination of them always results in a single phase. Somewhat less water is tolerated at lower temperatures. For E10 it is about 0.5 per cent v/v at 70 F and decreases to about 0.23 per cent v/v at –30 F.

In many countries cars are mandated to run on mixtures of ethanol. Brazil requires cars be suitable for a 25 per cent ethanol blend, and has required various mixtures between 22 and 25 per cent ethanol. The United States allows up to 10 per cent blends, and some states require this (or a smaller amount) in all gasoline sold. Other countries have adopted their own requirements. Beginning with the model year 1999, an increasing number of vehicles in the world are manufactured with engines which can run on any fuel from 0 per cent ethanol up to 100 per cent ethanol without modification. Many cars and light trucks (a class containing minivans, SUVs and pickup trucks) are designed to be flexible-fuel vehicles (also called dual-fuel vehicles). In older model years, their engine systems contained alcohol sensors in the fuel and/or oxygen sensors in the exhaust that provide input to the engine control computer to adjust the fuel injection to achieve stochiometric (no residual fuel or free oxygen in the exhaust) air-to-fuel ratio for any fuel mix. In newer models, the alcohol sensors have been removed, with the computer using only oxygen and airflow sensor feedback to estimate alcohol content. The engine control computer can also adjust (advance) the ignition timing to achieve a higher output without pre-ignition when it predicts that higher alcohol percentages are present in the fuel being burned. This method is backed up by advanced knock sensors—used in most high performance gasoline engines regardless of whether they are designed to use ethanol or not—that detect pre-ignition and detonation.

Fuel economy

In theory, all fuel-driven vehicles have a fuel economy (measured as miles per US gallon, or litres per 100 km) that is directly proportional to the fuel's energy content. In reality, there are many other variables that come into play that affect the performance of a particular fuel in a particular engine. Ethanol contains approximately 34 per cent less energy per unit volume than gasoline, and therefore in theory, burning pure ethanol in a vehicle will result in a 34 per cent reduction in miles per US gallon, given the same fuel economy, compared to burning pure gasoline. This assumes that the octane ratings of the fuels, and thus the engine's ability to extract energy from the fuels, are the same. For E10 (10 per cent ethanol and 90 per cent gasoline), the effect is small (~3 per cent) when compared to conventional gasoline, and even smaller (1–2 per cent) when compared to oxygenated and reformulated blends. However, for E85 (85 per cent ethanol), the effect becomes significant. E85 will produce lower mileage than gasoline, and will require more frequent refueling. Actual performance may vary depending on the vehicle. Based on EPA tests for all 2006 E85 models, the average fuel economy for E85 vehicles resulted 25.56 per cent lower than unleaded gasoline. The EPA-rated mileage of current USA flex-fuel vehicles should be considered when making price comparisons, but it must be noted that E85 is a high performance fuel, with an octane rating of about 104, and should be compared to premium. In one estimate the US retail price for E85 ethanol is 2.62 US dollar per gallon or 3.71 dollar corrected for energy equivalency compared to a gallon of gasoline priced at 3.03 dollar. Brazilian cane ethanol (100 per cent) is priced at 3.88 dollar against 4.91 dollar for E25 (as July 2007).

Alcohol: The renewable fuel

Ethyl alcohol, commonly called alcohol and technically termed ethanol, is one such fuel. Its importance lies in the ease with which it can be prepared from an astonishingly wide range of raw materials, some of which are to be found in every habitable country on the globe. These raw materials include vegetable matter, growing crops, farm waste, tropical grasses, waste organic products such as straw and saw dust, molasses, water gas, industrial wastes like sulphite liquor from the paper and pulp industry, and many others.

Its use may be regarded as a direct method of obtaining energy from the sun without the intermediary of storage in earth for a long period of time. As long as the sun shines, plants will perform their synthesis of starch from the abundant carbon dioxide and water that bathe our planet. From this annually-renewed store of raw materials, ethanol can be readily produced in quantities sufficient to meet the world demand. It thus has attributes of perennial renewal.

Alcohol as automobile fuel

Ethanol, if used as an automobile engine fuel, offers certain advantages. The chief amongst them is the possibility of high compression operation without knock. It is an anti-knock fuel and has the ability to stand very high compression ratios. Its octane rating is above 100 and it could operate safely at compression ratios around 12.

It has a high latent heat of vapourisation. This property can be utilised to achieve lower charge temperature during induction, higher charge density; hence higher volumetric efficiency and cooler engine operation.

The absence of pre-ignition and knock resistance makes it suitable for high-output engines and opens the option of supercharging of the engine, which is seriously restricted with gasoline fuel.

Ethanol is also safer than gasoline due to its higher flash point. Its vapours are not quite half as heavy as those of gasoline, so that it does not flow and accumulate in dangerous quantities at low levels; and a higher proportion is needed to form an explosive mixture with air. Hence the fuel tank is less likely to catch fire in case of accident.

Its uniformity of composition and much cleaner combustion are some other advantages. It tends to produce less carbon deposits than normal gasoline and the deposits are softer and easier to remove.

Its lower calorific value; higher viscosity, greater surface tension and hygroscopic nature are some of the difficulties in its use as a complete fuel in the present-day combustion engines. It can however be mixed with other fuel or fuel mixtures so as to impart to the resulting blend some of its important properties, namely higher compression operation without knock, cleaner combustion and cooler engine operation.

Alcohol and vehicular emissions

There is another aspect of automative engine operation. Its exhaust contains atmospheric pollutants like carbon monoxide, carbon dioxide, unburned hydrocarbons, oxides of nitrogen, lead salts, soot, aldehydes, ketones, etc. An automobile discharges around 0.66 tons of carbon monoxide over a period of a year and it is estimated that automobile exhaust is the source of ninety per cent of carbon monoxide found in the atmosphere of the USA. Oxides of nitrogen and unburned hydrocarbons from automobile exhaust create air pollution problems by forming photochemical smog. Their interaction involves formation of certain formaldehydes, peroxides, peroxyacyl nitrate, etc. which cause eye irritation, plant damage, and contribute to poor visibility.

Present day gasoline contains lead, added to raise its octane number. 98.8 per cent gasoline sold in the world market today contains tetraethyl lead. This lead ultimately finds its way, in the form of lead salts, in the exhaust effluent discharged through the tail-pipe of the vehicles; and causes lead poisoning of the environment. It is estimated that a few thousand tons of organic lead are spewed out of auto-exhausts every year.

Thus, pollutants like carbon monoxide, oxides of nitrogen, unburned hydrocarbons and lead salts from vehicular exhausts are posing a very serious health hazard. The concentration of these pollutants in the automobile exhaust effluent depends, apart from other things, on the nature of the fuel.

Ethanol and its blends, unlike gasoline, provide 'clean burning fuels'. Their use is likely to reduce the air pollution caused by automobile exhaust emissions. With its inherently high octane rating ethanol can be used as a blending agent to raise the octane rating of gasoline and eliminate thereby the need of lead additives. Its use as automobile fuel can thus eliminate the hazard of exhaust lead poisoning of the environment.

Alcohol Utilisation in Light Vehicular Engines

Experimental and theoretical investigations have been carried out to assess the effects of ethanol blending on the performance and exhaust emission characteristics of spark ignition engines of various types, such as E6/T Ricardo Variable Compression Engine, CFR Engine, EMC four-cylinder engine. Extensive laboratory experiments have been followed by field trials using automobiles of a popular make. During these investigations, ethanol-gasoline blends, with ethanol content varying from 0 to 100 per cent, have been tried in various engines in the laboratory and in the field. Engine operation with various blends has been studied with and without engine modifications. In addition to engine performance, we have also looked into the consumption characteristics, smoothness of operation, exhaust emissions and various other aspects such as engine component compatibility with various ethanol-gasoline blends.

Apart from these aspects of engine performance and compatibility, Smith and others have also examined the problems of stabilisation of blend against separation due to absorption of moisture, denaturing the blend to prevent misuse of its alcohol content, cold starting and engine response with various ethanol-gasoline blends. In the following sections are briefly summarised some of the major inferences drawn on the basis of these studies.

Knock resistance

Ethanol-gasoline blends permit a higher compression operation without knock. The 'optimum' compression ratio increases with the increase of ethanol percentage in the blend. Thus, for example, a 30 per cent ethanol-gasoline blend can operate effectively at a compression ratio about 23 per cent higher than the optimum compression ratio for gasoline. This shows that ethanol is a very effective knock suppressor, like TEL is, and has the additional advantage that it is a fuel in itself. Figure 24.12 shows the effect of adding ethanol to a typical regular gasoline with a research Octane number of 91.0. Addition of ethanol upto 10 per cent raises the octane rating of gasoline by 3 while blending 25 per cent ethanol raises the octane number of gasoline from 91 to 99. The octane number appears to increase linearly with the increase of ethanol content in the blend upto 25 per cent ethanol addition. It has also been observed that this useful effect of ethanol blending is more marked if the starting stock is low grade gasoline, while improvement in octane rating is relatively less in case of high-octane gasoline.

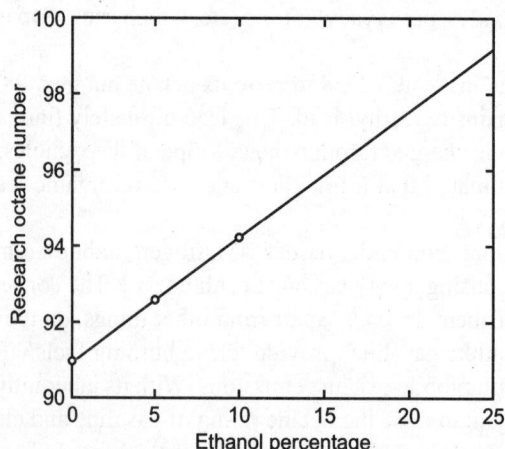

Fig. 24.12. Variation of octane rating with the ethanol percentage in the blend.

The high knock resistance of ethanol can be utilised in three ways: (i) as a blend constituent for improving straight-run or other spirit of low octane number, (ii) as a complete fuel in special 'ethanol' engines of higher compression ratio of the order of 12 or so, and (iii) as a dual-fuel for separate injection when required. The ordinary motor engine makes full use of the high knock rating of the fuel only during a small portion of its service. If it were operated on a cheaper fuel of relatively low rating but with automatic means of ethanol injection under high loads, the biofuel combination might make for greater economy.

'Optimum' blend

From intensive tests carried out on unmodified engines, the 'optimum' blend has been found. This blend gives improved engine performance, less exhaust emissions and smoother operation of the engine as compared to gasoline. This blend can be utilised in existing automobiles without any major modifications.

Water tolerance of the blend

The 'optimum' blend has been stabilised against separation due to absorption of moisture by providing some additives. 'Water tolerance' at various temperatures has been determined and often found within the prescribed limits set by the Indian power alcohol rules. The 'optimum' blend does not show any turbidity or any other sign of separation when cooled even below 0°C. During the course of many years of the use of this blend in the laboratory and in the field not a single case of separation has come to light.

Denaturing of the blend

The blend has been denatured to prevent illegal diversion of ethanol. Various denaturing agents were considered and tried in laboratory. The one finally selected satisfies most of the requirements of the denaturants. This, when used in very small quantities, effectively denatures the blend, gives a pungent smell and burning taste. No trouble has been found with this denaturing agent so far.

Engine wear and deposits with the blend

After 200 hours run using the blend, the wear of engine components was in no way more than that with gasoline while the 'optimum' blend showed carbon deposit which was about 115 of the carbon deposits obtained with gasoline.

Corrosion with the blend

The prolonged use of the blend may at times cause corrosion of surface components due to the production of acid bodies. The silencer has been found to suffer most. In some experiments, this problem was overcome by neutralising the acid products which cause corrosion by using small amounts of additives.

Copper and iron, as also rubber gaskets, are susceptible to attack by ethanol. However, this problem is encountered only when the percentage of ethanol in the blend is very high. Suitable measures such as 'tinning' can prevent this problem *vis-à-vis* the fuel tank. With the small percentage of ethanol in the 'optimum' blend recommended, this problem is not serious.

As a matter of fact, this type of problem does occur even with the use of leaded gasoline. For example, the use of gasoline tends to build up deposits on spark plugs and attack the mica or porcelain. None of these difficulties can arise with the use of the ethanol blend. In some experiments it was observed that the temperature of the spark plugs is reduced with the 'optimum' blend and this has the effect of prolonging their life.

Ease of starting with the blend

No greater difficulty than that experienced with gasoline has been encountered in starting up the engine with the 'optimum' blend. In fact, the startability of the engine improves with ethanol addition upto a maximum of about 20 per cent of ethanol. Even at 0°C the addition of a small amount of ethanol (as recommended for 'optimum' blend) improves the startability of the engine. At 10°C, somewhat similar results are obtained except that the difference in starting time with 'optimum' blend and gasoline becomes less marked.

Vapour lock and the blend

Increase of the vapour pressure of the ethanol-gasoline blend (having low ethanol content) with temperature is not significantly different from that of gasoline and consequently blends containing a small percentage of ethanol (as recommended for the 'optimum' blend) should not be more susceptible to vapour lock than gasoline. Experiments have shown that the 'ten per cent' point on the distillation curve is at more or less the same temperature for the 'optimum' blend as for gasoline.

Engine warm-up with the blend

The 'warming up' of the engine from start appears to be slower and greater acceleration has to be given just after the start to encourage rapid warming up. This characteristic of the blend should not be considered a disadvantage. In fact, when starting from cold it is not advisable to accelerate the engine to top speed and power in the shortest possible time.

Power and consumption with the blend

During the road tests it has been noted that power as also fuel consumption is not affected while using the 'optimum' blend. Slight adjustment in ignition timing is necessary to ensure the complete combustion to the blended fuel. With proper adjustments made in the ignition system, generally the same mileage was recorded as for gasoline, although theoretically the blend has slightly lower calorific value. This may be possible due to better combustion characteristics of the blend.

Alcohol blends and engine performance

Blends having more than 25 per cent of ethanol have no advantage over gasoline when used in the engine without modifications; hence they are of little practical value so far as the present-day vehicular engines are concerned.

At 'optimum' conditions for each blend, the gain in power output is very marked. With 30 per cent blend the maximum BHP is about 11 per cent more than that with gasoline. Thus, by taking advantage of increase in ignition advance with ethanol blends and using higher compression ratios made available by the antiknock nature of ethanol, marked improvement in the power output can be achieved.

Figure 24.13 shows that at any given compression ratio the engine brake mean effective pressure (indicative of engine power output) increases as the 'ethanol content increases' from 0 to 30 per cent. The increase in power output that is obtained as the compression ratio of the engine is increased is also apparent. When the compression ratio reaches 9:1 the octane number of the regular grades of fuel is insufficient to prevent knocking. Hence the power falls off rapidly in this area of knock with ethanol concentrations of less than about twenty per cent.

Figure 24.14 shows the effect of ethanol concentration on the specific fuel consumption of the engine. There is a clear improvement in fuel consumption associated with increasing the compression ratio of the engine made possible by ethanol blending. It may be observed from the figure that the fuel consumption is initially reduced as ethanol concentration is raised to a level of 10 to 20 per cent. At compression ratio 9:1 the detrimental effect of knock is again apparent as indicated by the curve at ethanol concentrations of less than about 20 per cent.

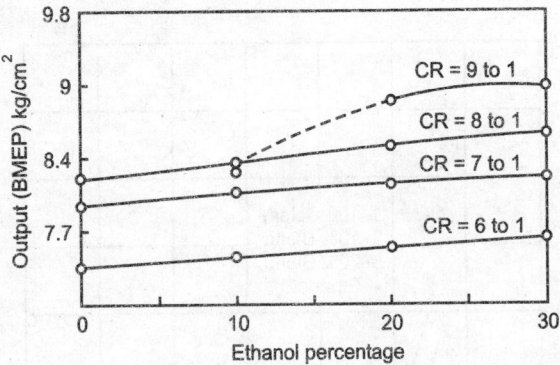

Fig. 24.13. Variation of engine power output with ethanol percentage in the blend at various compression ratios.

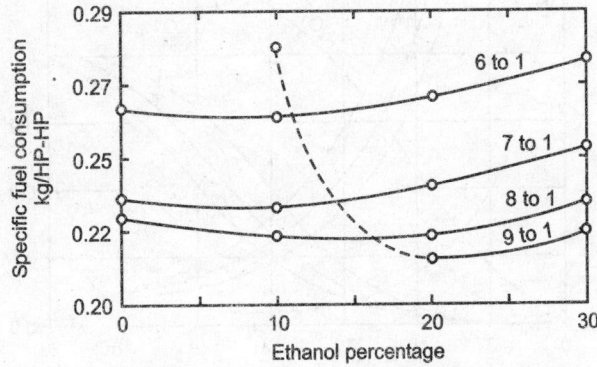

Fig. 24.14. Variation of specific fuel consumption with ethanol percentage in the blend at various compression ratios.

Alcohol blends and exhaust emissions

A change to ethanol blends without modifications or adjustment results in less carbon monoxide in the exhaust effluent than with gasoline as a fuel. This provides a simple way of reducing or completely eliminating carbon monoxide from the engine exhaust by the mere addition of ethanol to gasoline. Thus ethanol addition upto about 20 per cent removes even traces of carbon monoxide in exhaust gas, at the best power ratio for gasoline, when under similar conditions, operation with gasoline would result in about 3 per cent carbon monoxide in the exhaust effluent. Figure 24.15 shows the exhaust CO and NO_x concentrations computed for various ethanol-gasoline blends of practical utility, using a special computer programme, HBMR, developed by Smith. The theoretically predicted results confirm the conclusions drawn from the experimental results.

The addition of ethanol reduces unburned hydrocarbons in the exhaust effluent of an unmodified gasoline engine by a sustantial amount. Thus, the addition of ethanol upto 15 per cent or so reduces exhaust hydrocarbon concentrations upto 30 per cent depending on the air-fuel ratio. Figure 24.16 summarises the effect of ethanol blending on exhaust hydrocarbon concentrations determined experimentally using gas-chromatographic analysis technique. A typical gas chromatogram obtained during the test is shown in Fig. 24.17.

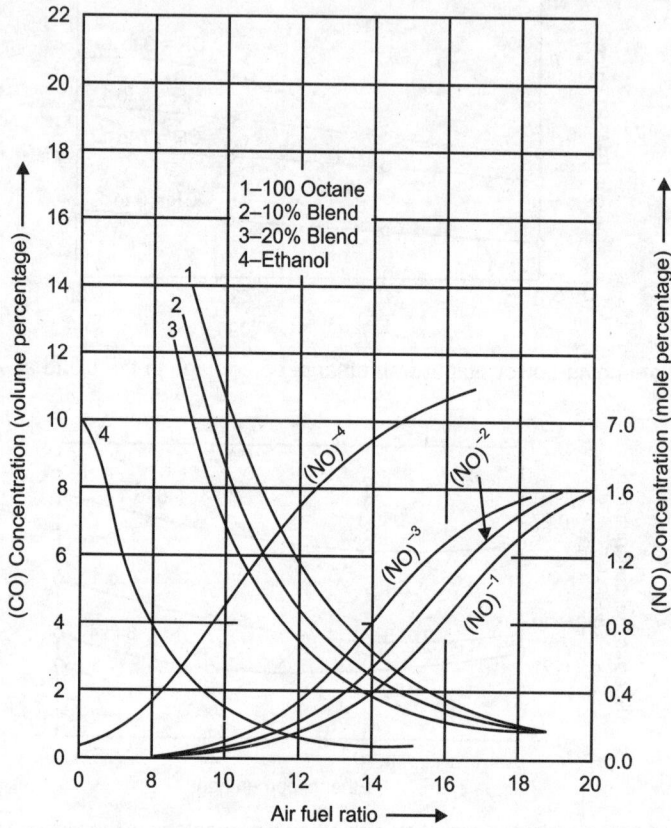

Fig. 24.15. Calculated (NO) concentration and (CO) percentage *vs* air fuel ratios for various fuels.

Ethanol/alcohol engine

Neat ethanol can be utilised as a complete fuel in 'ethanol engines' specially designed for this purpose. Such engines would have a high compression ratio of the order of 12 or so, a high-energy ignition source such as a magneto, and a carburettor specially designed for ethanol with larger jet sizes. Computerised design data have been obtained and designs have been prepared for the major components of an 'ethanol engine' by the Smith for future use. Computerised predictions show that such an engine would give much more specific output and around 10 to 15 per cent higher thermal efficiency.

Although an existing automobile can be modified to demonstrate its operation with ethanol neat, its reliability and life would be seriously jeopardised unless all the major components such as crank shaft, piston, connecting rods, etc. are replaced with much stronger units to withstand the higher peak pressure associated with the increase of compression ratio, every one unit increase of which causes peak cycle pressure to increase by about 120 psi.

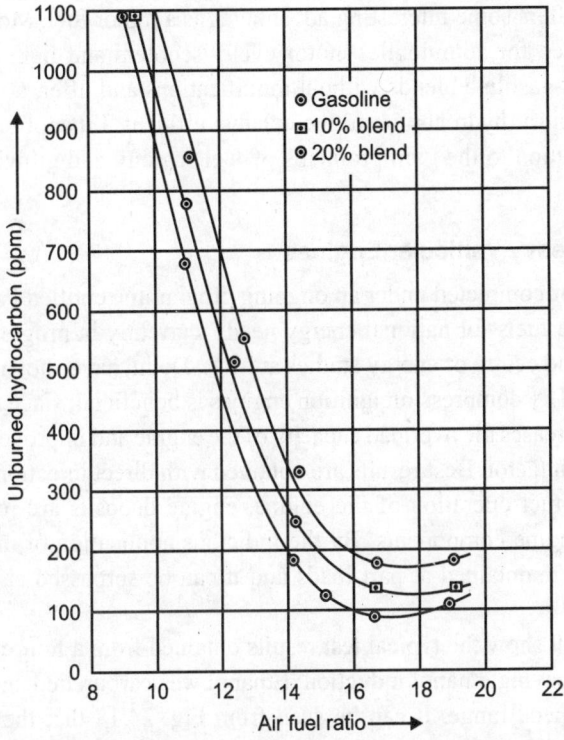

Fig. 24.16. Unburned hydrocarbon concentration in engine exhaust *vs* air-fuel ratio.

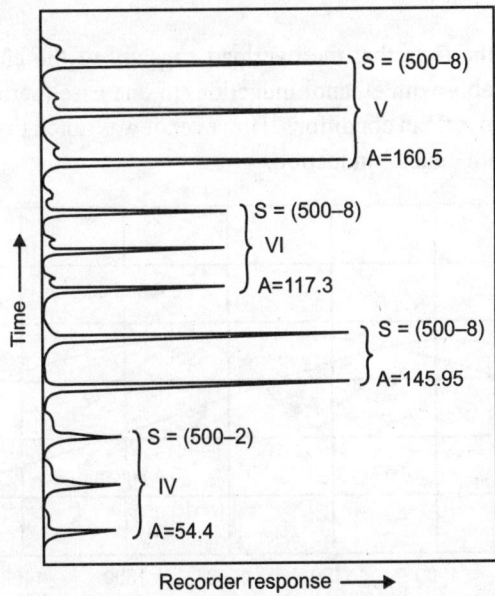

Fig. 24.17. Chromatograms showing unburned hydrocarbon concentration at various air-fuel ratios. Fuel, 10 per cent ethanol-gasoline blend.

In summary, ethanol offers some interesting advantages as a motor fuel. Modern high-compression spark ignition engines used for automobiles/motor cycles/scooters and light trucks can, apparently, make good use of ethanol-gasoline blends without modifications and offer, at the same time, reduced carbon monoxide and unburnt hydrocarbon in the exhaust effluent. Ethanol blending thus provides a partial but immediate solution to the twin problems of fuel scarcity and growing automobile exhaust pollution.

Alcohol Utilisation in Heavy Vehicular Engines

Experimental studies so far completed under an ongoing programme entitled Project U: 'Utilisation of unconventional alternative fuels for national energy needs' currently in progress at the department of mechanical engineering and centre of energy studies at I.I.T., Delhi, have shown that the use of ethanol in heavy vehicles powered by compression ignition engines is beneficial, since it reduces the vehicular exhaust smoke density, increases the overload capacity of the engine and improves the thermal efficiency as well as the air utilisation factor. Best results are obtained with direct injection engines. By inducting ethanol so as to have biofuel operation of the engine, engine deposits are reduced and there is no increase of wear of the engine components. By the judicious application of mixture heating, normal thermal efficiency can be maintained at part loads and it can be surpassed at full load and overload conditions.

Figures 24.18 and 24.19 show the typical test results obtained from a four-cylinder direct injection automotive diesel engine having ethanol induction. Ethanol was carburetted and tests were conducted to cover the entire load-speed range. It can be seen from Fig. 24.18 that the percentage of ethanol inducted at full load is sensibly the same over most of the speed range. Figure 24.19 shows that above half-load operation, the thermal efficiency is not adversely affected by induction of ethanol over the working speed range.

It was observed during the tests that the overload capacity of the engine as well as its thermal efficiency increased appreciably with ethanol induction. In one case thermal efficiency as high as 43 per cent was obtained under overload conditions. However, it was noted that the part-load performance of the engine deteriorated with ethanol induction.

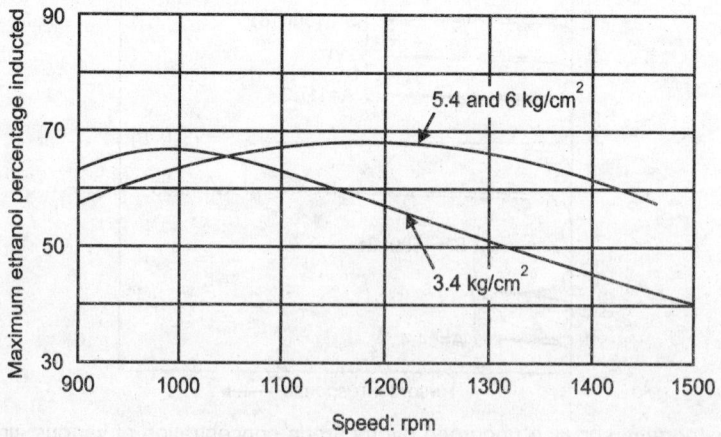

Fig. 24.18. Variation of maximum ethanol percentage induced at various speeds.

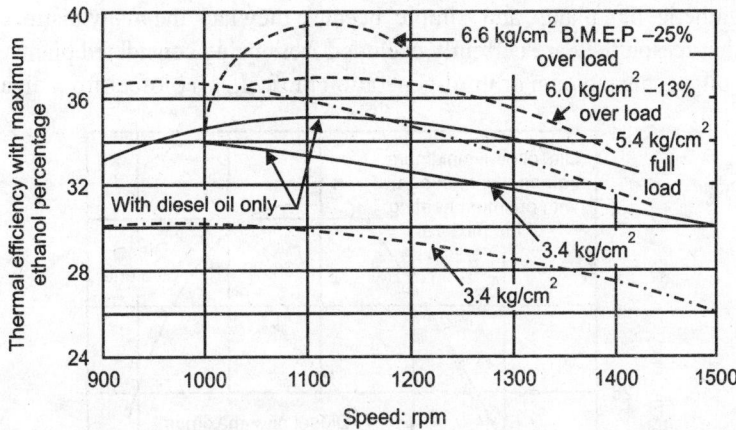

Fig. 24.19. Performance of a four-cylinder direct injection engine with ethanol induction.

The presence of ethanol in the inducted charge increases the delay period considerably at part-load, impairing the combustion process and hence engine performance. This malady can be overcome by the addition of heat to the air-ethanol mixture before admission to the engine. Heating of the inducted mixture to the optimum value restores the delay period almost to the normal value. By judicious application of mixture heating on lines similar to that in S.I. engines, the normal thermal efficiency can be maintained at part loads and surpassed at full and overload conditions as shown in Fig. 24.20 which is based on results obtained in test trials carried out with induction heating.

Detailed studies and extensive tests on alcohol-based fuels, carried out by various scientists in the last 20 years or so, have convincingly shown that in ethanol we have a fuel which, despite its drawbacks, can provide a low knock fuel with power to stand high compression ratios.

Capable of being produced in any country that can support growing crops, or with access to by-products of tropical zones, it enables countries with no indigenous oil deposits to provide a satisfactory motor spirit at minimum cost.

Its use in present-day automobiles in the form of ethanol-gasoline blends can be an immediate short-term measure which can stretch the available fuel supplies and help meet the energy crisis. As a long-term solution to the present-day fuel oil scarcity, vehicular engines can be designed to accommodate ethanol neat as fuel. Carburation of ethanol in heavy vehicles powered by diesel engines can increase their power ratings by 20 to 50 per cent depending upon the type of combustion chamber. This has an added attraction for road transport engines in that it reduces the noise level and exhaust smoke density.

Ethanol/ethyl alcohol can thus go a long way to provide a solution to the twin problems of fuel oil scarcity and growing air pollution due to vehicular engine exhaust emission.

ALGAE FOR BIOFUELS

Algae biofuels need long-term R&D (more R than D) in all areas: algae culture, productivity, harvesting and processing. Even if successful, resource limitations restrict potential due to need for CO_2, water, land, climate, all at same site. Closed photobioreactors do not seem not possible (except for inoculums) at the moment. The problem is not making algae biodiesel, but making algae biomass with high oil content, productively, and doing so cheaply.

Algae are a large and diverse group of simple, typically autotrophic organisms, ranging from unicellular to multicellular forms. The largest and most complex marine forms are called seaweeds.

They are photosynthetic, like plants, and 'simple' because they lack the many distinct organs found in land plants. For that reason they are currently excluded from being considered plants. Algae fuel, also called algal fuel, oilgae, algaeoleum or third-generation biofuel, is a biofuel from algae.

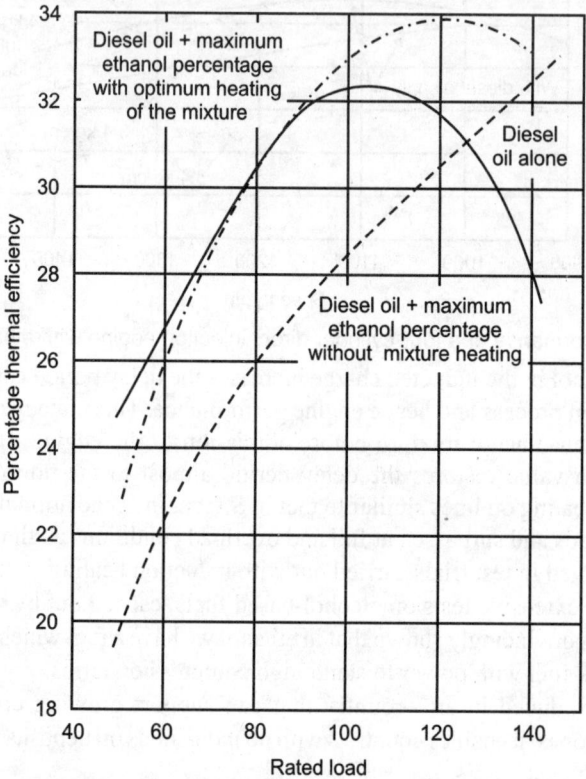

Fig. 24.20. Effect of mixture heating (with induction of maximum quantity of ethanol) on engine performance.

High oil prices, competing demands between foods and other biofuel sources and the world food crisis have ignited interest in algaculture (farming algae) for making vegetable oil, biodiesel, bioethanol, biogasoline, biomethanol, biobutanol and other biofuels. Among algal fuels' attractive characteristics: they do not affect freshwater resources, can be produced using ocean and wastewater, and are biodegradable and relatively harmless to the environment if spilled.

Algae cost more per pound yet can yield over 30 times more energy per acre than other, second-generation biofuel crops. One biofuels company has claimed that algae can produce more oil in an area the size of a two car garage than a football field of soyabeans, because almost the entire algal organism can use sunlight to produce lipids, or oil.

The United States Department of Energy estimates that if algae fuel replaced all the petroleum fuel in the United States, it would require 15,000 square miles (40,000 square kilometres), which is a few thousand square miles larger than Maryland.

Algae is a term that encompasses many different groups of living organisms. Many different species and strains occur—micro algae to macro algae (pond scum to giant kelp); and small, single-celled organisms to multi-cellular organisms, some with fairly complex differentiated form (giant kelp).

The main branches/lines of algae are:
1. Chromista: Brown algae, golden brown algae and diatoms.
2. The red line: red algae.
3. Dinoflagellates: Ciliated protists.
4. The euglenids: single celled organisms including both photosynthetic and non-photosynthetic species.
5. The green line: Plants and green algae.

Algae are among the original sources of fossil hydrocarbons found in geological formations. They account for more than 50 per cent of the ocean's biomass and provide 50 per cent of the world's photosynthesis. It grows in very dilute suspensions and is difficult to dewater.

Algal biomass contains lipids, proteins, carbohydrates and other nutrients.

More than 99.5 per cent of commercial algae biomass produced worldwide currently macro-algae, mainly seaweeds farmed near-shore. Microalgae production levels are only ~10,000 tons per year and 99 per cent of commercial micro-algae biomass production is based on open ponds.

Algae as a Source of Biofuels

Interests in algae as source of energy came in the wake of the oil crisis back in 1970s. The interest from the point of manufacture of fuels is in microalgae, some of which are highly productive of lipids (natural oils)-up to 80 per cent by cell weight, but normally 20 per cent. Algae to oil chain is given in Fig. 24.21.

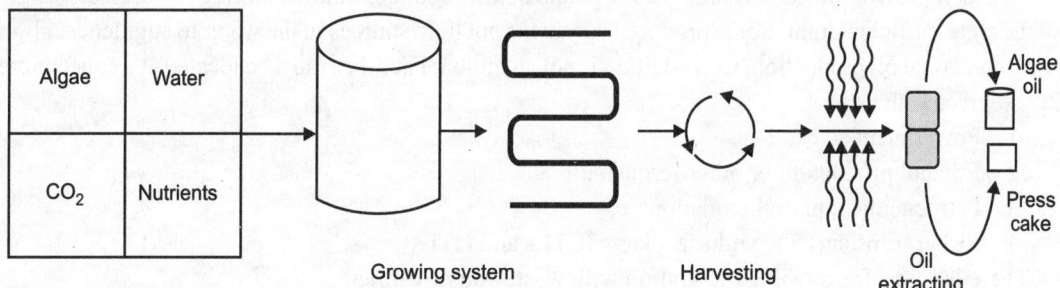

Fig. 24.21. The algae to oil chain

The interest in algae as a source of oil is due to a number of reasons including:
1. Their ability to grow on marginal land and both in fresh and sea water.
2. Seemingly higher yield per hectare, compared to most conventional agricultural crops.
3. High oil content—claims of up to 80 per cent, in most cases usually up to 20 per cent.
4. Lipids are, in general, good quality.
5. Carbon neutral.
6. Valuable coproducts are obtained—high protein content can be used as animal feed, fertilisers and methane gas for bio-gas.

Cultivation and Harvesting of Algae

Simply put, algal biomass production requires:
1. Water (sea, brackish or fresh-water).
2. Nutrients (nitrate, phosphate, iron and some trace elements).
3. Growth media.

4. Carbon dioxide.

5. Light.

Different strains of algae need different cultivation methods, but the techniques can be broadly classified into two categories:

1. Open pond systems, e.g. raceway type ponds.

2. Closed systems—photo-bioreactors (PBRs).

Algae grow in open, closed or semi-closed systems in round, long or tubular tanks that maximise access of the entire biomass to sunlight. Growth occurs only in the top layer, about two inches, of the growing medium, usually water. Application of microalgae is given in Table 24.9.

Table 24.9. Applications of micro-algae.

Sector	Applications
Food	Sushi, beer
Pharmaceutical	Health supplements, personal care
Agricultural	Fertilisers, aquaculture
Environmental	Recultivation of wasteland, e.g. water treatment plants and carbon capture in a power plant
Industrial	Biofuels

New cell growth blocks the sunlight for plants below. Semicontinuous mixing is necessary to give all the algae sufficient light. Some production systems put light sources in the water to augment sunlight. For commercial oil production, CO_2 addition is not an option. Facilities must be located at a concentrated CO_2 source, such as:

1. Power plant stacks.

2. Ethanol production or other fermentations.

3. Petrochemical partial oxidations.

4. Fisher tropsch (FT) synthesis plants (CTLs and GTLs).

There is scope for possible integration with wastewater treatment.

Open cultivation

Open ponds can be categorised into natural waters (lakes, lagoons, ponds) and artificial ponds or containers. The most commonly used systems include shallow big ponds, tanks, circular ponds and raceway ponds. One of the major advantages of open ponds is that they are easier to construct and operate than most closed systems. However, major limitations in open ponds include poor light utilisation by the cells, evaporative losses, diffusion of CO_2 to the atmosphere, and requirement of large areas of land. Furthermore, contamination by predators and other fast growing heterotrophs have restricted the commercial production of algae in open culture systems to only those organisms that can grow under extreme conditions. Also, due to inefficient stirring mechanisms in open cultivation systems, their mass transfer rates are very poor resulting to low biomass productivity.

The ponds in which the algae are cultivated are usually what are called the 'raceway ponds' (Fig. 24.22). In these ponds, the algae, water and nutrients circulate around a racetrack. With paddlewheels providing the flow, algae are kept suspended in the water, and are circulated back to the surface on a regular frequency.

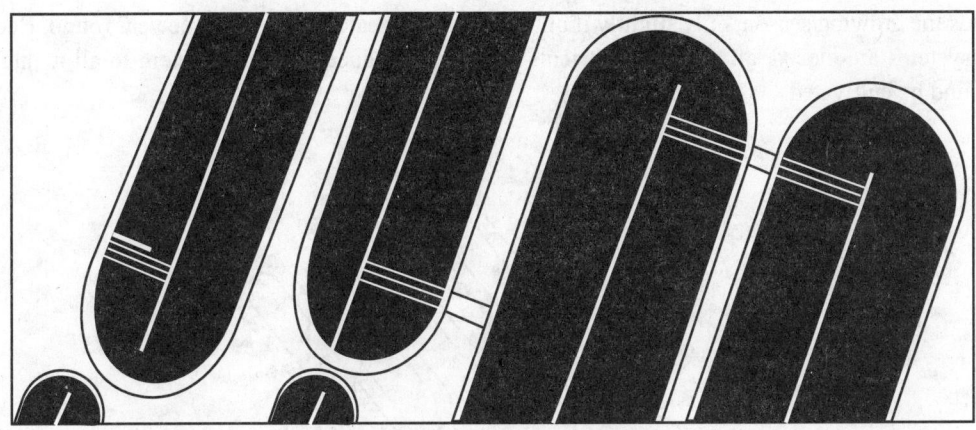

Fig. 24.22. Raceway ponds.

The ponds are usually kept shallow because the algae need to be exposed to sunlight, and sunlight can only penetrate the pond water to a limited depth. The ponds are operated in a continuous manner, with CO_2 and nutrients being constantly fed to the ponds, while algae-containing water is removed at the other end. The biggest advantage of these open ponds is their simplicity, resulting in low production costs and low operating costs. While this is indeed the simplest of all the growing techniques, it has some drawbacks owing to the fact that the environment in and around the pond is not completely under control. Bad weather can stunt algae growth. Contamination from strains of bacteria or other outside organisms often results in undesirable species taking over the desired algal growing in the pond.

The water in which the algae grow also has to be kept at a certain temperature, which can be difficult to maintain. Another drawback is the uneven light intensity and distribution within the pond. Comparison of open and closed systems for growing algae is given in Table 24.10.

Table 24.10. Comparison of open and closed systems for growing algae.

Description	Photo bioreactor	Open pond
Control of gas transfer	+ +	−
Light transmission	+ +	− −
Evaporation	+ +	− −
Uniform growing conditions	+ +	− −
Contamination risk	+ +	− −
Algae cell density	+ +	−
Process control	+ +	− −
Capital	−	+ +
Overall yield (Return/$)	+ +	−

Photo-bioreactors

Algae can also be grown in a photo-bioreactor (PBR). A PBR is a bioreactor, which incorporates some type of light source. Virtually any translucent container could be called a PBR; however the term is more commonly used to define a closed system, as opposed to an open tank or pond (Fig. 24.23). It allows more species to be grown, it allows the species that are being grown to stay dominant, and it extends the growing season, only slightly if unheated, and if heated it can produce year round. Because PBR systems are closed, all essential nutrients must be introduced into the system to allow algae to grow and be cultivated.

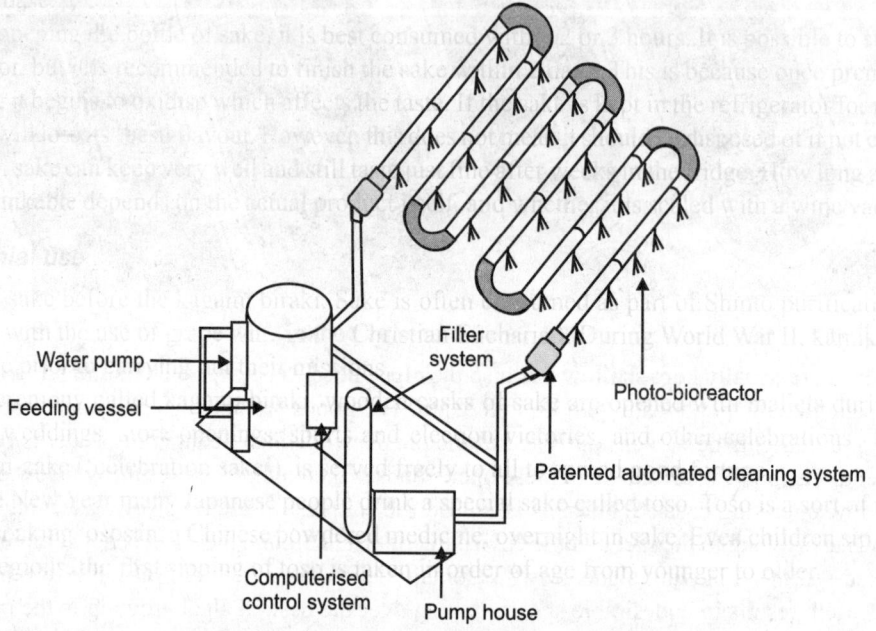

Fig. 24.23. Schematic of an algal photo-bioreactor.

A PBR can be operated in 'batch mode', but it is also possible to introduce a continuous stream of sterilised water containing nutrients, air and CO_2. As the algae grows, excess culture overflows and is harvested. If sufficient care is not taken, continuous PBRs often collapse very quickly; however once they are successfully started, they can continue operating for long periods.

Challenges in Production of Algal Biomass

There are many critical R&D issues and challenges for commercial algae production. These include:
1. Biological: Ability for sustainable cultivation.
2. Agricultural: Cultivation and harvesting.
3. Technology: Processing and contamination.
4. Economics: Current higher value applications.
5. Engineering: Plant scale-up.
6. Competition: Other second generation technologies, such as biomass to liquids (BTL).

Scalability presents the primary production challenge. Laboratory conditions that enable algae to grow many times more productively than land plants simply have not been realised in field settings.

Experiments in modestly scaled production have consistently shown that in field settings the biomass cannot withstand ambient temperatures, are inconsistent in production, too easily become unstable and simply stop growing. Fast growing pure algal cultures do not remain clean indefinitely, and 'weed' algae must be removed. Comparison of biomass production methods is given in Table 24.11. There are many exuberant algae productivity claims, some of which go as high as 1,000,000 litres/hectare-year and even violate the First Law of Thermodynamics. The maximum yield is likely to be of the order of ~2000 gal oil/acre-year with current technology.

Extracting the Oil

The extraction of oil from algae is one of the more costly processes, which determines the sustainability of algae-based biodiesel. Breakthroughs are anticipated to effectively extract oil from marine algae.

Table 24.11. Comparison of biomass production methods (year 2008).

Description	Raceway ponds	Tubular photobioreactors
Capital cost	$1,549 per ton	$15,500 per ton
Productivity	~82 tons/ha-yr	~158 tons/ha-yr
Biomass recovery cost	0.5 kg/m^3	4 kg/m^3
Process control	Poor	Good
Loss of carbon dioxide	~35%	< 5%
Susceptibility to weather/contamination	High	Less prone
Area	2.1-ha per 1000 tons	6.3-ha per 1000 tons

The breaking-down of algae cells to release oil, known as lysing, has long represented a challenge for the algae-to-oil industry. Algae cell walls are difficult to break down and while mechanical methods are energy-intensive, commonly used chemical solvents are toxic and require special handling.

Biomass residue from extraction can be used as protein animal feed; a source of other valuable microalgal products; or as a raw material for biogas production using anaerobic digestion.

The conventional methods of extraction are:

1. Oil expeller/press.
2. Solvent extraction.
3. Supercritical fluid extraction.

More recent developments include:

1. Enzymatic extraction.
2. Osmotic shock.
3. Ultrasound assisted extraction.

Oil expeller/press

Oil contained in dried algae is forced out under high mechanical pressure in an expeller or press. It utilises the same principle that is widely used in vegetable oil manufacturing. Large percentage of oil (70–75 per cent) can be extracted. A flow diagram of algal biorefinery concept is shown in Fig. 24.24.

Press configurations include screw, expeller, piston type, etc. It is often used in conjunction with chemical extractions.

Solvent extraction

It is always used in combination with oil expeller/press as a pre-treatment stage. The combined process extracts more than 95 per cent of oil present in algae. Solvents used include hexane, benzene, petroleum distillates, ethers, etc. The disadvantages of the process are:

1. Toxicity of solvents and issues related to solvent residues in the cake and oil.
2. Explosion hazard, which requires stringent safety standard and higher cost in investment.

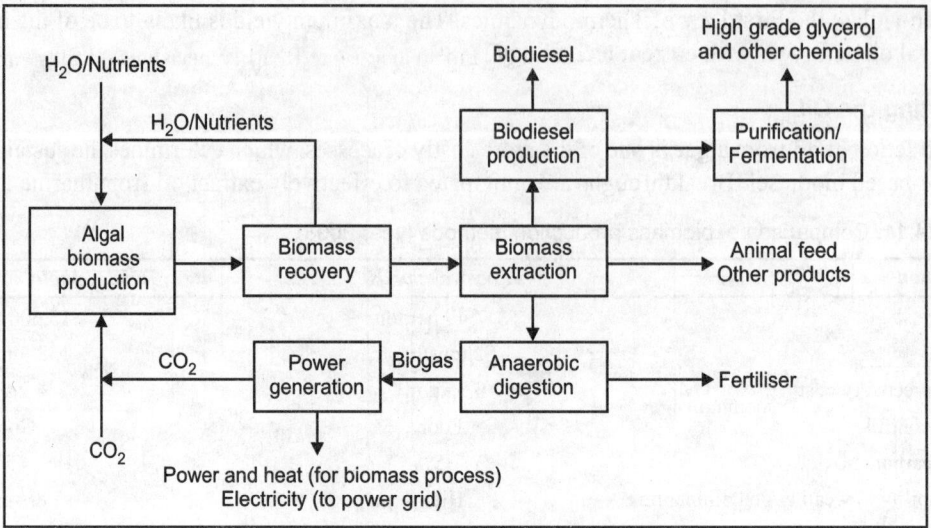

Fig. 24.24. Algal biorefinery concept.

Supercritical fluid extraction

CO_2 is liquefied under pressure and heated to critical point, the liquefied fluid then acts as the solvent in extracting the algae oil. The process extracts almost 100 per cent of the oils, but requires special equipment for containment and pressure. Water-based supercritical extraction processes have also been developed, as an alternative to CO_2-based processes and have the following advantages:

1. Low extraction times.
2. Higher quality of the extracts.
3. Lower costs of the extracting agent.
4. Environmentally compatible.
5. Extraction yield similar to conventional techniques.

Enzymatic extraction

Enzymatic extraction uses enzymes to degrade the cell walls with water acting as the solvent to facilitate the fractionation of the oil.

Osmotic shock

Osmotic shock is a sudden reduction in osmotic pressure. This can cause cells in a solution to rupture. Single-celled organisms such as algae are more vulnerable to osmotic shock, and hence the process is considered a potential method to release oil from algae species.

Ultrasonic extraction

The principle of ultrasonic extraction is based on acoustic cavitation effect when sound waves propagate through a liquid media with suitable vapour pressure and viscosity. The cavitation introduces strong shear force that easily ruptures the cell wall of algae, facilitating the extraction of oil content.

This is a safe and environmental friendly technology, which has minimum side effects due to its 'mild' extraction conditions. Efficiency and productivity can be easily enhanced in combination with other extraction techniques.

Algal Biorefinery

A biorefinery is a facility that integrates a variety of conversion processes to produce multiple product streams. A biorefinery maximises the value derived from a biomass feedstock. For example, it can produce one or more low-volume, high-value chemical products; a low-value high-volume liquid transportation fuel; and electricity and process heat for its own use and/or export.

It has been identified as the most promising route to the creation of a sustainable bio-based economy. Feedstock costs remain the primary driver of competitive biodiesel production costs. While biodiesel economics have improved following the drop in palm oil pricing in 2008 (CPO prices plunged by over 65 per cent since March 2008), uncertainty continues to plague these markets and margins in the industry remain volatile, depending on commodity pricing and government policies.

Commercial Developments

More than a 100 firms across the world are reported to be working on cultivation and harvesting of algal biomass. Some of these include: Algaen, arare, aquaflow, biodiesel, biofuels digest, biofuel review, bionavitas, carbon capture corp, cell tech, diversified energy, EnAgri, energy farms, energy update, ethanol India, genergetics, green energy, global green solutions, green shift, green start products, GS cleantech, infinifuel, inventure, Kent Sea Tech, Kiwikpower, OriginOil, PetroAlgae (XL TechGroup), plaatts, pelletbase, raytheon, texas clean fuels, simplexity and world oil (Table 24.12).

Table 24.12. Current status of algae development.

Company	Development
Live fuels	Seeking to produce fuel from bio-crude by 2010
Green fuel technologies	Emissions to biofuels. Algae bioreactor fitted to fuels stacks
BFS (Spain)	Plankton to oil using solar energy, photosynthesis, electro-magnetics
Veridium	Bioreactors convert carbon dioxide from fermentation
DeBeers fuels (South Africa)	Partner with Green fuel. Targeting 16–24 billion litres by 2012
Sapphire energy	Produced renewable gasoline in 2008; Targeting commercial production by 2012–13
PetroSum	Arizona field testing in 2007, followed by refinery. Targeting 10 million gpy; Exploring other sites in Australasia and China
Solazyme	Algae fermentation and oil recovery processes; Detailed plant design completed
A2BE	Fully enclosed, bio-isolated photo bio-reactors; Pilot plant expected to be operational by 2011

Thus, algae could play an important role as a potential feedstock for biofuels, as it offers significant advantages in terms of yield and productivity compared to conventional feedstocks. It may even have an advantage over other emerging 2nd generation technologies since it sequesters carbon in CO_2 emissions. It is able to utilise other pollutants such as NO_2, an added environmental advantage. Comparison between existing and next generation biofuels is given in Table 24.13. However, its success will be dependent on advancements of current research and developments to commercialisation.

Algae could have a key biofuels role, but scale of its potential role remains uncertain and will be determined by the rate of advancement in technology and, most importantly, its economics. Factors and their relevance in microalgae is given in Table 24.14.

Table 24.13. Comparison between existing and next generation biofuels.

Crop	Feedstock Availability	Sustainability	Yield	Quality relative to petroleum diesel	Technology	Availability of infrastructure	Capital intensity	Cost of production	By-product credit	Regional development	Time to commercialisation
Vegetable oils	Yes	Low to moderate	Low to moderate	Similar	Yes	Yes	Low	Low	Moderate	High	Established
Sugarcane	Yes	Moderate	High	Similar	Yes	Yes	Low	Low	Moderate	High	Established
Starch				Similar	Yes	Yes	Moderate	Low	Moderate	Moderate	Established
Corn	Yes	Low to moderate	Low								
Wheat	Yes		Low								
Jatropha	–	Moderate	Moderate	Similar	Yes	–	Low	Low	Moderate	High	Not there yet
Algae	–	–	–		–	–	–		High	Very low	5–10 years
2nd generation BTL	Very high	Yes	Yes	High	Yes	–	Very high	Very high	High	Very low	~5–10 years
2nd generation cellulosic ethanol	Very high	Yes	Yes	High	Yes	–	Very high	Very high	High	Very low	~5–10 years

Table 24.14. Micro-algae: A reality check.

Factor	Relevance
Grow faster	Not all that relevant (except for R&D)
More productive	Possible, but not proven (need R&D!)
Use power plant flue gas	CO_2—a need, not a virtue
Have high oil content	OK, but must be productive (R&D)
Use saline, brackish, waste-waters	Yes, use less water
Not compete with agriculture	OK, but we could eat algae!
Low cost of production/processing	Not true!
Closed photobioreactors can be used	Absolutely not true
Very large production potential	Many, many limitations

Chapter 25

Food Microbiology and Public Health

INTRODUCTION

Although food is indispensible to the maintenance of life, it can also be responsible for ill health. A simple insufficiency will lead to marasmus (protein-energy deficiency) while over-reliance on staples low in protein, such as cassava, produces the condition known as kwashiorkor. A diet may provide adequate protein and energy but be lacking in specific minerals or vitamins giving rise to characteristic deficiency syndromes such as goitre (iodine deficiency), pellagra (nicotinic acid), beriberi (thiamine) and scurvy (ascorbic acid).

Foods are complex mixtures of chemicals and often contain compounds that are potentially harmful as well as those that are beneficial (Fig. 25.1). Several vitamins are toxic if consumed in excessive amounts and many food plants produce toxic secondary metabolites to discourage their attack by pests.

Potatoes contain the toxic alkaloid solanine. Normally this is more concentrated in aerial parts of the plants and the peel which are not eaten, but high levels are also found in green potatoes and potato sprouts which should be avoided.

Cassava contains cyanogenic glycosides which produce hydrogen cyanide on hydrolysis. Similar compounds are also present in apple seeds, almonds, lima beans, yams and bamboo shoots. The body's detoxification pathway converts cyanide to thiocyanate which can interfere with iodine metabolism giving rise to goitre and cretinism. Traditional methods of preparing cassava eliminate the acute toxicity problem from hydrogen cyanide, but the increased incidence of goitre and cretinism in some areas where cassava is a staple may be a reflection of chronic exposure. Legumes or pulses contain a number of anti-nutritional factors such as phytate, trypsin inhibitors and lectins (haemagglutinins). Many of these are destroyed or removed by normal preparation procedures such as soaking and cooking. Even so, red kidney beans are still responsible for occasional outbreaks of food poisoning when they have been insufficiently cooked to destroy the lectins they contain. Lathyrism is a more serious condition associated with a toxin in the pulse *Lathyrus sativa* which can be a major food item in North African and Asian communities during times of famine. In favism, an enzyme deficiency predisposes certain individuals to illness caused by glycosides in the broad bean, *Vicia faba*.

To some extent toxic or antinutritional characteristics can be bred out of cultivars intended for human consumption, although the problem cannot be eliminated completely. For affluent consumers in the developed world, particularly toxic foods can be avoided since alternatives are normally available in plenty. This is not always the case in poorer countries where these diet-related conditions are far more common. It is however important to keep a sense of proportion in this. Eating inevitably exposes us to natural chemicals whose long-term effects on health are not known at present. Provided such foods form part of a balanced diet and are correctly prepared, the risks involved are generally acceptable, particularly when compared to the certain outcome should immoderate fear of food lead to complete abstinence.

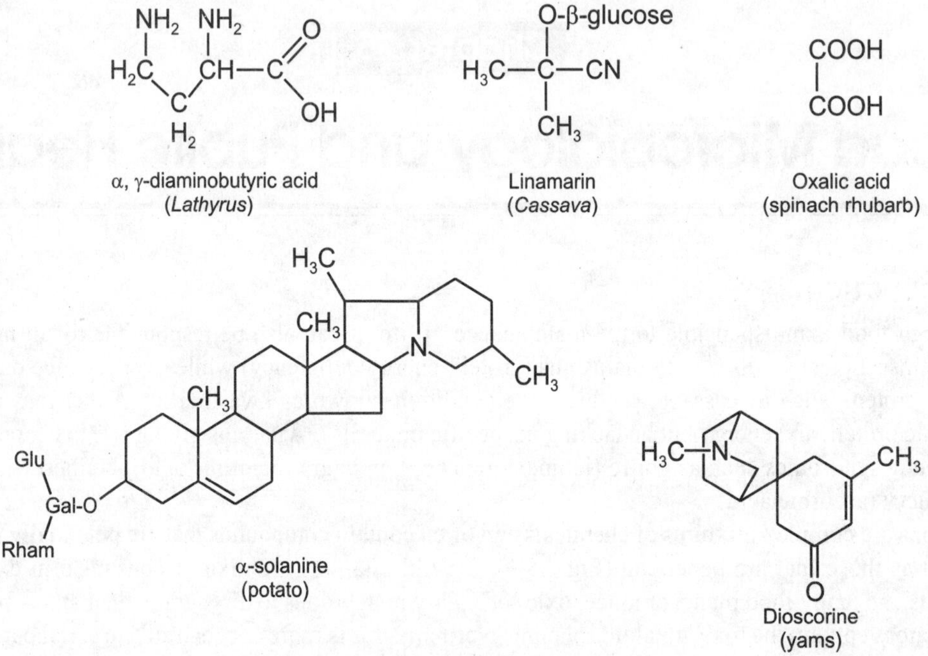

Fig. 25.1. Some natural food toxicants.

In addition to the hazards posed by natural toxins that are an intrinsic feature of their composition, foods may also act as the vehicle by which an exogenous harmful agent may be ingested. This may be a pesticide, some other chemical contaminant added by design or accident, a micro-organism or its toxin. Various causes of foodborne illness are summarised in Table 25.1.

Table 25.1. Possible causes of foodborne illness.

Chemical
Intrinsic, natural toxins, e.g. red kidney bean poisoning, toxic mushrooms
Extrinsic contamination
Algae, e.g. paralytic shellfish poisoning
Bacteria (infection and intoxication)
Fungi (mycotoxins)
Parasites
Protozoa
Viruses

Here we are concerned primarily with microbiological hazards (Table 25.2). These are considered in some detail subsequently, but to justify this attention, we must first provide some assessment of their importance.

Table 25.2. Some microbiological agents of foodborne illness.

Agents	Important reservoir/carrier	Transmission[a] Water food	Transmission[a] Person to person	Multiplication in food	Examples of some incriminated foods
Bacteria					
Aeromonas	Water	+	+	–	+	
Bacillus cereus	Soil	–	+	–	+	Cooked rice cooked meats
						Vegetables, starchy puddings
Brucella species	Cattle, goats, sheep	–	+	–	+	Raw milk, dairy products
Campylobacter jejuni	Chickens, dogs, cats, cattle, pigs, wild birds	+	+	+	–[b]	Raw milk, poultry
Clostridium botulinum	Soil, mammals, birds, fish	–	+	–	+	Fish, meat, vegetables (home preserved)
Clostridium perfringens	Soil, animals, man	–	+	–	+	Cooked meat and poultry, gravy, beans
Escherichia coli						
Enterotoxigenic	Man	+	+	+	+	Salads, raw vegetables
Enteropathogenic	Man	+	+	+	+	Milk
Enteroinvasive	Man	+	+	0	+	Cheese
Entero-haemorrhagic	Cattle, poultry, sheep	+	+	+	+	Undercooked meat, raw milk, cheese
Listeria monocytogenes		+	+	+	+	Soft cheeses, milk, coleslaw, pate
Mycobacterium bovis	Cattle	–	+	–	–	Raw milk
Salmonella Typhi	Man	+	+	±	+	Dairy produce, meat products, shellfish, vegetable salads
Salmonella (non-Typhi)	Man and animals	±	+	±	+	Meat, poultry, eggs, dairy produce, chocolate
Shigella	Man	+	+	+	+	Potato/egg salads
Staphylococcus aureus (enterotoxins)	Man	–	+	–	+	Ham, poultry and egg salads, cream-filled bakery produce, ice-cream, cheese

(Contd ...)

Agents	Important reservoir/carrier	Transmission[a]		Multip-lication in food	Examples of some incriminated foods
		Water food	Person to person		
Vibrio cholerae O1	Man, marine life	+	+	±	+	Salad, shellfish
Vibrio cholerae, non-O1	Man and animals marine life	+	+	±	+	Shellfish
Vibrio para-haemolyticus	Sea water, marine life	−	+	−	+	Raw fish, crabs, and other shellfish
Yersinia enterocolitica	Water, wild animals, pigs, dogs, poultry	+	+	−	+	Milk, pork and poultry
Viruses						
Hepatitis A virus	Man	+	+	+	−	Shellfish, raw fruit and vegetables
Norwalk agents	Man	+	+	0	−	Shellfish
Rotavirus	Man	+	0	+	−	0
Protozoa						
Cryptosporidium parvum	Man, animals	+	+	+	−	Raw milk, raw sausage (non-fermented)
Entamoeba histolytica	Man	+	+	+	−	Raw vegetables and fruits
Giardia lamblia	Man, animals	+	±	+	−	0
Helminths						
Ascaris lumbricoides	Man	+	+	−	−	Soil-contaminated food
Taenia saginata x and T. solium	Cattle, swine	−	+	−	−	Undercooked meat
Trichinella spiralis	Swine, carnivora	−	+	−	−	Undercooked meat
Trichuris trichiura	Man	0	+	−	−	Soil-contaminated food

[a]Almost all acute enteric infections show increased transmission during the summer and/or wet months, except infections due to rotavirus and Yersinia enterocolitica, which show increased transmission in cooler months.
[b]Under certain circumstances some multiplication has been observed. The epidemiological significance of this observation is not clear.
+ = Yes.
± = Rare.
− = No.
0 = No information.

SIGNIFICANCE OF FOODBORNE DISEASE

Foodborne disease has been defined by the world health organisation (WHO) as:

'Any disease of an infectious or toxic nature caused by, or thought to be caused by, the consumption of food or water.'

This definition includes all food and waterborne illness and is not confined to those primarily associated with the gastro-intestinal tract and exhibiting symptoms such as diarrhoea and/or vomiting. It, therefore, encompasses illnesses which present with other symptoms such as paralytic shellfish poisoning, botulism and listeriosis as well as those caused by toxic chemicals, but excludes illness due to allergies and food intolerances. The essential message of this section can be summarised by the conclusions of a WHO expert committee which pointed out that foodborne diseases, most of which are of microbial origin, are perhaps the most widespread problem in the contemporary world and an important cause of reduced economic productivity.

A number of assessments of the relative significance of hazards associated with food have concluded that micro-organisms are of paramount importance. A study conducted in the United States found that, although the attention given to different food hazards by the media, pressure groups and regulatory authorities might differ, as far as the food industry was concerned microbial hazards were the highest priority. Similarly, it has been estimated that the risk of becoming ill as a result of microbial contamination of food was 1,00,000 times greater than the risk from pesticide contamination.

For otherwise healthy, well-nourished people in the developed world, most food poisoning is an unpleasant episode from which recovery is normally complete after a few days. For society as a whole though, it is increasingly being recognised as a largely avoidable economic burden. Costs are incurred in the public sector from the diversion of resources into the treatment of patients and the investigation of the source of infection. To the individual the costs may not always be calculable in strictly financial terms but could include loss of income, costs of medication and treatment. Studies conducted by the communicable disease surveillance centre (CDSC) in London have even identified as a cost the 'trousseau effect', where an individual who is hospitalised incurs additional expense as a result of having to purchase items such as new night-attire for the occasion. On the larger scale, absence from work will also constitute a cost to the national economy.

For the food industry, the costs can be huge and it is not unusual for the company producing a product implicated in an outbreak of food poisoning to go bankrupt as a result. Companies not directly involved in an outbreak can also suffer. There is often a general decline in demand for a product prompted by public concern that the same problem could occur with similar products from other manufacturers. There was, for instance, a marked downturn in all yoghurt sales after the hazelnut yoghurt botulism outbreak in England in 1989.

Increased vigilance by companies to ensure that the same process failures responsible for an outbreak do not occur elsewhere, also has its attendant costs. For instance, it was estimated that the costs of checking the integrity of spray-drier cladding by dried-milk manufacturers following a salmonella outbreak caused by dried milk were of the order of hundreds of thousands of pounds.

Food retailers can also be affected as a result of a decline in sales, particularly if a suspect product is associated with one particular store.

In the less developed world the consequences of foodborne illness are even more serious. Diarrhoeal disease is a major cause of morbidity and mortality in poor countries, particularly among children. It has been estimated that some 1500 million children under 5 suffer from diarrhoea each year and that over 3 million die as a result. Diarrhoea can occur repeatedly in the same individual leading to malnutrition which in turn predisposes them to more severe diarrhoeal episodes and other serious infections. This can produce a downward spiral of increasingly poor health which can seriously impair a child's mental and physical development and can lead to its premature death (Fig. 25.2).

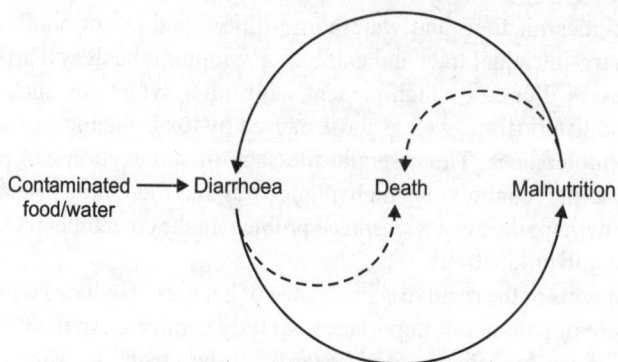

Fig. 25.2. The malnutrition and diarrhoea cycle.

Weaning is a particularly hazardous time for the infant. The anti-infective properties of maternal breast milk are lost or diluted and are replaced by foods which often have a low nutrient density. At the same time, the immature immune system is exposed to new sources of infection in the environment. Poor hygienic practices in the preparation of weaning foods and the use of contaminated water are often implicated in weaning diarrhoea and it has been estimated that 15–70 per cent of all diarrhoea episodes in young children are food associated.

INCIDENCE OF FOODBORNE ILLNESS

Statistics covering food borne illnesses are notoriously unreliable. Simply quantifying the problem of those diseases initiated by infection through the gastrointestinal tract is difficult enough, but to determine in what proportion food acted as the vehicle is harder still.

Many countries have no system for collecting and reporting data on gastrointestinal infections and even where these exist the reported data is acknowledged to represent only a fraction of the true number of cases. Studies have suggested that the ratio of actual to reported cases can be between 25:1 and 100:1. One should also be circumspect about using published national statistics for comparative purposes since apparent differences can often simply reflect differences in the efficiency of the reporting system. In the United States, reporting of foodborne illness outbreaks to the Centre for Infectious Diseases, is not compulsory so that some States report rates 200 times those of other States. In the early 1990s reported outbreaks of foodborne disease for the United States were roughly twice those reported by Canada which has a population only one tenth the size.

It seems unlikely that Canadians are markedly more susceptible to foodborne illness or more careless about food hygiene than their neighbours; more probably the disparity reflects a higher level of under-reporting in the United States. Some support for this appears if the statistics for all gastrointestinal disease are compared. These are a much closer reflection of the relative population sizes since these figures are officially notifiable in the USA.

Such statistical problems are not unique to North America. The WHO Surveillance Programme for Control of Foodborne Infections and Intoxications in Europe which reports data from more than 30 countries has noted the different national systems of notification and reporting. These include:

1. Notification of cases of foodborne disease without any specification of the causative agent or other epidemiologically important details.
2. Reporting only laboratory-confirmed cases of foodborne disease collated by a central agency.

3. Reporting cases of gastrointestinal infection which, in some cases, are regarded as being foodborne regardless of whether the involvement of food has been established.

4. Reporting only cases of salmonellosis.

If all these different types of data are treated as equivalent, 2,76,469 cases of foodborne disease became known to official health agencies in participating countries in 1993 and 1994. This amounted to a mean overall incidence in 1994 of 38.3 cases per 1,00,000 inhabitants. However, because of differences in the reporting systems between countries, this figure ranges from 2.0 to 915.8 per 1,00,000.

Most cases of foodborne illness are described as sporadic; single cases which are not apparently related to any others. Sometimes two or more cases are shown to be linked to a common factor in which case they constitute an outbreak. Outbreaks can be confined to a single family or be more generalised, particularly when commercially processed foods are involved.

In England and Wales, information on sporadic cases of foodborne, disease comes from a number of different sources. The office for national statistics publishes statistics on clinical cases of food poisoning which comprise notifications by medical practitioners and those cases identified during the course of outbreak investigations but not formally notified by a doctor. Although notification is statutory, i.e. required by law, these data are acknowledged to be incomplete as a result of significant under reporting. Diagnosis is often made purely on the basis of symptoms, without recourse to any microbiological investigation which could establish both the causative agent and the food vehicle. Some of the bacterial gastrointestinal agents causing food poisoning with the notable exception of clostridium botulinum are: (i) *salmonella*, (ii) *clostridium perfringens*, (iii) *bacillus sp.*, (iv) *staph. aureus*, (v) *E. coli* 0157, (vi) *shigella sonnei*, (vii) *clostridium botulinum*, (viii) *campylobacter*, and (x) *V. cholerae*.

It is reasonable to assume that the more ill you feel the more likely you are to seek medical attention and the more likely your case is to figure in official statistics. The situation can be represented as a pyramid, where the large base reflects the true incidence of food poisoning which is reduced to a small apex of official statistics by the various factors that contribute to under-reporting (Fig. 25.3).

The infectious intestinal disease (IID) study which collected data in England in the period 1999–2002 aimed to estimate some of these uncertainties. Based primarily around 70 representative doctor's practices, volunteers were recruited to notify the doctor each week whether or not they had symptoms of gastrointestinal illness during that week and, in cases where they had been ill, to submit a faecal specimen to the laboratory. Surveys were also made on the number of people visiting the doctor complaining of IID and the proportion from which faecal specimens were taken, the long-term medical sequelae of IID and the numbers of cases presenting to hospitals rather than to their local doctor. The results, published in the British Medical Journal, were broadly similar to those found in an earlier Dutch study and indicated that infectious intestinal disease occurs in 1 in 5 people each year amounting to an estimated 9.4 million cases. Of those people affected, only 1 in 6 went to the doctor. The proportion of cases that were not recorded by official statistics was large and varied widely by organism. For example, the degree of under reporting for salmonella was relatively low with 1 in 3.2 cases being reported. It was worse with campylobacter where the ratio was 1 in 7.6 cases.

Under reporting of viral IID was much more severe with national surveillance picking up only 1 in 35 cases of diarrhoea caused by rotavirus and 1 in 1562 caused by small round structured viruses. There were also many cases for which no causative organism was identified. An additional source of statistics is the CDSC of the public health laboratory service which collects information under a voluntary, nonstatutory reporting system from public health and hospital laboratories on isolations of gastrointestinal pathogens.

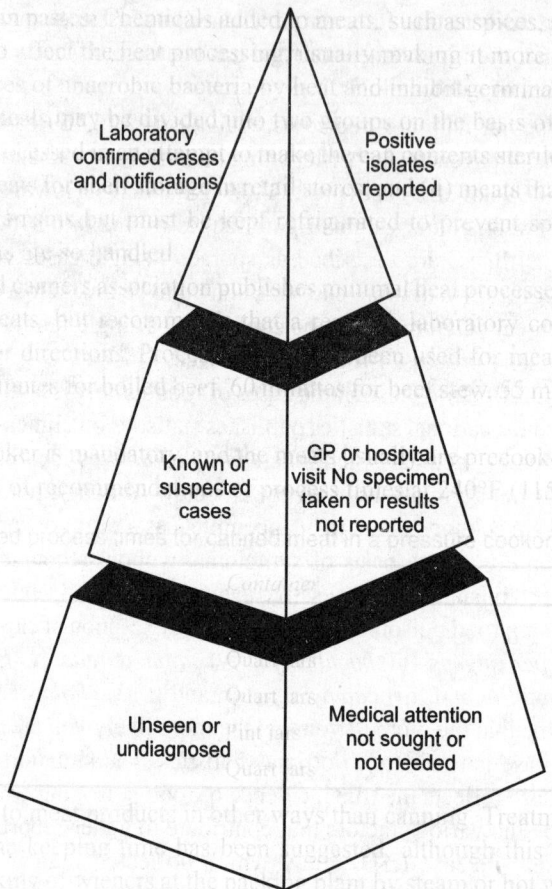

Fig. 25.3. The food poisoning pyramid.

The statistics generated in this way include cases where food was not the vehicle but the pathogen was acquired by some other means such as person-to-person spread or from domestic pets.

Information on outbreaks is collected by the CDSC from microbiologists and environmental health officials around the country. Sometimes the existence of an outbreak is impossible to ignore if it involves a large number of people or a readily defined commercial or institutional context, for example a large public reception, diners at the same restaurant or passengers in the same airliner. Sometimes the existence of an outbreak may emerge from followup investigations on sporadic cases. This is often possible where highly discriminating typing schemes are available that enable the pathogen strain causing an outbreak to be distinguished from strains responsible for the statistical background 'noise' of sporadic cases. Even so, it is probable that many outbreaks remain undetected, submerged in the numbers for sporadic cases.

RISK FACTORS ASSOCIATED WITH FOODBORNE ILLNESS

Outbreaks of food poisoning involve a number of people and a common source and are consequently more intensively investigated than the more numerous sporadic cases that occur. Valuable information is derived from these investigations about the most common contributory factors and faults in food hygiene that lead to outbreaks of foodborne illness. Specific examples will be given in the following section when bacterial pathogens are considered individually, but analysis of this information does allow a number of generalisations to be made.

The foods that are most frequently incriminated in foodborne disease in Europe and North America are those of animal origin: meat, poultry, milk, eggs and products derived from them. This is particularly true of illness caused by *Salmonella* and *Clostridium perfringens*. The same general picture is true of most industrialised countries although the relative importance of some animal products does differ. For example, in Spain between 1985 and 1989 eggs and egg products such as mayonnaise were incriminated in 62 per cent of outbreaks for which a cause was established. In the Netherlands in 1991 and 1992 Chinese food was the most common vehicle associated with outbreaks, ahead of both poultry and eggs and other meats.

Fish and shellfish are less commonly implicated but can be an important vehicle in some countries, often reflecting local dietary habits. Between 1973 and 1987, 20 per cent of food-poisoning outbreaks in the USA and 10 per cent of outbreaks in France in 1988 were associated with fish and shellfish, though for most other countries the figures are lower. Outbreaks can result from the distribution of a contaminated food product or from situations where meals are being produced for large numbers of people. Evidence from numerous countries has shown that mass-catering is by far the most frequent cause of outbreaks, whether it comes under the guise of restaurants, hotels, canteens, hospitals or special events such as wedding receptions. There are a number of reasons why this should be, but inadequacies of management, staff training and facilities are often identified.

Analyses of the specific failures in food hygiene that have contributed to outbreaks have been conducted on a number of occasions and results of two of these, from the United States and from England and Wales are presented in Table 25.3. Comparing the two is not entirely straightforward since, in most outbreaks more than one contributory factor has been identified so that the columns do not add up neatly to 100 per cent. Also, the surveys differ in the categories used and even where they are nominally the same they may still not be equivalent in all respects. Even so, inspection of Table 25.4 reveals two major contributory factors; temperature and time. Failure to cool foods and hold them at temperatures inimical to microbial growth, or to heat them sufficiently to kill micro-organisms, coupled with prolonged storage giving micro-organisms time to multiply to dangerous levels. An interesting difference between the two sets of data is the lower incidence of infected food handlers contributing to illness in England and Wales.

Table 25.3. Factors contributing to outbreaks of food poisoning.

Factor	England and Wales	USA
Preparation too far in advance	57	29
Storage at ambient temperature	38	63
Inadequate cooling	32	63
Contaminated processed food	17	–
Undercooking	15	5
Contaminated canned food	7	–
Inadequate thawing	6	–

(Contd ...)

Factor	England and Wales	USA
Cross contamination	6	15
Food consumed raw	6	–
Improper warm handling	5	27
Infected food handlers	4	26
Use of left overs	4	7
Extra large quantities prepared	3	–

Figures are expressed as percentages. Since several factors may contribute to a single outbreak columns do not total 100 per cent.

SITE OF FOODBORNE ILLNESS AND ALIMENTARY TRACT: ITS FUNCTION AND MICROFLORA

In most of the cases of foodborne illness we consider, the pathogenic (disease producing) effect occurs in the alimentary tract giving rise to symptoms such as diarrhoea and vomiting. Since these are essentially a dysfunction of the gut, a useful starting point would be to outline its normal operation and the role micro-organisms play in this process. The alimentary or gastrointestinal tract is not an internal organ of the body but a tube passing through it from the mouth to the anus (Fig. 25.4). Its principal functions are the digestion and absorption of food and the excretion of waste.

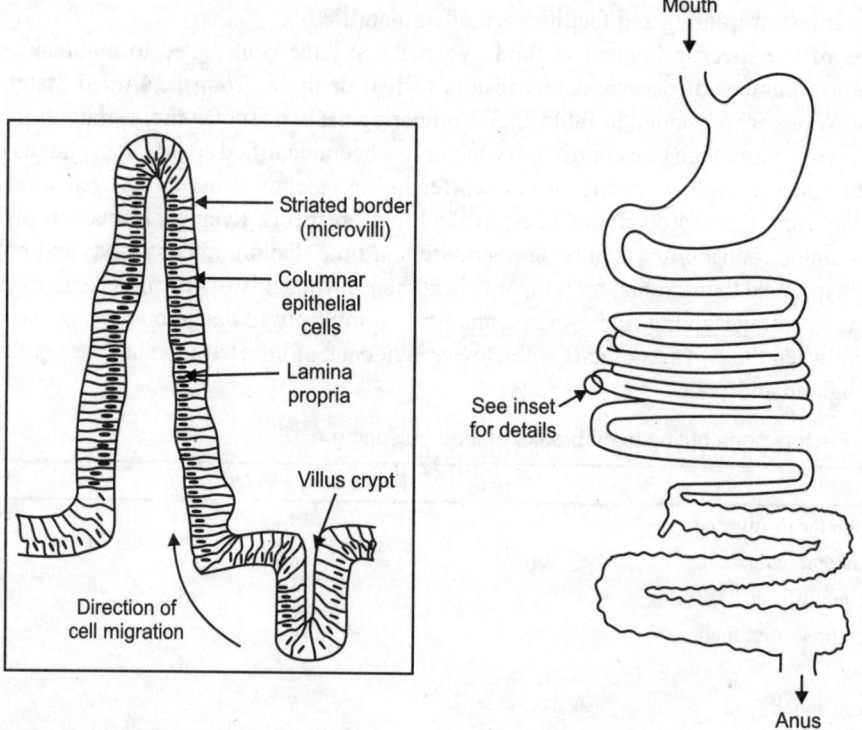

Fig. 25.4. The gastrointestinal tract. Inset: expanded view of inner surface of small intestine.

Unlike most of the body's other external surfaces, it is not lined with a dry protective skin and so, although it possesses some protective features, it offers a more congenial environment for micro-organisms and an easier route by which they can penetrate the body.

In the mouth, food is mixed with saliva and broken down mechanically to increase the surface area available for attack by digestive enzymes. Saliva is an alkaline fluid containing starch-degrading (amylase) enzyme and the antimicrobial factors immunoglobulin (IgA), lysozyme, lactoferrin and lactoperoxidase. It provides lubrication to assist chewing and swallowing and performs a cleansing function, rinsing the teeth and mouth to remove debris. On average, an adult secretes and swallows about 1.5 l of saliva each day. The variety of foods consumed and the range of micro-environments in the mouth result in a diverse and continually changing microflora. On the teeth, bacteria are associated with the formation of dental plaque an organic film in which bacteria are embedded in a matrix derived from salivary glycoproteins and microbial polysaccharides. The microbial composition of plaque varies with its age but filamentous *Fusobacterium* species and streptococci are common components. Plaque offers a protective environment for bacteria and its development is often a prelude to conditions such as dental caries and periodontal disease.

Swallowed food descends via the oesophagus into the stomach; a bulge in the alimentary tract which serves as a balance tank from which food is gradually released into the small intestine for further digestion. In the stomach, food is blended with gastric juice, an acidic fluid containing hydrochloric acid. Stomach pH can range from 0.8–5.0 (typically 2.0–3.0) and has a marked effect on ingested micro-organisms, killing most. Normally only acid-tolerant vegetative cells and spores survive and the microbial count in the stomach is low, although lactobacilli are frequently found in association with the stomach wall. Gastric acidity generally provides very effective protection for subsequent sections of the intestine but is not, as we shall see, an invulnerable defence. Bacteria can evade prolonged exposure to the acid by being sheltered in food particles or as a result of accelerated passage through the stomach as occurs, for instance, when the stomach is full. Alternatively, acidity may be neutralised by the food or absent as a result of illness.

The digestive functions of the stomach are not confined to those of a mechanical churn with antimicrobial features. Proteases, such as pepsin, and lipase which can operate at low pH partially digest the stomach contents. The gastric mucosa also secretes a protein responsible for efficient absorption of vitamin B_{12}. Little absorption of nutrients occurs in the stomach, with the notable exception of ethanol, but some material-transfer is often necessary to adjust the osmotic pressure of the stomach contents to ensure they are isotonic with body fluids. From the stomach, small quantities of the partially digested mixture of food and gastric juice, known as chyme, are released periodically into the small intestine. In this muscular tube over 6 metres long most of the digestion and absorption of food occur. Its internal lining is extensively folded and the folds covered with finger-like projections or villi which are themselves covered in microvilli. This gives the inner surface the appearance and texture of velvet and maximises the area available for absorption (Fig. 25.4).

In the first section of the small intestine, the duodenum, large-scale digestion is initiated by mixing the chyme with digestive juice from the pancreas and bile from the gallbladder which neutralise the chyme's acidity. The pancreatic juice also supplies a battery of digestive enzymes, and surfactant bile salts emulsify fats to facilitate their degradation and the absorption of fat soluble vitamins. Further digestive enzymes that break down disaccharides and peptides are secreted by glands in the mucous lining of the duodenum called, with evocations of a Gothic horror, the crypts of Lieberkühn.

The duodenum is a relatively short section of the small intestine, accounting for only about 2 per cent of its overall length. Food is swept along by waves of muscle contraction, known as peristalsis, from the duodenum into the jejunum and thence into the ileum. During this passage, nutrients such as amino acids, sugars, fats, vitamins, minerals and water are absorbed into capillaries in the villi from where they are transported around the body. Absorption is sometimes a result of passive diffusion, but more often involves the movement of nutrients against a concentration gradient; an active process entailing the expenditure of energy.

The microbial population increases down the length of the small intestine: counts of 10^2–10^3 ml^{-1} in the duodenum increase to around 10^3–10^4 in the jejunum, 10^5 in the upper ileum and 10^6 in the lower ileum. This corresponds with a decreasing flux of material through the small intestine as water is absorbed along its length.

In the higher reaches of the duodenum, the flow rate is such that its flushing effect frequently exceeds the rate at which micro-organisms can multiply so that only those with the ability to adhere to the intestinal epithelium can persist for any length of time. As the flow rate decreases further along the small intestine, so the microbial population increases, despite the presence of antimicrobial factors such as lysozyme, secretory immunoglobulin, IgA, and bile.

In the healthy individual, the microflora of the small intestine is mainly comprised of lactobacilli and streptococci, although, as we shall see, other bacteria have the ability to colonise the epithelium and cause illness as a consequence.

Extensive microbial growth takes place in the colon or large intestine where material can remain for long periods before expulsion as faeces. During this time active absorption of water and salts helps to maintain the body's fluid balance and to dry faecal matter. Bacterial cells account for 25–30 per cent of faeces, amounting to 10^{10}–10^{11} cfu g^{-1}, the remainder is composed of indigestible components of food, epithelial cells shed from the gut, minerals and bile.

Obligate anaerobes such as *Bacteroides* and *Bifidobacterium* make up 99 per cent of the flora of the large intestine and faeces. Members of the Enterobacteriaceae, most commonly *Escherichia coli*, are normally present at around 10^6 g^{-1}, enterococci around 10^5 g^{-1}, *Lactobacillus*, *Clostridium* and *Fusobacterium*, 10^3–10^5 g^{-1}, plus numerous other organisms, such as yeasts, staphylococci and pseudomonads, at lower levels.

The interaction between the gut microflora and its host appears to have both positive and negative aspects and is the subject of much current research and conjecture. Addition of antibiotics to feed has been shown to stimulate the growth of certain animals, suggesting that some gut organisms have a deleterious effect on growth.

A normal gut microflora confers some protection against infection. One example of this effect is the inflammatory disease pseudomembranous colitis caused by *Clostridium difficile*. Normally this organism is present in the gut in very low numbers, but if the balance of the flora is altered by antibiotic therapy, it can colonise the colon releasing toxins.

Similarly, the infective doses of some other enteric pathogens have been shown to be lower in the absence of the normal gut flora.

It appears that protection is not simply a result of the normal flora occupying all available niches, since enterotoxigenic *E. coli* adheres to sites that are normally vacant. Some direct antagonism through the production of organic acids and bacteriocins probably plays a part, but stimulation of the host immune system and its capacity to resist infection also appear to be factors.

In monogastric animals such as humans, gut micro-organisms do not play the same central role in host nutrition as they do in ruminants. Some facultative anaerobes found in the gut, such as *E. coli* and *Klebsiella aerogenes* are known to produce a variety of vitamins *in vitro* and studies using animals reared in a germ-free environment and lacking any indigenous microflora have shown that *in vivo* vitamin production by micro-organisms can be important on certain diets. In humans, however, the evidence is less convincing.

Some have questioned the efficiency of absorption of vitamins produced in the large intestine pointing to the fact that vegans have developed vitamin B_{12} deficiency despite its production in the gut and excretion in the faeces. It appears that an adequate balanced diet will probably meet all the body's requirements in this respect and that, short of coprophagy, which is practised by some herbivores such as rabbits, access to vitamins produced *in situ* is limited.

PATHOGENESIS OF DIARRHOEAL DISEASE

Several foodborne illnesses, such as typhoid fever, botulism and listeriosis, involve body sites remote from the alimentary tract which serves simply as the route by which the pathogen or toxin gains entry to the body.

A more common conception of foodborne illness, often described as food poisoning, is where symptoms, like the causative agent, are confined to the gut and its immediate vicinity. The patient presents an acute gastroenteritis characterised by diarrhoea and vomiting. Individual pathogens will be described in some detail subsequently, but for now we will consider some common features of the mechanisms involved.

Diarrhoea is the excessive evacuation of too-fluid faeces (Table 25.4). Any process which seriously interferes with the gut's capacity to absorb most of the 8–10 l of fluid it receives each day, or increases secretion into the intestinal lumen, will produce this condition.

Consequently, the aetiology of diarrhoea can be quite complex and a number of different mechanisms have been identified.

Table 25.4. Clinical classification of infectious diarrhoea[a].

Type	Symptoms	Typical causative organisms
Acute watery diarrhoea	Loose or watery stools without visible blood. Duration generally less than 7 days	Vibrio cholerae, Enterotoxigenic *E. coli*. Small round structured viruses
Acute bloody diarrhoea	Loose or watery stools with visible blood. Duration generally less than 7 days	*Shigella, Campylobacter jejuni* Enteroinvasive *E. coli*. Small round structured viruses
Persistent diarrhoea	Loose or watery stools with or without visible blood with a duration of 14 days or more	Multifactorial: enteric infection, malnutrition, impaired immunity, lactose intolerance

[a]Definition: passage of loose or watery stools three or more times in a 24-hour period.

Toxins frequently play a role in this process. As their nomenclature often causes students some confusion, one or two preliminary definitions are probably in order. *Exotoxin* is the term used to describe toxins that are released extracellularly by the living organism. These include:

1. Enterotoxins which act on the intestinal mucosa generally causing diarrhoea.
2. Cytotoxins which kill host cells.

3. Neurotoxins which interfere with normal nervous transmission.
4. Endotoxins are pyrogenic (fever producing) lipopolysaccharides released from the outer membrane of the Gram-negative cell envelope by bacterial lysis.

Bacterial food poisoning can be divided into three principal types:

Ingestion of preformed toxin

Toxins may be produced in and ingested with the food as in *Staphylococcus aureus* food poisoning and the *Bacillus cereus* emetic syndrome. Botulism is similar in this respect though in this case gastrointestinal symptoms are of minor importance. The absence of person to person spread and a relatively short incubation period between ingestion of food and the onset of symptoms are usual characteristics of this type of food poisoning.

Non-invasive infection

In a non-invasive infection, viable bacteria ingested with food, colonise the intestinal lumen. This is principally associated with the small intestine where competition from the endogenous microflora is less intense. To prevent their removal by the flushing action of the high flow rates in this section of the gut, the pathogen generally attaches to and colonises the epithelial surface. It does this by producing adhesins, molecules often associated with fimbriae on the bacterial cell surface, which recognise and attach to specific receptor sites on the microvilli. Loss of the ability to adhere to the gut wall will dramatically reduce a pathogen's virulence—its ability to cause illness.

Once attached, the pathogen produces a protein enterotoxin which acts locally in the gut changing the flow of electrolytes and water across the mucosa from one of absorption to secretion. Several enterotoxins act by stimulating enterocytes (the cells lining the intestinal epithelium) to overproduce cyclic nucleotides.

Most extensively studied in this respect is the cholera toxin produced by *Vibrio cholerae*. The toxin (MW 84,000) comprises five B subunits and a single A subunit. The B subunits bind to specific ganglioside (an acidic glycolipid) receptors on the enterocyte surface. This creates a hydrophilic channel in the cell membrane through which the A unit can pass. Once inside the cell, a portion of the A unit acts enzymically to transfer an ADP-ribosyl group derived from cellular NAD to a protein regulating the activity of the enzyme adenylate cyclase. As a result, the enzyme is locked into its active state leading to an accumulation of cyclic adenosine monophosphate (cAMP) which inhibits absorption of Na^+ and Cl^- ions while stimulating the secretion of Cl^-, HCO_3^- and Na^+ ions. To maintain an osmotic balance, the transfer of electrolytes is accompanied by a massive outflow of water into the intestinal lumen. This far exceeds the absorptive capacity of the large intestine and results in a profuse watery diarrhoea (Fig. 25.5).

A number of other enterotoxins have been shown to act in the same way as the cholera toxin including the heat labile toxin (LT) produced by some types of enterotoxigenic *E. coli*. Other toxins such as the heat stable toxin of *E. coli* are similar in the respect that they stimulate the production of a cyclic nucleotide in enterocytes. In this case it is cyclic guanosine monophosphate (cGMP) which differs slightly from cAMP in its activity but also produces diarrhoea as a result of electrolyte imbalances.

A different enterotoxin is produced by *Clostridium perfringens* as it sporulates in the gut. The toxin binds to receptors on the surface of cells of the intestinal epithelium, producing morphological changes in the membrane which affect absorption/secretion processes thus precipitating diarrhoea. It does not increase intestinal cAMP levels.

A traditional method of analysing for the presence of enterotoxins is based upon their *in vivo* action. The ileum of a rabbit under anaesthesia is tied off to produce a number of segments or loops which serve as test chambers. These are injected with cultures, culture filtrates or samples under test. If an enterotoxin is present it produces, after about 24 hours, an accumulation of fluid in the loop which becomes distended. A number of alternative assays, based on the effects of enterotoxins on cells in tissue culture are also used. These have the advantages of being more economical, more humane and easier to quantify than the ligated ileal loop assay but are less directly related to the clinical action of the toxin.

Invasive infection

Other diarrhoea-causing pathogens invade the cells of the intestinal epithelium but do not normally spread much beyond the immediate vicinity of the gut. Some, such as *Salmonella* preferentially invade the ileum to produce a profuse watery diarrhoea. Bacterial cells invade and pass through the epithelial cells to multiply in the *lamina propria*, a layer of connective tissue underlying the enterocytes. The precise mechanism of fluid secretion into the intestinal lumen is not known and is probably multifactorial. A heat-labile enterotoxin which stimulates adenylate cyclase activity has been identified in some salmonellas as well as a cytotoxin. It has also been suggested that the local acute inflammation caused by the infection and responsible for the fever and chills that are often a feature of salmonellosis, causes an increase in levels of prostaglandins, known activators of adenylate cyclase.

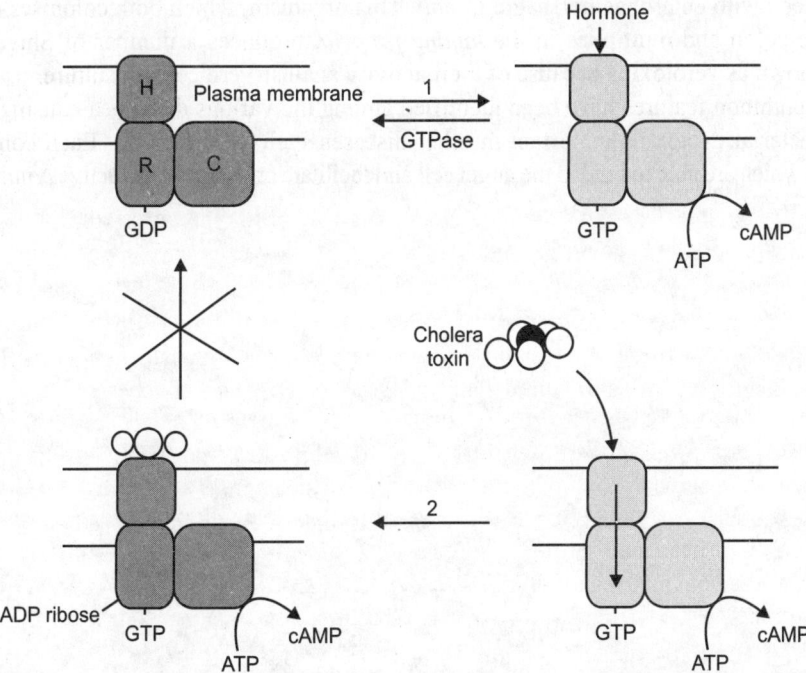

Fig. 25.5. Cholera toxin and its mode of action. (1) Reversible physiological activation of adenylate cyclase (C) through hormone binding to receptor (H) and (2) cholera toxin binding and translocation of A subunit leads to ADP ribosylation of regulatory subunit (R) and irreversible activation.

Other enteroinvasive pathogens like *Shigella* and enteroinvasive *E. coli* invade the colonic mucosa and produce a dysenteric syndrome characterised by inflammation, abscesses and ulceration of the colon and the passage of bloody, mucus- and pus-containing stools. Bacterial cells adhere to the enterocytes via outer membrane protein adhesins. They are then engulfed by the enterocytes in response to a phagocytic signal produced by the bacterium and multiply within the cytoplasm invading adjacent cells and the underlying connective tissue. The strong inflammatory response to this process causes abscesses and ulcerations of the colon.

Invasiveness can be diagnosed by examination of the fluid accumulated and the mucosal surface in rabbit ileal loops. A less definitive test for invasiveness is the Sereny test which measures the ability of an organism to cause keratoconjunctivitis in the eye of guinea pigs or rabbits.

Some shigellas also produce a protein exotoxin, known as Shiga toxin, which has a range of biological activities. It inhibits protein synthesis by inactivating the 60S ribosomal subunit and is a powerful cytotoxin. It has neurotoxic activity causing paralysis and death in experimental animals and is an enterotoxin capable of causing fluid accumulation in ligated rabbit ileal loops. As an enterotoxin, it appears unrelated to cholera toxin since it does not stimulate adenylate cyclase or cross-react with antibodies to cholera toxin. Its role in the pathogenesis of shigellosis is unclear since strains incapable of producing Shiga toxin remain pathogenic. Enteroinvasive *E coli* causes a similar syndrome but does not produce Shiga toxin.

Some authors have linked the enterotoxin activity of Shiga toxin with the watery diarrhoea which often precedes dysentery. Interestingly, a similar sequence of watery diarrhoea with supervening bloody diarrhoea is seen with enterohaemorrhagic *E. coli*. This organism, which both colonises the epithelial surface in the colon and multiplies in the *lamina propria*, produces a number of Shiga-like toxins, sometimes known as verotoxins because of their activity against Vero cells in culture.

Recently, common features have been identified among the various diarrhoea-causing toxins and a number of bacterial exotoxins important in other diseases such as diphtheria. Each consists of five, linked B units which are able to bind to the target cell and facilitate transport of the active A unit into the cell.

Chapter 26

Microbiology in Food Plant Sanitation

INTRODUCTION

The food industry sanitarian is concerned with aseptic practices in the preparation, processing and packaging of the food products of a plant (or plants), the general cleanliness and sanitation of plant and premises, and the health of employees. The duties of microbiologist in connection with the food products may involve quality control and storage of raw products, the provision of a good water supply, prevention of the contamination of the foods at all stages during processing from equipment, personnel and vermin, and supervision of packaging and warehousing of finished products. The supervision of cleanliness and sanitation of plant and premises includes not only the maintenance of clean and well-sanitised surfaces of all equipment touching the foods but also generally good housekeeping in and about the plant and adequate treatment and disposal of wastes. Duties affecting the health of the employees include provision of a potable water supply, supervision of matters of personal hygiene, regulation of sanitary facilities in the plant and in plant-operated housing units, and contact with sanitary aspects of plant lighting, heating, and ventilation. The microbiologist must also participates in the training of employees in sanitary practices. Only bacteriological aspects of plant sanitation will be discussed here.

For the most part, the sanitarian concerns himself chiefly with general aspects of sanitation, making inspections, consulting with personnel responsible for details of sanitation and executives directing such work, and training personnel in sanitation. He may or may not be connected with a plant laboratory.

BACTERIOLOGY OF WATER SUPPLIES

The water for drinking purposes and for plant use may be from the same source or from different sources.

Drinking Water

The water that the employees drink must meet public health standards. Coliform bacteria must not be present at levels indicating contamination of the water by sewage. Total plate counts of the water sometimes are made to indicate when trouble may be incipient so that such trouble can be forestalled.

Plant Water

All water that comes into contact with foods should meet the bacteriological standards for drinking water, and preferably all freshwater at the plant should be that good. But this water also should be satisfactory from a bacteriological standpoint for use with the particular food being processed. A water supply may be adjudged potable, yet be unsatisfactory for use with a food. Thus, for example, water containing appreciable numbers of psychrophiles of the genera *Pseudomonas*, *Achromobactel* or *Alcaligenes* might be unsatisfactory without treatment in a dairy plant making butter or cottage cheese. The slimy growth of iron bacteria in water supplies often leads to trouble in the food plant.

More likely to be important is the chemical composition of the water, which must be suited to the use to be made of it. Thus hard water is undesirable in pea canning and in brewing; iron and manganese are bad in beet canning and in brewing; excessive organic matter may lead to off-flavours, etc.

Of special interest in canning factories is the bacteriology of the water in which the cans of processed foods are cooled after their heat treatment. If this water contains micro-organisms able to spoil the food, it will, after entering defective cans through minute leaks, increase the percentage of cans of food spoiling during storage. Many canneries routinely chlorinate the cooling water to reduce or eliminate this trouble.

The shortage of water in many food plants has necessitated reuse of part of the water, and micro-organisms may build up in such reused water. Water employed for the final rinse of a food must be fresh and potable, but after use may be returned for soaking, first wash or fluming, preferably after treatment with chlorine, chlorine dioxide or a similar germicide.

In-plant or continuous chlorination beyond the break point (the point where the chlorine demand has been satisfied) to a residual of 5 to 7 ppm of chlorine is employed for continuous application to areas and equipment where slime bacteria may be a problem, e.g. conveyors or belts, can coolers, product washers and flumes. The chlorinated water may be applied as a spray, or parts of equipment may be immersed. When operations cease, chlorinated water may be applied to fillers, peelers, dicers, and similar equipment. Contaminated or polluted water lines are held filled with chlorinated water containing 50 to 100 ppm of chlorine for 12 to 48 hours the strength of chlorine and length of time depending on the extent of pollution.

Ice used in contact with foods should meet the bacteriological requirements for potable water. Much work has been done on the incorporation of bacteriostatic or bactericidal chemicals in water and in ice to aid in food preservation. It has been noted previously that a chlortetracycline or oxytetracycline dip for dressed poultry has been approved, and that these antibiotics may be incorporated in ice to be applied to fish and other seafood.

Sewage and Waste Treatment and Disposal

The food sanitarian is concerned directly or indirectly with the adequate treatment and disposal of wastes from his industry. Solid and concentrated wastes ordinarily are kept separate from the watery wastes, and may be used directly for food, feed, fertiliser or other purpose, may first be concentrated, dried or fermented (e.g. pea-vine silage), or may be carted away to available land as unusable waste. Care is taken to keep out of the waste waters as much wasted liquid or solid food material as possible, by taking precautions to avoid introduction into the watery wastes of drip, leakage, overflow, spillage, large residues in containers, foam, frozen-on food, and food dust during the handling and processing of the food. It is recommended that sewage of human origin be kept separate from other plant waters because of the possible presence of human intestinal pathogens and the necessity for a guarantee of their removal or destruction. Such sewage may be turned into a municipal system, if one is available, for adequate treatment and disposal or may be treated separately at the food plant. Other food-plant wastes should not contain human pathogens.

Wastes from food plants ordinarily contain a variety of organic compounds, which range from simple and readily oxidisable kinds to those that are complex and difficult to decompose. The strength of the sewage or food waste containing organic matter is expressed in terms of biochemical oxygen demand (BOD), which is the quantity of oxygen used by aerobic micro-organisms and reducing compounds in the stabilisation of decomposable matter during a selected time at a certain temperature. A period of 5 days at 20°C is generally used, and results are expressed as 5-day BOD. The BOD is determined by dilution of a measured quantity of waste with water that has been saturated with oxygen and incubation of the mixture at 20°C, along with a control of dilution water alone. After 5 days, the residual oxygen in both control and test sample is measured by titration. The difference represents the oxygen-consuming capacity of the waste, and is calculated to be expressed as parts per million of oxygen taken up by the waste. To calculate the strength of the waste in terms of pounds of BOD:

$$\frac{\text{ppm 5-day BOD} \times \text{gallons of waste} \times 8.34}{10,00,000} = \text{pounds BOD}$$

This value can be converted to population equivalent (P.E.) by assuming that the domestic sewage of one person is equivalent to one-sixth of a pound of BOD per day.

Whenever appreciable amounts of wastes high in oxidisable organic matter (high BOD) are emptied into natural waters, such as streams, ponds or lakes, the 7 to 8 ppm of free oxygen normally present in the waters is used up soon by oxidation processes carried out by aerobic or facultative micro-organisms. When the oxygen drops below 3 ppm, the fish either leave or die, and when anaerobic conditions have been attained, hydrolysis, putrefaction and fermentation by micro-organisms will follow, with the result that the body of water will become malodorous and cloudy and hence unsuited for recreational use and unfit for drinking and for use in the food plant. Wastes from a food plant, then, to be emptied into a body of water, must either be so greatly diluted by that water as to be innocuous or must be treated first to reduce the oxidisable compounds to a harmless level. Even the effluent from an efficiently operated sewage treatment system will encourage the growth of algae and higher aquatic plants in the water and make it less attractive for recreational purposes.

Preliminary treatments of food-plant wastes by chemical means may be employed, but most systems of treatment and disposal depend upon (i) screening out of large particles, (ii) floating off of fatty and other floating materials, (iii) sedimentation of as much of the remaining solids as is practicable, (iv) hydrolysis, fermentation, and putrefaction of complex organic compounds and finally (v) oxidation of the remaining solids in the water to a point where they can enter a municipal sewage treatment and disposal system, a plant disposal system, a lake or stream or soil. The completeness of oxidation required will depend upon the disposal to be made. Thus less oxidation might be required for feeding to a municipal system or for irrigating soil than for entering a stream or lake.

Chemical Treatment

In chemical pretreatments, a chemical or mixture of chemicals is added to the sewage or waste so as to cause formation of a flocculent precipitate, which, in settling, carries with it much of the suspended and colloidal material, including bacteria. The effluent then is run into a body of water, onto soil or into a biological treatment system. The chemicals commonly used are soluble aluminum or iron salts, such as alum or ferrous sulphate, plus lime, giving a flocculent precipitate of aluminum or ferric hydroxide. Disposal of the sludge (settlings) so obtained may be difficult.

Biological treatment and disposal

The general biological methods for waste disposal and/or treatment include (i) dilution, by running waste waters into a large body of water, (ii) irrigation, in which waste-waters are sprayed onto fields of open-textured soil, (iii) lagooning, by running the waste waters into shallow artificial ponds (with or without other treatments), (iv) use of trickling filters, made of crushed rock, coke, filter tile, etc. (v) use of the activated sludge method, in which waste water is inoculated heavily with sludge from a previous run and is actively aerated in tanks, and (vi) use of anaerobic tanks of various kinds, where settling, hydrolysis, putrefaction and fermentation take place, usually to be followed by some aerobic treatment.

The dilution method seldom is practicable because a sufficiently large or rapidly moving volume of water rarely is available or because the location is such that sewage decomposition cannot proceed without objections from nearby populations. Irrigation is increasing in popularity and is especially adaptable to use by plants located in rural areas and near open-textured soil. Lagooning has been used · especially for seasonal wastes, as from canning factories. The wastes are decomposed slowly in these shallow ponds or lagoons until the liquid part can be run into a stream or other body of water during the rainy season or time of melting snow, when there is a good volume of water. Usually, sodium nitrate is added to reduce obnoxious odours. Sometimes the liquid is pumped from and returned to a lagoon, or it may be pumped from one lagoon to another in a series of lagoons. Trickling filters and activated sludge systems are probably the most effective of the systems listed, but they are expensive to run and require supervision by an expert. Anaerobic tanks yield an effluent that needs further treatment and should be either turned into a municipal system or given an aerobic treatment.

Types of Food Wastes

An extended discussion of the nature and composition of wastes from the different food industries cannot be given here. It should be noted, however, that each type of waste has a characteristic BOD that may be high, low or intermediate and each presents its own problems of treatment and disposal. Dairy wastes, for example, are usually high in protein and lactose and contain many micro-organisms. Such wastes, if not already acid, will turn acid if kept under anaerobic conditions and then will be more difficult to treat. Some wastes may be acid originally-wastes from fruit canneries, for instance. Malthouse, brewery, distillery, sweet-corn cannery and corn-products plant wastes are high in carbohydrates and likely to become acid under anaerobic conditions. Wastes high in proteins, e.g. pea or fish cannery or packing-plant wastes, are likely to putrefy under anaerobic conditions. Other wastes may contain antiseptic chemicals, such as the sulphite in waste sulphite liquors from paper mills, and therefore may be difficult to decompose by means of micro-organisms. Ranges of 5-day BOD values reported for wastes from various types of food-processing plants are given in Table 26.1.

Table 26.1. Range of 5-day BOD values for wastes from various food-processing plants.

Source of waste	5-day BOD, ppm	Source of waste	5-day BOD, ppm
Dairy plants	500–2000	String-bean cannery	160–600
Meat-packing plants	Up to 2500	Lima-bean cannery	190–450
Poultry plants	300–7500	Sweet-corn cannery	625–6000
Sugar processing	500–1500	Pea cannery	380–4700
Fruit cannery	200–2100	Pumpkin cannery	2800–6900
Tomato cannery	180–4000	Spinach cannery	280–730
Brewery	420–1200	Sauerkraut cannery	Up to 6300

MICROBIOLOGY OF THE FOOD PRODUCT

To reduce contamination with micro-organisms to a minimum and obtain good keeping quality of the product, the raw materials are examined, the equipment contacting the food is adequately cleansed, sanitised and tested, the preserving process is checked, and packaging and storage are supervised.

Ingredients

The raw product is inspected and tested for quality, but this does not necessarily involve bacteriological laboratory testing in all instances. Some of the ingredients of some products may contain numbers and kinds of micro-organisms that can affect the keeping quality of the product or even its acceptability. Some ingredients, such as sweetening agents, starch and spices, can be purchased on specification as to maximal allowable content of micro-organisms or of numbers of certain kinds. The numbers of bacteria in ingredients are important in foods for which there are bacterial standards, e.g. ice cream, which must not contain more than 50,000 bacteria per gram in some areas. Large numbers of spores of aerobes are undesirable in dry milk to be used in breadmaking because of the increased risk of ropiness developing; heat-resistant spores in sugar and starch may add to the difficulty in adequately heat-processing canned vegetables to which sugar or starch is added; and large numbers of bacteria in spices may favour the spoilage of summer sausage.

The microbiology of the main raw product often is important. Excessive mould mycelium in the raw fruit, which is indicative of the presence of rotten parts, may lead to condemnation of the canned or frozen product. Large numbers of thermoduric bacteria in raw milk may yield a pasteurised milk that will not meet the bacterial standards for numbers as estimated by the standard plate-count method. Large numbers of bacteria on vegetables or in fruits may indicate inferiority that will carry over into the frozen product. Laboratory examination may be employed to detect these undesirable organisms and estimate their numbers.

Often there is opportunity for micro-organisms to grow in a food product during handling and processing in the plant. Examples are the build-up of thermophiles where foods are kept hot, as in forewarmers and blanchers, and increases in total numbers of bacteria in vegetables between blanching and freezing. Line samples may be tested in the laboratory to ascertain where appreciable growth of micro-organisms is taking place.

Packaging Materials

Packaging materials are a possible source of contamination of foods with micro-organisms, but ordinarily the penetrability of nonmetallic materials to moisture and to gases is of more significance in the preservation of foods than the microbiology of these materials, for they harbour mostly low numbers of innocuous micro-organisms or no organisms. Also, as has been indicated previously, wrappers may be treated or impregnated with bacteriostatic or fungistatic compounds, e.g. cheese wraps with sorbic or caprylic acid.

Paper and paperboard used for milk cartons contain mostly bacilli and micrococci, and occasionally other rods, actinomycetes and mould spores, but no organisms of public health significance. Treatment with hot paraffin kills most of the organisms present, provides an almost sterile surface, and prevents bacteria within the cardboard, mostly bacterial spores, from reaching the food. Wax paper is practically sterile as produced, as are most plastic packaging materials. All packaging materials should be protected from contamination with dust or other sources of micro-organisms in handling.

According to Federal regulations a food is deemed to be adulterated 'if its container is composed, in whole or in part, of any poisonous or deleterious substance which may render its contents injurious to health'.

Equipment

Unless the equipment that comes in contact with foods is adequately cleansed and sanitised, it may be an important source of contamination of foods with micro-organisms. Not only may organisms persist on equipment, but they may increase in numbers when treatment has been inadequate. Microbiological standards for plant sanitation have been suggested but to date have not been applied officially. Thatcher has proposed that standards be based on counts of total numbers of micro-organisms per unit surface area of equipment coming in contact with foods as an indication of the effectiveness of cleaning and sanitising, and on special tests for bacteria of human origin, e.g. coliform bacteria and streptococci of fecal origin, staphylococci from nasopharyngeal or suppurative sources, and *Streptococcus salivarius* from the mouth, to indicate contamination from personnel.

Cleansing

Cleansing from a bacteriological viewpoint, cleansing of equipment is primarily to remove as much food for micro-organisms as is practicable. Equipment may be disassembled for cleaning and sanitising, although this is difficult with some pieces. To aid in the cleansing action of water, cleansing agents called detergents are employed. These agents may serve to soften or condition the water, improve the wetting ability of the cleansing solution, emulsify or saponify fats, solubilise minerals, deflocculate or disperse suspended materials, and dissolve as much soluble material as possible. At the same time the detergents should be noncorrosive and readily rinsed from the surfaces. Among the detergents used alone or in mixtures are the alkaline varieties, such as lye, soda ash, sodium metasilicate, trisodium phosphate and the polyphosphates; acid detergents, usually organic acids, such as hydroxy acetic, gluconic, citric, tartaric and levulinic acids; and wetting agents, which may be anionic (NaR), such as the hydrocarbon sulphonates; nonionic, e.g. polyether alcohol; or cationic (RCl), for example, the quaternary ammonium compounds. Cleaning may be aided by the employment of brushes and of water under pressure.

Sanitising

The sanitising process is an attempt to kill most or all of the micro-organisms on equipment surfaces. The kind of sanitiser, the concentration employed, the temperature of the sanitiser, and the method of application will vary with the kind of sanitising agent, the conditions during use, the type of equipment to be treated, and the micro-organisms to be destroyed. Among the sanitising agents in common use are hot water, flowing steam or steam under pressure, halogens (chlorine or iodine) and halogen derivatives, and the quaternary ammonium compounds.

Steam under pressure is the most effective way of applying heat as a sanitising agent, but its use is limited to closed systems that can withstand pressure. Steam jets, flowing steam or hot water may be used, but jets are ineffective except at very short distances, flowing steam may condense and drop in temperature as it passes through equipment, and hot water may undergo a similar drop in temperature. All micro-organisms and their spores can be killed by adequate treatment with high-pressure steam. Effectively applied 'flowing steam' and boiling water will kill all but some of the more resistant bacterial spores. The lower the temperature of 'hot' water, the less effective it will be in killing organisms.

Chlorine, iodine and their compounds (hypochlorites, chloramines, iodophors, etc.) are effective germicides if in proper concentrations and if given enough time to act. Usually, more sanitiser is necessary in the presence of organic matter. Bacterial spores are especially resistant to these sanitisers. Chlorine is used to destroy undesirable bacteria in water for drinking, for use in foods, for washing foods or equipment and for cooling. Hypochlorites are more labile but more effective at acid pH values than at alkaline ones. As stated earlier, in-plant or continuous chlorination beyond the break point (where chlorine demand has been satisfied) to a residual of 5 to 7 ppm is employed for continuous application to areas where slime bacteria may be a problem, e.g. on conveyors, belts or product washers. Chlorine (50 to 100 ppm) also is used to treat contaminated or polluted water lines.

Quaternary ammonium compounds are, in general, more effective against Gram-positive than Gram-negative bacteria. These compounds have a residual effect, that is, they adhere to equipment surfaces and deter bacterial growth; but they rinse off onto foods coming into contact with these surfaces, and, if they are present in detectable concentrations, might be considered undesirable. Many of these compounds are active under alkaline conditions. Most are affected by hardness of water.

Detergent sanitisers, which usually are a combination of an alkaline detergent and a quaternary ammonium compound, sometimes are used to cleanse and sanitise utensils or equipment in one operation.

Cleaned-in-place systems

Some industries, especially the dairy industry, leave pipelines permanently connected and clean and sanitise them in place. Apparatus is available for accomplishing this automatically. Different sequences of treatments are recommended for different cleaned-in-place (CIP) systems. Milk pipelines, for example are rinsed first with tepid water, which is pushed or pulled through the system. Then hot (160°F or 71°C) detergent solution may be passed through, followed by rinsing water and finally a sanitising agent, such as hot water (170°F or 77°C or over), chlorine solution (200 ppm), or a quaternary ammonium compound (200 ppm). Often a sanitising treatment is given immediately before use.

Fungistatic paints

There also is the possibility of contamination of foods and equipment from walls, ceilings and other parts of the food plant. Most troublesome are the moulds, whose spores are readily air-borne and may travel considerable distances in the plant. Cleanliness, of course, will retard mould growth, but at the present time, fungistatic paints are used on walls and ceilings likely to be subject to mould growth. Commonly used in paints are copper-containing compounds such as copper naphthanate or copper-8-quinolinolate or phenol derivatives, e.g. pentachlorophenol or other chlorophenols, oxyquinoline sulphate, phenyl mercurial, etc. Occasionally, drip from overhead ceilings, pipes, etc. introduces organisms other than moulds and must be prevented.

Preservation Process

The sanitarian usually has little to do with the processing of the foods except to check through the laboratory, if one is available, for the effectiveness of the processing. The laboratory, for example, might run keeping quality tests on canned foods and bacterial counts on frozen foods, pasteurised milk, dry milks, etc.

Vending Machines for Foods and Beverages

With the rapid expansion of the use of vending machines to dispense perishable foods has come increased interest in the sanitation of these machines and dispensed foods. The United States Public Health Service

Ordinance and Code (The Vending of Foods and Beverages) covers sanitation of foods and machines, operation of machines and inspection. 'Readily perishable foods' are defined as those consisting in whole or in part of milk, milk products, eggs, meat, fish, poultry, etc. These are foods which can support rapid growth of micro-organisms and can cause food infections or intoxications. Adequately dried or canned foods are excepted. Perishable foods include sandwiches, pastries, hot coffee, tea or chocolate, malted milk, fluid milk, ice cream, frozen desserts and hot-food plates (meat, stews, soup, baked beans, poultry, fish, etc.).

During transportation from the commissaries and in the machine, perishable foods should be kept either cold (below 50°F or 10°C, usually at 38° to 40°F, or 3.3° to 4.4°C) or hot (150°F or 66°C or above). Slow growth of psychrophiles can take place at the lower temperatures and of thermophiles in the hot foods if these recommendations are barely met, and excessive heat will deteriorate many foods. All parts of vending machines in contact with readily perishable foods should be cleaned and sanitised periodically, daily if the above temperature limitations are not met. Water used in connection with the foods should be potable, and waste disposal should be adequate. Most machines dispensing perishable foods are equipped with safety devices to stop the dispensing of food when refrigeration or heating fails.

Food Handling on a Large Scale

Food handling on a large scale by caterers, commissaries, restaurants, institutions, airlines, camps, etc. are subject to similar considerations. The ordinance defines 'safe' temperatures for storage of foods as 45°F (7.2°C) or below or 140°F (60°C) or above, except during necessary periods of preparation and service. It requires the washing of raw fruits and vegetables, and the thorough cooking of stuffing, poultry, stuffed meats and poultry (heating to at least 165°F or 74°C), and pork and pork products (all parts heated to at least 150°F or 66°C) before being served. The ordinance has regulations concerning the health and cleanliness of personnel, the cleanliness, sanitisation, and protection of food utensils, and the potability of water. It specifies foods that are clean, wholesome, unspoiled, free from adulteration and misbranding, safe for consumption, and meeting any standards of quality or inspection. Also described is the handling of pastry fillings and of puddings.

Sandwiches

Sandwiches and other foods may be retailed without vending machines. Such foods may be a potential food-poisoning hazard, for they often are held at ambient temperatures for 18 to 24 hours before being sold. One survey indicated that the wrapped sandwiches examined showed signs of contamination during preparation and of growth of bacteria prior to vending. All sandwiches showed high total numbers of bacteria per gram, no salmonellae or *Clostridium perfringens*, and considerable numbers of staphylococci (most of which, however, were coagulase-negative), with higher numbers in the moist sandwiches than in the dry, and appreciable numbers in those heated to 55.5°C (132°F) and served hot. Similar results were obtained by McCroan who concluded that spiced ham sandwiches and cheese sandwiches were more hazardous than sandwiches containing mayonnaise, e.g. egg salad and chicken salad sandwiches, for contact with the acid dressing helped repress the staphylococci.

Microbiological standards for foods

It is evident from previous discussion that microbiological standards for foods may be of three types: (i) those on the raw product and ingredients, (ii) those concerned with plant sanitation and methods of packaging, storage and handling, and (iii) those on the finished product as marketed. Standards must be adapted to the types of food for which they are intended. They probably would be different for a food to be consumed raw than for the same food to be cooked or subjected to heating or other processing before being marketed. The type of spoilage organism to be feared and, therefore, watched for will vary with the food and the method of processing. Standards for ingredients of soft drinks, for example, include those for numbers of yeasts; for low acid foods to be canned, numbers and kinds of heat-resistant bacterial spores are significant; and numbers of aerobic spore formers in flour may indicate the likelihood of the development of ropiness in bread. The type of pathogen most likely to be present will be different in different foods. Tests for coliform bacteria to indicate the possible presence of intestinal pathogens are useful in setting standards for oysters but have little meaning when made on frozen orange juice. Salmonellae might be looked for in eggs or egg products and trichinae in raw pork.

The chief purposes of microbiological standards for foods are to give assurance (i) that the foods will be acceptable from the public health standpoint, i.e. will not be responsible for the spread of infectious disease or for food poisoning, (ii) that the foods will be of satisfactory quality, that is, will consist of good original materials that have not deteriorated or become unduly contaminated during processing, packaging, storage, handling, or marketing, (iii) that the foods will be acceptable from an esthetic viewpoint, in that the introduction of filth in the form of fecal material, parts of vermin, pus cells, mould mycelium, etc. has been prevented, and (iv) that the foods will have keeping qualities that should be expected of the product.

Many difficulties are encountered in establishing and applying microbiological standards for foods. Sampling for tests is a problem, for the lack of homogeneity in most foods makes location, size and number of samples significant. Standards usually are based on total numbers of organisms, numbers of an indicator organism, or numbers (or total absence) of pathogens; but there has been some disagreement as to what counts should be considered significant, what the indicator organism should be, and whether pathogens can be demonstrated. Counts are statistically uncertain, and dye reduction tests do not necessarily test for the important organisms. Finally the numbers and kinds of organisms in most foods decrease during storage in the dry or frozen condition. If an 'average standard' is adopted, half of the food samples are eliminated. If legal action is involved, the level of a standard must be justified; and counts or results on a sample by prosecutor, defendant and a neutral agency may not necessarily agree.

It has been recommended that: (i) testing procedure and standards be adapted to the particular kind of food, (ii) a numerical relationship be demonstrated between the standard and the hazard, (iii) tolerances be allowed for admitted inaccuracies of sampling and analysis, i.e. all samples would not be required to meet the standard, and results from successive samples, taken at stated intervals, would be considered in setting and interpreting standards, and (iv) any suggested standard be tried out first on a voluntary basis. It has been found, however, that setting a standard usually results in better plant sanitation within the industry and in lower average bacterial counts and better keeping quality for the product.

HEALTH OF EMPLOYEES

As has been pointed out, duties of the sanitarian that affect the health of employees include provision of potable drinking water, supervision of matters of personal hygiene, regulation of sanitary facilities within the plant and of sewage treatment and disposal, and supervision of sanitation in plant eating establishments and in plant-operated housing units. Most of these duties involve the sanitary aspects of plant and housing construction, selection of qualified personnel to direct operations of the facilities and training of employees in sanitary practices.

The bacteriology of drinking water and of sewage treatment and disposal has been discussed briefly. However, sanitation in eating places in the plant deserves special mention. Special places should be designated for eating carried lunches, and such places should be kept neat and sanitary. If the plant serves meals to employees in a cafeteria or restaurant, the sanitarian should be responsible for supervision of sanitation in the preparation, handling, serving and storage of the food so as to avoid the spread of infectious micro-organisms and to prevent outbreaks of food poisoning. To prevent the spread of disease food equipment and utensils should be handled, washed and sanitised thoroughly.

Before washing, all food equipment and utensils should be presoaked, if necessary, and preflushed or prescraped. Washing should be by means of a solution of a suitable detergent, which must be at 110°F (60°C) or higher (160°F or 71°C, or over for single tank conveyor machines). When hot water is employed in sanitising it should be at 170°F (77°C) or over, with exposure for at least ½ minute. The final rinse water should be at that temperature or at 180°F (82°C) or over at the entrance of the manifold. With chemical sanitisers, immersion should be for at least 1 minute at not less than 75°F (24°C), and the solutions should contain at least 50 ppm of available chlorine or 12.5 ppm of available iodine or have an equivalent bactericidal effect. Very large pieces of equipment may be treated with live steam, rinsed with boiling water or sprayed or swabbed with a chemical sanitising solution at least twice as strong as that used for immersion treatment.

Transient bacteria are removed from hands of workers by soap and water, with scrubbing aiding in the removal; but the permanent organisms remain, such as staphylococci, streptococci, coliforms and pseudomonads. Chemicals in soaps or used as detergents, e.g. bisphenols, iodophors and quaternary ammonium compounds, are effective in reducing numbers of bacteria, if used daily in successive hand washings.

Chapter 27

Analytical Techniques in Food Biochemistry

INTRODUCTION

An analytical technique is a method that is used to determine the concentration of a chemical compound or chemical element. There are a wide variety of techniques used for analysis, from simple weighing (gravimetric) to titrations (titrimetric) to very advanced techniques using highly specialised instrumentation.

Without question, food can be considered as a very complex and heterogeneous composition of hundreds, if not thousands, of different biochemical compounds. In the area of food biochemistry, the isolation and quantitative measurement of these chemical components has posed, and continues to pose, immense challenges to the analytical biochemist. Without the ability to measure both specifically and quantitatively those biochemical components in food matrices, further advancements in the understanding of how foods change during maturation or processing would not be possible.

Although it is impossible to address the quantitative analysis of all the different food components, the major techniques for the analysis of protein, lipids, carbohydrates, minerals, vitamins, and pigments will be addressed in detail in this chapter. The principles behind their analysis are the building blocks for other analytical determinations, including techniques such as gas chromatography, high performance liquid chromatography (HPLC) and spectroscopy, including infrared and mass spectroscopy.

PROTEIN ANALYSIS

Proteins are considered to be among the most abundant cell components and, except for storage proteins, and important for biological functions within the organism—plant or animal. Many food proteins have been purified and characterised over the years and found to range from approximately 5000 to more than a million Daltons. In general, they are all composed of various elements including carbon, hydrogen, nitrogen, oxygen and sulphur. These elements are formed into twenty different amino acids, which are linked together by peptide bonds to form proteins. In general, nitrogen is the most distinguishing element in proteins, varying from approximately 13 to 19 per cent due to variations in the specific amino acid composition of proteins.

For the past several decades, protein analysis has been performed by determining the nitrogen content of the food product after complete acidic hydrolysis and digestion by the Kjeldahl method and subsequent conversion to protein content using various conversion factors. As far back as the turn of the century, colorimetric protein determination methods such as the Biuret procedure (which exploited the development of the violet-purplish colour that is produced when cupric ions complex with peptide bonds under alkaline conditions) became available. The colour absorbance is measured at 540 nm, with

649

the colour intensity (absorbance) being proportional to the protein content with a sensitivity of 1–10 mg protein/ml. Over the years, further modifications were made with the development of the Lowry method, which combines the Biuret reaction with the reduction of the Folin-Ciocalteau phenol reagent (phosphomolybdic-phosphotungstic acid) by tyrosine and tryptophan residues in the proteins. The resulting bluish colour is read at 750 nm, which is highly sensitive for low protein concentrations (sensitivity 20–100 µg). Other methods exploit the tendency of proteins to absorb strongly in the ultraviolet spectrum (i.e. 280 nm), primarily due to tryptophan and tyrosine residues. Since the tryptophan and tyrosine contents in proteins are generally constant, the absorbance at 280 nm has been used to estimate the concentration of proteins using Beer's law. Because each protein has a unique aromatic amino acid composition, the extinction coefficient (E_{280}) must be determined for each individual protein for protein content estimation.

Although these methods are appropriate for quantitating the actual amounts of proteins available within a sample or commodity, they do not possess the ability to differentiate and quantitate the actual types of proteins within a mixture. The most currently used methods for detecting and/or quantitating specific protein components can be catalogued in the fields of spectrometry, chromatography, electrophoresis or immunology or a combination of these.

Electrophoresis is defined as the migration of charged molecules in a solution through an electrical field. Although several forms of this technique exist, zonal electrophoresis (in which proteins are separated from a complex mixture into bands by migrating in aqueous buffers through a solid polymer matrix called a polyacrylamide gel) is perhaps the most common. In nondenaturing/native electrophoresis, proteins are separated based on their charge, size and hydrodynamic shape. In denaturing polyacrylamide gel electrophoresis (PAGE), an anionic detergent, sodium dodecyl sulphate (SDS), is used to separate protein subunits by size. Isoelectric focusing is a modification of electrophoresis in which proteins are separated by charge in an electrophoretic field on a gel matrix in which a pH gradient has been generated using ampholytes. Proteins will focus or migrate to the location in the pH gradient that equals the isoelectric point (pI) of the protein. Resolution is among the highest of any protein separation technique and can separate proteins with pI differences as small as 0.02 pH units. More recently, with the advent of capillary electrophoresis, proteins can be separated on the basis of charge or size in an electric field within a very short period of time. The primary difference between capillary electrophoresis and conventional electrophoresis is that a capillary tube is used in place of a polyacrylamide gel. Unlike a gel, which must be made and cast each time, the capillary tube can be reused over and over. Electrophoresis flow within the capillary also can influence separation of the proteins in capillary electrophoresis.

High performance liquid chromatography (HPLC) is another extremely fast analytical technique that possesses excellent precision and specificity as well as the proven ability to separate protein mixtures into individual components. Many different kinds of HPLC techniques exist, depending on the nature of the column characteristics (chain length, porosity, etc.) and the elution characteristics (mobile phase, pH, organic modifiers). In principle, proteins can be analysed based on the polarity, solubility or size of their constituent components.

Reversed-phase chromatography was introduced in the 1950s and has become a widely applied HPLC method for the analysis of both proteins and a wide variety of other biological compounds. Reversed-phase chromatography is generally achieved on an inert column packing, typically covalently bonded with a high density of hydrophobic functional groups, such as linear hydrocarbons with 4, 8 or 18 residues in length, or the relatively more polar phenyl group. In fact, reversed-phase HPLC has proven itself useful and indispensable in the field of varietal identification. It has been shown that the processing quality of various grains depends on their physical and chemical characteristics, which are at least partially genetic in origin, and that a wide range of qualities exists within varieties of each species. The selection of the appropriate cultivar is therefore an important decision for a farmer, since it greatly influences the return he receives on his investment.

Size-exclusion chromatography separates protein molecules based on their size or, more precisely, their hydrodynamic volume, and it has become very popular in recent years. Size-exclusion chromatography utilises uniform rigid particles whose uniform pores are sufficiently large for the protein molecules to enter. Large molecules do not enter the pores of the column particles and are therefore excluded, that is, they are eluted in the void volume of the column (i.e. elute first), whereas smaller molecules enter the column pores and therefore take longer to elute from the column. An application example of size-exclusion chromatography is the separation of soyabean proteins. In one particular study, nine peaks were eluted for soyabean, corresponding to different protein size fractions; one peak showed a high variability for the relative peak area and could serve as a possible differentiation among different cultivars. Differences, qualitatively and quantitatively, in peanut seed protein composition were detected by size-exclusion chromatography and contributed to evaluation of genetic differences, processing conditions and seed maturity. Basha found that size-exclusion chromatography was an excellent indicator of seed maturity. Basha discovered that the area of one particular component (peak) decreased with increasing maturity and remained unchanged towards later stages of seed maturity. The peak was present in all studied cultivars, all showing a 'mature seed protein profile' with respect to this particular peak, which was therefore called 'Maturin'.

LIPID ANALYSIS

By definition, lipids are soluble in various organic solvents but insoluble in water. For this reason, lipid insolubility in water becomes an important distinguishing and analytical factor used in separating lipids from other cellar components such as carbohydrates and proteins. Fats (solids at room temperature) and oils (liquid at room temperature) are composed primarily of tri-esters of glycerol with fatty acids and are commonly called triglycerides. Other major lipid types found in foods include free fatty acids, mono and diacylglycerols and phospholipids.

Fats and oils are widely distributed in nature and play many important biological roles, especially within cell membranes. In general, many naturally occurring lipids are composed of various numbers of fatty acids (one to three) with various chain lengths, usually greater than 12 carbons, although the vast majority of animal and vegetable fats are made up of fatty acid molecules of greater than 16 carbons.

The total lipid content of a food is commonly determined using various organic solvent extraction methods. Unfortunately, the wide range of relative hydrophobicity of different lipids makes the selection of a single universal solvent almost impossible for lipid extraction and quantitation. In addition to various solvent extraction methods (using various solvents), there are nonsolvent wet extraction methods and other instrumental methods that utilise the chemical and physical properties of lipids for content determination.

Perhaps one of the most commonly used and easiest to perform methods is the Soxhlet method, a semicontinuous extraction method that allows for the sample in the extraction chamber to be completely submerged in solvents for 10 minutes or more before the extracted lipid and solvent are siphoned back into the boiling flask reservoir. The whole process is repeated numerous times until all the fat is removed. The fat content is determined either by measuring the weight loss of the sample or the weight of lipid removed.

Another excellent method for total fat determination includes supercritical fluid extraction. In this method, a compressed gas (usually CO_2) is brought to a specific pressure-temperature combination that allows it to attain supercritical solvent properties for the selective extraction of lipid from a matrix. In this way specific types of lipids can be selectively extracted while others remain in the matrix. The dissolved fat is then separated from the compressed, liquified gas by a drop in pressure, and the precipitated lipid is then quantified as per cent lipid by weight.

Another method often used for total lipid quantitation is the infrared method, which is based on the absorption of infrared energy by fat at a wavelength of 5.73 µm. In general, the more energy is absorbed at 5.73 µm, the higher the lipid content in the material. Near-infrared spectroscopy has been successfully used to measure the lipid content of various oilseeds, cereals and meats; it has the added advantage of being nondisruptive to the sample, in contrast to other previously reviewed methods.

Although the above-cited methods are appropriate for quantitating the actual amounts of lipids within a given sample, they do not offer the ability to characterise the types of fatty acids within a mixture. Gas chromatography, however, does offer the ability to characterise these lipids in terms of their fatty acid composition. First of all, mono-, di- and triglycerides need to be isolated individually if a mixture exists, usually by simple adsorption chromatography on silica. The isolated glycerides can then be hydrolysed to release individual fatty acids, which are subsequently converted to their ester form; that is, the glycerides are saponified and the fatty acids thus liberated are esterified to form fatty acid methyl esters. The fatty acids are now volatile and can be separated chromatographically using various packed and capillary columns using a variety of temperature-time gradients.

Separation of the actual mono-, di- and triglycerides is usually much more problematic than determining their individual fatty acid constituents or building blocks. Although gas chromatography has also been used for this purpose, such methods give insufficient information to provide a complete triglyceride composition of a complex mixture. Such analyses are important for the edible oil industry for process and product quality control purposes as well as for the understanding of triglyceride biosynthesis and deposition in plant and animal cells.

With HPLC analysis, Plattner was able to establish that, under isocratic conditions, the logarithm of the elution volume of a triacylglycerol was directly proportional to the total number of carbon atoms (CN) and inversely proportional to the total number of double bonds (X) in the three fatty acyl chains. The elution behaviour is controlled by the equivalent carbon number (ECN) of a triacylglycerol, which may be defined as $ECN = CN - Xn$ where, n is the factor for double bond contribution, normally close to 2.

The IUPAC commission on oils, fats and derivatives undertook the development of a method for the determination of triglycerides in vegetable oils by liquid chromatography. Materials studied included soyabean oil, almond oil, sunflower oil, olive oil, rapeseed oil and blends of palm and sunflower oils and almond and sunflower oils. AOAC International adopted this method for determination of triglycerides (by partition numbers) in vegetable oils by liquid chromatography as an IUPAC-AOC-AOAC method. In this method, triglycerides in vegetable oils are separated according to their equivalent carbon number by reversed-phase HPLC and detected by differential refractometry. Elution order is determined by calculating the equivalent carbon numbers. $ECN = s$ and $CN - 2n$, where CN is the carbon number and n is the number of double bonds.

CARBOHYDRATES ANALYSIS

Carbohydrates play several important roles in foods, including among other things, imparting important physical properties to the foods as well as constituting a major source of energy in the human diet. In fact, it has been estimated that carbohydrates account for greater than 70 per cent of the total daily caloric intake in many parts of the world.

Carbohydrates found in nature are almost exclusively of plant origin, with at least 90 per cent of them occurring in the form of polysaccharides. Interestingly, although the most carbohydrates are in the form of polysaccharides, starches are about the only polysaccharide that is digestible by humans. The vast majority of polysaccharides are therefore nondigestible, and they have been divided into two classes, soluble and insoluble, which form what is commonly called dietary fibre.

For decades total carbohydrate was determined by exploiting the tendency of carbohydrates to condense with various phenolic-type compounds including phenol, orcinol, resorcinol, napthoresorcinol, and α-naphthol. The most widely used condensation was with phenol, which offered a rapid, simple and specific determination for carbohydrates. Virtually all types of carbohydrates, mono-, di, oligo- and polysaccharides, could be determined. After reaction with phenol in acid in the presence of heat, a stable colour is produced that can be read spectrophotometrically. A standard curve is usually prepared with a carbohydrate similar to these being measured.

Although the above method was, and still is, used to quantitate the total amount of carbohydrate in a given sample, it does not offer the ability to determine the actual types and/or building blocks of individual carbohydrates. Earlier methods, which included paper chromatography, open column chromatography, and thin-layer chromatography, have largely been replaced by HPLC and/or gas chromatography. Gas chromatography has been established as an important method in carbohydrate determinations since the early 1960s, and several unique applications have since then been reported.

For carbohydrates to be analysed by gas chromatography, they must first be converted into volatile derivatives. Perhaps the most commonly used derivatising agent is trimethylsilyl (TMS). In this procedure, the aldonic acid forms of carbohydrates are converted into their TMS ethers. The reaction mixtures are then injected directly into the chromatograph, and temperature programming is utilised to optimise the separation and identification of individual components. A flame ionisation detector is still the detector of choice for carbohydrates. Unlike gas chromatography, HPLC analysis of carbohydrates requires no prior derivatisation of carbohydrates and gives both qualitative (identification of peaks) and quantitative information for complex mixtures of carbohydrates. HPLC has been shown to be an excellent choice for the separation and analysis of a wide variety of carbohydrates, ranging from monosaccharides to oligosaccharides. For the analysis of larger polysaccharides, a hydrolysis step is required prior to chromatographic analysis. A variety of different columns can be used, with bonded amino phases used to separate carbohydrates with molecular weights up to about 2500, depending upon carbohydrate composition and, therefore, solubility properties. The elution order on amine-bonded stationary phases is usually monosaccharide and sugar alcohols followed by disaccharides and oligosaccharides. Such columns have been successfully used to analyse carbohydrates in anything from fruits and vegetables all the way to processed foods such as cakes, confectionaries, beverages, and breakfast cereals. With larger polysaccharides, gel filtration becomes the preferred chromatographic technique, as found in the literature. Gel filtration media have been successfully used to characterise polysaccharides according to molecular weight.

MINERAL ANALYSIS

Minerals are extremely important for the structural and physiological functioning of the body. It has been estimated that 98 per cent of the calcium and 80 per cent of the phosphorous in the human body are bound up within the skeleton. Those minerals that are directly involved in physiological function (e.g. in muscle contraction) include sodium, calcium, potassium and magnesium. Certain minerals (or macrominerals) are required in quantities of more than 100 mg per day; these include sodium, potassium, magnesium, phosphorous, calcium, chlorine and sulphur. Another 10 minerals (trace minerals) are required in milligram quantities per day; these include silica, selenium, fluoride, molybdenum, manganese, chromium, copper, zinc, iodine, and iron. Each of the macro- and trace-minerals has a specific biochemical role in maintaining body function and is important to overall health and well-being.

Although minerals are naturally found in most food materials, some are added to foods during processing to accomplish certain objectives. An example of this is salt, which is added during processing to decrease water activity and to act as a preservative (e.g. pickles and cheddar cheese). Iron is added to fortify white flour, and various other minerals such as calcium, iron and zinc are added to various breakfast cereals. In fact, salt itself is fortified with iodine in North America in order to control goiter.

It should also be noted that food processing can decrease the mineral content (e.g. the milling of wheat removes the mineral-rich bran layer). During the actual washing and blanching of various foods, important minerals are often lost. It can, therefore, be concluded that accurate and specific methods for mineral determination are in fact important for nutritional purposes as well as for properly processing food products for both human and animal consumption.

In order to determine the total mineral content of a food material, the ashing procedure is usually performed. Ash refers to the inorganic residue that remains after ignition, or in some cases complete oxidation, of organic material. Ashing can be divided into three main types: (i) dry ashing (most commonly used), (ii) wet ashing (oxidation), for samples with high fat content (such as meat products) or for preparation for elemental analysis, and (iii) plasma ashing (low temperature) for when volatile elemental analysis is conducted.

In dry ashing, samples usually are incinerated in a muffle furnace at temperatures of 500°–600°C. Most minerals are converted to oxides, phosphates, sulphates, chlorides or silicates. Unfortunately, elements such as mercury, iron, selenium and lead may be partially volatised using this procedure.

Wet ashing utilises various acids to oxidise organic materials and minerals that are solubilised without their volatilisation. Nitric and perchloric acids are often used, and reagent blanks are carried throughout the procedure and are subtracted from sample results. In low-temperature plasma ashing, samples are treated in a similar way to those in dry ashing, but under a partial vacuum, with samples being oxidised by nascent oxygen formed by an electromagnetic field.

Although the above three methods have been proven to be appropriate for quantitating the total amount of mineral within a sample, they do not possess the ability to either differentiate or quantitate actual mineral elements within a mixture.

When atomic absorption spectrometers became widely used in the 1960s and 1970s, they paved the way for measuring trace amounts of mineral elements in various biological samples. Essentially, atomic absorption spectroscopy is an analytical technique based on the absorption of ultraviolet or visible radiation by free atoms in the gaseous state. The sample must be first ashed and then diluted in weak acid. The solution is then atomised into a flame. According to Beer's Law, absorption is directly related to the concentration of a particular element in the sample.

Atomic emission spectroscopy differs from atomic absorption spectroscopy in that the source of radiation is, in fact, excited atoms or ions in the sample other than from external source, has in part taken over. Atomic emission spectroscopy does have advantages with regard to sensitivity, interference, and multielement analysis.

Recently, the use of ion-selective electrodes has made online testing of the mineral composition of samples a reality. In fact, many different electrodes have been developed for the direct measurement of various anions and cations such as calcium, bromide, fluoride, chloride, potassium, sulphide and sodium. Typically, levels down to 0.023 ppm can be measured. When working with ion-selective electrodes it is common procedure to measure a calibration curve.

VITAMIN ANALYSIS

By definition, vitamins are organic compounds of low molecular weight that must be obtained from external sources in the diet and are also essential for normal physiological and metabolic function. Since the vast majority of vitamins cannot be synthesised by humans, they must be obtained from either food or dietary supplements. When vitamins are absent or at inadequate levels in the diet, deficiency disease commonly occurs, (e.g. scurvy and pellagra from a lack of ascorbic acid and niacin, respectively).

Analyses of vitamins in foods are performed for numerous reasons; for example, to check for regulatory compliance, to obtain data for nutrient labelling, or to study the changes in vitamin content attributable to food processing, packaging and storage. Therefore, numerous analytical methods have been developed to determine vitamin levels during processing and in the final product.

Vitamins have been divided into two distinct groups: (i) those that are water soluble (B vitamins, vitamin C), and (ii) those that are fat soluble (vitamins A, D, E and K).

The scientific literature contains numerous analytical methods for the quantitation of water-soluble vitamins including several bio-, calorimetric and fluorescent assays that have been proven to be accurate, specific and reproducible for both raw and processed food products. The scientific literature also contains an abundance of HPLC-based methodologies for the quantitation of water-soluble vitamins. High performance liquid chromatography (HPLC) has become by far the most popular technique for the quantitation of these water-soluble vitamins. In general, it is the nonvolatile and hydrophilic nature of these vitamins that make them excellent candidates for reversed-phase HPLC analysis. The ability to automate these analyses using autosamplers and robotics makes HPLC an increasingly popular technique. Since the vast majority of vitamins occur in food in trace amounts, detection sensitivity is paramount to their detection. Although ultraviolet absorbance is the most common detection method, both fluorescence and electrochemical detection are also used in specific cases. Refractive index detection is seldom used for vitamin detection due to its inherent lack of specificity and sensitivity.

During the 1960s, gas chromatography using packed columns was widely applied to the determination of various fat-soluble vitamins, especially vitamins D and E. Unfortunately, thin-layer chromatographic and open-column techniques were still necessary for preliminary separation of the vitamins, followed by derivatisation to increase the vitamins' thermal stability and volatility. More recently, the development of fused-silica, open tubular capillary columns has revived the use of gas chromatography, leading to a number of recent applications for the determination of fat-soluble vitamins, especially vitamin E. This being said, the method of choice for determining fat-soluble vitamins in foods is HPLC. The interest in this chromatographic technique is due to the lack of need for derivatisation and the greater separation and detection selectivity this technique offers. Various HPLC methods of analysis were introduced for the first time in the 1995 edition of the Official Methods of Analysis of AOAC International; these include vitamin A in milk (AOAC 992.04,) and vitamins A (AOAC 992.26), E (AOAC 992.03) and K (AOAC 992.27) in various milk-based infant formulas.

It should be noted that at present there is no universally recognised standard method for determining any of the fat-soluble vitamins that can be applied to all food types.

PIGMENT ANALYSIS

Colour is a very important characteristic of foods and is often one of the first quality attributes used to judge the quality or acceptability of a particular food. There are a vast number of natural and synthetic pigments, both naturally occurring and added to foods, that contribute to food colour. Of the naturally occurring pigments in foods, the vast majority can be divided into five major classes, four of which are distributed in plant tissues and one in animal tissues. Of those found in plants, two types are lipid soluble (i.e. the chlorophylls and the carotenoids), and the other two are water soluble (i.e. anthocya-nins and betalains). Carotenoids are found in animals but are not biosynthesised; that is, they are derived from plant sources.

Several analytical methods have been developed for the analysis of chlorophylls in a wide variety of foods. Early spectrophotometric methods allowed for the quantitation of both chlorophyll *a* and chlorophyll *b* by measuring absorbance at the absorbance maxima of both chlorophyll types. Unfortunately, only fresh plant material could be assayed, as no pheophytin could be determined. This became the basis for the AOAC International spectrophotometric procedure, which provides results for total chlorophyll content as well as for chlorophyll *a* and chlorophyll *b* quantitation.

Schwartz described a simple reversed-phase HPLC method for the analysis of chlorophylls and their derivatives in fresh and processed plant tissues. This method simplified the determination of chemical alterations in chlorophyll during the processing of foods and allowed for the determination of pheophytins and pyropheophytins.

For carotenoid analysis, numerous HPLC methods have been developed, particularly for the specific separation of various carotenoids found in fruits and vegetables. Both normal and reversed-phase methods have been used, with the reversed-phase methods predominating. Reversed-phase chromatography on C-18 columns using isocratic elution procedures with mixtures of methanol and acetonitrile containing ethyl acetate, chloroform, or tetrahydrofuran have been found to be satisfactory. Detection of carotenoids usually range from approximately 430 to 480 nm. Since β-carotene in hexane has an absorption maximum at 453 nm, many methods have detected a wide variety of carotenoids in this region.

Measurements of anthocyanins have been performed by determining absorbance of diluted samples acidified to about pH 1.0 at wavelengths between 510 and 540 nm. Unfortunately, absorbance measurements of anthocyanin content provide only for a total quantification, and further information about the amounts of various individual anthocyanins must be obtained by other methods. Reversed-phase HPLC methods employing C-18 columns have been the methods of choice due to the water-soluble nature of anthocyanins. Mixtures of water and acetic, formic or phosphoric acids are usually employed as part of the mobile phase.

Charged pigments such as betalains can be separated by electrophoresis, but HPLC has been found to provide for more rapid resolution and quantitation. Betalains have been separated on reversed-phase columns by using various ion-paring or ion-suppression techniques. This procedure allows for more interaction of the individual molecules of betaine with the stationary phase and better separation between individual components.

Appendix

Miscellaneous Fermentation Products

Foodstuff	Details	Origin
Acidophilus milk	Skim or full fat milk, sterilised, incubated with *Lactobacillus acidophilus* or *Bifidobacterium bifidum* < 48 hours). Therapeutic value: lowering pH of intestine	Europe and North America
Aperitif wine	Bitter tasting, high alcohol wine, often red, drunk before meals. Red wine or white wine strengthened with added grape spirit or alcohol, flavourings. For example, Campari from Italy = red and flavoured with quinine. Dubonnet–France = red or white, flavoured with quinine and herbs	International
Bacon	Pork sides cured-curing salts containing some or all of sodium chloride, potassium nitrate, sodium nitrite, sugars, ascorbic acid. Covered in curing pickle –3°–6°C for 2–10 days. Taken away from brine and stored at same temperature for up to 2 weeks. May be cold smoked at 25°–35°C or cooked to internal temperature of 50°–55°C. Bacteria - Micrococcus or Staphylococcus-reduce nitrate to nitrite, which is active form in producing active pink nitroso compounds. Lactobacillus active in maturing. Shorter process may find chemical curing more important than microbial curing	International
Bagel	Traditional Jewish bread. Baker's yeast and sometimes egg added to wheat flour dough, fermenting and proofing 40–50 min, knocked back to original size by expelling gas, dividing and rolling into balls, grilled 4–5 minutes at 200°C, dropped into boiling water for 15–20 minutes, drained and baked in oven at 200°C for 15 minutes until crisp	Middle East, North America
Bagoong	Fermented salty fish paste. Condiment with rice dishes in Asia. Remove heads and eviscerate fish. May be sun dried for 3–4 days and then pounded. One part salt to 3 parts fish. Fermented in earthenware vats for 1–4 months. Final NaCl of 20–25%, by weight. May be further pounded and coloured up with Angkak (a red colouring agent made from rice by action of mould *Monascus purpureus*). Pickle appearing at surface of fermenting mass removed and may be used as fish sauce. Proteolysis by autolytic enzymes releases peptides, amino acids, amines and ammonia. Minor role for salt-tolerant bacteria of Micrococcus, Staphylococcus, Pediococcus and Bacillus	East Asia, South East Asia

(Contd...)

Foodstuff	Details	Origin
Basi	Alcoholic wine from sugar cane juice. Extracted by pressing cane, stored up to year, concentrated by boiling, leaves from guava may be immersed late in boiling. Filter into earthenware containers. Cooled to 40°–45°C. Starter may be added, perhaps dried rotting fruit. 30°–35°C, 4–6 days, or left 3–9 months. Starter comprises yeasts (Saccharomyces and Endomycopsis) and bacteria-lactic acid bacteria, especially Lactobacillus	East Asia, South East Asia, Africa
Bongkrek	Coconut press cake, bound by mould mycelium into solid mass. Fried in oil and eaten with soup. Press cake remaining after coconut oil extract, for example, from copra is soaked for several hours in water. Vinegar may be added to lower pH. Pressed, sun-dried, steamed, cooled, inoculated with mould. Fermented on banana leaves, plastic sheets, mats or trays in dark, 24–48 hours 30°–35°C. Mould mycelium penetrates and knits everything together. Mould *Rhizopus oligosporus* or *Neurospora sitophila*	South East Asia
Cachaca	Sugar cane spirit, +38% alcohol	Brazil
Chicha	Effervescent sour alcoholic beverage. Yellow to red in colour made from maize or other starch crops, for example, cassava or beans. Dates to Inca. Chewed (normally women) but these days amylases may be developed via malting. Boiled with water, left 24 hours to extract soluble materials, re-boiled. Sugars and molasses may be added. Filtered and the wort left to ferment in previously used containers. 20°–30°C for 1–5 days. Lactic acid bacteria especially Lactobacillus, yeast, Acetobacter. Limit the life of the product to the time until which excess acetic acid is produced	South America
Corned beef	Usually from brisket-canned. Curing, but some mild fermentation. Name derives from large grains of salt used, which were called 'corns'. Beef salted in brine or pickle or the pickle is injected in more modern processes. Curing pickle sodium chloride, potassium or sodium nitrate or sodium nitrite, spices and herbs. These may include laurel, allspice, celery and onions. Placed in covered pickle for up to 2–3 weeks. Cooked in water or steamed to internal temperature of 68°–71°C, cooled. May be canned and recooked. Micrococcus and some lactic acid bacteria	International
Country ham	Semi-dried cured pork. Salted and dried usually uncooked, may be smoked. Matured several months. For example, Cumberland, Kentucky, Parma (seasoned with pepper, allspice coriander and mustard and rubbed with pepper). Smithfield ham heavily smoked with hickory. Salts used are sodium chloride and potassium or sodium nitrate. Sometimes sugar used. Flavourings added to curing salt. Left at 5°–15°C for 2–4 weeks and further pickling added, more weeks or months before cold smoking at 30°–40°C over 1–5 weeks. Matured at 20°–25°C for up to 2 years. Ham dries in this period. Nitrate to nitrite by Micrococcus and Staphylococcus. Some lactic acid bacteria, especially *Lactobacillus casei, Lactobacillus plantarun*. Some moulds especially *Penicillium nalgiovense* or Aspergillus spp. may coat surface of dried hams	International

(Contd...)

Foodstuff	Details	Origin
Dried fish	Salted low-fat fish dried to various degrees. Storage and preservation in hot countries. Eviscerate and salt to 30–35 per cent of weight with sodium chloride, loaded into barrels left at ambient (20°–35°C) for 5–128 days. Removed from containers and sun- or air-dried for several weeks or even months. May be smoked in this period. Only salt-tolerant Micrococcus, Staphylococcus, Bacillus and lactic acid bacteria (Pediococcus and Lactobacillus) will survive	International
Dried meat	For example, salt beef, pastrami. Semi-dried uncooked meat (beef, lamb, goat, etc.) that has been cured, smoked and dried. Pieces of meat heavily salted with sodium chloride, potassium or sodium nitrate or sodium nitrite. Sugars, spices and seasonings. 5°–15°C at high humidity (80–90% RH) at first, later high temperature and low humidity to encourage drying. Cold smoking 32°–38°C for 2–8 days before maturing for several weeks. Chemical curing with nitrates aided by Micrococcus and Staphylococcus reducing nitrate to nitrite. Also some fermentative lactic acid bacteria and yeast may develop. Pastrami (as an example) beef usually, black pepper, nutmeg, paprika, garlic and allspice. Smoked	International
Fermented egg	Whole eggs (especially duck) coated in salt and ash paste and coated in rice hulls. The salt coating likely to comprise sodium chloride, sodium carbonates, tea leaves, calcium oxide and ash from burning grass. Eggs rolled over hull mixture, packed into earthenware or porcelain jars. Tightly sealed with mud and salt. 20°–30°C for 15–50 days. Sodium hydroxide made from reaction of lime and sodium carbonate enters through eggshell and denatures and coagulates the egg protein, that is, a chemical as opposed to a microbial 'fermentation'	East Asian, South East Asia
Fish sauce	Brown salty liquid produced by breakdown of fish by fish enzymes. Small marine or fresh waterfish, shrimps used whole, cereal (usually rice) added and koji. 1–2 parts salt to 5 parts fish. Packed into jars, concrete tanks or wooden vats. Left to ferment 20°–35°C for 3–15 months. Liquid separated by filtration. Solid residues may be used to make Bagoong. Autolytic breakdown of fish protein. Sometimes fresh pineapple juice or koji added as source of proteinases. Trimethylamine and ammonia key products. Salt-tolerant Staphylococcus, Micrococcus and Bacillus may play a minor role in flavour development	East Asia, South East Asia, Europe
German salami	Dry, smoked uncooked sausage usually medium chopped and medium seasoning. Cold (–4° to –2°C) lean meat chopped and mixed with sodium chloride, potassium nitrate or sodium nitrite. Sodium ascorbate, spices, seasonings, sugar and sometimes glucono-δ-lactone. Pork fat chopped in. Stuffed at –4°C into casings or reformed collagen or artificial cellulose. Transferred to 'green room' where fermentation takes place at 20°–32°C under high RH for 18–48 hours if starter culture added. Or 5–9 days if not. Usually hot smoked to an internal temperature of 55°–63°C, dried slowly at 15°–24°C. Micrococcus and *Staphylococcus carnosus* important in early stages, converting nitrate to nitrite and stabilising colour. Pediococcus and Lactobacillus become dominant and may be added as starters	Germany

(Contd...)

Foodstuff	Details	Origin
Ghee	Clarified butter, usually from cow, goat, buffalo or sheep. Keeps well without refrigeration. Butter, cream or kaffir heated to 110°–140°C to melt and evaporate water. Filtered through muslin. Cooled to solidify. Antioxidants added. Lactic acid bacteria-Leuconostoc, Streptococci, Lactobacillus. Severe heating kills lactic acid flora	Indian subcontinent Middle East, South East Asia, Africa
Jerky	Lean meat, salted and sun or air dried in strips or thin sheets. Hot climates-dry product with good keeping properties. Snack or crumbled into soups or stews. Meat pieces salted with sodium chloride and perhaps nitrate. Left several days. Micrococci and Staphylococci reduce nitrate. Some development of lactic acid bacteria for flavour	America, Africa
Kanji	Strong flavoured red alcoholic beverage made from beet juice or carrot. Refreshing. Usually consumed in hot weather. Roots peeled and shredded, 100 parts root, 5–6 parts salt, 3–4 parts mustard seed, 400–500 parts water. Ferment at 26°–34°C for 4–7 days. Liquid drained for drinking. Portions of previous kanji may be added as a starter. *Hansenula anomala* and *Candida guilliermondii, Candida tropicalis* and *Geotrichum candidum* are active in fermentation	India, Israel
Kefir	Acidic and mildly alcohol effervescent milk from cows, buffalo goat milk. Heated to 90°–95°C for 3–5 min. Cooled. Put into earthenware vessels. Inoculated with 5% kefir grains or 2–3% other starter. Ferment at 20°–25°C for 10–24 hours, cooled to 12°–16°C for a further 14–18 hr, 'ripened' at 6°–10°C for 5–8 days. Foamy and creamy. Diverse lactic acid bacteria: *Lactobacillus casei, Lactobacillus acidophilus, Steptococcus lactis.* Produce lactic acid from lactose. *Lactobacillus bulgaricus* produces acetaldehyde, *Leuconostoc cremoris* produce diacetyl and acetoin and *Lactobacillus brevis* makes acetoin, acetic acid, ethanol and CO_2. *Candida kefyr* and *Kluyveromyces fragilis* convert lactose to ethanol and CO_2 during the cooler ripening period	Middle East, Europe, North Africa
Kimcin	Mildly acidic carbonated vegetables-radish, Chinese cucumber, Chinese cabbage. Essential dish at most Korean meals. Vegetables mixed with small amounts of onion, chilli pepper, garlic, ginger or other flavouring agent and 4–6% salt or brine. Large earthenware vessels. Fish (shrimps, oysters) may be added to flavour. Left in a cool place to ferment often in cellar 10°–18°C for 5–20 days. Maturation may be continued for many weeks if cool. Facultative lactic acid bacteria including *Leuconostoc mesenteroides, Streptococcus fecalis,* Pediococcus, *Lactobacillus plantarum, Lactobacillus brevis.* Aerobic bacteria Alcaligenes, Flavobacterium, Pseudomonas and *Bacillus megaterium* also grow. Later stages some yeast and moulds. Diverse organic acids	East Asia
Mead	Sweet alcoholic beverage from fermentation of honey with water or fruit juice. Often spiced. Honey added to 3–4 volumes of water or sometimes fruit juice often with addition of hops, herbs or spices. Usually boiled together. Surface froth skimmed off 2–3% brewer's yeast added as starter. Ferment 15°–25°C for 3–6 weeks. Usually aged in oak casks at 10°–15°C for up to 10 years. Periodically transferred between casks or racked to remove deposits. Usually pasteurised, clarified and filtered. Lactic acid bacteria also involved-Lactobacilli with production of lactic and other compounds and lowering of pH	International

(Contd...)

Foodstuff	Details	Origin
Nata	Thick white or cream-coloured gelatinous film growing on surface of juice from coconut, pineapple, sugar cane or other fruit waste. Eaten as dessert. Fruit juice mixture and pulp ground to a mash and diluted with water, 2%, glacial acetic acid, 15% sucrose plus 0.5% ammonium dihydrogen phosphate. 10% inoculum of 48 hours culture of acetic acid bacteria added to mixture in jars 28°–31°C for 12–15 days. The thick layer of cells plus polysaccharide which forms on surface is washed to remove acetic acid, boiled and candied with 50% sucrose. Stored in barrels till needed. *Acetobacter aceti* ssp. Xylinum produces an extracellular polymer that can hold 25–30 times own water in gel	Philippines
Papadum	Thin dried sheets of legume, cereal or starch crop flour. Stiff paste made by pounding legume flour, for example, *Phaseolus aureus* or Mung bean, *Phaseolus mungo*. Or rice flour, potato, sago or mix. Salt, spices including cardamom, caraway, pepper may be added. Dough made into long cylinder then portions cut and greased and rolled very thinly. Ferment in sun for several hours. Usually stored in tins until needed. Served after baking in hot fire or deep-frying in oil. Saccharomyces, Candida and lactic acid bacteria all involved	Indian subcontinent
Pepperoni	Dried meat sausage-production closely similar to German salami. Moulds of *Penicillium nagliovense* and Aspergillus grow on surface and impact flavour	Europe, North America, Oceania
Pickled fish	Fatty fish, for example, herring pickled in salt sugar and acid brine. Up to 1.5 hours. Usually whole or head removed, 15–17% salt, 5–7%, sugar plus added spices and put in barrels. Left to ferment for several months 5°–15°C. More salt and sugar may be added. After perhaps more than 1 year, fish washed and filleted and cut into pieces and packed in pickles of salt, sugar and acid (5–12% acetic). Proteolysis by cathepsins (endogenous proteinases). Softening of texture. Lactic acid bacteria of Pediococci. Leuconostoc and Lactobacillus and salt tolerant Micrococcus and Bacillus and yeasts play a minor role in flavour development	International
Pickled fruit	For example, cucumber, dill, but also lime pickle. Pick fruit under-ripe keeping sugar low and acidity high. Wash, dry, 2–3% or brine (5–10% salt). Sometimes inoculated with salt by needle. Herbs and spices may be added. Large earthenware jars filled, covered and scaled. 10°–15°C for 2–6 weeks. Vinegar, salt and sugar may be added in modern commercial operations to replace traditional fermentation process. Gram-negative Enterobacter grow first, then lactic acid bacteria Leuconostoc, Streptococci, Pediococci, Lactobacillus dominate, producing lactic acid, acetic, ethanol, CO_2. Yeast then start to dominate, converting some of the acid to ethanol. If containers opened, oxidative growth occurs	International
Pisco	Distilled alcoholic beverage from South American wines	South America
	Leaves and shoots of evergreen tree *Camellia sinensis*. Pruned to bush. Leaves rolled and fermented. Young leaves and shoots picked by hand. Wither 18–24 hours partly fermented. First for Oolong tea or for black tea, rolled directly, cells broken, release contents including enzymes and gives leaf a characteristic twist. Leaves spread in layers 10–15 mm deep	East Asia, South East Asia, Indian subcontinent, Africa

(Contd...)

Foodstuff	Details	Origin
	in high humidity rooms to ferment 3–6 hours. Colour goes from green to light brown. Fired by placing on trays through hot air (70°–95°C) and colour goes dark brown. Sorted and classified and packed as dried tea. Black tea can be classified into top quality orange pekoe, from young shoots and leaf tips and souchong, medium quality and made from lower leaves. Green tea: fresh leaves are streamed to make them more pliable and to prevent fermentation, then rolled and fired. Oolong tea-leaves partially fermented before being dried. Fermentation primarily by enzymes released in rolling process. Especially oxidation. Perhaps minor role by bacteria and yeasts	
Tempe	Beans, mostly soya, bound together by mould mycelium into cake, sliced and dipped into soya or fish sauce or cooked in batter. Or in soups. Soyabeans or other legume beans cleaned and soaked in water for 1–12 hours. Some fermentation takes place. Then boiled for 1–3 hours. Cooled, de-hulled, drained, inoculated with mould or a previous batch of tempe, wrapped in banana leaves or perforated polythene bags allowed to ferment at 27°–32°C for 36–48 hours. Mycelium penetrates. In initial soaking some early growth of Enterobacteriacea including *Klebsiella pneumoniae,* which makes Vitamin B_{12}, then lactic acid bacteria dominate, making lactic acid and lowering pH to 4.6–5.2. Helps establish mould *Rhizopus oligosporus* used in second stage. It releases proteinases. Ammonia produced, ergo pH rises again to 6.5–7. Some lipase released-with up to 25 per cent lipid converted to free fatty acids	South East Asia
Tequila	Mexican. Juice from *Agave tequilara* fermented by *Saccharomyces cerevisie* and distilled and matured in oak	South America
Thickeners	Various microbially derived thickeners are now available to go alongside more traditional agents such as starch, pectins, alginates, plant gums and cellulose derivatives. Examples are xanthan (*Xanthomonas compestris* growing on glucose switches to gum production when the supply of nitrogen is depleted), gellan (*Pseudomonas elodea*), pullulan (*Aureobasidium pullulans*)	International
Vermouth	Fortified herb and spice-flavoured wine. Usually Muscat flavoured by mixing in approximately 0.5% of macerate of herbs and spices for 1–2 weeks. Daily mixing. When desired flavour reached, the wine is drawn off and filtered. Refrigerated and cold stored for >1 year. Now herb essences and extracts may be used. French vermouths lower in sugar content and higher in colour and alcohol when compared to Italian. Dry vermouths incorporate more wormwood and bitter orange peel, *Citrus auranticum* while sweet ones contain coriander, cinnamon and cloves	Europe
Worcestershire sauce	Soyabeans, anchovies, tamarinds, shallots, garlic, onion, salt, spices and flavouring added to vinegar, molasses and sugar. Allowed to ferment 4–6 months with occasional agitation. After maturation, the mix is pressed through a mesh screen that allows just the finer particles to pass. Pasteurised to stop fermentation, then bottled	England

References

Allen, C.L., *Basic Concepts of Microbiology*, Butterworths, London.

Alvarez, A.J., *Microbiology of Food and Allied Products*, John Wiley & Sons, New York.

Arceivala, K.J., *Chemistry and Biology of Yeasts*, Marcel Dekker Inc., New York.

Batterman, S.A., *Yeasts and their Importance*, McGraw-Hill, Tokyo.

Benaim Pinto, C., *Sampling and Analysis of Airborne Micro-organisms*, Prentice-Hall, London.

Betina, V.K., *Dairy Microbiology*, Applied Science Publishers, London.

Bradley, R.S., *Pollution Prevention through Biotechnology*, Academic Press, London.

Brown, M.H., *Environmental Microbiology*, Cambridge University Press, Cambridge.

Budyko, M.I., *Food Processing Waste,* Progress Publishers, Moscow.

Cambell, K.E. and Lemer, H.A., *Microbial Technology*, Academic Press, London.

Cook, K., *Introduction to Environmental Microbiology*, John Wiley & Sons, New York.

Commoner, B., *Chemistry and Ecotoxicology of Pollution*, John Wiley & Sons, New York.

Considine, D.A., *Chemical Process Technology Encyclopedia,* McGraw Hill Book Co., New York.

Coolingwood, R.W., *Biological Indicators of Water Quality,* John Wiley & Sons, New York.

Cox, C.S., *Dioxin-Toxicological and Chemical Aspects*, S.P. Medical and Scientific Books, New York.

Daniel, F.L., *Biological Risk Engineering*, Pergamon Press, Oxford.

Downe, S.A., *Biochemistry of Industrial Micro-organisms*, John Wiley & Sons, New York.

Dugan, P.R., *Fungi, Food and Fermentation*, Plenum Publishing Corporation, London.

Goldman, M., *Yeast from Molasses Alcohol*, Gordon and Breach, Science Publishers, New York.

Gould, G.W., *Ecology of Micro-organisms*, D. Van Nostrand, New York.

Harding, G., *Acetic Acid Bacteria*, Prentice-Hall, London.

Hidy, G.M., *Biohazards,* Heinemann, London.

Huff, C.B., *Applied Environmental Microbiology*, Elsevier Scientific Publishing Co., Amsterdam.

Jackson, M.L., *Vinegar Fermentation*, Prentice-Hall, London.

Jackwerth, E., *Encyclopedia of Biotechnology and Industrial Microbiology*, Academic Press, London.

James, A. and Evison L., *Production of Industrial Enzymes*, John Wiley & Sons, New York.

Jarvis, B., *Micro-organisms in Food*, John Wiley & Sons, New York.

Jencks, W.P., *Encyclopedia of Environmental Microbiology*, John Wiley & Sons, New York.

Kim, C.K., *Water and Waste-water Disinfection*, Marcel Dekker, New York.

Lechevallier, M.W., *Modern Brewery Technology*, Academic Press, London.

References

Index

Adsorption, Absorption and Ion Exchange